HarperCollins*Publishers*
1 London Bridge Street
London SE1 9GF

www.harpercollins.co.uk

First published as *The Illustrated Encyclopedia of Healing Remedies*
by Harper Element in 1998.

This revised edition published by HarperCollins*Publishers* in 2018.

5 7 9 10 8 6 4

Cover photographs © iStock
Interior photographs © Shutterstock except 74L Botbin,
135L Roger Culos, 136L Melburnian, 151R Lwalsh84,
174L John Tann, 180R Olivier Pichard.

A catalogue record of this book is available from the British Library

ISBN 978-0-00-826821-3

General Editor of revised edition: Claudia Martin
Designer: Peter Clayman
Proofreader: Anne Rieley
Indexer: Geraldine Beare

Printed and bound in China

Note from the Publisher
Any information given in this book is not intended to be taken as a
replacement for medical advice. Any person with a condition requiring
medical attention should consult a qualified practitioner or therapist.

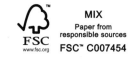

MIX
Paper from
responsible sources
FSC
www.fsc.org **FSC™ C007454**

This book is produced from independently certified FSC™ paper
to ensure responsible forest management.

For more information visit: www.harpercollins.co.uk/green

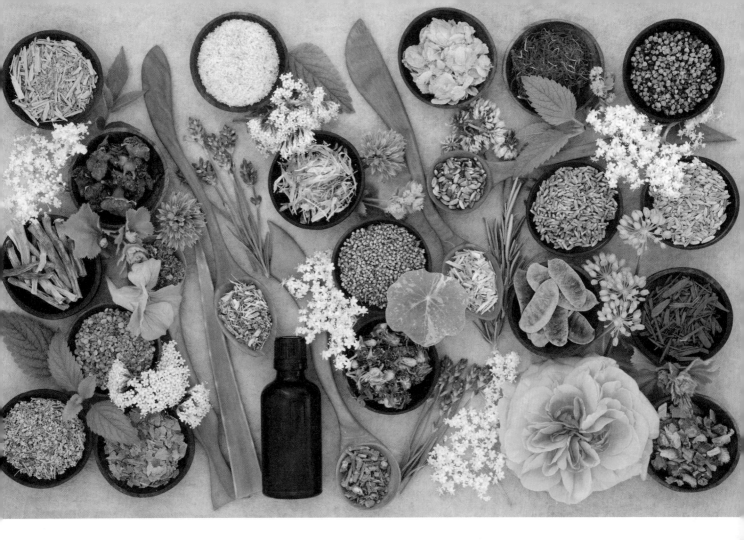

ABOUT THE CONTRIBUTORS

C. Norman Shealy M.D., Ph.D. is the founder of the International Institute of Holistic Medicine and a world-renowned neurosurgeon. He is the director of Shealy Wellness in Fair Grove, Missouri, a center for comprehensive healthcare and pain and stress management. He has written many books, including *Blueprint for Holistic Healing* and *Medical Intuition*.

Karen Sullivan is a nutritionist as well as the author and editor of numerous books on alternative health and nutrition, including *The Natural Home Remedies Guide* and *Eat Yourself Smart*. She lectures widely on women's health and general health issues.

Mary Clark has been a practitioner of healing for over 30 years. She has studied Ayurveda, nutrition, herbalism, aromatherapy, and stress management. She provides a unique combination of approaches in her work for various corporations in the U.S.A., including Forbes, Sony, and Barnes & Noble.

Eve Rogans began studying traditional Chinese medicine in 1981, starting with acupuncture and moving into herbalism. She has undergone clinical training in China, as well as working in both private and public practice, where she specializes in pediatric acupuncture and the field of substance abuse.

Non Shaw trained in the Western herbal tradition. She is the author of numerous articles and books about herbs and flower essences, including *The Complete Illustrated Guide to Herbs, Illustrated Elements of Herbalism*, and *Bach Flower Remedies: In a Nutshell*.

Sheila Lavery has written widely on healthcare for magazines and newspapers, as well as being the author of books including *Your Pregnancy Companion, Aromatherapy: In a Nutshell*, and *The Healing Power of Sleep*. Her work often focuses on children's health issues.

Pippa Duncan is former editor of one of the U.K.'s leading health magazines and the author of books including *Meditations for Your Pregnancy* and *A Parent's Guide to Complementary Healthcare for Children*.

Rachel Newcombe is an award-winning health writer and editor with a particular interest in natural medicine. She's a regular contributor to publications in the U.K. and internationally and has written several health books.

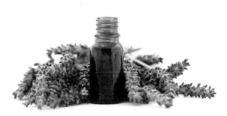

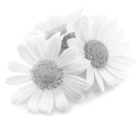

CONTENTS

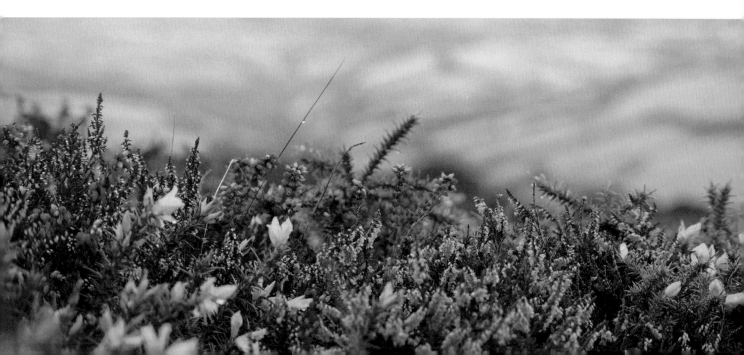

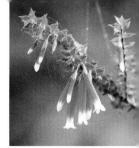

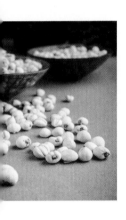

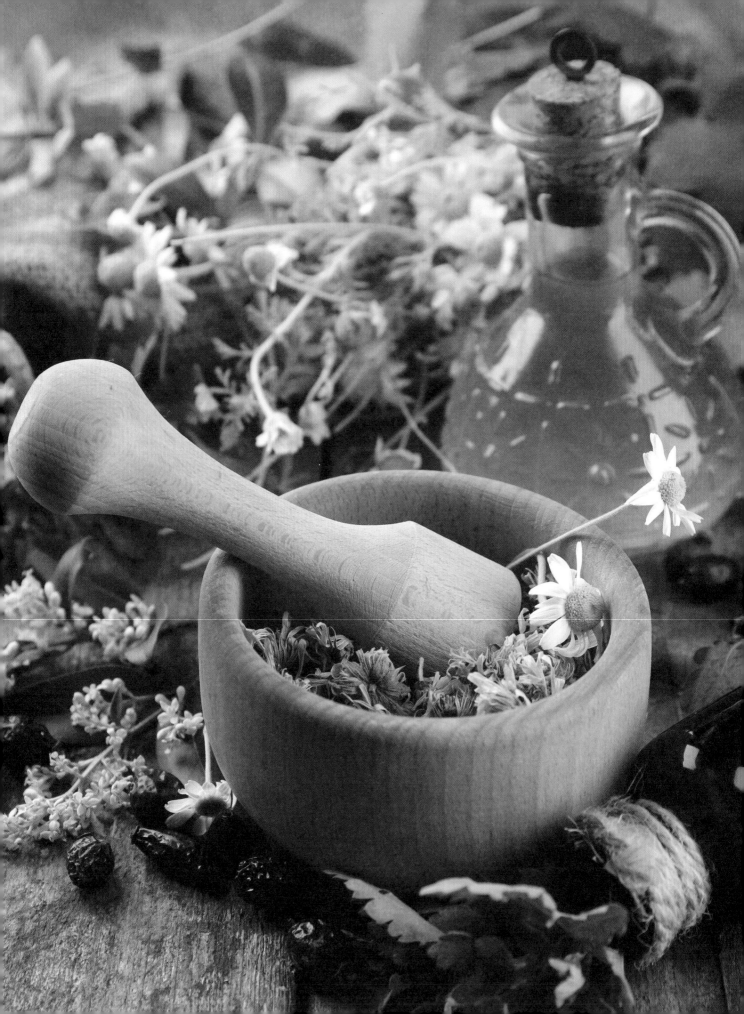

FOREWORD

The "Father of Medicine" is generally considered to be Hippocrates, who was born around 460 B.C.E. on the island of Cos, and died around 370 B.C.E. The body of work that is attributed to Hippocrates consists of 79 books and 59 treatises on which modern medicine is said to be founded. It is particularly interesting that a great deal of his writing addresses the role model of the physician – he should look healthy and well nourished, wear decent clothes, and have a degree of friendliness. Other than that, the most consistent commentary is on attention to anatomical detail, and precautions about the limitations of therapy, especially surgery.

In terms of theory, modern medicine dates from the work of Hippocrates, although the history of natural therapy extends back to long before his time. From those early days in Greece, two major schools of thought have dominated Western medicine – on the one hand rationalism, and on the other empiricism. Essentially the rationalists believe that science can ultimately know all the answers about life, and even create it. The "success" of experiments into cloning has certainly appeared to give credence to this view. In contrast, empiricists, or naturalists, believe in the ineffable quality of the universe, the natural order of life, and a concept of the divine, or vital force. Interestingly, empiricism has been embraced to a greater extent by the general public and rationalism by the Western medical society. Individuals seem to feel much more at home with a way of understanding health and disease that relies on sensory input and personal experience.

The dramatic increase in popularity of Ayurveda and traditional Chinese medicine in the West can be seen as a return to what is in essence a naturalist or empiricist approach, although both these therapies have developed into organized systems. Homeopathy was developed very much later, at a time when Western medicine was in a remarkably non-scientific pit of superstition and useless therapy which was often worse than no therapy at all. These therapies, and the others covered in this book, put the reader back in touch with empirical approaches to health, giving him or her the opportunity to grasp and use insights that Western physicians have largely ignored. The idea is to choose remedies from this book according to intuition, with the introductory chapter, entitled "Healing Therapies," as a guide, and judge their results according to your own sensory perception.

When I asked my Professor of Medicine, Eugene A. Stead Jr., M.D., in 1978 what he considered to be the role of a physician, he answered that it is to be a triage officer. "Triage" is a term that is often used in connection with battle or disaster victims, and means the allocation of treatment to patients according to the principle of maximizing the number of survivors. A triage officer would stand at the door when a patient was significantly ill and advise when medicine or surgery was truly needed to save life or function. Dr. Stead advised that when life and function are not at risk, as in the vast majority of symptomatic illnesses, the patient should "go into the department stores and choose that which most appeals."

In this wonderful and comprehensive book, you have a remarkable department store of choices. May your browsing be healing.

C. NORMAN SHEALY M.D., Ph.D.
Missouri

INTRODUCTION

The increased use of natural medicines and remedies over the past decades has prompted one of the most exciting developments in healthcare in our time. Many of the tenets of modern medicine have been challenged. The main premise of conventional medicine is that curing disease will lead to good health. This ignores the fundamental concept that pathology is individual to the sufferer, and that prevention is ultimately more important than treatment for the population at large. The modern clinical emphasis on separating different aspects of our physical, mental, and spiritual health has resulted in a dehumanizing of medicine.

Yet, by treating the whole person, holistic therapies can restore the proper balance and promote a sense of complete well-being, inside and out.

We, in the West, have been encouraged to adopt a "pill-popping" approach to health – taking an average of 26.5 million pills per hour. Sleeping tablets, analgesics (painkillers), antihistamines, sedatives, and antidepressants rank among the top 20 drugs prescribed by physicians, and more than 52 million aspirin or paracetamol tablets are taken each day in the U.S. Perhaps the most alarming result of this overdependence upon drugs is the fact that we have stopped taking responsibility for our own health. When we have a headache, we take a painkiller; when we have a cold, we might take an antihistamine.

We suppress the symptoms of health conditions because we want to feel better; we no longer accept the logic that pain or discomfort is a message from our body that something is wrong. We have become used to the idea that someone or something else can deal with our health problems.

By taking a pill or conventional medicine in some form, we do experience a relief from symptoms, but what is important to remember is that the cause of the pain or illness remains. By treating the symptoms, or suppressing them, we are doing nothing to treat the root cause. Eczema sufferers

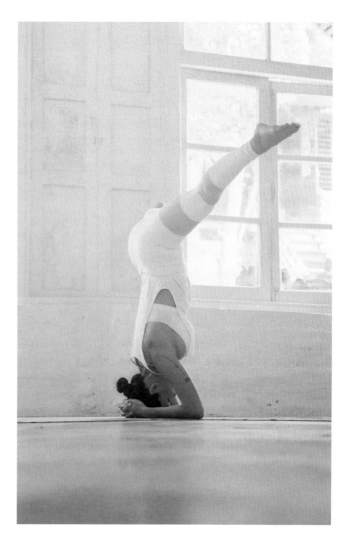

apply ointments and creams to the surface of the skin; they may take anti-inflammatories or antihistamines to ease the itching, but the cause of the eczema is still there, and the body's reaction has been masked by drugs. They have not been cured; their illness has merely been controlled.

In the past twenty years, this trend has begun to change. Concerns about the overuse of painkillers, antihistamines, and antibiotics have proved that conventional medicine, despite its many miracles, has its drawbacks. Many of us are no longer happy to accept the risks of prescription drugs, and are realizing that there are natural, healthy alternatives. With the increased interest in diet, emotional health and well-being, and exercise, we are becoming more

Exercise therapies such as yoga are becoming more and more popular as a way of combating the stress of Western lifestyles.

in tune with our bodies and are choosing to listen to the messages they give. Even more importantly, we are taking steps to prevent illness rather than simply treat it when it does arise, and for this reason we are willing to try natural substances that not only treat health conditions, at cause level, but work with the body to keep it well.

Natural remedies are more likely to make you feel better, more vital, and more alert; they have fewer side-effects and because they work actively to prevent illness, they are, perhaps, the answer to the healthcare crisis that has been spiraling out of control in the Western world.

Our understanding of how different cultures approach healthcare is blossoming, and figures show that many of the most common Western illnesses, such as eczema, asthma, cancer, chronic fatigue syndrome, and digestive problems simply do not exist to the same degree in other countries.

We have a cornucopia of information at our fingertips, and a greater understanding of how disease can be prevented and cured using exercise, herbs, oils, superfoods, vitamins and nutritional supplements, and other substances that encourage our bodies to work at their optimum level.

Our approach to our health is changing dramatically, and this increased interest is being fed by a broad range of products from around the world that are now available in our local shops and stores. Our growing understanding of holistic treatment has encouraged us to examine the healing practices of cultures from around the world, and from each we can gather invaluable information about diet, lifestyle, illness, health, and wellbeing.

A well-stocked herb garden, used with care and skill, may be more therapeutic than any number of proprietary medicines.

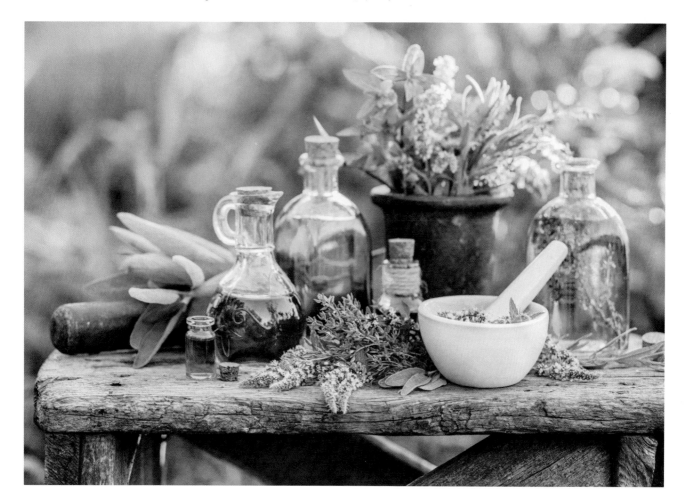

This book concentrates on the remedies that form the basis of eight international therapeutic disciplines: Ayurveda, Chinese herbal medicine, folk or traditional medicine (also called home remedies), herbalism, aromatherapy, homeopathy, flower essences, and nutrition. In addition, it also addresses the key field of mind–body healing and how we can work on our happiness and peacefulness through talking therapies, meditation, or prayer, ultimately benefiting both mind and body. The book also addresses the vital importance of exercise, from Pilates to yoga, from children playing in the park to elderly people enjoying armchair exercises. All these remedies can be used to encourage and enhance good health and to treat and prevent illnesses, both chronic and acute. Many of these remedies are derived from plants, which have a wide variety of therapeutic uses; indeed, up to 140 conventional drugs in use today are based on plants and herbs.

A large percentage of these remedies have been in use for thousands of years, and it was the practice of herbalism and other disciplines that made it possible for so many of our conventional drugs to be created. However, in practice, pharmaceutical companies isolate and often synthesize the active ingredient of a plant or herb, and many natural practitioners believe that this causes side-effects and other problems that do not occur when the substance is taken in its whole, natural form. They believe that medical herbalism offers a gentler, safer, and less disruptive effect, allowing the body to undertake its own natural healing process.

There are over 1,000 remedies outlined in this book, many of which you can grow in your own garden or on the windowsill, or purchase from a reputable health shop. Others will be items from your larder or store cupboard – everyday goods with healing and therapeutic properties that may surprise you. Each of the ingredients listed in the "Healing Remedies" chapter has a data file of features, cautions, and other useful information, and there are often recipes for practical applications. Each of the main disciplines is also introduced in the "Healing Therapies" chapter, which

helps you to understand how, for instance, the use of something like cinnamon or ginseng differs between Western and Chinese herbalism, and between folk medicine and Ayurveda. You'll learn how a rose aromatherapy oil is different from a rose flower essence, and how vitamin C and healthy bacteria can encourage good health. You'll discover natural alternatives to caffeine and sleeping pills, laxatives, and antacids, in remedies that strengthen your mind and body, lift your mood, calm your nerves, and enhance your resistance to infection and illness. In the "Treating Common Ailments" chapter, over 200 common ailments are also discussed in detail, with practical examples of how you can use the remedies from around the world to cure or prevent them.

Ayurvedic tea is a simple form of healing remedy.

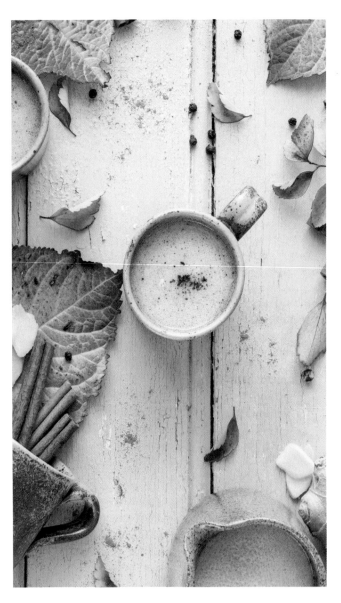

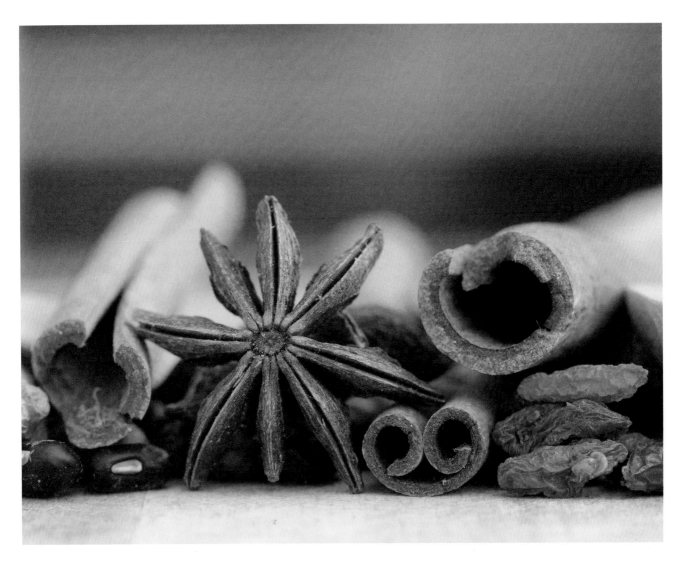

Throughout the book, you will come across "Caution" boxes that give advice on possible side-effects, maximum dosages, and the extra care that must be taken when giving natural remedies to children, the elderly, pregnant women, and breastfeeding mothers. In addition, advice is given on when it is inadvisable to combine natural remedies with conventional medication, and when it is best to consult with your physician, such as when you are undergoing treatment for cancer or HIV/AIDS.

On pages 238–241, "A Guide to Treatment," advice is offered on how to self-diagnose and when to self-treat, so that you know you are always taking the best care of your own and your family's health.

We are on the brink of an exciting new era in healthcare, and with the benefit of these remedies, presented in easy-to-follow files, you and your family can experiment with safe substitutes to conventional medicines by following the comprehensive instructions. The remedies in this book form the basis of a "stay-well" philosophy, with substances and exercises to boost immunity, help prevent heart disease, encourage emotional wellbeing and relaxation, enhance your strength, and keep your body's systems functioning the way they should. These remedies are the medicine of the future, and this is the essential guide for anyone who wants to take responsibility for their own health. By using only a few of these remedies, you can live longer and with a better quality of life. These are the secrets of good health from around the world; experiment with care and you'll be amazed at the results.

Karen Sullivan
London

Traditional Chinese medicine is one of the most popular natural therapies.

HOW TO USE THIS BOOK

This comprehensive reference work covers the origins, methods, principles, and remedies of Ayurveda, Chinese herbal medicine, traditional or folk medicine (also called home remedies), herbalism, aromatherapy, homeopathy, flower essences, nutrition, and mind–body healing.

CHAPTER ONE:
HEALING THERAPIES

—

Nine sections cover the different therapies. In each case, the background and history of the therapy are covered together with how it works, information on visiting a practitioner, and extensive guidelines for self-help.

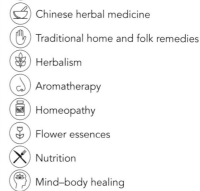

THERAPY SYMBOLS
For ease of reference, each of the nine therapies covered in this book is represented by a symbol:

- Ayurveda
- Chinese herbal medicine
- Traditional home and folk remedies
- Herbalism
- Aromatherapy
- Homeopathy
- Flower essences
- Nutrition
- Mind–body healing

Introduction to the history and background of each therapy

The principles behind the therapy and how it works

Cross-referencing directs the reader to all the remedies linked with this therapy

Information on preparations and on harvesting and sourcing remedies

Methods for preparing remedies, and safe dosages for adults and children

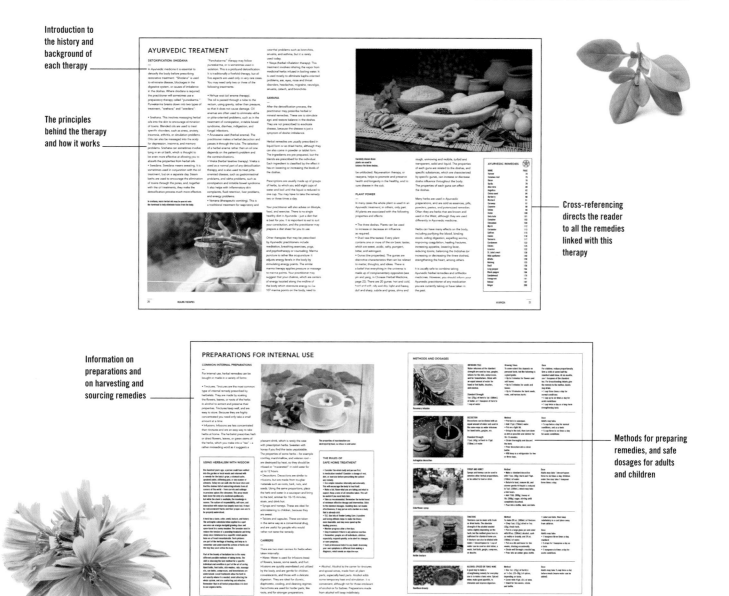

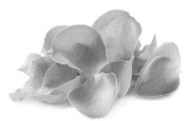

CHAPTER TWO:
HEALING REMEDIES
—

More than 200 healing ingredients are listed in alphabetical order of their Latin name. In each ingredient's data file, details are provided on which therapies use the substance, what it treats, how it should be taken, and how the substance is obtained or made. The chapter ends with a listing of vitamins, minerals, and dietary supplements.

Symbols show which therapies make use of this remedy

The remedy is described and illustrated

How to use the remedy source in particular treatments

Dosages, sources, and remedy combinations are listed

Bullet points highlight the properties of the remedy

Cautions warn when it is inadvisable to use a particular remedy

Step-by-step recipes describe how to prepare the remedy

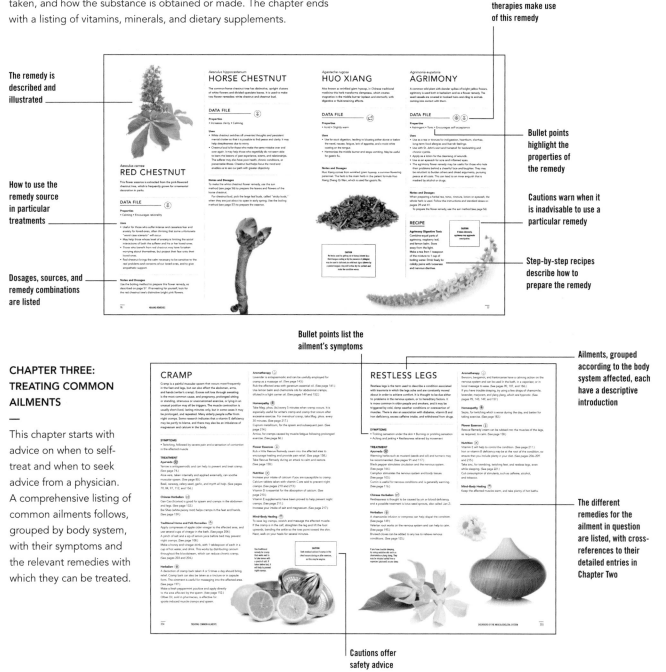

CHAPTER THREE:
TREATING COMMON AILMENTS
—

This chapter starts with advice on when to self-treat and when to seek advice from a physician. A comprehensive listing of common ailments follows, grouped by body system, with their symptoms and the relevant remedies with which they can be treated.

Bullet points list the ailment's symptoms

Ailments, grouped according to the body system affected, each have a descriptive introduction

The different remedies for the ailment in question are listed, with cross-references to their detailed entries in Chapter Two

Cautions offer safety advice

CHAPTER FOUR:
REFERENCE
—

Here you will find advice on sourcing ingredients both locally and online, as well as tracking down qualified practitioners. There is also a full glossary of terms, and a list of useful websites, addresses, and books for further reading.

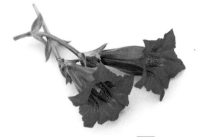

HEALING
THERAPIES

CHAPTER ONE

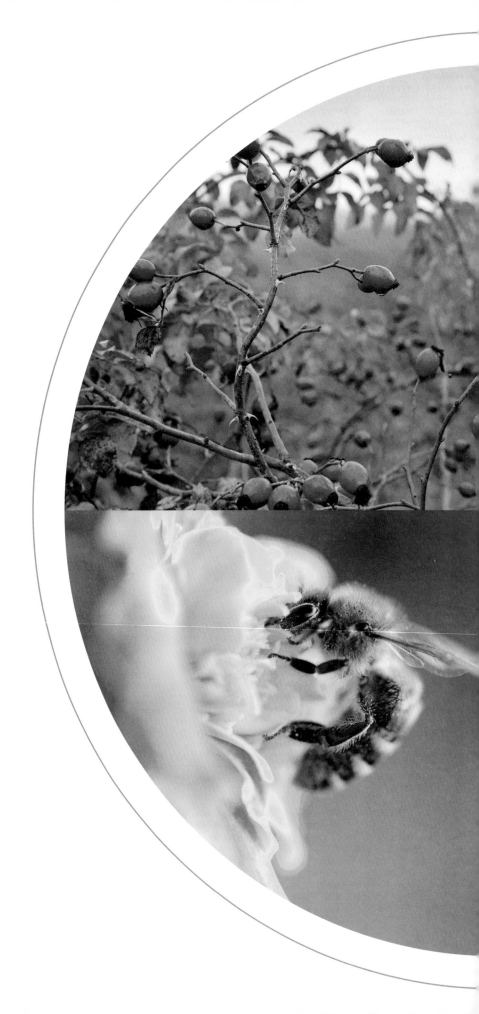

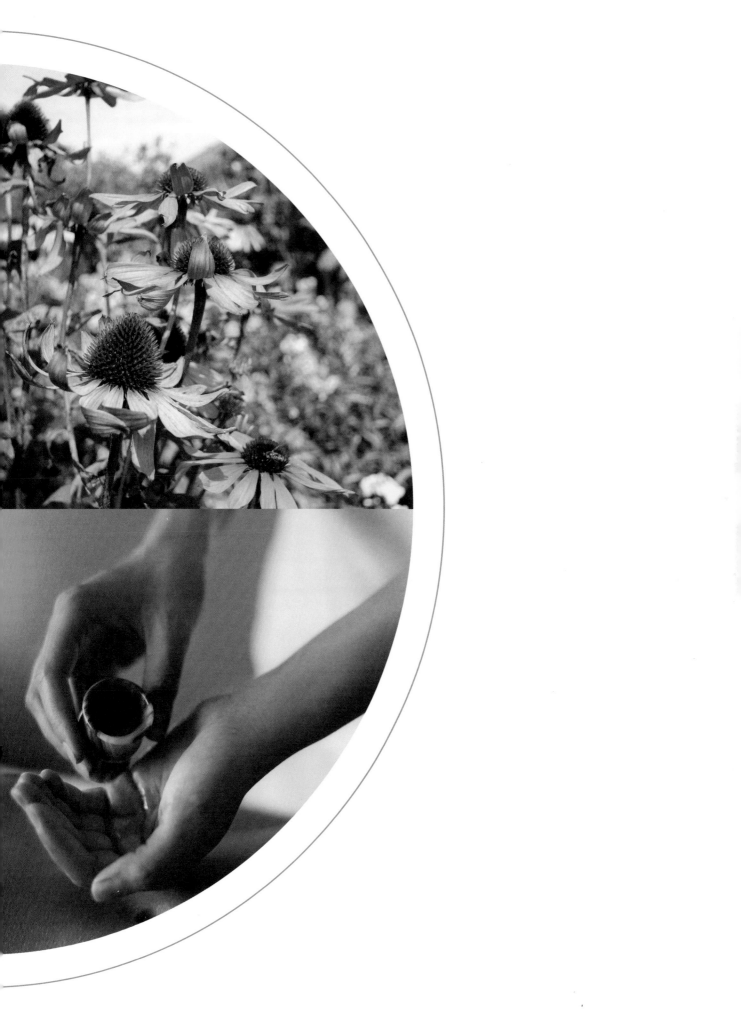

AYURVEDA

Ayurveda is a holistic system of medicine, meaning that our mind, body, and spirit are all taken into consideration in the diagnosis and treatment of illness. In the West we have long believed that each of us has the same anatomy, physiology, and disease process, but it has become increasingly clear that this approach does not take into account our differences – including our mental attitudes, our lifestyles, and our fundamental energy or spirit. Ayurveda is based on the philosophy that we are all unique, so it addresses each of these things in its treatment of people as individuals, and teaches that all illnesses affect the body and the mind, which should not be treated in isolation from each other.

WHAT IS AYURVEDA?
—

Ayurvedic medicine is the traditional system of medicine practiced in India and Sri Lanka. Like traditional Chinese medicine, Ayurveda is a complete system of healthcare, designed to contribute to a way of life, rather than an occasional treatment.

The word "Ayurveda" means "science" or "wisdom" of life, and it embraces elements as diverse as medicine, philosophy, science, spirituality, astrology, and astronomy. Although Ayurveda has been practiced for over 3,000 years, it is an advanced system of living as relevant today as it was so many years ago. In fact, as we realize the limitations of our conventional Western approach, it becomes clear that Ayurveda can offer much to treat and prevent many modern diseases that conventional medicine has been unable to treat. These include ME (myalgic encephalomyelitis), stress-related disorders, arthritis, impotence, asthma, eczema, and chronic illness. It offers natural herbal remedies to counter imbalances in the body, and detoxification, diet, exercise, meditation, spiritual guidance, and wide-ranging techniques to improve mental and emotional health.

PRANA: THE ENERGY OF LIFE
—

The fundamental belief in Ayurveda is that everything within the universe is composed of energy, or "prana." Like everything else, we too are comprised of energy, which changes according to our circumstances, our environment, our diets and lifestyles, and the world around us. Some of these changes can be positive, and others negative, and in order to ensure that most of the changes are positive, we must live in a way that encourages energy balance. Energy controls the functions of every cell, thought, emotion, and action, so every aspect of our lives, including the food we eat and the thoughts we think, affects the quality of our energy, and consequently our health.

Ayurvedic medicine teaches that there is no single prescription for health that is appropriate for everyone. In Ayurveda every person must be treated individually. The skill of the practitioner lies in his ability to correctly identify each individual's constitution, diagnosing the causes of imbalance and then treating the patient accordingly.

A HISTORY OF AYURVEDA
—

Over 3,000 years ago, 52 great Rishis, or seers, of ancient India discovered through meditation the "Veda," or the knowledge of how our world and everything within it works. Contained within the knowledge of the Veda were the secrets of sickness and health. These secrets were organized into a system called Ayurveda, the sophistication of which is apparent in the most famous of all ancient Ayurvedic texts, the *Charaka Samhita*. Its believed author was the first great Hindu physician known, Charaka, who practiced about 1000 B.C.E. The knowledge of the Rishis had three main components: etiology (the science of the cause of illness and disease), symptomatology (the study of symptoms), and finally medication (the process of treating individuals to cure disease or relieve pain).

Throughout much of their history, the Indians came into contact with the Persians, Greeks, and Chinese, with whom they exchanged information. Ayurvedic beliefs were founded on Hindu philosophy, but were enlarged and enhanced by the teachings of the Lord Buddha (d. 483 B.C.E.), who taught that the mind could be enriched through correct thinking. Today Buddhism is one of the fastest-growing belief systems in the West. The eightfold path of Buddhism encompasses:

- Right understanding
- Right concentration
- Right livelihood
- Right mindfulness
- Right action
- Right thought
- Right effort
- Right speaking.

Another important Ayurvedic text, the *Sushruta Samhita*, offers guidance on surgery, surgical equipment, suturing, and the importance of hygiene during and after an operation. Detailed medical information is teamed with commonsense advice on how to live a healthy and meaningful life. Its author, Sushruta, who lived in the 5th century C.E., noted the relationship of malaria to mosquitoes, and of plague to rats. He knew of more than 700 medicinal plants, and described more than 100 surgical instruments. He treated fractures, removed tumors and kidney stones, and delivered babies by cesarean section.

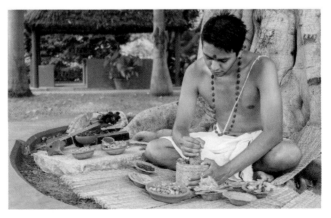

The word "Ayurveda" means "wisdom of life." Life encompasses body, mind, and soul.

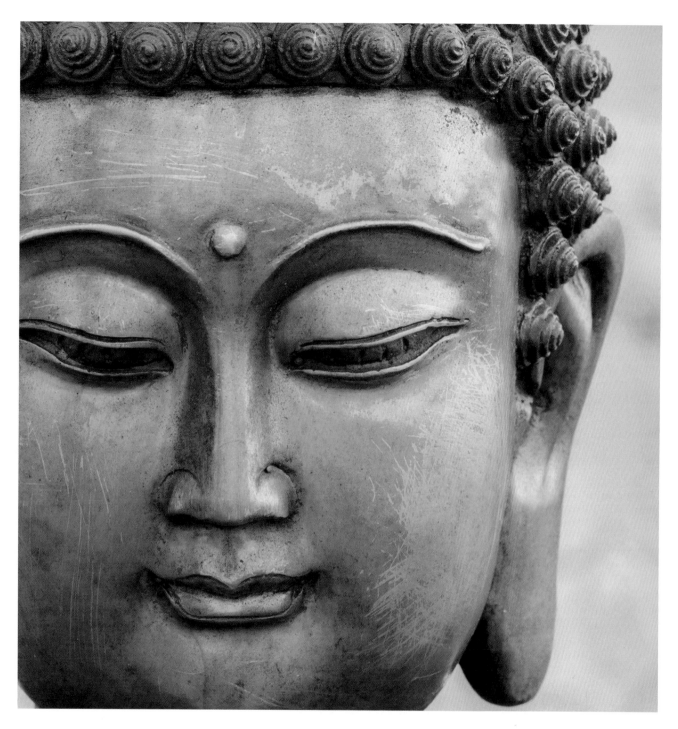

In Vedic philosophy our lives become meaningful when we strive to fulfill our potential, but that cannot be achieved without basic good health.

CAUSES OF DISEASE
—

Ayurvedic practitioners believe that disease may be triggered by many external causes, including planetary influences, acts of god, fire and accidents, harmful gases (which we would today call pollution), poisons and toxins, and evil spirits. As well as this, there are two other main causes of illness, an imbalance of the "tridoshas" (vátha, pitta, and kapha; see page 19) and mental imbalance.

The purpose of Ayurveda is to enable people to avoid serious illness by understanding how we become ill. For the most part, it works on a preventive basis, but when we do become ill it offers a wide range of treatments to help the

The teachings of the Buddha were integrated into the philosophy of Ayurveda.

body heal itself. Every Ayurvedic remedy is free of side-effects, is made from natural substances, and is nontoxic. In order to benefit from Ayurveda, it is not necessary to understand or believe in the complex spirituality that goes hand-in-hand with the system. All that is necessary is an open mind and a desire to be healed.

HOW DOES AYURVEDA WORK?

THE FIVE ELEMENTS
—

The universe consists of five elements, or pancha-mahabhutas: Ether (space), Air, Earth, Fire, and Water. All five elements exist in all things, including ourselves:

• Ether corresponds to the spaces in the body: the mouth, nostrils, thorax, abdomen, respiratory tract, and cells.
• Air is the element of movement so it represents muscular movement, pulsation, expansion and contraction of the lungs and intestines, even the movement in every cell.
• Fire controls enzyme functioning. It shows itself as intelligence, fuels the digestive system, and regulates metabolism.
• Water is in plasma, blood, saliva, digestive juices, mucous membranes, and cytoplasm, the liquid inside cells.
• Earth manifests in the solid structures of the body: the bones, nails, teeth, muscles, cartilage, tendons, skin, and hair.

THE THREE DOSHAS
—

There are three further bio-energies, called doshas or the tridoshas, which exist in everything in the universe, and which are composed of different combinations of the five elements. The three doshas affect all body functions, on both a mental and a physical level. Good health is achieved when all three doshas work in balance. Each one has its role to play in the body:

• Vátha is the driving force; it relates to the nervous system and the body's energy.
• Pitta is Fire; it relates to the metabolism, digestion, enzymes, acid, and bile.
• Kapha is related to Water in the mucous membranes, phlegm, moisture, fat, and lymphatics.

We will be made up of a combination of two or all three types of dosha, although we may tend to be predominantly one. Some subgroups include vátha-pitta, vátha-kapha or pitta-kapha.

Your constitution is determined by the state of your parents' doshas at the time of your conception, and each individual is born in the "prakruthi" state, which means that you are born with levels of the three doshas that are right for you. But, as we go through life, environment, stress, trauma, poor diet and exercise, poor digestion, poor elimination of body wastes, and injury cause the doshas to become imbalanced, a state known as the "vikruthi" state. When levels of imbalance are excessively high or low it can lead to ill health. Ayurvedic practitioners work to restore individuals to their "prakruthi" state.

Turmeric reduces kapha and vátha, and increases pitta.

THE FUNDAMENTAL QUALITIES
—

The principle of qualities in Ayurveda is similar to the Chinese concept of yin and yang, in that every quality has its opposite, and good health depends on finding a balance between the two extremes of qualities such as slow and fast, wet and dry, cloudy and clear, hot and cold. For example, heat relates to pitta, an imbalance of which can cause problems such as fevers, heartburn, or emotional disturbances such as anger or jealousy. If you have an excess of pitta you need to reduce your heat quality by eating fewer pitta foods, such as onions, garlic, and beef, and introduce more "cooling" foods, such as eggs, cheese, and lentils.

DIGESTION AND ELIMINATION
—

In Ayurveda, good digestion is the key to good health. Poor digestion produces "ama," a toxic substance that is believed to be the cause of illness. Ama is seen in the body as a white coating on the tongue, but it can also line the colon and clog blood vessels. Ama occurs when the metabolism is impaired as a result of an imbalance of "agni." Agni is the Fire which, when it is working effectively, maintains normality in all the functions of the body. Uneven agni is caused by imbalances in the doshas, and such factors as eating and drinking too much of the wrong foods, smoking, and repressing emotions.

Malas represent the effective elimination of waste products and there are four main types: sharkrit or pureesha (feces), mootra (urine), sweda (sweat), and ama, which cannot be eliminated and an accumulation of which causes disease.

THE SEVEN TISSUES
—

Imbalance in the doshas also causes imbalance in the seven body tissues, or "dhatus." These are: plasma (rasa), blood (raktha), muscle (mamsa), fat (madas), bone (asthi), marrow and nerves (majja), and reproductive tissues (shukra). The dhatus support and derive energy from each other, so when one is affected the others also suffer.

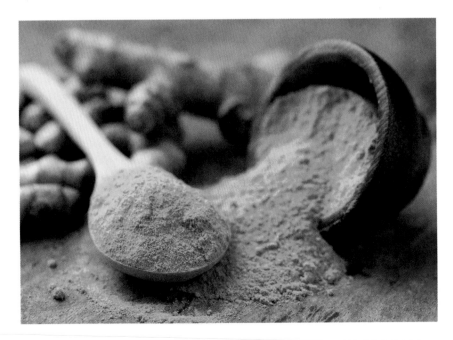

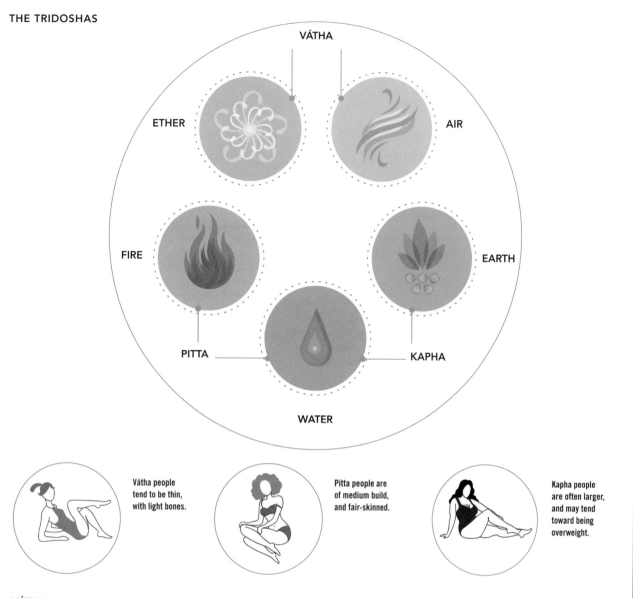

VÁTHA

AIR

ETHER

FIRE

EARTH

PITTA

KAPHA

WATER

Vátha people tend to be thin, with light bones.

Pitta people are of medium build, and fair-skinned.

Kapha people are often larger, and may tend toward being overweight.

VÁTHA

Vátha is a combination of the elements Air and Ether, with Air being the most dominant. Its qualities are light, cold, dry, rough, subtle, mobile, clear, dispersing, erratic, and astringent. Predominantly vátha people are thin with dry, rough, or dark skin; large, crooked or protruding teeth; a small, thin mouth, and dull, dark eyes.

Characteristics:
• Often constipated
• Frequent but sparse urine and little perspiration
• Highly original and creative mind
• Poor long-term memory
• Rapid speech
• Tendency to anxiety and depression
• High sex drive (or none at all)
• Love of travel
• Dislike of cold weather

PITTA

Pitta is mostly Fire with some Water. Its qualities are light, hot, oily, sharp, liquid, sour, and pungent. Pitta types seem to conform to a happy medium, and are of medium height and build, with soft, fair, freckled, or bright skin; soft, fair, light brown, or reddish hair that goes prematurely gray; small, yellowish teeth, and an average-sized mouth.

Characteristics:
• Speaks clearly, but often sharply
• Enjoys light but uninterrupted sleep
• Intelligent
• Clear memory
• Jealous
• Ambitious
• Passionately sexual
• Interested in politics
• Dislikes heat
• Loves luxury
• Loose stools and a tendency to diarrhea
• Strong appetite
• Great thirst

KAPHA

Kapha is a combination of mostly Water and some Earth. Its qualities are heavy, cold, oily, slow, slimy, dense, soft, static, and sweet. Kapha people tend to be large-framed and often overweight, with thick, pale, cool, and oily skin; thick, wavy and oily hair, either very dark or very light; strong white teeth, and a large mouth with full lips.

Characteristics:
• Speaks slowly and monotonously, and needs plenty of deep sleep
• Sluggish or slow but steady appetite
• Heavy sweating
• Large soft stools
• Businesslike
• Good memory
• Passive, bordering on lethargic
• Dislikes cold and damp
• Delights in good food and familiar places

AYURVEDIC TREATMENT

DETOXIFICATION: SHODANA
—

In Ayurvedic medicine it is essential to detoxify the body before prescribing restorative treatment. "Shodana" is used to eliminate disease, blockages in the digestive system, or causes of imbalance in the doshas. Where shodana is required, the practitioner will sometimes use a preparatory therapy called "purwakarma." Purwakarma breaks down into two types of treatment, "snehana" and "swedana":

• Snehana. This involves massaging herbal oils into the skin to encourage elimination of toxins. Blended oils are used to treat specific disorders, such as stress, anxiety, insomnia, arthritis, or circulation problems. Oils can also be massaged into the scalp for depression, insomnia, and memory problems. Snehana can sometimes involve lying in an oil bath, which is thought to be even more effective at allowing you to absorb the properties from herbal oils.
• Swedana. Swedana means sweating. It is sometimes used in conjunction with the oil treatment, but on a separate day. Steam baths are used to encourage the elimination of toxins through the pores, and, together with the oil treatments, they make the detoxification process much more effective.

In snehana, warm herbal oils may be poured onto the forehead to help eliminate toxins from the body.

"Panchakarma" therapy may follow purwakarma, or is sometimes used in isolation. This is a profound detoxification. It is traditionally a fivefold therapy, but all five aspects are used only in very rare cases. You may need only two or three of the following treatments:

• Nirhua vasti (oil enema therapy). The oil is passed through a tube to the rectum, using gravity, rather than pressure, so that it does not cause damage. Oil enemas are often used to eliminate vátha or pitta-oriented problems, such as in the treatment of constipation, irritable bowel syndrome, diarrhea, indigestion, and fungal infections.
• Ánuvasana vasti (herbal enema). The practitioner makes a herbal decoction and passes it through the tube. The selection of a herbal enema rather than an oil one depends on the patient's problem and the contraindications.
• Vireka (herbal laxative therapy). Vireka is used as a normal part of any detoxification therapy, and is also used to treat pitta-oriented disease, such as gastrointestinal problems, and vátha problems, such as constipation and irritable bowel syndrome. It also helps with inflammatory skin complaints, fluid retention, liver problems, and energy problems.
• Vamana (therapeutic vomiting). This is a traditional treatment for respiratory and catarrhal problems such as bronchitis, sinusitis, and asthma, but it is rarely used today.
• Nasya (herbal inhalation therapy). This treatment involves inhaling the vapor from medicinal herbs infused in boiling water. It is used mostly to eliminate kapha-oriented problems, ear, eyes, nose and throat disorders, headaches, migraine, neuralgia, sinusitis, catarrh, and bronchitis.

SAMANA
—

After the detoxification process, the practitioner may prescribe herbal or mineral remedies. These are to stimulate agni and restore balance in the doshas. They are not prescribed to eradicate disease, because the disease is just a symptom of doshic imbalance.

Herbal remedies are usually prescribed in liquid form or as dried herbs, although they can also come in powder or tablet form. The ingredients are pre-prepared, but the blends are prescribed for the individual. Each ingredient is classified by the effect it has on lowering or increasing the levels of the doshas.

Prescriptions are usually made up of groups of herbs, to which you add eight cups of water and boil until the liquid is reduced to one cup. You may have to take the remedy two or three times a day.

Your practitioner will also advise on lifestyle, food, and exercise. There is no single healthy diet in Ayurveda – just a diet that is best for you. It is important to eat to suit your constitution, and the practitioner may prepare a diet sheet for you to use.

Other therapies that may be prescribed by Ayurvedic practitioners include meditation, breathing exercises, yoga, and psychotherapy or counseling. Marma puncture is rather like acupuncture: it adjusts energy levels in the body by stimulating energy points. The similar marma therapy applies pressure or massage to marma points. Your practitioner may suggest that your chakras, which are centers of energy located along the midline of the body which distribute energy to the 107 marma points on the body, need to

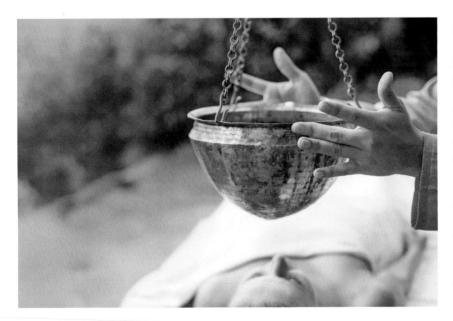

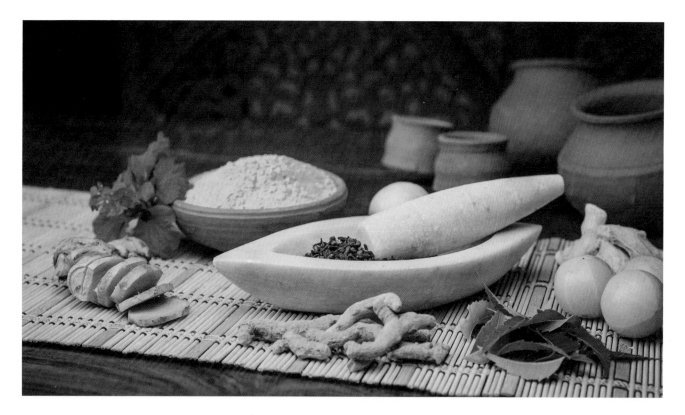

Carefully chosen Asian plants are used to balance the three doshas.

be unblocked. Rejuvenation therapy, or rasayana, helps to promote and preserve health and longevity in the healthy, and to cure disease in the sick.

PLANT POWER
—

In many cases the whole plant is used in an Ayurvedic treatment; in others, only part. All plants are associated with the following properties and effects:

• The three doshas. Plants can be used to increase or decrease an influence as required.
• Shad rasa (the tastes). Every plant contains one or more of the six basic tastes, which are sweet, acidic, salty, pungent, bitter, and astringent.
• Gunas (the properties). The gunas are distinctive characteristics that can be related to matter, thoughts, and ideas. There is a belief that everything in the universe is made up of complementary opposites (see yin and yang, in Chinese Herbal Medicine, page 22). There are 20 gunas: hot and cold, hard and soft, oily and dry, light and heavy, dull and sharp, subtle and gross, slimy and

rough, unmoving and mobile, turbid and transparent, solid and liquid. The properties of each guna are related to the doshas, and specific substances, which are characterized by specific gunas, can increase or decrease dosha influence throughout the body. The properties of each guna can affect the doshas.

Many herbs are used in Ayurvedic preparations, and are sold as essences, pills, powders, pastes, and potencized remedies. Often they are herbs that are known and used in the West, although they are used differently in Ayurvedic medicine.

Herbs can have many effects on the body, including purifying the blood, binding stools, aiding digestion, expelling worms, improving coagulation, healing fractures, increasing appetite, lowering fever, reducing toxins, balancing the tridoshas (or increasing or decreasing the three doshas), strengthening the heart, among others.

It is usually safe to combine taking Ayurvedic herbal remedies and orthodox medicines. However, you should inform your Ayurvedic practitioner of any medication you are currently taking or have taken in the past.

AYURVEDIC REMEDIES	
NAME	PAGE
Yarrow	74
Calamus root	75
Onion	78
Garlic	79
Aloe vera	80
Angelica	82
Celery seed	84
Barberry	90
Mustard	91
Caraway	97
Cayenne	98
Senna	99
Cedar	100
Gotu kola	101
Camphor	103
Cinnamon	104
Myrrh	112
Coriander	113
Saffron	115
Cumin	116
Turmeric	117
Cardamom	122
Cloves	125
Licorice	132
St. John's wort	138
Wild sunflower	140
Alfalfa	150
Nutmeg	153
Basil	156
Long pepper	164
Black pepper	164
Sandalwood	179
Fenugreek	191
Vetiver	197
Ginger	200

CHINESE HERBAL MEDICINE

Chinese medicine is an ancient system of healing – acupuncture and Chinese herbal medicine grew up in tandem over 2,000 years. It is based on the philosophy of a very different civilization from our own, a civilization that perceived people as either "in harmony" or "out of harmony" with themselves and their surroundings. Traditional Chinese medicine (TCM) sees disease in terms of patterns of disharmony, and so attempts to restore the balance in the person who is sick. Energy is believed to flow through channels called meridians, through which disease may be treated.

WHAT IS CHINESE HERBAL MEDICINE?
—

TCM uses terminology that sounds strange to most Westerners. Instead of talking about rheumatic diseases or neurological diseases, it classifies diseases as being caused by wind, heat, dampness, or cold. Instead of talking about rheumatism in the knee joint, it may classify it as cold–damp in the stomach meridian (see page 23). Western medicine focuses on a specific cause for a specific disease, and when it isolates that cause or agent it tries to control or destroy it. Chinese medicine is also concerned with the cause, but it focuses on the patient's response to that disease entity, both physiological and psychological. All the

relevant information, including symptoms that may not seem related to the patient's main complaint, is collected together to enable the practitioner to discover the pattern of disharmony within that person, which can then be addressed by Chinese medicine. For instance, two patients coming with asthma may have completely different diagnoses according to Chinese medicine. The one with a pale face, prone to catching colds (lung qi deficiency) will be given a completely different herbal formula from the patient who has a dry cough, thirst, and breathlessness on exertion (lung yin deficiency). TCM does treat the same diseases – to a large extent people have the same problems the world over – it just perceives them in an entirely different way.

YIN AND YANG
—

Chinese medicine is based on the philosophy of yin and yang. These are the dual forces in the universe, seen both within nature and in human beings. They are used to explain the ongoing process of natural changes – yang is more prevalent during the day, while yin forces are more prevalent at night. Everything has a yin and a yang aspect. For instance: fall and winter have a yin aspect, while spring and summer have a yang aspect. When it comes to breathing, inhalation is yin while exhalation is yang. There is no absolute yin or yang in living things – a cold yin-type illness may have aspects of yang, such as sharp, forceful contractions. Yin and yang both depend on each other and keep each other under control. However, it is when they go seriously out of balance and do not correct themselves that there is disease.

A SHORT HISTORY
—

The earliest known herbal formulas in China were written down in the 3rd century B.C.E. The main book of the theory of Chinese

The symbol for yin and yang shows them to be interdependent.

medicine – the Yellow Emperor's *Inner Classic* – was compiled in the 1st century C.E., and is still taught in schools of TCM. Over the centuries, leading physicians have written down both herbal and acupuncture formulas. The *Imperial Grace Formulary* of the Tai Pang Era (around 985 C.E.) for example, contains 16,834 entries, many of which are still commonly referred to today. The early herbal formulas were very simple and elegant, while the later ones are much more complicated. Either type can be useful, depending on the patient and the physician's preferred manner of working.

THE CHINESE THEORY OF LIFE
—

The Chinese believe that every living being is sustained by a basic life force, called "qi" (pronounced "chee"). Human beings receive their qi from a mixture of the influences of both Heaven and Earth. Therefore, we do have an element of the divine in us, which separates us from the animals. Chinese medicine works with the qi that we have to make us better. It may unblock the flow of qi in the body if it is stuck, or it may nourish qi if it is deficient.

We are born with a fixed amount of qi inherited from our parents (yuan qi – source or genetic qi). This is used both as our "reserve tank" and as a catalyst in most of the chemical processes of the body. We can nourish our yuan qi, though we cannot add to it. We may, however, deplete it through bad living practices – long-term lack of sleep or good food, drugs, drink, or years of excessive sex. The Chinese believe that this source qi is stored in the kidneys (where its substance is called jing or essence), and its functions include the control of sexual and reproductive activity in the body. We get our day-to-day qi from the air we breathe (gong qi) and the food we eat (gu qi).

Qi permeates the entire body; it directs the blood, nerve, and lymphatic systems (ying qi). It protects us from catching viruses (wei qi), and fights them if they get into the body. It transforms the food we eat into bodily substances – blood, tears, sweat, and urine – keeps organs in their proper place, and prevents excessive loss of sweat. Qi keeps the body warm and is naturally the source of movement and growth, as it has all these functions. We also use it in TCM to describe the functions of any organ – for instance, lung qi may be "weak" or liver qi "blocked."

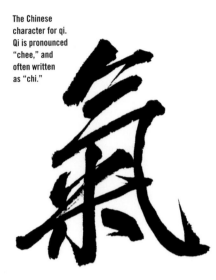

The Chinese character for qi. Qi is pronounced "chee," and often written as "chi."

MERIDIANS AND ORGANS
—

Although qi is everywhere in the body, it has main pathways along which it flows, nourishing and warming the organs and body parts, and harmonizing their activity. These channels are called the meridian system (jing-luo). Most acupuncture points are sited along these channels, and most herbs that a practitioner of Chinese medicine prescribes enter one or more of the meridian pathways. There are 12 main meridians, and these correspond to the 12 main organs in the body. These meridians are bilateral – there is an identical pair on each side of the body. Some are more yin meridians, with functions more to do with storing the vital essences of the body. These are the kidneys, liver, spleen, heart, lungs, and pericardium. The other six are more yang meridians, with functions more to do with transportation of fluids and food. These are the bladder, gall bladder, stomach, small intestine, large intestine, and the triple burner (a mechanism which regulates the overall body temperature and the upper, middle, and lower parts [jiaos] of the body). There are also six extra meridians, one of which runs up the front center line of the body (the ren mai or conception vessel), and one of which runs up the spine (the du mai or governor vessel).

Chinese herbs may nourish qi.

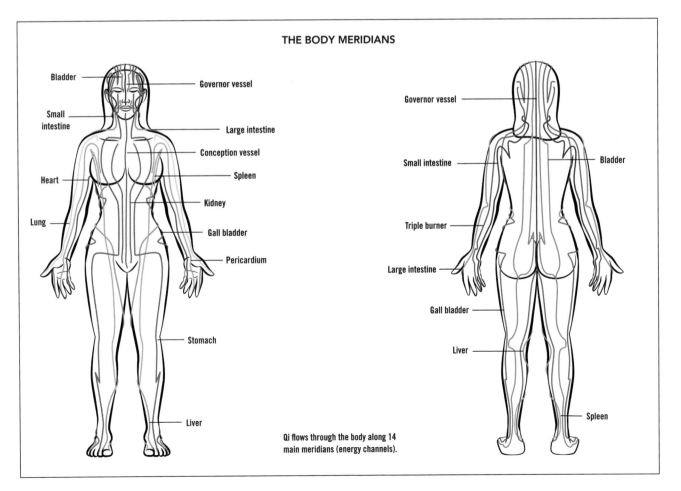

THE BODY MERIDIANS

Bladder
Small intestine
Heart
Lung
Governor vessel
Large intestine
Conception vessel
Spleen
Kidney
Gall bladder
Pericardium
Stomach
Liver

Governor vessel
Small intestine
Triple burner
Large intestine
Gall bladder
Liver
Bladder
Spleen

Qi flows through the body along 14 main meridians (energy channels).

CONSULTING A CHINESE HERBALIST

THE CONSULTATION

—

When you consult a practitioner of Chinese herbal medicine, he or she will first of all ask you in detail about your presenting condition – when it first appeared, your symptoms, what makes it worse or better. You will then be asked about your past medical history and your general health, for example:

• Your appetite, diet, digestion, stools, and urination
• Your sleep patterns, any pain – headaches, backache – and ear, nose, and throat (ENT) problems
• Intake of drugs, alcohol, and nicotine
• Body temperature (more hot or cold), circulation, and perspiration
• Energy levels, mental, and emotional states
• Gynecology – menstruation, pregnancies, and menopause.

Finally, your practitioner will take both radial (wrist) pulses and look at your tongue, in order to help him or her to make a diagnosis according to Chinese medicine.

UNDERSTANDING THE DIAGNOSIS

—

When a practitioner of Chinese medicine talks about an organ being out of balance, he or she usually refers to the meridian related to that organ, not necessarily the physical organ itself. For instance, the liver meridian runs from the big toe, up the inside of the leg, through the genitals, and then deep into the liver organ itself. There can be problems along the course of the meridian, and there is also a sphere of influence which each organ has within the body.

The liver controls the free flow of qi generally in the body, including the evenness of emotions, digestion, and menstruation. It also stores the blood, rules circulation in the tendons, has the major influence on the eyes, and manifests in the nails. It is therefore possible to see how diseases in these areas of the body may be treated via the liver meridian.

In illness, different meridians exhibit different tendencies of disharmony – for

PREPARATIONS AND TREATMENT

There are many ways of taking herbs. Individual herbs can be added to foods or taken as a tea, but Chinese herbs are rarely taken singly – they are much more effective when made into a composite prescription.

DECOCTIONS
Packets of dried herbs are boiled for around 30 minutes, down to 2 cups, and then often boiled again to last two days. They smell worse than they taste!

POWDERS
One teaspoon of cooked, freeze-dried herbs is taken two or three times a day, mixed with a little cold water to a paste; then a little boiling water is added.

TINCTURES
One teaspoon taken two or three times a day. More palatable but weaker than decoctions or powders.

PILLS AND CAPSULES
These are used for patent remedies (prescriptions which have not been changed to suit the individual). They are easy to swallow, but you have to take large quantities, up to eight tablets at a time.

SYRUPS
These are patent remedies, mainly good for coughs or children's tonics.

PLASTERS
These are used for rheumatic ailments (wind-damp); they are very effective for relieving local pain and stiffness. Treatment generally means taking herbs two or three times a day until the problem is gone.

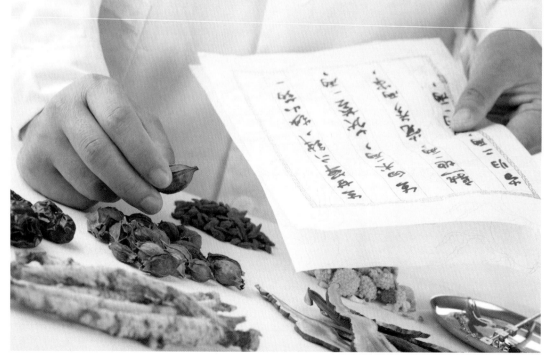

A practitioner of herbal medicine makes up a prescription.

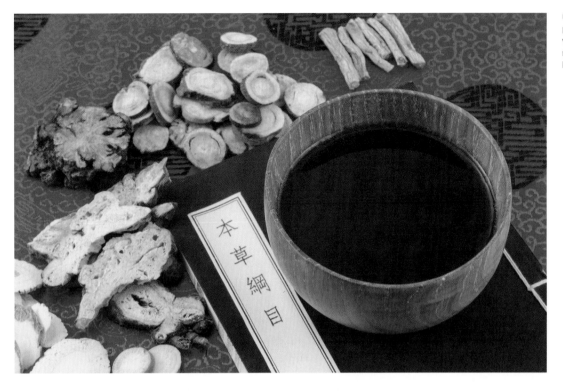

Chinese herbal preparations come in various forms, from raw and powdered herbs, to decoctions.

instance, the spleen has a tendency to deficiency causing damp. This creates symptoms such as diarrhea or lassitude (tiredness). The liver, on the other hand, has a tendency toward rising yang, creating red sore eyes, migraines, and high blood pressure. It is these disharmonies that Chinese herbal medicine can address.

THE PRESCRIPTION
—

The practitioner may search through some books to check on the herbal prescription most suited to your condition, and will then write down a personal prescription tailored to your needs. This will include anything from 4 to 20 herbs, and their dosages in ounces or grams, or in qian (Chinese measurements). The names of the herbs will be in English, Latin, Pinyin (anglicized Chinese), or in Chinese characters.

Your practitioner will then make up the prescription for you or refer you to a herbal supplier to have it made up elsewhere.

Chinese herbs are hardly ever used singly – they are used mainly in combination with other herbs to make a balanced prescription. Each herb also has a particular range of dosages assigned to it –

when comparing it to other herbs in a prescription, one can see whether it is used in an average dose, or whether one would use a smaller or larger dose in that prescription.

Both these features mean that it is important to consult a qualified herbalist before using the herbs suggested in this book. This book is, however, a useful resource for understanding and checking your prescriptions.

REPEAT VISITS
—

At first you will need to see your practitioner every one or two weeks so that he or she can alter the prescription as your symptoms improve. You may experience slight nausea, diarrhea, or digestive upset as your system becomes used to the herbs. In this case, you will need to halve your dosage and build it up again slowly; your practitioner may add more digestive herbs in order that you may tolerate it better. After that, you may be able to see or even telephone your practitioner once a month in order to report on progress, and so that the prescription can be changed accordingly. Herbal medicines should not be taken without review by a registered herbalist for more than 30 days.

TASTES

In the next chapter, "Healing Remedies," we will mention the taste of each herb used in Chinese herbalism. In traditional Chinese medicine, taste partly determines therapeutic function, so it is important to know what each taste signifies:

ACRID
Pungent or acrid substances disperse and move qi (energy). Acrid herbs mainly affect the lung functions.

BITTER
These herbs reduce excess qi, drain, and dry excess moisture. Bitter herbs mainly affect the heart organ.

SALTY
These herbs purge (drain through the bowels) and soften. Salty herbs mainly affect the kidney organ.

SWEET
Sweet substances tonify, harmonize, and strengthen qi, and may sometimes moisten. Sweet herbs mainly affect the spleen organ.

SOUR
Sour substances are astringent and prevent or reverse the abnormal leakage of fluids and energy. They mainly affect the kidney organ.

BLAND
Bland substances have none of these tastes. They primarily leach out dampness and promote urination. This helps both the spleen and the kidneys.

THE HERBS USED

PLANTS AND MINERALS
—

Chinese herbs are mostly made of plant parts – leaves, flowers, fruit, or fruit peel, twigs, roots, bark, or fungus. There are some minerals, such as gypsum, but these are less commonly used. There are also animal parts in traditional Chinese herbal medicine, such as snake, mammal bones, or deer horn. However, their importation has now been forbidden, and herbal practitioners find alternatives to prescribe. Some patent remedies containing animal products may still be sold. They are now illegal in this country, so please check with the pharmacy first. Always go to a reputable practitioner (see page 384). Some herbal patents for insomnia and mental disturbance contain mineral substances such as oyster shell or magnetite. In excess, these can cause indigestion, so use them for a limited amount of time and find alternative prescriptions.

The medicinal use of herbs in China is believed to date back to about 2000 B.C.E., when Emperor Chi'en Nung wrote a book called the *Pen Tsao*, which listed the medicinal properties of over 300 plants. The Chinese word for herbalism, "Ben cao," dates from about 500 B.C.E. "Ben" means a plant with a rigid stalk, and "cao" means a grass-like plant. Herbalism developed to include the use of mineral and animal ingredients.

PATENT HERBAL PREPARATIONS
—

These are sold as over-the-counter remedies for colds and flu, coughs and phlegm, even strep throat infections; also for rheumatic ailments, pain, and bruising from trauma. Patent remedies used for anything else must be diagnosed by a herbal practitioner, even tonics; for instance, do you need to tonify the qi, blood, yin, or yang? It is important to consult a herbal practitioner if you intend to use a patent remedy over a long period of time, such as a long-term tonic for an elderly person. Common preparations include:

• Tong Xuan Li Fei Wan. This is best for colds and flu where you feel chilled and achy, and there is sneezing, maybe with watery catarrh.

• Yin Qiao Jie Du Pian. Honeysuckle and forsythia febrifugal pills are best for colds and flu where you feel hot, have a sore throat, sneezing, and thick catarrh.
• Qing Qi Hua Tan Wan. Take for chest congestion and tightness in the chest, a cough, and coughing up thick yellow phlegm. It should produce an improvement in a couple of days, if it does not, seek professional help.
• Chuan Bei Pi Pa Lu. Use for an acute and chronic cough which produces thick phlegm.
• Huo Xiang Zheng Qi Wan. Also known as herba agastachis pills, these are useful for gastric flu and for vomiting caused by food poisoning. If there is no improvement within a day, seek professional advice.
• Die Da Wan Pills and Imperial Ted Da Wine. The remedy is taken internally for bruises, sprains, and healing fractures. It is not to be taken during pregnancy or if there is copious bleeding.
• Jing Wan Hung. This ointment is used for burns and bedsores.
• Dang Gui Pian (angelica tea), Shi Chuan Da Bu Wan (ten flavor tea), and Wu Ji Rai Feng Wan (white phoenix pills). These remedies are often prescribed for menstrual problems, depending on the nature and cause of the problem. For example, Dang Gui Pian is good for pain but not for excessive bleeding. All these remedies supplement qi and blood. For persistent problems, it is wise to consult a physician.

SAFETY NOTES
—

As mentioned on the previous page, it is important to consult a qualified practitioner before using herbs medicinally. If prescribing herbs over a long period of time, it is important that the practitioner pays particular attention to any liver or kidney symptoms which may arise during the course of treatment. A very few individuals may experience idiosyncratic reactions to herbs – these are usually due to genetic abnormalities and the herbs would not cause a reaction in most other individuals. Regular liver function tests are sometimes advised by practitioners, but their value in these cases is still a matter of debate.

Chinese herbal medicine may be very effective for children, when under the care of a qualified practitioner. Children's dosages are usually half or a quarter of those given for adults. There are ways of encouraging children to take the herbs, either by involving them in the preparation of the prescription, or by sweetening it with honey, or by offering a cookie afterward!

Many herbs are expressly forbidden in pregnancy, while some are especially good for pregnant women. Take only herbs prescribed by a qualified practitioner when pregnant.

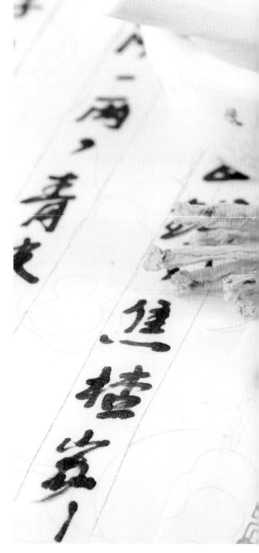

A prescription may contain an assortment of herbs.

PLANT PARTS

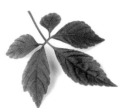

LEAF
Jiaogulan (*Gynostemma pentaphyllum*) leaf is sometimes used as a tonic.

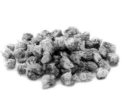

FLOWER
Ju Hua (chrysanthemum) is used therapeutically, for colds, dizziness, and headaches.

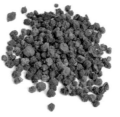

FRUIT
Wu Wei Zi (schisandra fruit) is sour and relieves sweating.

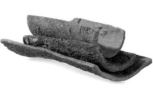

BARK
Rou Gui (cinnamon bark) is a warm herb and relieves cold.

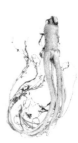

ROOT
Jie Geng (platycodon root) moves lung qi.

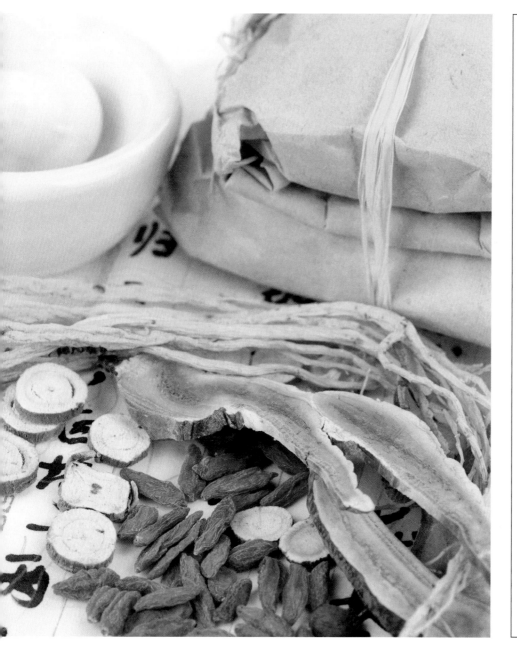

CHINESE REMEDIES

NAME	PAGE
Huo Xiang	77
Yi Zhi Ren	81
Bai Zhi	82
Dang Gui	82
Huang Qi	87
Bai Zhu	88
Mu Xiang	88
Huo Ma Ren	95
Hong Hua	97
Gui Zhi	104
Chen Pi	109
Dang Shen	110
Yi Yi Ren	111
Huang Lian	113
Shan Zhu Yu	114
Shan Zha	115
Tu Su Zi	118
Xiang Fu	120
Du Zhong	124
Zhe Bei Mu	129
Tian Ma	130
Gan Cao	132
Fang Feng	144
Chuan Xiong	145
Jin Yin Hua	146
Gou Qi Zi	147
Mai Men Dong	157
Bai Shao	159
Ren Shen	160
San Qi	160
Huang Bai	162
Ban Xia	163
Jie Geng	165
Yuan Zhi	166
He Shou Wu	167
Ye Jiao Teng	167
Fu Ling	168
Xing Ren	169
Tao Ren	170
Sheng Di Huang	172
Shu Di Huang	172
Da Huang	173
Wu Wei Zi	180
Huang Qin	181
Han Fang Ji	185
Suan Zao Ren	201

TRADITIONAL HOME AND FOLK REMEDIES

Every culture, across the centuries, has had its own understanding and ways of healing. Local plants, customs, and beliefs determined the form it took, which varied not only across countries but also between villages. Even today, away from the convenience of conventional physicians, local communities around the world practice their own form of medicinal healing using plants, age-old wisdom, and an instinctive and learnt knowledge of their bodies as the tools.

A RETURN TO OLD WAYS
—

With the advent of technology and the growing dependence upon the miracles of modern medicine, most of us have lost the art of looking after ourselves. We have become dependent upon physicians, prescription drugs, store-bought preparations, and, through that, have lost an understanding of our bodies and how they work. Somewhere along the line we have put not only our faith but our independence in the hands of others. When we have a cold, a rash, even painful joints, we go straight to the medicine cabinet, or ring to arrange an appointment at the physician's surgery. The use of natural preparations, and the number of people addressing minor complaints in their own homes, hit an all-time low over the past decades, and only now are we experiencing a renaissance of natural healing and home remedies, as it becomes clear that conventional medicine, for all its wonders, is not the answer to everything.

Busy Western physicians have little time to spend diagnosing their patients, and our Western approach to pathology and anatomy is based on the theory that we are all the same. Individual personalities, lifestyles, emotions, spirituality, and indeed physical bodies are not taken into consideration for most conventional treatment, but we have now learnt that it is the complex combination of these very things that can make us sick or well. Treatment, therefore, needs to examine a wider picture.

In the past, many of us had the knowledge and the wherewithal to treat ourselves, using foodstuffs in our larders, and plants growing in our yards and fields. There would have been a village healer or physician who could be called upon in times of emergency, but for day-to-day and common ailments, treatment was undertaken at home.

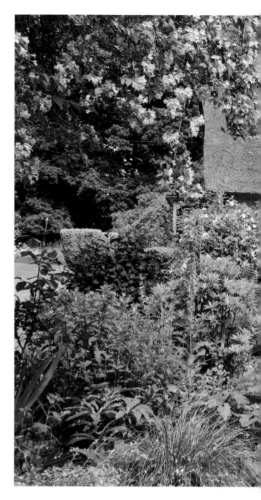

Folk and home remedies make use of local plants and store cupboard staples.

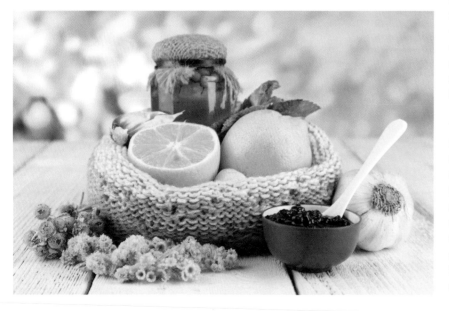

While our understanding of biochemistry could not match that of a modern physician, our knowledge of how plants and various substances work in our bodies, and, indeed, how our bodies respond in various situations, and to different treatments, was much more profound. Women instinctively treated their children and their families – recognizing a bad temper as the onset of illness, perhaps, and being capable of addressing the cause of an illness according to a more general knowledge of our holistic being.

Today, most drugs on the market tend to deal with symptoms, rather than the root cause of an illness. Conditions and symptoms such as asthma, eczema, ME (CFS), headaches, and menstrual problems are controlled rather than cured. We take a tablet to ease the pain of a headache, but we do not stop and consider why we have a headache. We apply creams to stop the itching of eczema, but we do nothing to address the cause. In the past, we had a

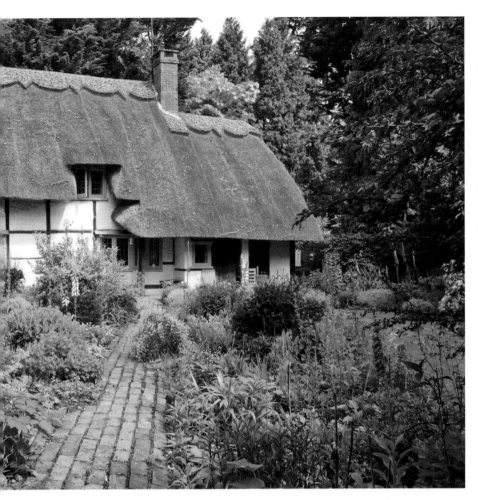

PREVENTING ILLNESS

—

Natural medicine in the home is more than just first aid for common and minor ailments. It can be preventive, using some of the most common items in the larder – onions, garlic, thyme, mint, sage, chamomile – to protect against many illnesses. Modern research – particularly over the last three decades – is now justifying the use of plants and household items, things that have been used for centuries in both folk medicine and traditional cookery. For example, mint calms the digestive system, lemon is a great detoxifier, helping the liver and kidneys to function effectively, rosemary has profound antiseptic powers and is a natural stimulant, and caraway seeds will prevent flatulence.

By incorporating some of these elements in your day-to-day meals, you not only add flavor and variety, but also provide the systems of your body with nourishment and support. These remedies have a beneficial effect on our general health and deal with specific problems, something that conventional drugs do not. Most available drugs work to address specific systems and do nothing for our overall health; many of them have side-effects that are more dangerous than the symptoms they are addressing.

Traditional folk and home remedies tend to work with our bodies, allowing them to heal themselves by keeping them strong and healthy.

much greater general understanding of the causes and effects of illness, and a much more instinctive approach to treatment. Folk medicine and home remedies kept the majority of people healthy and it is that tradition to which many people are increasingly returning today.

The cottage garden was designed to provide a source of medicinal plants, as well as vegetables and beautiful flowers.

Adding beneficial herbs, such as mint, sage, and thyme, to a salad, is an easy way to maintain health.

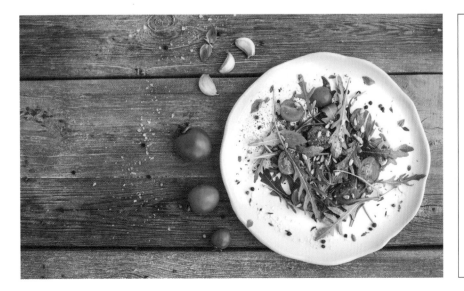

LEARNING ABOUT FOLK MEDICINE

Take time to learn about the various properties of the products available, and experiment until you find remedies that suit you and your family. Retrain yourself to consider the underlying causes of illness before seeking an instant relief from symptoms. Many of the home remedies work as fast as conventional drugs to bring relief, but the treatment of chronic disorders, such as bronchitis or rheumatism, will be slow, gentle, and cumulative, working to strengthen and stimulate various parts of the body over a long period of time. It is important to remember that the fresher or more recently picked the herb, the stronger its active properties. Dried herbs are more readily available and are about one-third as strong as the fresh product – and in some cases are better for the condition.

A HISTORICAL PERSPECTIVE

HAND IN HAND
—

Whenever possible, a system of folk medicine is best understood as dynamic in a historical context. The Aztecs in Mexico provide a good example of how conventional medical systems can go hand in hand with folk medicine, feeding from one another and allowing both to grow according to the needs of the population.

Aztec establishment (as opposed to folk) medicine was highly organized, with a herbarium, a zoo, an intellectual elite, and a training and certification academy. It was based on a complex theoretical structure and experimental research. Some segments of the population, however, had only limited access to this medicine. They relied instead on traditional treatments and medicines. Aztec establishment medicine was eliminated when the Spanish conquerors killed the medical personnel and introduced their own medicine. This intrusive system became the new medicine of the Aztec establishment.

The system still offered limited access. Some elements of the European approach, however, were compatible with the folk medical practice of the Native Americans and were therefore incorporated into a new folk system. Mexican folk medicine thrived and continued to incorporate elements of the new establishment medicine.

Similarly, Native North American systems, while not highly organized and academic, were the establishment medicine in their own societies before conquest. Europeans brought diseases that decimated populations and challenged indigenous medical systems. The social and moral bases of the systems came under attack by missionaries and governments, even as immigrants began to adopt the ideas and materials from native systems. Again, this intrusive medicine became the establishment medicine, and Native American medicine, incorporating some Euro-American elements, became folk medicine.

DISCOVERING PLANT BENEFITS
—

But the history of using plants for medicine and healing goes back to the beginning of humankind. In their search for nourishment, primitive humans sampled many kinds of plants. Those that were palatable were used for food, while plants with toxic or unpleasant effects were avoided or used against enemies. Other plants that produced physiological effects such as perspiration, defecation, healing, or hallucinations were saved for medicinal purposes and divination. Over the course of thousands of years, people have learnt to use a wide variety of plants as medicines for different ailments.

More than 4,000 years ago, the Chinese emperor Qien Nong (Chi'en Nung) put together a book of medicinal plants called *Ben Zao* (Pen Tsao). It contained descriptions of more than 300 plants, several of which are still used in medicine. The Sumerians, at the same time and later, were recording

The common foxglove (*Digitalis purpurea*) is the original source of the common heart medicine digoxin.

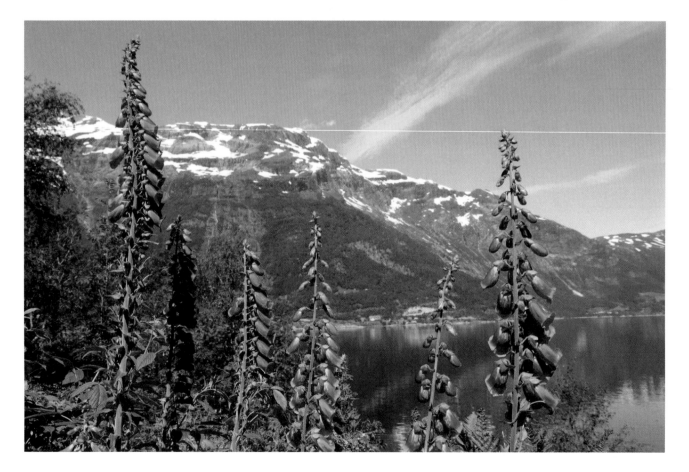

prescriptions on clay tablets, and the Egyptians were writing their medical systems on rolls of papyrus. The oldest such document, known as the *Papyrus Kahun*, dates from the time of King Amenemhet III (1840–1792 B.C.E.) and contains information about women's diseases and medical conditions.

The most famous of these medical papyri, the so-called *Ebers Papyrus*, reports voluminously on the pharmaceutical prescriptions of the era. It includes specific information on how plants are to be used, for example, in the treatment of parasite worms or of stomach ailments. Some of these plants are still used today – in folk and conventional medicine.

The Greeks and the Romans derived some of their herbal knowledge from these early civilizations. Their contributions are recorded in Dioscorides' *De Materia Medica* and the 37-volume natural history written by Pliny the Elder. Some of these works are known to us through translations into Arabic by Rhazes and Avicenna. The knowledge of medicinal plants was further nurtured by monks in Europe, who grew medicinal plants and translated the Arabic works. The first recognized apothecaries opened in Baghdad in the 9th century. By the 13th century, London had become a major trading center in herbs and spices.

In the Dark Ages, the belief of the Christian Church that disease was a punishment for sin caused a great setback in medical progress. Women in childbirth welcomed the pain as an opportunity to atone for their sins. Only in monasteries did herbals and other documented sources of natural medicine continue to be painstakingly translated.

The Renaissance provided a new forum for the development of the folk tradition. William Caxton printed dozens of medical manuals and Nicholas Culpeper translated the entire physicians' pharmacopeia *The English Physician* and *Complete Herbal* in 1653. It is still in print. The advent of alchemy, and the split between the "new philosophy" of reason and experiment, and the previous tradition of "science" (ancient medical doctrines, herbalism, astrology, and the occult) ended the golden age of

herbals. Witch hunts disposed of village "healing women"; women were forbidden to study and all nonprofessional healers were declared heretics. The use of herbs became associated with magic and the occult, an uneasy alliance that has been difficult to shake. Herbalism was effectively dropped from mainstream medical training, though folk advice and treatment from the apothecary herbalist continued to be available, especially in less well-off areas.

TRADITIONAL FOLK MEDICINE TODAY
—

The term "folk medicine" refers to the traditional beliefs, practices, and materials that people use to maintain health and cope with disease, outside of an organized relationship with academic, professionally recognized, and established medical systems and treatments. The beliefs and practices that make up a system of folk medicine are very closely related to the history, traditions, and life of a recognizable social group. Many people practice folk medicine today, generally working in an environment where they share the belief system of their patients, and their approach to maintaining health and treating disease.

As research into the active constituents of herbs continues, increasing numbers of ancient treatments and tonics are being rediscovered and recognized, and brought back into widespread use. The global transport network means that we now have access to treatments used in countries around the world – bringing us a variety of amazing plants such as ginseng, guarana, tea tree oil, aloe vera, and ginkgo biloba.

Much of the pharmacopeia of academic medicine – including aspirin (from the white willow) – has been derived from folk remedies, even as academic medicine has disparaged the folk reasons for their use. In the past this process has mostly been haphazard, but since the Second World War there has been an intensified, systematic investigation of tribal and folk medicines in the search for new preparations. More than 120 current prescription drugs are obtained from plants, and about 25 percent of all prescriptions contain one or more active ingredients from plants. There are plenty of herbal remedies already in use

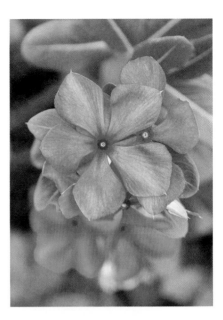

The rosy periwinkle (*Catharanthus roseus*) is a source of the conventional drugs vincristine and vinblastine, used to treat cancer.

within orthodox medicine; for example, components of the yew tree have been used successfully to halt cancer, and the rosy periwinkle is used to control leukemia, especially leukemia in children.

Comparison and evaluation of folk and academic medical systems and practices is difficult. On the one hand, indiscriminate interpretation of folk medicine may result in inappropriate rejection of proven establishment methods – for example, immunizations and drugs required to treat chronic and serious illness that may not have existed in the past. On the other hand, the dangerous aspects of folk medicine have often been emphasized, usually without recognizing the contributions of folk to conventional medicine and the similarities between them.

Today, there is a greater understanding of the power of natural remedies, and their use is being slowly accepted and indeed encouraged, particularly for ailments that people can safely and appropriately treat at home, such as headaches and upset stomachs, or sore throats. Disorders of the liver, heart, kidneys, etc., as well as severe illness – particularly in small children – are too serious for home treatment, and should be referred to a professional practitioner. For more advice on when to self-treat, turn to pages 238–241.

PREPARING FOLK REMEDIES

WHO CAN BENEFIT?
—

Folk medicine and home remedies do not provide a miracle cure, but almost anyone can benefit from the prudent use of herbs, plants, and household items as a form of restorative and preventive medicine. Most plants offer a rich source of vitamins and minerals, aside from having healing properties, and can be an important part of the daily diet, eaten fresh, or perhaps drunk as a tisane. A herbal tonic is useful, for example, in the winter months, when fresh fruit and green vegetables are not a regular part of our diets. Or plants like echinacea or garlic can be taken daily to improve the general efficiency of the immune system.

Some of the most common conditions that respond to home treatment include: hay fever, colds, and respiratory disorders, digestive disorders (like constipation and ulcers), cardiovascular disease, headaches, anxiety, depression, chronic infections, rheumatism, arthritis, skin problems, anemia, and many hormonal, menstrual, menopausal, and pregnancy problems. On top of that are scrapes, bruises, burns, swellings, sprains, and bites and stings.

Herbs do influence the way in which the body works, and although they are natural, they will have a profound effect on its functions. It is essential that you read the labels of any herbal products you have purchased, and follow carefully the advice of your herbalist. More is not better: although herbs don't have the side-effects of orthodox drugs, they have equally strong medicinal properties and can be toxic when taken in excess, causing liver failure, miscarriage, and heart attack, among other things.

REMEDY TYPES
—

There are a variety of forms in which treatment can be offered, depending on the condition and your individual needs:

• Powders. Plants in this form can be added to food or drinks, or put into capsules for easier consumption. Make your own powder by crushing dried plant parts.

• Tinctures. Powdered, fresh, or dried herbs are placed in an airtight container with alcohol and left for a period of time. Alcohol extracts the valuable or essential parts of the plant and preserves them.
• Infusions. Effectively another word for tea, an infusion uses dried herbs, or in some instances fresh, which are steeped in boiled water for about 10 minutes. Infusions may be drunk hot, which is normally best for medicinal teas, or cold, with ice.
• Decoctions. The roots, twigs, berries, seeds, and bark of a plant are used, and much like an infusion, they are boiled in water to extract the plants' ingredients. The liquid is strained and taken with honey or brown sugar as prescribed.
• Tisanes. Tisanes are mild infusions, usually pre-packaged and sold in the form of a tea bag, which are boiled for a much shorter period than an infusion.
• Pills. Plant remedies only rarely take this form since it is difficult to mix more than one herb and control the quantities. Some of the more common remedies will be available from professional herbalists or health food stores, or you can press your own with a domestic press.
• Ointments. For external use, ointments and creams are often prescribed. You can make your own by boiling the plant parts to extract the active properties, and adding a few ounces (grams) of pure oils (such as olive or sunflower).
• Poultices. Intended for external use, a poultice is made up of a plant that has been crushed and then applied whole to the affected areas. You can also boil crushed plant parts for a few minutes to make a pulp, which will act as a poultice, or use a powdered herb and mix with boiling water. Because they are most often applied with heat and use fresh parts of the plant, they are more potent than compresses. Poultices are particularly useful for conditions like bruises, wounds, and abscesses, helping to soothe and to draw out impurities.
• Compresses. A compress is usually made from an infusion or decoction, which is used

Infusions and decoctions can be taken hot or cold, sweetened with honey or brown sugar.

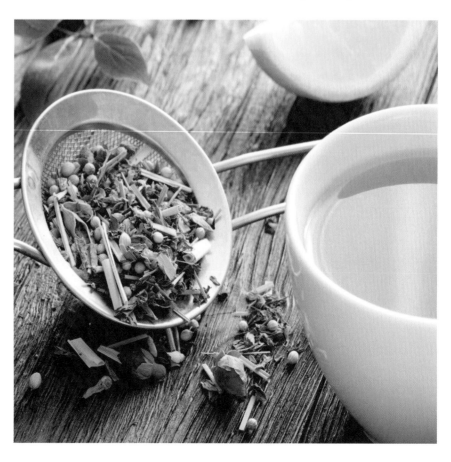

HOW TO MAKE FOLK REMEDIES

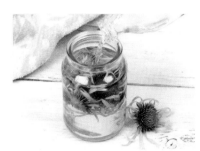

TINCTURE

1 You can make your own tincture at home by crushing the parts of the plants you wish to use (about 1oz. [25g.] will do).

2 Suspend the plants in alcohol (about 1pt. [600ml.] of vodka or any 40 percent spirit) for about two weeks, shaking occasionally. Dried or powdered herbs (about 4oz. [100g.]) may also be used, with the same amount of alcohol.

3 After straining, the tincture should be stored in a dark glass airtight jar. Doses are usually 5–20 drops, which can be taken directly or added to water.

DECOCTION

1 Put 1 teaspoonful of dried herb or 3 teaspoonfuls of fresh herb (for each cup) into a pan. Fresh herbs should be cut into small pieces.

2 Add some water to the herbs. If making large quantities, use 1oz. (30g.) dried herb for each 1pt. (600ml.) of water. The container should be glass, ceramic, or earthenware. Metal pans should be enameled. Do not use aluminum.

3 Bring to the boil and simmer for 10–15 minutes. If the herb contains volatile oils, cover the pan. Strain, cool, and refrigerate. The decoction will keep for about three days.

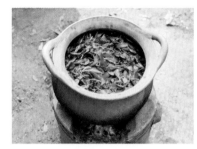

INFUSION

1 Infusions are most suitable for plants from which the leaves and flowers have been used, since their properties are more easily extracted by gentle boiling. Put 1 teaspoonful of the herb or herb mixture into a china or glass teapot, for each cup of tea that is required.

2 Add 1 cup of boiling water to the pot for each teaspoonful of herb that has been used. Keep the pot covered and always use the purest water available, which will ensure that the medicinal properties of the plant are effectively obtained.

3 Strain the infusion and drink hot or cold, sweetened if wanted with licorice root, honey, or brown sugar. Infusions should be made fresh each day, if possible.

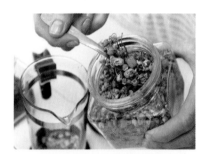

OINTMENT

1 Make 1pt. (600ml.) of infusion or decoction (depending on what is appropriate for the herb), and strain. Reserve the liquid.

2 Pour 3fl.oz. (90ml.) of oil into a pan. Mix 3oz. (90g.) of fat into the oil. If a perishable base fat is used (such as lard), a drop of tincture of benzoin should be added for each 1oz. (30g.) of base. Add the liquid.

3 Simmer until the water has evaporated. Stiffen the mixture with a little beeswax or cocoa butter to make a cream. Melt in slowly.

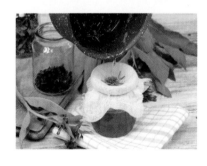

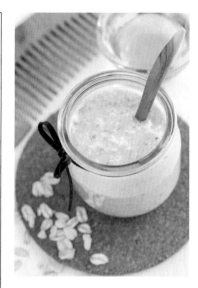

Oats can be used to prepare face masks, baths, and ointments.

TRADITIONAL HOME AND FOLK REMEDIES

to soak a linen or muslin cloth. The cloth is then placed on the affected area, where it can be held in place by a bandage or plastic wrap. Compresses can be hot or cold and are generally milder than poultices.

• Essential oils. Often used in other therapies, like aromatherapy (see page 42), the essential oils of a plant are those which contain its "essence," or some of its most active principles. Oils are useful for making tinctures and ointments.

• Baths. Plants and other items can be added to bath water for therapeutic effect – inhalation (through the steam) and by entering the bloodstream through the skin.

• Inhalations. Warm moist air can relieve many respiratory problems and allow the healing properties of plants and other products to enter the bloodstream through the lungs. To prepare an inhalation, half fill a big bowl with steaming water, and add a herbal infusion or decoction, or 2–3 drops of an essential oil.

HERBALISM

Since before recorded history, humans have used plants for food, medicines, shelter, clothing, dyes, weapons, musical instruments, and transportation. The cultural development of different countries and the rise and fall of empires have often been linked to the understanding and exploitation of plants. Herbalism, the use of plants for medicinal purposes, has been common to all peoples of the world. Our understanding of herbalism has been passed down by word of mouth from generation to generation.

HISTORY OF HERBALISM
—

It is the most natural thing in the world to use local flora for food and medicine, and list this knowledge for posterity. All native cultures have a well-developed understanding of local plants, and most of the world, even today, relies on herbal expertise for its primary healthcare. Shamans, wise women, bush doctors, traditional healers, and native medicine workers carry on a tradition thousands of years old.

Herbalism is the oldest, most tested, and proven form of medicine in the world. The *Ebers Papyrus* of the ancient Egyptians lists 85 herbs, some of which, like mint, are used in a similar way today. The Chinese herbal, *Pen Tsao*, contains over a thousand herbal remedies. The Assyrian and Babylonian scribes wrote herbal recipes on clay tablets.

The Greek Hippocrates (477–360 B.C.E.), known as the "father of medicine," mentions herbs, remedies, and treatment stratagems which are still valid. Indeed, there is much practical and theoretical knowledge to be rediscovered. Globally, herbal lore is a treasure chest beyond price.

In the West, the Saxons wrote the *Leech Book of Bald*, a mixture of remedies and ritual. Their nine sacred herbs included yarrow, marigold, and hawthorn. A modern practitioner of herbal medicine would rate them equally highly. The golden age of herbals was precipitated by the development of the printing press.

Nicholas Culpeper (1616–1654) printed the *London Dispensatory* (1649) in English (it had previously been printed in Latin), and later published his *Complete Herbal* – a book, he boasted, from which any man (or woman) could find out how to cure themselves for less than three pennies! Culpeper's *Complete Herbal* was immensely popular and is still available, having gone through over 40 reprints.

Botanical medicine was regarded as fringe medicine for many years. It was valued as a starting place for modern research, but thought to have nothing to offer Western society as a therapy in itself. Pharmaceutical companies identified the active therapeutic principles of many plants, synthesized commercial analogues, and patented new drugs. But in doing so they often missed the major principles of using natural sources for therapeutic purposes.

Herbalism, when practiced properly, is marked by a completely different attitude from orthodox medicine. It is a holistic system that uses plants, or plant parts, in a nonintrusive way. Herbalists believe that the constituents of a plant work synergistically to stimulate the natural healing process.

AS A SELF-HELP SYSTEM
—

Modern herbalism can be practiced on two levels: as a self-help system, and by a professional herbalist. These levels differ in the range of herbs that can be used,

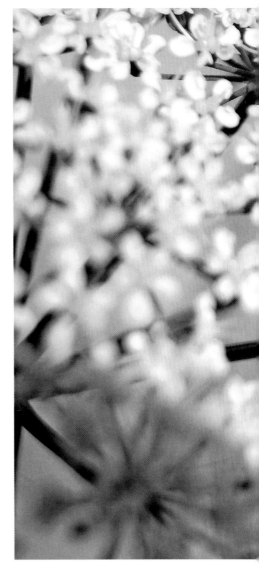

Really getting to know plants and the therapeutic actions of the remedies they provide is crucial to a sound practice of herbalism.

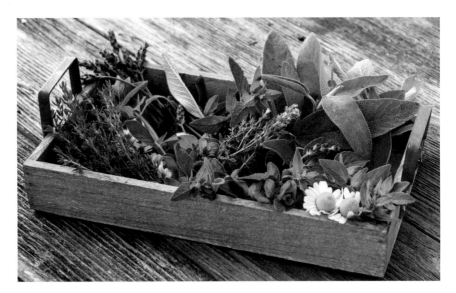

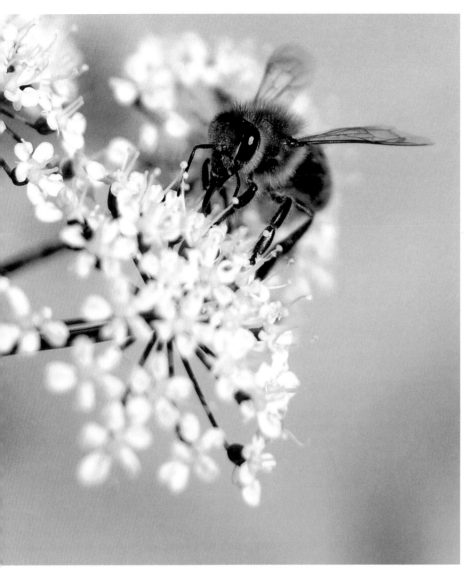

For the Saxons, yarrow was a sacred herb, used for rituals and the treatment of disease.

should the need arise. Such patients have yearly checks to maintain optimum health. Whole families register, as herbalism is especially suited to children and the elderly.

A consultation will take about an hour and consider all aspects of health, diet, exercise, and lifestyle. Your herbalist will take a "holistic" view, which means taking into consideration everything that affects your health on a physical, mental, and spiritual level. You will be asked questions about:

- Age
- Career
- Personality and what is important to you
- Concerns
- Appetite
- Sleeping patterns
- Previous medicines and illnesses
- Bowel movements
- Family
- Symptoms
- Any other aspect that is relevant.

As well as listening to what you say, your therapist will want to know how you feel and will note your appearance. The condition of your hair, skin, and facial expression, your posture, and how you move all provide important clues that will help with the diagnosis. There may also be a physical examination. Treatment will then be prescribed by the therapist.

Before a first visit it is worth spending some time considering your health and your expectations. It is useful to make a list of relevant points in your medical history and questions you want to ask, as these can easily be missed or forgotten in the stress of a first meeting. If for any reason you do not get on with the practitioner, try another one. It is important that there is a relationship of mutual trust and respect.

Many of the herbs prescribed will be familiar, but some will be unknown to you. After a consultation, a herbalist is able to prescribe herbs which are limited by law and not freely available over the counter to the general public.

the results that can be achieved, and the amount of responsibility taken for treatment. As a self-help system, herbs are ideal as a simple system of home care for first aid, everyday ailments, the management of chronic conditions, strengthening of the body, and preventive treatment. Herbs can be taken safely as long as a few simple rules are adhered to (see "The Tenets of Herbalism" on page 36, and "The Rules of Safe Home Treatment" on page 38). Unless advised otherwise, always stay within the standard dosages offered on pages 39 and 41.

SEEING A PROFESSIONAL
—

Professional consultant medical herbalists are usually trained in orthodox diagnosis and can treat all of the ailments treated by a family physician or general practitioner. Accredited members of organizations such as the National Institute of Medical Herbalists have undergone four years of university or university-standard study and two years of supervision. They will understand all the indications and contraindications of herbs, and any problems that may arise from taking orthodox drugs. They will refer to other specialists if necessary.

For a list of organizations that keep a register of qualified herbal practitioners, see "Useful Resources," pages 382–391.

It is becoming more common for a patient to register with a herbalist in the same way as one would register with a physician – for a check-up and then to be on the books

USING HERBS AT HOME

THE TENETS OF HERBALISM
—

To be able to care for yourself and your family by making natural remedies is a pleasure, and the benefits are legion. The organic chemistry of remedy-making is an extension of cooking, and the same principles and skills apply. For success, use the best-quality ingredients, practice absolute cleanliness, and follow the instructions carefully.

It is important to remember that several herbs may be recommended for a particular ailment; all are slightly different. For example, would rose, lavender, rosemary, or chamomile be best for your headache? Would a cool compress be best, or a long soak in a rosemary bath? Knowledge of the herb, the individual, and the different methods must be combined to prescribe remedies that will be really effective. Remember these basic tenets of herbalism:

• The whole plant is better than an isolated extract.
• Treat the whole person, not just the symptoms.
• Practice minimum effective treatment and minimum intervention.
• Strengthen the body and encourage it to heal itself.

WHERE TO GET HERBS
—

Many herbs and herbal products are freely available. Plants or seeds can be bought from garden centers (always check the Latin name) and online, then grown in the garden or in a windowbox. Dried herbs are available from herb stores and some wholefood outlets, as well as online. Always specify the herb (the Latin name if possible) and the part of the plant to be used – root, bark, leaf, or flower.

Herbal products, remedies, tinctures, tablets, etc. are available from wholefood stores, and some pharmacies and general food stores. Always read the label and the instructions very carefully.

Regarding plants picked from the wild, countries have different rules and some plants are protected by law. Check the legal situation and get permission from

A dedicated herb garden close to the house is the best way to grow herbs, such as echinacea.

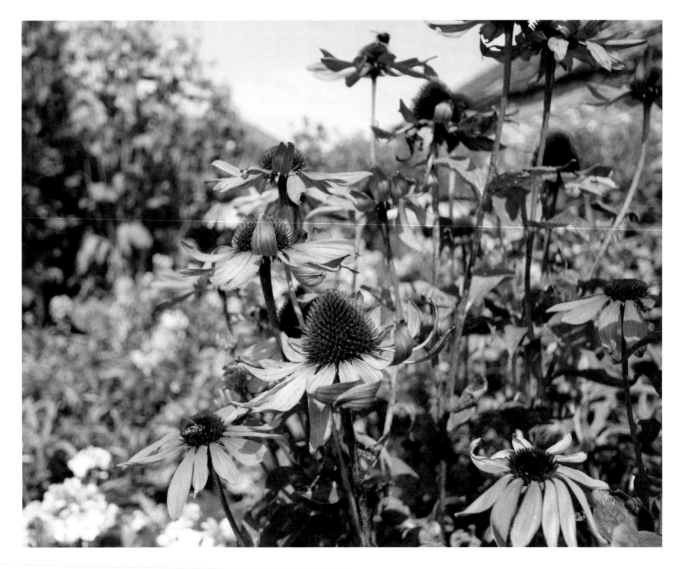

WHAT IS A HERB?

Herbage, like foliage, refers to plants with green leaves, but in herbal remedies more than leaves are used. Indeed, any part of a plant can be used, as well as fungi and algae:

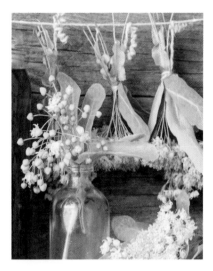

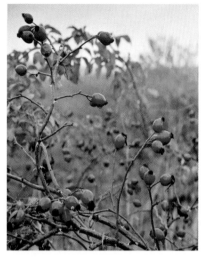

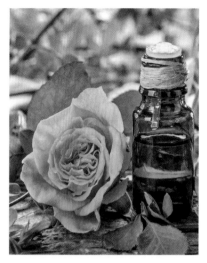

- Flowers: chamomile, marigold, linden (pictured)
- Leaves: peppermint, sage, thyme, comfrey
- Bark: willow, oak, cinnamon
- Buds: cloves
- Seeds: fennel, cardamom

- Fruits: cayenne, rosehips (pictured)
- Root: dandelion, marshmallow
- Inner sap or gel: clove, aloe vera
- Bulb: garlic
- Wood: pau d'arco

- Essential oil: rosemary, lavender, rose (pictured)
- Fixed oil: olive oil, St. John's wort
- Resin: myrrh, frankincense
- Seaweed: kelp, bladderwrack
- Mushrooms: ganoderma (reishi), oyster

the landowner. Check identification carefully and pick the minimum required, with proper regard for conservation. Never gather roots from the side of the road, by recently sprayed crops or foliage, or from sick-looking plants.

USING THE FRESH PLANT

—

The easiest way to take a herb is to pick it directly from the plant. Leaves can be used in salads, sandwiches, or soups. Chickweed, chicory, dandelion, and marigold make excellent salad additions. Nettle is traditional for green soup. Elderflower fritters are fun. Chewing a few fresh leaves of marjoram will help clear the head. Horseradish leaves will clear sinuses. Sage eases mouth sores and sore throats.

For cuts, grazes, and stings, pick four or five leaves (dock is traditional when stung on countryside walks as it is so readily available) and rub the leaves together between the hands to bruise them and release the juices. When damp, apply to the affected area and hold in place. Poultices can be made in the same way.

Fresh leaves can also be used to make water infusions (teas), decoctions, tinctures, infused oils, and creams. Follow standard recipes and dosages (see pages 39 and 41). Most recipes give the amounts for dried herbs. When using fresh material add one-third more, as fresh plants contain a considerable amount of water.

PREPARATIONS

—

Most herbs are sold in dried form. In this form they can simply be powdered and sprinkled onto food (half a flat teaspoon twice daily), but most are prepared further. Herbs are prepared for:

- Availability and preservation, so that seasonal plants are available to use all year round.
- Convenience, as compressed tablets are often more convenient to take than a cup of tea.
- To aid the action of the herb. For example infused oils for rubs, or with added honey to give a soothing and demulcent quality to thyme.

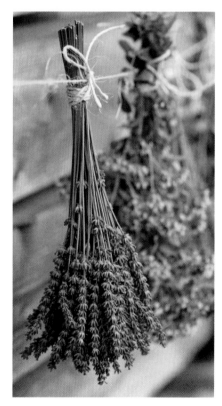

Dried herbs are most convenient for medicinal use, as they are readily available all year round.

PREPARATIONS FOR INTERNAL USE

COMMON INTERNAL PREPARATIONS
—

For internal use, herbal remedies can be bought or made in a variety of forms:

• Tinctures. Tinctures are the most common type of internal remedy prescribed by herbalists. They are made by soaking the flowers, leaves, or roots of the herbs in alcohol to extract and preserve their properties. Tinctures keep well, and are easy to store. Because they are highly concentrated you need only take a small amount at a time.
• Infusions. Infusions are less concentrated than tinctures and are an easy way to take herbs at home. The herbalist prescribes fresh or dried flowers, leaves, or green stems of the herbs, which you make into a "tea" – a rather misleading word as it suggests a

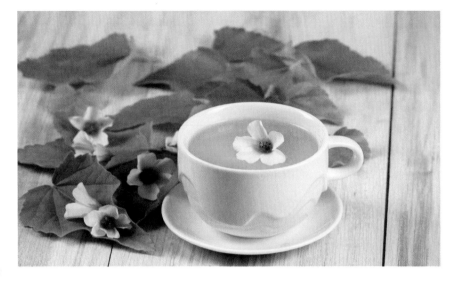

The properties of marshmallow are destroyed by heat, so infuse in cold water.

pleasant drink, which is rarely the case with prescription herbs. Sweeten with honey if you find the taste unpalatable. The properties of some herbs – for example comfrey, marshmallow, and valerian root – are destroyed by heat, so they should be infused or "macerated" in cold water for up to 12 hours.
• Decoctions. Decoctions are similar to infusions, but are made from tougher materials such as roots, bark, nuts, and seeds. Using the same proportions, place the herb and water in a saucepan and bring to the boil, simmer for 10–15 minutes, strain, and drink hot.
• Syrups and honeys. These are ideal for administering to children, because they are sweet.
• Tablets and capsules. These are taken in the same way as a conventional drug, and are useful for people who would rather not taste the remedy.

CARRIERS
—

There are two main carriers for herbs when taken internally:
• Water. Water is used for infusions (teas) of flowers, leaves, some seeds, and fruit. Infusions are quickly assimilated and utilized by the body, and are gentle for children, convalescents, and those with a delicate digestion. They are ideal for diuretic, diaphoretic, cooling, and cleaning regimes. Decoctions are used for harder parts, like roots, and for stronger preparations.

USING HERBALISM WITH WISDOM

One hundred years ago, a person could have walked into the garden or local woods and returned with a remedy for the baby's gripe, a stomach ache, sprained ankle, stiffening gout, or any number of ailments. Today we can walk into the local store and find the shelves full of natural ingredients from all corners of the world – from carrots and cabbage to precious spices like cinnamon. This array would have been the envy of a medieval apothecary; but while the stock is available, the knowledge is scarce. The culture of responsibility, self-care, and interaction with nature has largely been lost. It must be rediscovered if herbs and their proper uses are to be properly understood.

A herb has a taste, color, smell, texture, and history. The antiseptic calendula lotion applied to a spot was once an orange marigold growing clear and open-faced in a sunny meadow. The lavender used to reduce the tension of a pounding headache and bring sleep once shimmered in a soporific violet-purple haze on a French mountainside. Such pictures are part of the heritage of healing, and help us to remember and understand the actions of herbs and the way they work within the body.

Part of the beauty of herbalism lies in the many different possible methods of taking herbs. The skill in choosing the best method for a specific individual and condition is part of the art of caring. Hand baths, foot baths, skin washes, rubs, massage oils, eye baths, compresses, and fomentations are undervalued. Local treatments allow the herb to act exactly where it is needed, avoid affecting the whole system, and are comforting and effective. Remember that in all herbal preparations it is best to use organic herbs.

THE RULES OF SAFE HOME TREATMENT

• Consider the whole body and person first. Is medication needed? Consider a change of rest, diet, or exercise before prescribing the patient any remedy.
• Use simple remedies internally and externally. This will encourage the body to heal itself.
• Make a list. Know what you are taking and what to expect. Keep a note of all remedies taken. This will be useful if you need help later.
• Take as recommended. Remember the herbal tenet of minimum effective dosage and intervention. Stick to the standard dosages. Doubling does not double effectiveness; it may put an extra burden on a body that is already sick.
• TLC. Use lots of Tender Loving Care. A positive and loving attitude helps to make the illness more bearable, and may even speed up the healing process.
• Monitor progress after a few days.
• Stop treatment if there is any adverse reaction.
• Remember, people are all individuals; children, especially, respond quickly, so be alert for changes or new symptoms.
• Seek professional help if in any doubt. Assessing your own symptoms is different from making a diagnosis, which needs an objective eye.

• Alcohol. Alcohol is the carrier for tinctures and spiced wines, made from all plant parts, especially hard parts. Alcohol adds some temporary heat and stimulation. It is convenient, although not for those intolerant of alcohol or for babies. Preparations made from alcohol will keep indefinitely.

METHODS AND DOSAGES

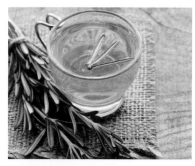

Rosemary infusion

INFUSION (TEA)
Water infusions at the standard strength are used as teas, gargles, lotions for the skin, compresses, and for fomentations. Dilute with an equal amount of water for hand or foot baths, douches, and enemas.

Standard Strength
1oz. (25g.) of herb to 1pt. (500ml.) of water; or 1 teaspoon of herb to 1 cup of water

Brewing Times
To some extent this depends on personal taste, but the following is a good guide:
- Up to 3 minutes for flowers and soft leaves
- Up to 5 minutes for seeds and leaves
- Up to 10 minutes for hard seeds, roots, and various barks

Dose
For children, reduce proportionally. Give a child of seven half the standard adult dose. At six months, use 1 teaspoon of the standard tea. For breastfeeding infants give the remedy to the mother. Adults may drink:
- 1 cup three times a day for normal conditions
- 1 cup up to six times a day for acute conditions
- 1 cup twice a day as a long-term strengthening tonic

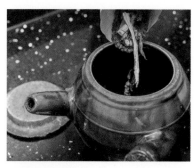

Astragalus decoction

DECOCTION
Decoctions can be diluted with an equal amount of water and used in the same ways as water infusions for hand baths, gargles, etc.

Standard Strength
1½oz. (40g.) of herb to 1½pt. (750ml.) of water

Method
- Put herb in saucepan.
- Add 1½pt. (750ml.) water.
- Put on a tight lid.
- Bring to the boil, then turn down as low as possible and simmer for 10–15 minutes.
- Strain thoroughly and discard the herb.
- Pour decoction into a clean bottle.
- Will keep in a refrigerator for two or three days.

Dose
Adults may take:
- ⅓ cup twice a day for normal conditions, and as a tonic
- ⅓ cup three to six times a day for acute conditions

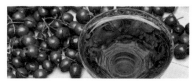

Elderflower syrup

SYRUP AND HONEY
Syrups and honeys can be used to sweeten other herbal preparations, or be added to food or drink.

Method
- Make a standard decoction with 1½oz. (40g.) herb and 1½pt. (750ml.) of water.
- Return to heat, remove lid, and simmer gently till liquid is reduced to ½pt. (250ml.), which may take a few hours.
- Add 1¼lb. (600g.) honey or 1lb. (500g.) sugar, stirring until completely dissolved.
- Pour into a bottle, label, and date.

Dose
Adults may take 1 dessertspoon three to six times a day. Children under five may take 1 teaspoon three times a day.

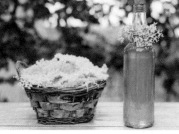

Nettle tincture

TINCTURE
Tinctures can be made with fresh or dried herbs. The absolute strength of the alcohol needed varies slightly depending on the herb, but the method given here is sufficient for standard home use. A tincture can also be diluted with water: 1 dessertspoon to 1 cup of water can be used as skin lotion, a wash, foot bath, gargle, compress, or douche.

Method
To make 9fl.oz. (300ml.) of tincture:
- Chop ½oz. (12g.) dried or 1oz. (25g.) fresh herb.
- Put in a large glass jar and cover with 6fl.oz. (200ml.) alcohol, such as vodka or brandy, and 3fl.oz. (100ml.) of water.
- Put on a lid and leave for two weeks, shaking occasionally.
- Strain well through a muslin bag.
- Pour into an amber glass bottle.

- Label and date, then keep indefinitely in a cool place away from children.

Dose
Adults may take:
- 1 teaspoon three times a day, standard
- 5 drops to 1 teaspoon a day as a tonic
- 1 teaspoon six times a day for acute conditions

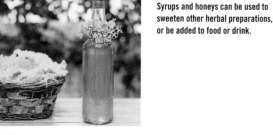

Hawthorn brandy

ALCOHOL-SPICED OR TONIC WINE
A good way to make a strengthening remedy for everyday use is to make a tonic wine. Spiced wines make good aperitifs, to stimulate and improve digestion.

Method
- Use 1oz. (25g.) of herb(s) or 1–2oz. (25–50g.) of spices, depending on taste.
- Cover with 4¼pt. (2l.) of wine.
- Stand for two weeks, strain, and bottle.

Dose
Adults may take ½ cup twice a day before meals (warm water can be added).

PREPARATIONS FOR EXTERNAL USE

COMMON EXTERNAL PREPARATIONS
—

Herbs may be prepared or bought in a variety of forms for external use:

• Creams and ointments. These are applied externally to soothe irritated or inflamed skin conditions, or ease the pain of sprains or bruises. Cream moistens dry or cracked skin, and massaging the ointment into bruises helps to ease the pain. In both cases the active ingredients of the herb pass through the pores of the skin into the bloodstream to encourage healing. Creams can be made from infused oils (see recipe in "Methods and Dosages" opposite).
• Liniments and rubs. These oil-based preparations may be used in massage to ease joints, or to soothe skin conditions.
• Compresses. Either hot or cold, compresses help with aches, pains, and swollen joints. Fold a clean piece of cotton into an infusion of the prescribed herb and apply to the point of pain. Repeat as the compress cools or, in the case of cold compresses, until the pain eases.

• Poultices. Made from bruised fresh herbs or dried herbs moistened into a paste with hot water, compresses are also good for painful joints or drawing out infection from boils, spots, or wounds. Place the herb on a clean piece of cotton and bandage onto the affected area. Leave in place for around two hours or until the symptoms ease.
• Suppositories and douches. These are sometimes prescribed for rectal problems such as piles, or vaginal infections, respectively. The suppositories will come ready-made for you to insert. Douches are made from an infusion or decoction that has been allowed to cool.
• Herbal baths. Perhaps the most pleasant of the herbal remedies, baths are a useful supplement to other forms of treatment. The heat of the water activates the properties of the volatile oils so that they are absorbed

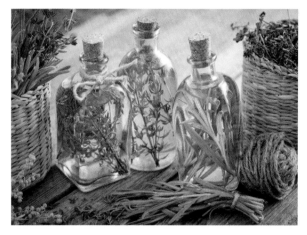

Herbal infused oils can be added to the bath, exerting a healing effect on both mind and body.

through the pores of the skin and inhaled through the nose. In both cases they pass into the bloodstream, and when inhaled they also pass through the nervous system to the brain.

Itchy skin can be soothed by calendula lotion, prepared from oil infused with marigold flowers.

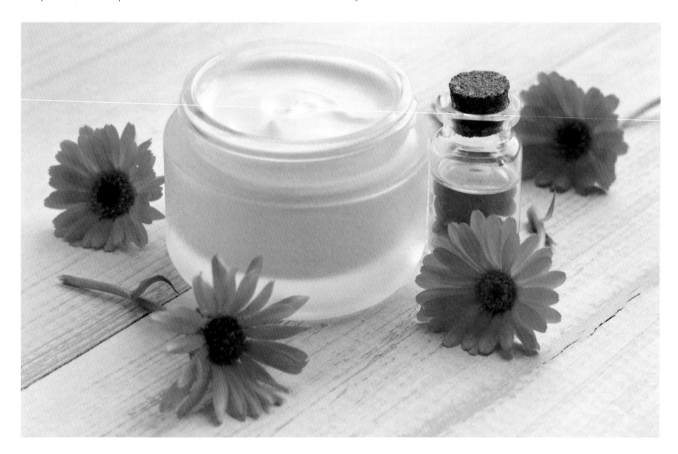

METHODS AND DOSAGES

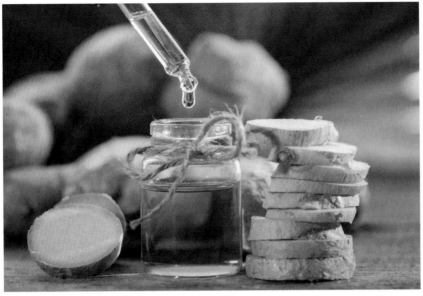

Ginger liniment

LINIMENT

A liniment is a soothing rub to relieve fatigued and stiff muscles and joints.

Method
- Put the fresh herb in a jar and cover with olive oil.
- Leave for up to 6 weeks.
- Strain the mixture through a cloth.
- Stand until the oil separates off: use this.

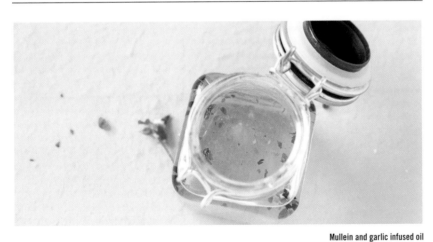

Mullein and garlic infused oil

INFUSED OIL

Oil is soothing and nourishing for the skin, and acts as a lubricant to carry the active principles of the herbs in rubs, massage oils, and salves. All parts of the plant can be infused in oil. There are two methods of infusion, hot and cold. Hot is used for thyme, rosemary, comfrey root, and spices such as cayenne, mustard, and ginger. Cold is used for flowers (see St. John's wort, page 138).

Method
This double method makes a strong infused oil which can be used as it is, mixed with tincture for a liniment, or thickened with beeswax (for a thin cream, use 1 part beeswax to 10 parts infused oil; for a thick salve, use 1 part beeswax to 5 parts infused oil).

To make ½pt. (250ml.):
- Chop 2–3oz. (50–75g.) dried herbs or spices, or 3–4oz. (75–l00g.) fresh herbs.
- Put half into a clean pan with a lid and cover with ½pt. (250ml.) pure vegetable oil (a light vegetable oil is best).
- Put in a water bath and simmer gently for 2 hours (it is important that direct heat is not used, as this might burn the oil).
- Strain, and throw away the used herbs.
- Put the remaining half of unused herbs in the pan.
- Cover these with the oil (it will have changed color, having picked up some of the quality of the herbs).
- Replace the lid and return the pan to the water bath for another couple of hours.
- Strain, then pour the oil into clean bottles, label, and date.

HERBALISM REMEDIES

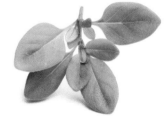

AROMATHERAPY

The word aromatherapy means "treatment using scents." It refers to a particular branch of herbal medicine that uses concentrated plant oils called essential oils to improve physical and emotional health, and to restore balance to the whole person. Unlike the herbs used in herbal medicine, essential oils are not taken internally, but are inhaled or applied to the skin. Each oil has its own natural fragrance, and a gentle healing action that makes aromatherapy one of the most pleasant and popular of all the available complementary therapies.

HOW AROMATHERAPY WORKS
—

Aromatherapy is subtle but effective when used correctly and given time to work. While one treatment may prove immediately relaxing or reviving, the effects tend to be short-lived. Regular treatments are needed to rebalance body systems and, if you have been stressed or ill, it could take several weeks of treatment before you notice an improvement. The practice of aromatherapy involves using more than just the aroma of certain plant oils to treat mind and body. It is concerned with getting essential oils into the body in order to alter body chemistry, support body systems, and improve moods and emotions. This is done most effectively by massaging oils into the skin. Manipulating the soft tissues of the body has been shown to release emotional and physical tension, relieve pain, promote healthy circulation, and restore the whole person to a balanced state of health. Massage is the method of choice for professional aromatherapists. However, for home use, oils can also be added to bath water, or applied on hot or cold compresses to swollen, painful, or bruised areas.

When applied to the skin, essential oils start to work immediately on body tissues. The molecules in the oils are so small that they can be absorbed through the pores of the skin and into the bloodstream, by which means they are carried to every part of the body.

However, aroma is important. Inhalation can reinforce the effects of oils applied to the skin, and it is a safe way to benefit from the healing properties of oils that could cause irritation. No one knows exactly how aromas affect the mind, but it has been theorized that receptors in the nose convert smells into electrical impulses which are transmitted to the limbic system of the brain. Smells reaching the limbic system can directly affect our moods and emotions, and improve mental alertness and concentration.

THE BENEFITS OF AROMATHERAPY
—

Aromatherapy benefits people rather than cures illnesses. It is gentle enough to be used by people of all ages and states of health. It is nurturing for babies and children, and offers comfort and care to the elderly. Pregnant women and even seriously ill patients with cancer or AIDS can benefit from professional treatment. Aromatherapy is not recommended as a cure for any disease. Its most potent effect is that it relaxes mind and body, relieves pain, and restores body systems to a state of balance in which healing can best take place. It is also most effective when used as a preventive or to alleviate subclinical symptoms before they escalate

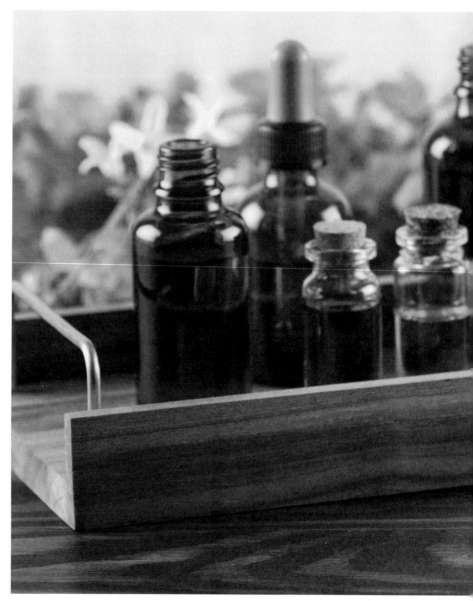

Aromatherapy is a safe, natural treatment that can benefit everyone, no matter what age or state of health.

into disease. The therapy has been shown to be particularly effective in preventing and treating stress and anxiety-related disorders, muscular and rheumatic pains, digestive problems, menstrual irregularities, menopausal complaints, insomnia, and depression.

SEEING A PROFESSIONAL
—

A first appointment with an aromatherapist lasts between 60 and 90 minutes. Every consultation begins with the therapist taking your case history. In order to provide safe, effective, holistic treatment he or she needs to know about your medical history and if you have come with a particular problem. As well as finding out which oils would be

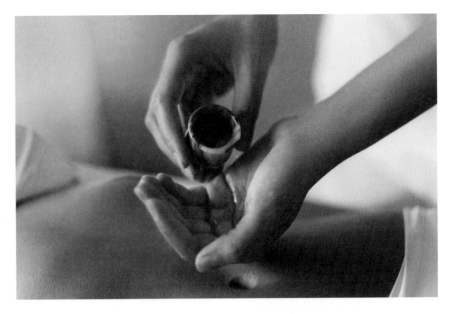

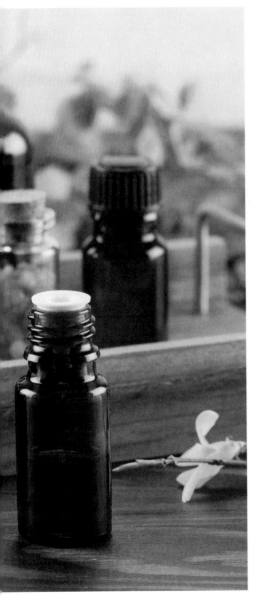

best to use, aromatherapists need to know which to avoid. If you are pregnant, have sensitive skin, high blood pressure, epilepsy, or have recently had an operation, some oils would be unsuitable to use. Pregnant women, for example, should avoid certain oils, including thyme, basil, rosemary, clary sage, and juniper, because they may harm the fetus or induce miscarriage. The therapist will ask about your stress levels, and if you are using medication or taking homeopathic remedies. It is also important for the aromatherapist to know what sort of mood you are in and what kind of day you have had. This interview takes about 20 minutes and you may be asked to sign a consent form at the end of it.

Treatment usually involves massage. For this you will be asked to undress down to your underwear and lie on a massage table covered with a towel to keep you warm and prevent you from feeling exposed. The aromatherapist will move the towel as he or she works around your body, but will not remove it completely. The therapist uses the information you have provided when deciding on a suitable blend of oils. Generally, the oils you like best are the ones that work best for you. Using the chosen blend, the aromatherapist will begin your massage using gentle massage strokes and may also work on pressure points of the body. During the 30–45 minutes that it takes to give a full body massage the therapist will talk very little, if at all, allowing you to relax completely. At the end of your

Essential oils are blended with a carrier oil for massage. In addition to being a relaxing experience in itself, massage ensures that the oils are effectively absorbed through the skin and into the bloodstream.

massage, you may be advised not to bathe for several hours so that the oils can be fully absorbed. The therapist may conclude the visit by giving you oils to use at home.

ANCIENT ORIGINS OF A MODERN THERAPY

Aromatic plant oils have been used therapeutically for thousands of years. The ancient Vedic literature of India, and historic Chinese and Arabic medical texts, document the importance of aromatic oils for health and spirituality. The Egyptians were the most noted of the ancient aromatherapists. Physicians from all over the world are reputed to have traveled to Egypt to learn aromatic techniques. Aromatherapy is believed to have come west at the time of the Crusades. It was not until the 18th and 19th centuries that scientists were able to identify many of the individual components of plant chemistry.

Research enabled scientists to extract the active components of medicinal plants. Ironically, this led to the development of pharmaceutical drugs and a rejection of plant medicine. However, in the 1920s the devotion of a French chemist, René Maurice Gattefosse, initiated a modest revival in plant oils. Gattefosse discovered that lavender oil quickly healed a burn on his hand. He coined the term "aromatherapie." Later, a French army surgeon, Dr. Jean Valnet, published *Aromatherapie*, still considered by many to be the bible of aromatherapy. In the 1950s, Marguérite Maury, an Austrian beauty therapist and biochemist, introduced the concept of using essential oils in massage, and established the first aromatherapy clinics, in Britain, France, and Switzerland.

HOW ESSENTIAL OILS WORK

ESSENTIAL OILS IN ACTION
—

Essential oils are extracted from the aromatic essences of certain plants, trees, fruit, flowers, herbs, and spices. They are natural volatile oils with identifiable chemical and medicinal properties. Over 150 essential oils have been extracted, each one with its own scent and unique healing properties. Oils are sourced from plants as commonplace as parsley and as exquisite as jasmine. For optimum benefits, essential oils must be extracted from natural raw ingredients and remain as pure as possible.

Despite considerable research, the chemistry of essential oils is not fully understood. Each oil is composed of at least 100 different chemical constituents, which are classified as aldehydes, phenols, oxides, esters, ketones, alcohols, and terpenes. There may also be many chemical compounds that have yet to be identified. The oils and their actions are extremely complex. All the oils are antiseptic, but each one also has individual properties; for example, they may be analgesic, fungicidal, diuretic, or expectorant. The collective components of each oil also work together to give the oil a dominant characteristic. It can be relaxing, as in the case of chamomile, refreshing, like grapefruit, or stimulating, like rosemary.

Within the body, essential oils are able to operate in three ways: pharmacologically, physiologically, and psychologically. From a pharmacological perspective, the chemical components of the oils react with body chemistry in a way that is similar to drugs, but slower, more sympathetic, and with fewer side-effects. Essential oils also have notable physiological effects. Certain oils have an affinity with particular areas of the body. For example, rose has an affinity with the female reproductive system, while spice oils tend to benefit the digestive system. The oil may also sedate an overactive system, or stimulate a different part of the body that is sluggish.

Some oils, such as lavender, are known as adaptogens, meaning they do whatever the body requires of them at the time.

The psychological response is triggered by the effect that the aromatic molecules have on the brain.

Essential oils are not all absorbed into the body at the same rate. They can take 20 minutes or several hours, depending on the oil and the individual body chemistry of the person being treated. On average, absorption takes about 90 minutes. After several hours, the oils leave the body. Most oils are exhaled; others are eliminated in urine, feces, and perspiration.

METHODS OF EXTRACTION
—

Essential oils are extracted from plants by a simple form of pressure known as expression, or by distillation. Most oils are extracted by steam distillation. This involves steaming the parts of the plant to be used in order to break down the walls of the cells that store the essence. The released essence, combined with the steam, passes to cooling tanks, where the steam condenses to a watery liquid, and the essential oil floats on top. The oil is skimmed off and bottled, and the remaining liquid is sometimes used as flower or herbal water.

BLENDING AND USING ESSENTIAL OILS
—

Essential oils can be used alone or blended together. Oils are blended for two reasons: to create a more sophisticated fragrance, or to enhance or change the medicinal actions of the oils. Blending changes the molecular structure of essential oils, and when they are blended well therapists can create a "synergistic" blend, where the oils work in harmony and to great effect. To create a blend, the therapist considers not only the symptoms and underlying causes of a patient's particular problem, but also the individual's biological and psychological make-up, and personal fragrance preferences. For therapeutic purposes it is usual to mix only three or four oils together.

If you want to blend oils at home, choose two or three oils that you believe complement each other. In general, oils from

Most essential oils are extracted by steam distillation. In the final cooling tank, the oil is skimmed from the surface.

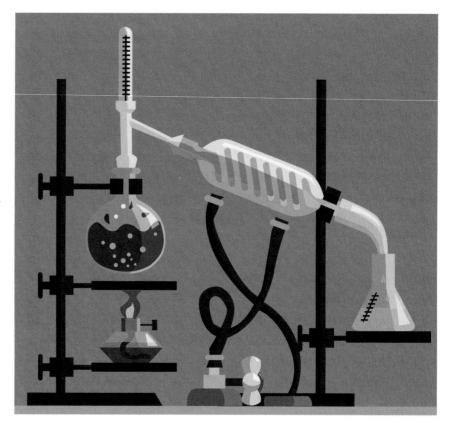

the same groups (citrus, floral, spicy, etc.), and those which share similar constituents, blend well. Using the proportions detailed overleaf, mix a blend using small amounts of the strongest scented oils and more of the lighter fragrances. You can use the recipes for suggested blends in the "Healing Remedies" chapter, or create some of your own. Be guided by your own likes and dislikes – the best blend for you is often the one you find most appealing.

To use oils on the skin, choose a light cold-pressed vegetable oil such as grapeseed, sweet almond, or sunflower oil as a base. For hair treatments, choose a more penetrative oil, such as olive oil or jojoba. Where you need a slightly astringent oil, try hazelnut. Add your essential oils to the base oil a little at a time. Shake the bottle well and rub a little on the back of your hand to test the scent. Adjust the quantities until you achieve the blend you want. Add about 5 percent wheat germ oil to preserve the blend. Store blended oils in labeled dark bottles, out of children's reach, and use within three months.

Lavender is one of the most versatile essential oils because it responds to the body's particular needs at the time.

USING ESSENTIAL OILS SAFELY
—

Aromatherapy is compatible with conventional medicine and most other forms of holistic treatment. However, if you are taking medication, consult your physician. Some oils are not compatible with homeopathic treatment. Aromatherapy is safe to use at home for minor or short-term problems, providing you follow certain guidelines:

• Do not take essential oils internally.
• Do not put essential oils in the eyes.
• Keep all oils away from children.
• Do not apply oils undiluted to the skin, unless it is stated that it is safe to do so.

You should consult a qualified aromatherapy practitioner for advice and treatment, and discuss your intended aromatherapy treatment with your conventional healthcare team, if you:

• Are pregnant
• Have an allergy
• Have a chronic medical condition such as high blood pressure or epilepsy
• Are receiving any medical or psychiatric treatment
• Are taking homeopathic remedies
• Have a chronic or serious health problem, or if a problem becomes severe or persistent
• Intend to treat babies or very young children.

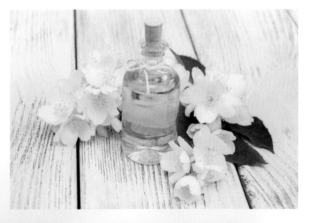

Jasmine, highly valued for its exquisite floral fragrance, is widely used in cosmetics and perfumes.

AROMATHERAPY TECHNIQUES

AROMATHERAPY MASSAGE
—

The most common form of treatment among professional aromatherapists is massage. The techniques of massage as we know it today in the West were developed in the 19th century by a Swedish professor, Pier Heidrich Ling, and his work is the basis for massage treatment today. Different strokes are appropriate to different areas of the body. Gentle strokes are used to commence a session to relax the superficial muscles, and more vigorous strokes then stimulate the deeper muscles. Key techniques include:

• Effleurage. Effleurage is designed to sensitize your partner and prepare for the later strokes. It is particularly effective for the face. Place your hands on your partner's cheeks, fingers downward. Then stroke gently toward the ears, using the minimum pressure required to maintain contact. You can use this sliding stroke to massage the whole body if you vary the pressure and speed.
• Circling. Place both hands on your partner, a few inches apart, and stroke in a wide circular movement. Press into the upward

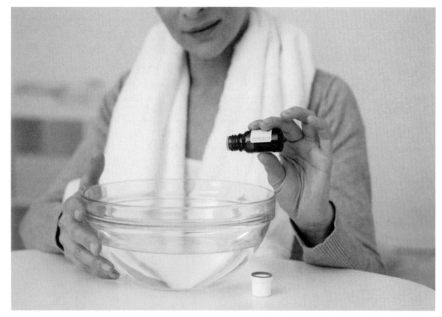

Steam inhalation is useful for colds and headaches.

stroke and glide back down. Your arms will cross as you make the circle, so just lift one hand over the other to continue. Circle lightly in a clockwise direction over the stomach to aid digestion.
• Kneading. Place both hands on the area to be massaged with your fingers pointing away

from you. Press into the body with the palm of one hand, pick up the flesh between your thumb and fingers, and press it toward the resting hand. Release and repeat with the other hand, as if you were kneading dough.

Aromatherapy massage can be given by a registered practitioner, or experiment with a partner or friend.

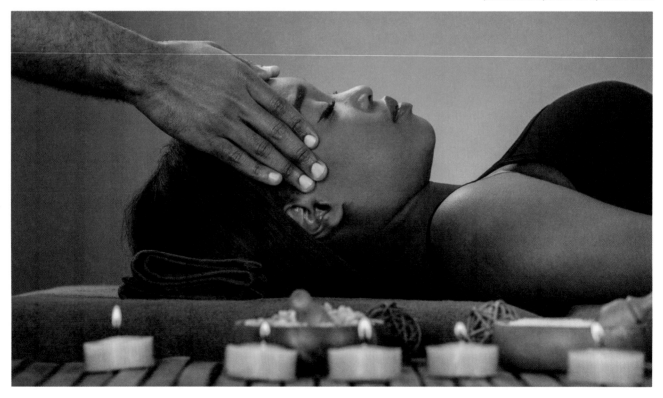

TECHNIQUES AND MEASUREMENTS

MASSAGE
Massage in itself is nurturing and therapeutic, and the rubbing action releases the fragrance of the oils and ensures that they are well absorbed into the skin. When combined with the medicinal properties of the oils, massage forms a potent healing treatment that can be relaxing or energizing; it can soothe the nervous system, or stimulate the blood and lymphatic systems to improve physical and psychological functioning. It eases pain and tension from tired, taut, or overworked muscles, and lifts the spirits. Whenever possible, try to include massage in your home aromatherapy treatments.

Basic Measurements
Dilute the essential oil in a cold-pressed vegetable carrier oil such as grapeseed, sweet almond, or sunflower oil. Use up to 5 drops of essential oil to a teaspoon of carrier oil for adults, half that strength for children under seven, and a quarter of the strength for children under three. The only essential oils suitable for babies are chamomile, rose, or lavender. Use only 1 drop to 1 teaspoon of carrier oil.

BATHS
Aromatic baths are a simple, useful, and versatile way to use essential oils at home. They can be used to enhance moods, relax or stimulate body systems, treat skin disorders, and ease musculoskeletal pain. Essential oils do not dissolve in water, but form a thin film on the surface. The heat of the water releases their vapor and aids absorption into the skin.

Basic Measurements
Fill the bath with warm water before you add the oils. For adults, add 5–10 drops of essential oil to a full bath. Use less than 4 drops for children over two, and 1 drop for babies. Stir through the water with your hand.

VAPORIZERS
These can be electric, or a ceramic ring that is heated by a light bulb, but most are ceramic pots warmed by a small candle. They are a natural way to scent, deodorize, or disinfect a room, and are one of the best ways to use oils for enhancing mood and balancing the mind. Vaporizers are also useful for when young children have breathing difficulties.

Basic Measurements
Add water and 6–8 drops of oil to the vaporizer. Alternatively, add the oil to a bowl of water and place by a radiator.

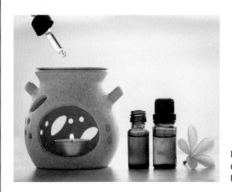

STEAM INHALATIONS
Inhalations are most beneficial for throat and respiratory infections, sinus and catarrhal congestion, and headaches. They are also effective for those oils that could cause irritation if applied to the skin. The steam releases the vapors of the oils. Steam inhalations are not always suitable for asthmatics or people with breathing difficulties, and they are not appropriate for treating children and infants.

Basic Measurements
Add 3–4 drops of oil to a bowl of boiling water. Bend over the bowl, cover your bead with a towel, and breathe deeply for a few minutes. You can also use this method as a facial sauna.

CREAMS, LOTIONS, SHAMPOOS, AND GELS
One of the best ways to use oils for skin care and chronic skin complaints is to add them to a cream or lotion. This is more convenient and less greasy than massage, and it also means the oils can be applied when needed to wounds, bruises, or itchy skin. Adding oils to shampoos helps with everyday hair-care problems, and using essential oils with shower gels is excellent for fatigue and hangovers.

Basic Measurements
Add 1 or 2 drops of essential oil to creams, lotions, and shampoos, and massage into the skin or scalp. Choose unscented products that are lanolin-free and made from good-quality natural ingredients.

GARGLES AND MOUTHWASHES
Although essential oils should not be swallowed, mouthwashes and gargles are excellent ways to use antiseptic oils to treat mouth ulcers, gum disease, throat infections, and bad breath. These methods are not suitable for children.

Basic Measurements
Dilute 4–5 drops of essential oil in a teaspoon of brandy. Mix into a glass of warm water and swish around the mouth or use as a gargle. Do not swallow.

HOT AND COLD COMPRESSES
Compresses are an effective way of using essential oils to relieve pain and inflammation. They can be either hot or cold. Hot compresses are good for muscle pain, arthritis, rheumatism, toothache, earache, boils, and abscesses. Cold compresses benefit headaches, sprains, and swelling.

Basic Measurements
Add 4–5 drops of essential oil to a bowl of hot or cold water. Soak a folded clean cotton cloth in the water, wring it out, and apply over the affected area. If using a hot compress, cover with a warm towel and repeat when it cools. A few essential oils – such as lavender, tea tree oil, and sandalwood – can be applied undiluted to the skin. Most oils should not be used neat as they can cause irritation.

In an aroma lamp, the essential oil is usually heated by a tea light candle.

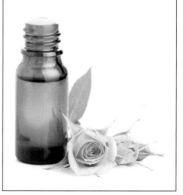

HOMEOPATHY

Homeopathy is based on the principle that "like cures like," meaning the treatment given is similar in substance to the illness it is helping. Although it has roots that go back many centuries, it began in its present form a mere 200 years ago. Many physicians are skeptical about homeopathy's effectiveness, so it is up to you to decide if the therapy works for you.

THE ORIGINS OF HOMEOPATHY
—

It was the Greek physician Hippocrates, known as the "father of medicine" who, in the 5th century B.C.E., was the first to understand the principle of treating the body with a remedy that will produce similar symptoms to the ailment suffered. He also believed that symptoms specific to an individual, that person's reactions to an ailment, and a person's own powers of healing were important in diagnosing and choosing a cure. On this basis, he built up his own medicine chest of "homeopathic" remedies. But it was the German physician

Samuel Hahnemann (1755–1843) who first developed homeopathy as it is known and practiced today. A prominent physician, chemist, and author, Hahnemann had become increasingly disillusioned with the methods of treatment of the day. These included harsh practices such as blood-letting and purging, and large doses of medicines that were often more debilitating than the illness itself. Yet it was obvious these practices were not working – disease was rampant. Hahnemann was one of the first physicians to advocate the improvement of poor hygiene, both in the home and in public places, and he stressed the importance of a good diet, fresh air, and higher standards of living for all. But disillusionment with the lack of response to his initiatives meant that he eventually decided to give up medical practice. In 1789 he moved to Leipzig, where he became a translator of medical texts.

Homeopathy is based on the principle of stimulating the body's defense mechanism by treating it with minute doses of a substance similar to those of the illness.

While translating one of these texts in 1790, *A Treatise on Materia Medica*, by Dr. William Cullen of London University, Hahnemann noticed an entry that was to set him on a path which would lead him all the way to the founding of homeopathic practice.

Cullen wrote that quinine (an extract of Peruvian bark) was an effective treatment for malaria because of its astringent qualities. As a chemist, Hahnemann knew quinine was effective against the disease, but doubted this was due to its astringency. He decided to explore this further and for days took doses of quinine himself and recorded his reactions. He found that he developed all the symptoms of malaria – palpitating heart, irregular pulse, drowsiness, and thirst – although he did not have the disease. Each time he took a new dose, the symptoms recurred. He speculated that it was the quinine's ability to induce the malarial symptoms that made it effective as a treatment. To back up his theory, he gave doses of quinine to volunteers, whom he called "provings," recorded their reactions, and found similar results.

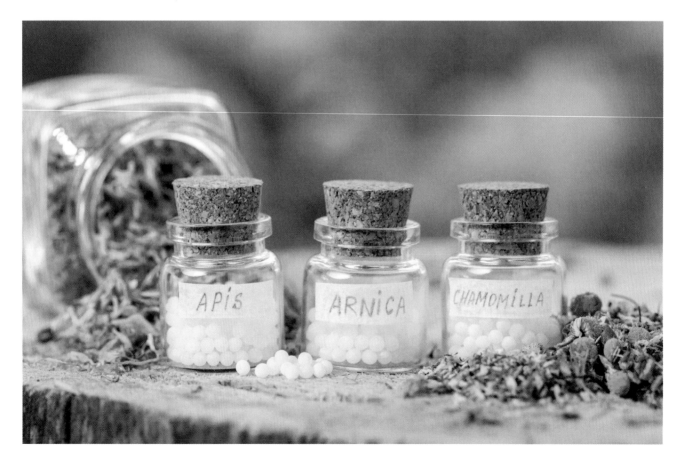

Hahnemann experimented with other substances, as well as quinine, which were used as medicines at the time, such as arsenic, belladonna, and mercury. With each new substance given, he noted that individuals differed in their severity of symptoms and how they healed. Some showed few symptoms, while others suffered badly. Hahnemann believed he had developed a new system of medicine – a system that worked on the principle that a substance and a disease that produce similar symptoms can negate each other, resulting in the full health of the patient. He called his new system "homeopathy," from the Greek words *homios*, meaning like, and *pathos*, meaning suffering.

HOMEOPATHY TODAY
—

There are now more than 2,000 homeopathic remedies available, with new ones continually being added. The remedies are made from animal, vegetable, and mineral sources, which are as varied as honey bees (including the sting), snake venom, poison ivy leaves, onions, coffee beans, and daisies. But the amounts used are so minute that no substance can be tasted or side-effects experienced, however poisonous or toxic the substance might be. In this book, however, we have not included remedies that are poisonous or toxic, as they should be administered only under the care of a qualified homeopath.

In his "provings," Hahnemann had been worried by some patients who got worse before they got better after taking the substances given to them. To prevent this happening, he developed a new system of diluting the remedies. He diluted each remedy and then "succussed" or shook it. He believed that doing this released the energy of the substance. He found not only that the new system of diluting prevented the worsening of symptoms, but also, to his astonishment, that the more diluted the substance, the better its effects. He called this method "potentization."

The process of making the remedies is very precise. Soluble substances such as plant and animal extracts are dissolved in a solution of about 90 percent alcohol and 10 percent distilled water, depending on

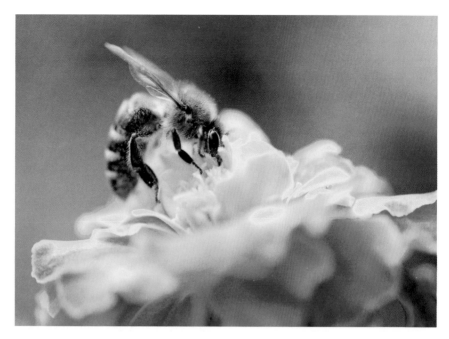

the substance. The mixture is kept in an airtight container and left to stand for two to four weeks, occasionally being shaken. Insoluble substances, such as gold, are first ground down into a fine powder until they become soluble, and then undergo the same process. The mixture is then strained, and the resulting solution is known as the mother tincture.

The mother tincture is then diluted again to produce the different potencies which make up the homeopathic remedies. The dilution is measured as either decimal (x) or centesimal (c). Decimal remedies are diluted to the ratio 1:10, while the centesimal ratio is 1:100. So to produce a 1c potency, one drop of the mother tincture is added to 99 drops of an alcohol and water solution, and then succussed. To produce a 2c potency, one drop of the 1c solution is mixed with an alcohol and water solution, and then succussed. By the time the remedy reaches a 12c potency it is unlikely that any of the original substance remains in the solution. This is why most physicians find it difficult to accept the efficacy of homeopathy. But the therapy's supporters believe that physics is not yet developed enough to explain the phenomenon. Once the solution has been succussed and diluted to a certain level, the potentized remedy is then added to lactose, or milk sugar, in the form of tablets, pilules, granules, or powder, and stored in a dark glass bottle, away from direct sunlight.

Whole bees and their stings are used to produce a remedy known as Apis mellifica. This is prescribed for patients with rashes, especially where there is burning or stinging.

For treatment purposes, different potencies are prescribed. For an acute illness, a low-potency remedy is recommended; for a chronic disease, a higher potency is more useful.

THE 12 TISSUE SALTS
—

Biochemic tissue salts are homeopathically prepared ingredients that were introduced at the end of the 19th century by a German physician, Wilhelm Schussler. He believed that many diseases were caused by a deficiency of one or more of 12 vital minerals. A deficiency in each salt would manifest as particular symptoms. Lack of calcarea phosphorica (Calc. phos.), for example, would show up as teething problems or an inability to absorb nutrients properly, while lack of magnesium phosphate (Mag. phos.) would affect nerve endings and muscles. Replacing the missing mineral with a minute dose of the tissue salt can correct the problem. Tissue salts are prepared only from mineral sources such as calcium, iron, and salt, but homeopathic remedies are made from animal, vegetable, and mineral sources. In all cases they are diluted to such an extent that there can be no possible side-effects from even the most toxic substances.

HOMEOPATHIC TECHNIQUES

THE PRINCIPLES OF HOMEOPATHY
—

Homeopathy sees symptoms of disease as a positive outward sign that the body is trying to heal itself. Therefore, it holds that the symptoms should not be suppressed (as they are in allopathic medicine), and remedies are used which will help stimulate and support the healing process. In some cases, the symptoms will worsen before they improve.

A homeopath prescribes remedies for the "whole" person, basing his or her decision on Hahnemann's principles – the "law of similars," the principle of minimum dose, and prescribing for the individual:

• The law of similars. Formulated in 1796, it states that a substance that, in large doses, can produce symptoms of illness in a healthy person can cure similar symptoms in a sick person if used in minute doses. Hahnemann believed this was because nature allows for the existence of two similar diseases in the body at the same time. Homeopathic remedies work by introducing a similar artificial disease that negates the original disease, and yet its own effects are so minimal it causes no suffering.
• The minimum dose. This states that successive dilutions enhance the curative properties of a substance, while eradicating any side-effects. This means only the most minute dose of the substance is needed to help heal.
• Whole-person prescribing. Homeopaths believe that symptoms, pain, or diseases do not occur in isolation, but are an overall reflection of a person. They therefore do not just look at the problem presented to them, but at the person as a "whole." Each person is treated as an individual, and the homeopath will consider the patient's personality, temperament, emotional and physical state, and likes and dislikes before prescribing a treatment. In this way, a homeopath might see two people with similar symptoms, but would treat them totally differently.

Homeopaths also believe treatment works according to a set of three rules known as the "laws of cure." These are:

• A remedy starts healing from the top of the body and works downward.
• It starts from within the body, working outward, and from major to minor organs.
• Symptoms clear up in reverse order to their manner of appearance.

Homeopaths also believe that treatment should be prescribed according to a person's constitution, which is made up of inherited and acquired mental, physical, and emotional characteristics. These are matched to a remedy that will improve all-round health, no matter what illness the individual is suffering. This constitutional profile corresponds to a particular remedy, and a person might therefore be known as a Sepia type, or a Lachesis type.

The homeopathic remedy Chamomilla may be prescribed for low pain threshold and nervous afflictions.

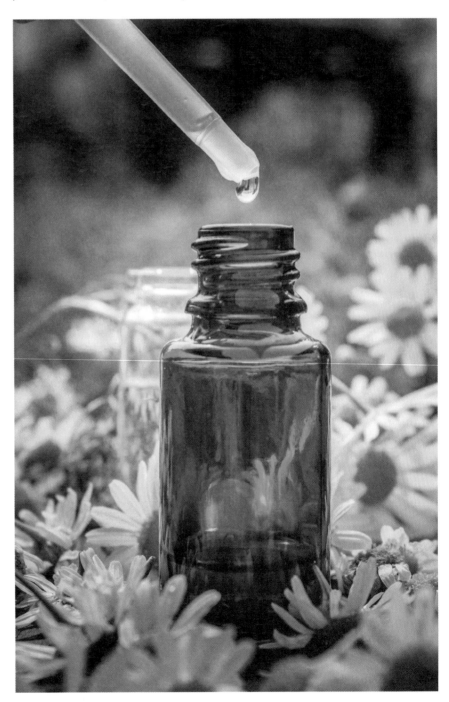

VISITING A HOMEOPATH

—

A first visit may last around an hour, as the homeopath asks detailed questions to build up an overall picture of your mental, physical, emotional, spiritual, and general health. As well as questions about any inherited problems, past illnesses, and diet, you may also be asked which side you sleep on, what type of weather you prefer, and whether you have food preferences. Only then will the homeopath prescribe a remedy specifically to suit you. One remedy at a time is usually given, although the prescription may change as your symptoms change. You may not be told which remedy has been prescribed. This is because some people are not happy with the constitutional character type attributed to them. Diet and lifestyle changes may also be recommended.

The remedies should be handled as little as possible, so are usually taken on a spoon and slipped under the tongue to dissolve. Food and drink should be avoided for a half-hour before and afterward. You may also be advised to avoid coffee and peppermints as they may counteract the remedies.

A follow-up appointment will be made for about a month later to assess progress. You may only need two appointments, but chronic conditions tend to take longer. If there is no improvement after around four visits, think about trying alternative treatment. Once symptoms improve, the remedy should be stopped. The remedies are perfectly safe, and although "overdosing" will do no harm, as with any medicine it is best avoided. With the approval of your physician, treatment can be given alongside conventional medicine, although some drugs may affect the efficacy of homeopathic remedies.

HOME USE

—

The remedies can be used at home for simple ailments and first aid, but should not be taken as a substitute for professional care. As a general rule, low potencies (e.g. 6c) are used for chronic conditions, and higher potencies (e.g. 30c) for acute conditions such as a cold. Remedies for acute conditions are usually taken on a half-hourly basis at first, and then the intervals spread out to about 8–12 hours. More chronic conditions may combine both low and high potencies.

HOW TO TAKE AND STORE REMEDIES

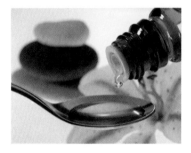

Remedies should not be touched by hand. Tap them out into the container lid or transfer them to a clean teaspoon.

• Take only one remedy at a time.
• Do not touch the remedies; empty them onto a teaspoon and put under the tongue, or tip them into the cap of the bottle to transfer them to the mouth.
• Take in a "clean mouth" at least 30 minutes after meals. If you need to take them sooner, rinse your mouth out first with water. Avoid alcoholic drinks and cigarettes, spicy or minty foods while taking the remedies.
• Store in a cool dark place in tightly closed bottle away from strong smells such as perfumes, air fresheners, or essential oils. Stored correctly, remedies will keep for around five years.

Homeopathic remedies are often offered as globules, which makes them very easy to take.

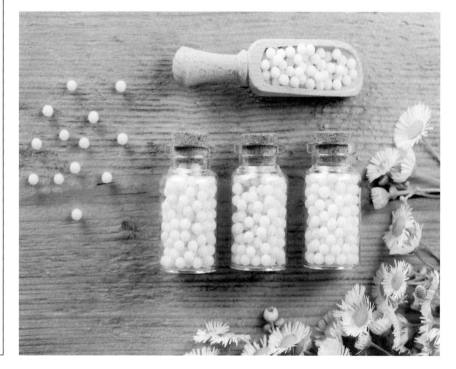

FLOWER ESSENCES

Flower essences, or flower remedies, as they are more commonly known, are used therapeutically to harmonize the body, mind, and the spirit. The essences are said to contain the life force of the flowers used to make them. Thousands of essences are available in health food stores, and they work "vibrationally" on a mental and emotional level, to relieve negative feelings, encourage the healing process, and to balance the energy in the body.

WHAT ARE FLOWER ESSENCES?
—

Flower essences are ideal for home use, being simple to make and use. They are prepared in water and preserved with alcohol. Historically, flower water and the morning dew collected from flower petals were thought to be imbued with magical properties. That flower remedies work is indisputable for those who are regular users; but no one knows how, so there is still an element of magic associated with their use

Dr. Edward Bach, the originator of the Bach Flower Remedies, sought his ingredients in the English countryside and tested them all on himself.

– even today, when our understanding of vibrational medicine is growing.

Flower remedies are so simple that they are often dismissed as a placebo. They do not work in any biochemical way, and because no physical part of the plant remains in the remedy, its properties and actions cannot be detected or analyzed as if it were a drug or herbal preparation. Therapists believe the remedies contain the energy, or imprint, of the plant from which it was made and work in a way that is similar to homeopathic remedies. In this way a remedy is believed to provide the stimulus needed to kick-start your own healing mechanism.

DR. BACH
—

Until recently, the name Dr. Edward Bach was almost synonymous with flower remedies. His set of 38 remedies became the inspiration for the worldwide development of remedies. They are still the cornerstone of flower remedy therapy and easily available. While working in the London Homeopathic Hospital, just after the First World War, he noticed that people with similar attitudes often had

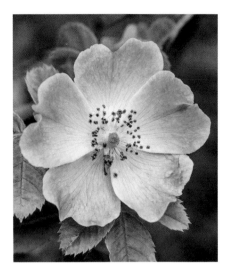

Flower remedies draw on the vibrational power of flowers like wild rose.

similar complaints. He concluded that, independently of other factors, mood and a negative attitude predisposed people toward ill health, and that illness was a manifestation of a deeper disharmony or an indication that the personality was in conflict. Between 1928 and 1932 he identified seven main negative states and found the first 12 of the flower remedies he needed to address them.

Over the subsequent few years, Dr. Bach dedicated himself to finding natural remedies from the countryside, and at his death had made 38 separate remedies. His successors at his house in Oxfordshire, England, called Mount Vernon, continue to make his remedies today, and they are sold under the brand name of Bach Flower Remedies.

OTHER REMEDIES
—

The Bach Flower Remedies are made from the trees and flowers Dr. Bach saw on his travels, which are native to England, with the exceptions of olive and vine. In the last 20 years, remedies from the U.S. and Australia have also been made. Sometimes they are called flower essences (do not confuse them with essential oils), but they are said to work in the same way as the original flower remedies. They address the emotional self, unlocking repressions, liberating negativity, and encouraging positive wellbeing.

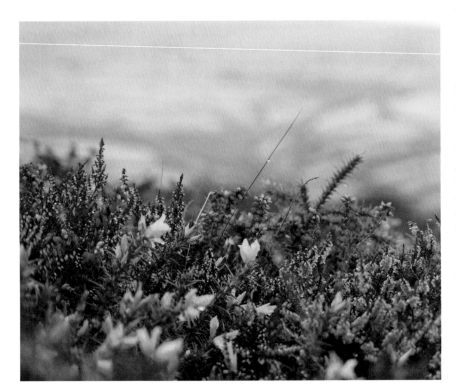

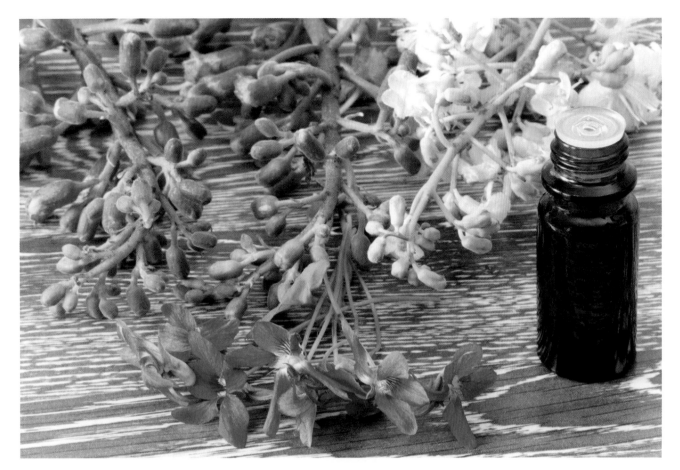

All of the 38 original flower remedies are included in this book, with the addition of 11 others: kangaroo paw, bush fuchsia, Sturt's desert rose, gray spider flower, hibbertia, mulla mulla, wedding bush, waratah, black-eyed Susan, bluebell, and wisteria.

SEEING A PROFESSIONAL
—

Flower remedies were created to be so simple to use that people could treat themselves. However, many practitioners of other disciplines – such as herbalism, homeopathy, and aromatherapy – use flower remedies to complement their own remedies, and a few flower essence therapists use the remedies exclusively.

Most therapists have their own ways of working. But every consultation should begin with an interview between you and the therapist. This can last from as little as 15 minutes to over an hour. During this time the therapist will explain the system to you if you do not already know how it works.

He or she will ask why you have come to see a therapist and will listen while you talk about yourself and your worries. The therapist will observe your posture and appearance, and will listen to the tone of your voice and the way you say things, as these can be as revealing as what you say. While you chat, the therapist may take notes and ask questions to work out, by a process of elimination, which remedies would be best for you. He or she might ask questions about your fears, how you feel about your children or other family members, or how easily you give up when something you attempt does not work out. It is not enough for the therapist to know that you have a problem at home or at work.

At the end of the consultation the therapist will help you select the remedies. The number of remedies prescribed depends on the individual, but it is unlikely to be more than six, and will often be much fewer. Most people feel at least a little better at the end of the consultation because they have been able to talk through their problems.

Flower essences can be bought in health stores or prepared at home.

The Dr. Edward Bach Foundation maintains an international register of qualified practitioners in the Bach Flower Remedies. A list of practitioners may be obtained from the Bach Centre (see page 389).

NEGATIVITY MAY CONTRIBUTE TO ILL HEALTH

Negative emotions depress the mind and immune system, repress activity, and may contribute to ill health. All are rooted in one or more of the following, which are headings under which Dr. Bach grouped his 38 remedies:

• Fear
• Uncertainty
• Insufficient interest in present circumstances
• Loneliness
• Oversensitivity to influences and ideas
• Despondency or despair
• Over-care for the welfare of others.

By learning the healing capacity of peace, hope, joy, faith, certainty, wisdom, and love it is possible to develop a positive outlook and a sense of wellbeing.

USING FLOWER REMEDIES

WHEN TO USE
—

Flower remedies are simple and effective, and they can be used to treat all types of mental or emotional problems:

• To support in times of crisis
• To treat the emotional outlook produced by illness
• To address a particular recurring emotional or behavioral pattern
• To give strength during a temporary emotional setback
• As a preventive remedy when things start to go out of balance.

Remedies act swiftly for passing moods and there should be an improvement very quickly, although it may take months to start to change a long-standing pattern.

CHOOSING REMEDIES
—

Successful treatment depends on accurate diagnosis. Get to know the different essences available and then aim to match the

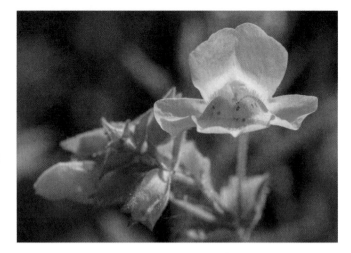

The mimulus, or monkey plant, can be used to prepare a remedy that offers freedom from fear.

remedies to the individual character. If you find it hard to decide on a remedy, make a note of the one you think you need and then ask yourself the same questions you would ask anyone for whom you were prescribing:

• How do you feel?
• Why are you feeling like that?
• How do the symptoms affect you?
• What could have caused the problem?

Some people recommend that an appropriate affirmation is written down several times a day for a week while taking a remedy. An example of a positive affirmation for the clematis daydreamer would be: "I am awake (or becoming awake) and open to the experience of here and now."

ARE THEY SAFE?
—

The remedies are not addictive or dangerous, nor do they interfere with any other form of treatment. They are suitable for people of all ages. Pregnant women and children can take them with confidence. Flower remedies are safe for young babies, should they need them, and they can also be given to animals and plants.

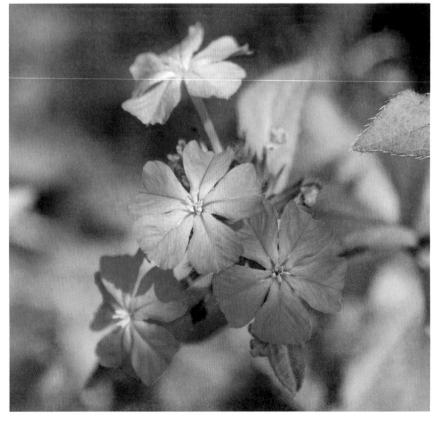

REMEDIES AND ALCOHOL

Flower remedies and essences are preserved in alcohol. The amount of alcohol in a personal remedy made solely with water is minute, but it is enough to upset those who are alcohol intolerant or recovering from alcoholism. Always check the status of those to whom you give a remedy. Thoughtlessness can do untold damage.

It is possible to remove the alcohol by putting the diluted drops of remedy in a boiling hot drink – the steam will evaporate the alcohol. Leave the remedy to cool before taking. Sip throughout the day.

If you find it hard to trust your intuition, cerato may be the right choice of remedy.

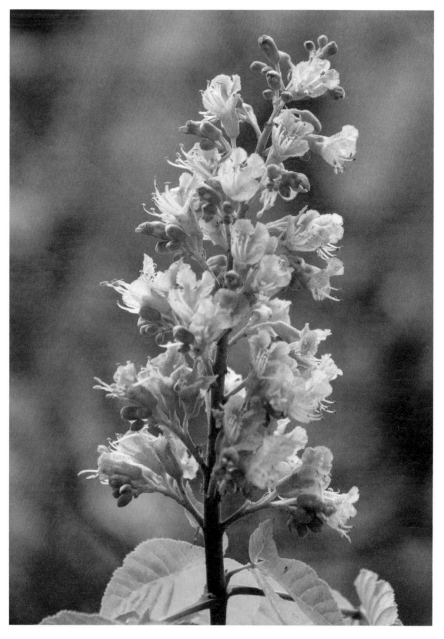

The flowers of red chestnut are a good remedy for parents who are over-anxious about their family's welfare.

The flower remedies or essences bought in a store are sold in stock bottles. They can be used straight from the bottle, but it is better to make a personal remedy mix. Sometimes a single flower remedy is needed, but in most cases two or more are combined.

Method

1 Decide on the remedies that are most applicable. If you think you need several, simplify to a maximum of seven covering immediate issues, and check again in a few weeks.

2 Put 2 drops of each remedy into a clean 1fl. oz. (30ml.) amber glass dropper bottle. This is the standard amount, but read the label, as occasionally some of the newer essences suggest you use 4 or 7 drops.

3 If the remedies are to be used within a week, fill the bottle with clean spring water. If the remedies are to be taken for a prolonged period, add 1 teaspoonful (5ml.) of brandy to the bottle and then fill with spring water.

4 Label the bottle with your name and the date. Give the remedy a title or a few words to remind you of the purpose. Keep remedies, like other medicines, out of the reach of children.

Dose

• The standard dose is 4 drops, on or under the tongue, 4 times a day.

• At times of crisis, 2 drops from the stock bottle can be put into a glass of water (or, in an emergency, any drink) and sipped as needed.

• If it is impossible to take anything by mouth, put the drops on the skin or in washing water.

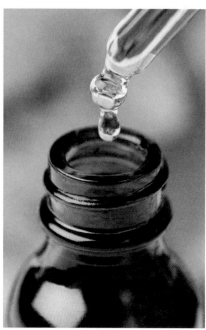

When making a personal remedy, put 2 drops of each chosen essence into an amber glass dropper bottle.

CHILDREN AND FLOWER ESSENCES
—

Flower remedies are ideal for children. However, physical symptoms must be professionally treated. Consult a physician if in doubt. When treating children:

• Listen and do not trivialize children's emotional lives. Be calm and methodical. Notice the mood or address a previously known pattern. Give the remedy for a day or two, then reassess. Moods in children may change rapidly.

• If worried about a child (or other family member) take red chestnut, Rescue Remedy (see page 158), or any other remedy that seems relevant, to settle yourself before deciding on treatment.

• If the child is of breastfeeding age, give the remedy to the mother. It may also be put in the bath: for example, use impatiens to treat the hot and restless frustration of a teething baby.

• Support the parents if their child is unwell. For example, give Rescue Remedy and walnut if the child is hospitalized.

• Treat the parents. Their emotional problems (even if suppressed) may be the root of a child's distress.

MAKING THE REMEDIES

BASIC RULES
—

Before you begin to make your own remedies, consider these basic rules:

• Correct identification. Find the plant and site well before the day of picking. Make sure that it is legal to pick it or that you have the landowner's permission.

• Preparation. Collect the essential tools. Absolute cleanliness is vital. Wash your hands and rinse them several times. Utensils can be cleaned by boiling in spring or rain water for 20 minutes and then allowing them to drain dry. Wrap them in a clean cloth to keep them ready for a suitable day.

• The right day. For sun method remedies (see right), choose a warm, sunny day with no clouds. For boiling method remedies (see far right) any bright, sunny day is good.

• On the day. Pick with respect. Pick flowers that you are drawn to. Pick from all sides of the plant, from the top and bottom branches of trees, or from a wide area with meadow plants. Work quickly so there is only a little time between picking the flowers and putting them into the water to make the remedy. If you need to carry the flowers, cover your palm with a large leaf (preferably from the plant being picked) to prevent the heat and oils from your hand contaminating the blossoms.

• Labeling. When you have finished making your remedy, label and date it clearly. Keep it in a cool, dark place, away from direct sunlight.

FLOWER REMEDIES AND ANIMALS

It is possible to successfully treat animals with flower remedies. Get to know the different essences available and then aim to match the remedies to the individual character of your pet. You need to know the animal's nature and note how differently it behaves when ill. For example, a dog that looks sorry for itself needs willow; an aggressive one needs holly or vine; and cats often need water violet for their pride and independence. Add 4 drops to a small animal's drinking water, and 10 drops for large animals such as horses and cows. Add more drops whenever the water is replaced.

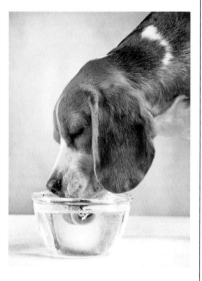

Flower essences can be added to your pet's drinking water.

Chicory is best picked in late summer.

THE SUN METHOD

This method is used for flowers other than tree blossoms. Pick when the flowers are coming into full bloom. This will depend on the climate, but the following can serve as a general guide:

• Early spring: oak, gorse, olive, vine
• Late spring: white chestnut, water violet
• Summer: rock water, mimulus, agrimony, rock rose, centaury
• Late summer: scleranthus, wild oat, impatiens, chicory, vervain, clematis, heather
• Fall: cerato, gentian

A 3fl.oz. (100ml.) bottle of mother tincture will last the average family many years. This recipe can make more, up to six bottles. Each 3fl.oz. (100ml.) should contain 1½fl.oz. (50ml.) of brandy and be made up as outlined below:

You'll Need:
• Bottle of spring or mineral water
• Plain glass bowl
• 3fl.oz. (100ml.) amber bottle(s)
• 1½ fl.oz. (50ml.) brandy
• Natural and unbleached filter paper
• Pen and label

1 Decide beforehand on the plants, where to pick from, and where to place the bowl (as close to the plants as possible, but away from shadows and possible contamination), then wait for a suitable sunny day.
2 The best time for harvesting the plants is between 9a.m. and midday. The flowers are dry from the dew, but not yet exhausted by the sun.
3 Pick the flowers and put in the water as quickly as possible. Float the flowers on the water until the whole surface is covered. Use a twig or leaf to arrange them, not your fingers.
4 Leave the bowl out in the open where it will receive direct sunshine for 3 hours.
5 Remove the flowers with a twig and filter the liquid.
6 Pour 1½fl.oz. (50ml.) of the water into the bottle with the brandy. Shake and label with the name, "flower essence mother tincture," and date. This mother tincture will be used to prepare stock bottles and it will keep for many years. To prepare a stock bottle, put 2 drops of mother tincture into a 1fl.oz. (30ml.) dropper bottle, and top up with brandy.

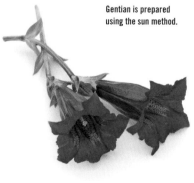

Gentian is prepared using the sun method.

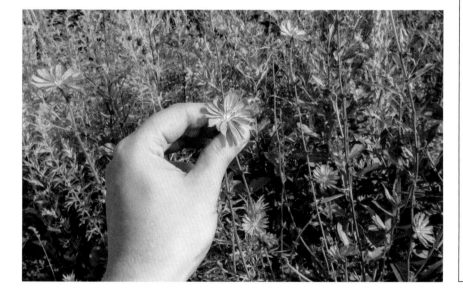

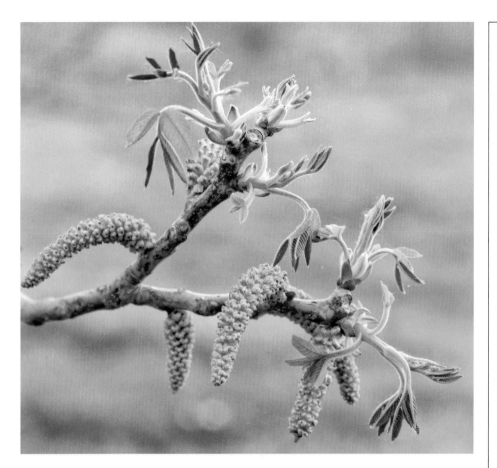

Pick the twigs and flowers of
walnut blossom in late spring.

THE BOILING METHOD

The boiling method is mainly used for the flowers of trees. In addition to the flowers, it is necessary to collect twigs that have a few leaves on them. Pick when the flowers are at their best:

- Early spring: cherry plum
- Mid-spring: elm, aspen
- Late spring: beech, chestnut bud, hornbeam, larch, walnut, star of Bethlehem, holly, crab apple, willow
- Early summer: red chestnut, pine, mustard
- Summer: honeysuckle, sweet chestnut, wild rose

You'll Need:
- 6pt. (3l.) saucepan with lid (use an enamel, glass, or stainless steel pan; avoid copper, aluminum, and Teflon-coated pans)
- A glass measuring jug
- 2pt. (1l.) of cold water (rain water or mineral water)
- 3fl.oz. (100ml.) amber glass bottle(s) (up to six)
- 1½fl.oz. (50ml.) of brandy
- Natural and unbleached filter paper
- Pen and label

1 If you are going to boil the remedy outside, check your camping stove and equipment.
2 Take everything into the field between 9a.m. and 11a.m. on a sunny day.
3 Touch as little as possible. Pick twigs or flowers until the saucepan is three-quarters full. Put on the lid and take to the heat source as quickly as possible.
4 When the pan is on the heat, cover the flowers and twigs with the cold water and bring to the boil.
5 Simmer for a half-hour. Use a twig from the tree to push the twigs under the water.
6 Remove the pan from the heat, and stand it outside to cool, with the lid on.
7 When cool, remove the twigs, then carefully filter the water into the jug.
8 Put 1½fl.oz. (50ml.) of the flower water into the 3fl.oz. (100ml.) bottle(s) with the brandy. Label with the name, "flower essence mother tincture," and date. This is the mother tincture from which a stock bottle is made, as described under "The Sun Method" opposite.

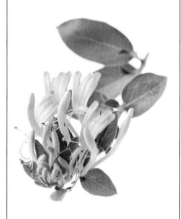

NUTRITION

The use of nutrition for health, or nutritional therapy, can help with almost anything, since food is the basic fuel of all the chemical processes that take place in the body. Almost all ill health of body and mind can have a basis in nutritional elements that are missing or insubstantial within the diet – or in unhealthy additions to our diet, such as large quantities of saturated fat, sugar, and salt. All the systems in the body will be improved by a healthy diet. In a fit state, you are much more likely to fight off infection and deal efficiently with any health problems or injury.

A HEALTHY DIET
—

Our diet should be made up of complex carbohydrates (5–9 portions per day), fruits and vegetables (4–9 portions), proteins (3–5 portions), and fat (under 1oz. [30g.] per day is recommended for a healthy diet). We also need to drink plenty of fluids, particularly water. But eating the right foods doesn't necessarily mean that you are getting enough nutrients. Refining and processing foods takes out much of the nutritional value, and pesticides and other agents used in the growing process place extra demands on our bodies. Before our food ever reaches the grocery store it may be nutritionally deficient. Therefore, take extra steps to preserve the nutritional content of your food whenever possible:

• Eat the skins of vegetables.
• Don't cut, wash, or soak fruit and vegetables until you are ready to eat them. Exposing their cut surfaces to air destroys many nutrients.
• Eat brown, unpolished rice and whole grains.
• Choose fresh fruit and vegetables first, but remember that nutritional value decreases with age. Frozen is a better option if you aren't going to eat the food immediately. Eat raw whenever possible; if cooking, use as little water as possible. If you do boil fruit or vegetables, use the water remaining after cooking in your sauces or gravy.
• Eat organic food whenever possible. It may be more expensive, but you can be sure that the food you are eating has not been processed, and has been grown without the use of pesticides and other chemicals.

DIETARY FIBER
—

Dietary fiber, also known as bulk and roughage, is an essential element in the diet, even though it provides no nutrients. It consists of plant cellulose and other indigestible materials in foods, along with pectin and gum. The chewing it requires stimulates saliva flow, and the bulk it adds in the stomach and intestines during digestion provides more time for absorption of nutrients. A diet with sufficient fiber produces softer, bulkier stools, and helps to promote bowel regularity and avoid constipation and disorders such as diverticulosis. Other health benefits of fiber include:

• Reduces the production of cholesterol in the body
• May protect against some coronary heart diseases
• Helps to control diabetes
• Helps to control weight
• Protects against cancers of the colon.

Fruits and vegetables should make up at least one-third of the food we eat. People who eat five portions a day have a lower risk of heart disease, stroke, and some cancers.

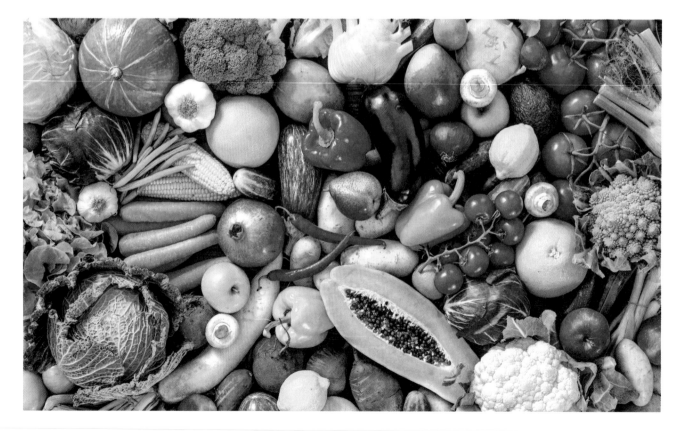

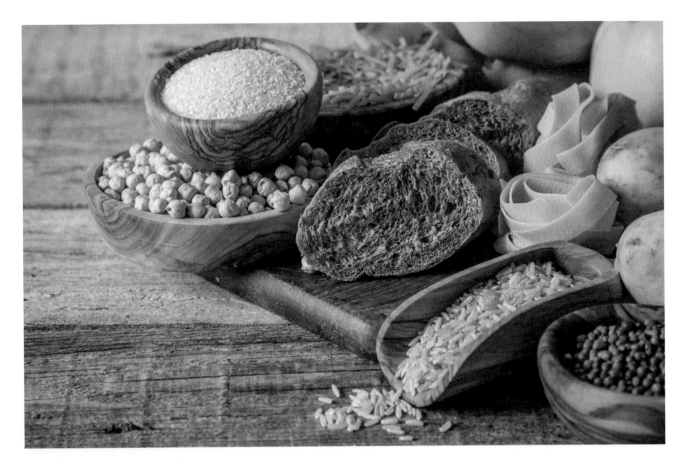

Complex carbohydrates, such as wholegrain cereals, potatoes, and pulses, should make up one-third of our daily diet. They are good sources of energy, fiber, vitamins, and minerals.

The best sources of fiber are fruit and vegetables, wholegrain breads and cereals, and products made from nuts and legumes. An intake of 0.7–2oz. (20–60g.) of fiber per day is ideal. A diet overly abundant in dietary fiber can cut down on the absorption of important trace minerals during digestion. Take a good multivitamin and mineral tablet if you increase your fiber intake significantly.

FOODS TO AVOID
—

Aim to reduce the amount of saturated fat, sugar, and salt in your diet. We all need to consume some fat, yet we need to pay attention to the amount and type of fat we eat. There are two main types of fat: saturated and unsaturated. Too much saturated fat can increase the cholesterol in your blood, which increases your risk of heart disease. Saturated fat is found in foods such as cakes, biscuits, chips,

butter, cream, cheese, and fatty meats. Replace these foods with those that contain unsaturated fats, such as oily fish (including tuna, salmon, mackerel, and trout), avocado and vegetable oils. Trim the fat off meat, drink skimmed milk, replace cream and ice cream with low-fat yogurt, and spread your bread with a reduced-fat spread.

Eating too many foods and drinks high in sugar increases your risk of obesity and related conditions. Swap drinks high in sugars for lower-calorie options. For example, swap a sugary soda for sparkling

Low-fat dairy products, meat, fish, eggs, beans, and pulses are good sources of protein.

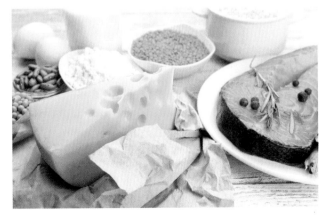

water with a slice of lemon. Reduce your alcohol intake. Avoid sugary breakfast cereals, cakes, biscuits, and pastries. Check the labels of packaged sauces and meals to make sure they are not high in sugar.

Too much salt in your diet can raise your blood pressure, which leaves you at greater risk of heart disease or stroke. Even if you do not add salt to your food, there are high levels of salt in many food products, such as breads, chips, cereals, soups, and sauces. Check food labels to help you reduce your salt intake.

VITAMINS AND MINERALS

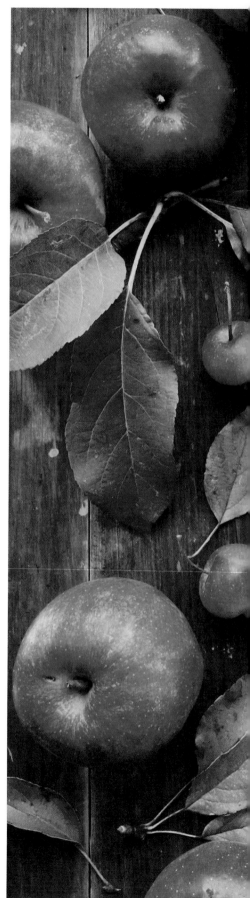

MICRONUTRITION
—

Our understanding of vitamins and minerals – and other micronutrients, compounds, and elements – and their role in our body has improved dramatically over the last decades. We now know that "micronutrition" – or the vitamins, minerals, and other health-giving components of our food, such as amino acids, fiber, enzymes, and lipids – is crucial to life, and that by manipulating our nutritional intake, we can not only ensure good health and address ailments, but prevent illness and some of the degenerative effects of aging.

VITAMINS
—

Vitamins are a group of unrelated organic nutrients which are essential to regulate the chemical processes that go on in the body – such as releasing the energy from food, maintaining strong bones, and controlling our hormonal activity. Ideally, vitamins are present in roughly the same quantity in various foods.

MINERALS
—

Minerals are inorganic chemical elements, which are necessary for many biochemical and physiological processes that go on in our bodies. Inorganic substances that are required in amounts greater than 100mg. per day are called minerals; those required in amounts less than 100mg. per day are called trace elements. Minerals are not necessarily present in foods – the quality of the soil and the geological conditions of the area in which they were grown play an important part in determining the mineral content of foods. Even a balanced diet may be lacking in essential minerals or trace elements because of the soil in which the various foodstuffs were grown.

There is some evidence that "subclinical" deficiencies – in other words, a deficiency which is not extensive enough to be life-threatening or to produce large-scale symptoms – may be the cause of certain forms of cancer, heart disease, weight and skin problems, and a host of other health conditions.

AMINO ACIDS
—

An amino acid is any compound that contains an amino group and an acidic function. There are 20 amino acids necessary for the synthesis of proteins, which are essential for life. These 20 amino acids form the building blocks of all proteins and are involved in important biological processes, such as the formation of neurotransmitters in the brain. There are 10 essential amino acids:

- Arginine (essential for children but not adults)
- Histidine
- Isoleucine
- Leucine
- Lysine
- Methionine
- Phenylalanine
- Threonine
- Tryptophan
- Valine.

The remaining 10 are called "nonessential," which means that they can usually be made by the body from other substances. In some conditions, however, nonessential amino acids are necessary, for example in cases of extreme illness or a very poor diet.

LIPIDS AND DERIVATIVES
—

Lipids are commonly called "fats," and while many fats are now known to be unhealthy, there are many that are essential to body processes and actually work to prevent the effects of "unhealthy" fats in our bodies. Many lipids, including fish oils and evening primrose oil, and their derivatives are used to unclog arteries, work to retard the effects of aging, and to discourage heart disease and the build-up of cholesterol.

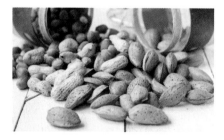

Peanuts, almonds, and hazelnuts are good sources of the essential amino acid phenylalanine.

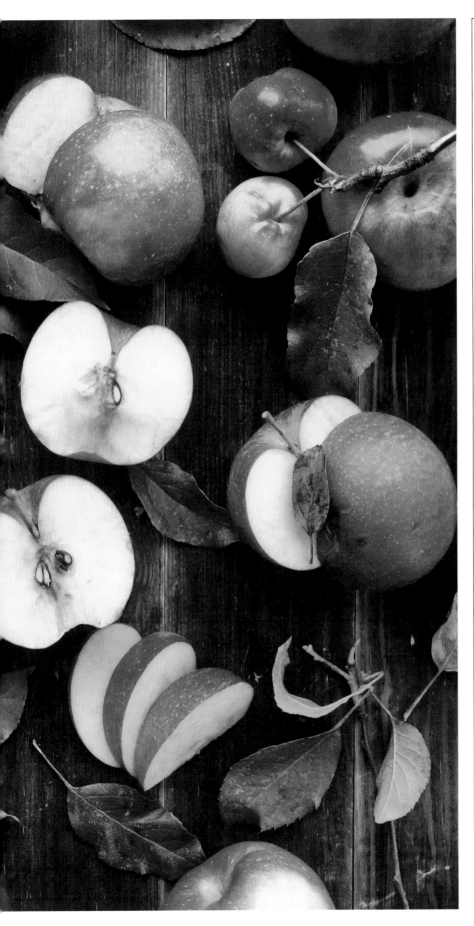

A HISTORY OF NUTRITION

18TH CENTURY

Although there was not yet any scientific understanding of what a "vitamin" was, in the 18th century, English sailors were given lime or lemon juice in order to prevent scurvy, a disease caused by lack of vitamin C, which occurred as a result of long periods of time away at sea without fresh fruit or vegetables.

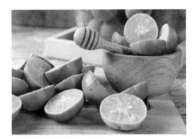

From the 18th century, English sailors ate limes as a protection against scurvy.

19TH CENTURY

In the late 19th century, naturopaths drew attention to the use of food and its nutritional elements as medicine, a concept that was not new, but which had not been acknowledged as a therapy in its own right until that time. Naturopaths used nutrition and fasting to cleanse the body, and to encourage its ability to heal itself. As knowledge about food, its make-up, and the effects it has on our body became greater with the development of biochemistry, the first nutritional specialists undertook to treat specific ailments and symptoms with the components of food.

20TH CENTURY

By the middle of the 20th century, scientists had put together a profile of proteins, carbohydrates, and fats, as well as vitamins and minerals, which were essential to life and to health. More than 40 nutrients were uncovered, including 13 vitamins. It was discovered that minerals were needed for body functions, and a new understanding of the body and its biochemistry fed the growing interest in the subject. By the 1960s, physicians began to treat patients with special diets and supplements, prescribed according to individual symptoms, problems, and needs, but while conventional medical physicians discussed nutrition in terms of food groups, nutritionists were prescribing vitamins in megadoses. Other elements and compounds were soon identified as necessary to human life, and we are now able to purchase substances such as amino acids, lipids, and dietary enzymes.

TODAY

Today, nutrition has changed from a mainly physician-led dietary therapy, also called clinical nutrition, to a more profound theory of health based on treating the patient as a whole (holistic health), and looking for deficiencies that may be causing illness, which are specific to each individual.

Apples contain vitamin C, which helps combat infection and boost immunity.

TAKING SUPPLEMENTS

SHOULD YOU TAKE SUPPLEMENTS?
—

Vitamins, minerals, and other elements work together within the body to ensure that all processes can be carried out. When even one element is missing, the body becomes unbalanced and unable to work at its optimum level. The best source of all micronutrients is food. Supplements are not a replacement for food, and most cannot be ingested without food. They cannot be taken in place of a good diet, but their beneficial effects will be optimized if combined with a balanced intake of nutritious foods. People suffering from chronic conditions or who smoke or drink regularly may need to take supplements to ensure optimum health.

Micronutrients work in conjunction with one another, and taking large doses of any one supplement can upset the balance within the body. A good vitamin and mineral supplement will ensure that you are getting the correct amounts of each, according to the relationships between them. Extra supplements should only be taken on the advice of a registered nutritionist or medical practitioner. Where supplements are taken to discourage the course of illness – for example vitamin C for colds or flu – it is safe to take larger doses than usual. Read the packet for further information.

Registered nutritionists have achieved great success with treating conditions like rheumatism and arthritis, high blood pressure, fatigue, constipation and other digestive disorders, the healing and recuperation processes following injury or surgery, skin problems, and many psychological and behavioral problems. Neuralgia, osteoporosis, PMS, postnatal illness, pregnancy problems, reduced immunities, stress, and viruses may respond to dietary treatment.

A nutritionist can advise on healthy diet and recipes, as well as any necessary supplements.

WHEN TO TAKE SUPPLEMENTS
—

The best time for taking most supplements is after meals, on a full stomach, although some vitamins and minerals work best on an empty stomach. Read the label on any supplement you plan to take to find out the best time to take it.

Time-release formulas need to be taken with food, as their nutrients are slowly released over a number of hours. If there is not enough food to slow their passage through the body, they can pass the sites where they are normally absorbed before they have had a chance to release their nutrients. Take supplements evenly throughout the day for best effect.

WHEN TO SEE A PRACTITIONER
—

Most supplements can be taken safely without input from a registered nutritionist, but if you suffer from chronic health problems, or a specific ailment, it is best to seek expert advice. Amino acids and other

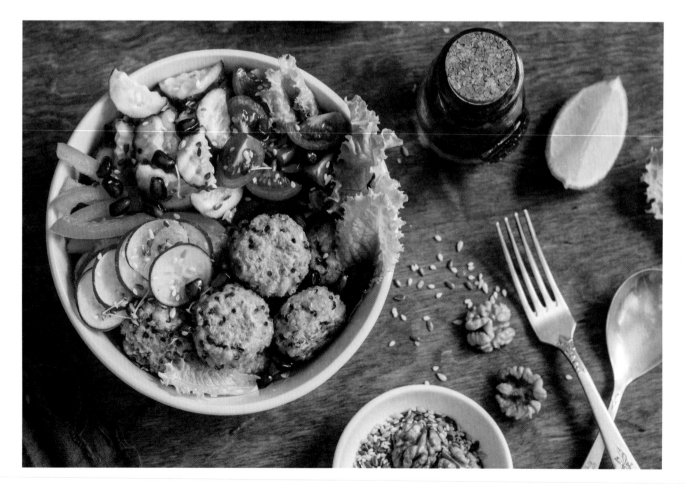

elements should only be taken with the advice of a professional. A nutritionist will make sure that you are taking a balanced combination of nutrients that will work together to make you healthy. Remember that everyone's needs are different, based on overall health, diet, whether or not you smoke or drink, are pregnant, and other influences. It is sensible to ensure that you receive advice that is tailored specifically to your individual needs.

Always take care to consult with a registered nutritionist or a dietician, as the term "nutritionist" is not legally protected in many states and countries. Any person can call themself a nutritionist even if they are wholly self-taught. Turn to page 384 for advice on finding a registered nutritionist.

Folic acid is found in dark green vegetables, citrus fruits, dried beans, peas, nuts, and lentils. A supplement containing folic acid is often suggested in pregnancy.

CHILDREN
—

Children need far lower doses than adults, and a healthy, organic diet should offer a large proportion of their nutritional needs. A good vitamin and mineral supplement will provide anything extra that is required, but if you feel your child needs further supplements, see a practitioner. If you are buying products yourself, read the label to ensure that the product is safe for children, and follow the advice carefully.

PREGNANCY
—

A growing baby puts heavy demands on your body when you are pregnant, and it is more important than ever to ensure that you have a good diet. Research has now proved that we need extra folic acid and iron

Children's supplements are often colored and flavored to make them attractive to children. However, care should be taken that children do not confuse them with candies. Supplements should be kept out of the reach of children.

during pregnancy, and a good multivitamin and mineral supplement is often suggested. Consult with your healthcare provider about which supplements are recommended during pregnancy. Do not take vitamin A supplements while pregnant (see page 206).

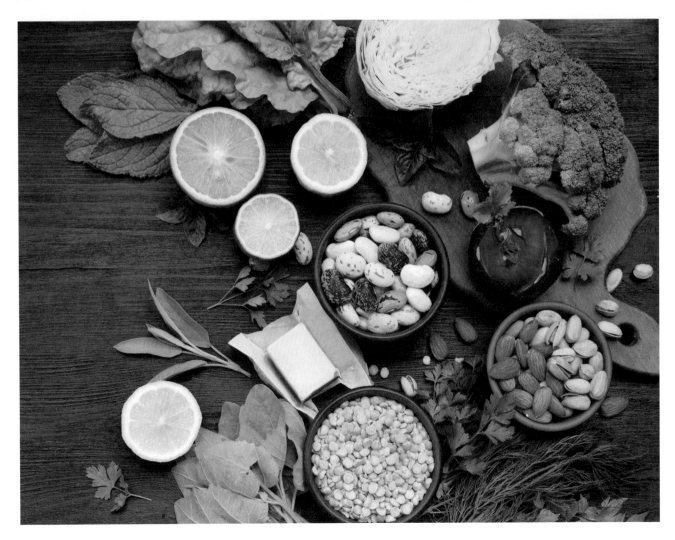

SUPPLEMENT FORMS

WHICH SUPPLEMENT?
—

Most supplements come in a variety of forms. They are also prepared with different quantities of the active ingredients, so read the label carefully to ensure that you are getting the correct quantity for your needs:

• Powders. Many supplements come in powder form, which will usually provide you with extra potency, with no binders or additives. This is useful for people with allergies, or those who find it difficult to swallow a tablet. Powders are particularly useful for children – sprinkle a little powder in their breakfast juice, or stir it into some yogurt or dessert.
• Capsules. These are convenient to take and easy to keep. Fat-soluble vitamins are normally taken in capsule form, but many contain vitamin and mineral powders which allow a higher potency. Garlic and evening primrose oil are commonly available as capsules, and the capsules can be broken apart and applied externally as necessary.

• Liquids. Liquids are appropriate for people who have difficulty swallowing tablets or capsules. Many children's formulas come in liquid form for easy administration. Liquids can be mixed with food or stirred into drinks. Liquid supplements can also be applied externally.
• Tablets. Many supplements come in tablet form and these are the most practical for many people because they can be easily stored and they will keep for a long time. Check the label to see what is added to your tablets in the form of binders or fillers, which are added to preserve or bulk out the active ingredient.

READING THE LABEL
—

Supplements work in different ways, and you will need to understand some of the key words that appear on the labels in order to choose which are most suitable for you.

Chelated is a term that appears on mineral supplements, and it means that the mineral is combined with amino acids to make assimilation more efficient. Most nutritionists recommend taking chelated minerals because they are 3 to 5 times more effective.

Time-release formulas are created with a process that allows them to be released into the body over an 8–10-hour period. These are particularly useful for water-soluble vitamins (see pages 207–210), any excess of which is excreted within 2 or 3 hours of taking the supplement. Time-release formulas are reputed to provide stable blood levels during the day and night.

RDA AND SUPPLEMENTS
—

Governments around the world have provided guidelines for how much of each vitamin or mineral we need in our diets. These are called RDAs (recommended daily allowance) or RDIs (recommended daily intake) and they apply to healthy individuals with a good, balanced diet. These levels

Some supplements come in a variety of forms, allowing the individual to choose between capsules, powders, liquids, or tablets.

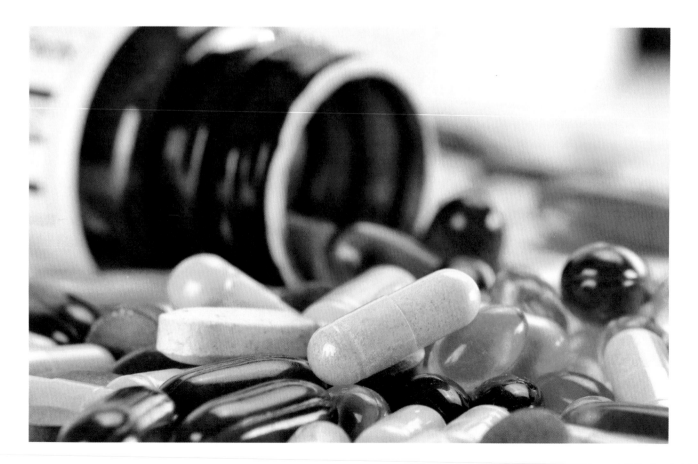

ANTIOXIDANTS AND SUPERFOODS

Much of the cell damage that occurs in disease is caused by highly destructive chemical groups known as free radicals. These are the products of oxidation, a process that occurs naturally in our body as we breathe. Today, because of the other elements in the air, there are more free radicals than ever. In small quantities, free radicals can fight bacteria and viruses; in larger quantities they encourage the aging process and cause damage to our cells.

Many nutritionists believe that free radicals can be combated by antioxidants – the ACE vitamins (vitamin A in the form of beta carotene, vitamin C, and vitamin E), the minerals selenium and zinc, and to a lesser extent manganese and copper. Antioxidants protect other substances from oxidation. Some trials have shown that additional antioxidant vitamins – such as 2,000mg. of C and 400mg. of E daily – can reduce the incidence of heart attacks, strokes, cataracts, and other diseases, and slow down the process of aging. However, some physicians believe that the jury is still out on antioxidants.

Many so-called "superfoods" are high in antioxidants, including blueberries, goji berries, pomegranate, and broccoli. Although not all physicians agree on the power of antioxidants, they do agree that these vitamin-rich, high-fiber foods are a good addition to a balanced diet. Other foods that are high in antioxidants, such as green tea and chocolate, are also high in fat or caffeine. These can be consumed as part of a healthy diet, but not to excess.

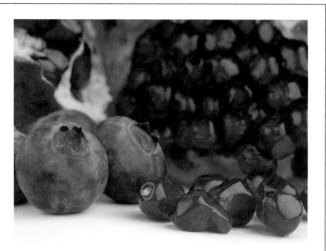

The "superfoods" blueberries and pomegranates are high in antioxidants, vitamins, and fiber.

are an "adequate" intake for the average person. In other words, they are not therapeutic levels and they do not take into account the varying needs of the population. People with illnesses, a stressful lifestyle, or who are on medication, or eat a highly refined diet may need much more than the RDA. RDAs are given in mg. (milligrams) or mcg. (micrograms).

The therapeutic dosage for different vitamins and minerals may be many times the RDA. For example, the RDA for vitamin C is 60mg., while the therapeutic dose is 2,000mg. The RDA for vitamin E is 10mg., while the therapeutic dose is 400mg. The RDA for zinc is 15mg. but the therapeutic dose is 30–60mg.

NUTRITIONAL REMEDIES

TYPE	PAGES
Vitamins	206–211
Minerals	212–221
Amino acids	222–227
Lipids and other supplements	228–235

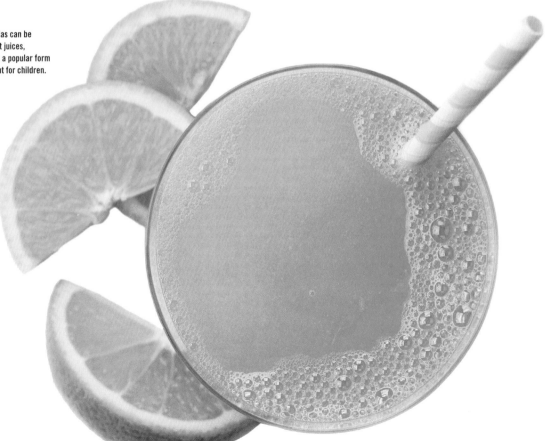

Liquid formulas can be added to fruit juices, making them a popular form of supplement for children.

MIND–BODY HEALING

In natural healing, the mind and body are inherently connected in a holistic manner – and healing one may help to heal the other. Traditional medicine takes a slightly different view from modern medicine on how to go about treating and healing illness and disease, but together traditional and modern ideas and practices can complement and balance each other.

THE MIND–BODY CONNECTION
—

The mind and body might seem like separate entities, but in terms of health and wellbeing, they are very connected. Mental states, such as thoughts, beliefs, emotions, and attitudes can affect how you feel physically, both in a positive and negative manner.

If you feel low, fed up, and negative about yourself and are not able to deal properly with your emotions, physical ill health may develop. In contrast, if you feel happy and enthusiastic about life, and are coping with things well, you are more likely to feel energized and well.

What you do physically, such as taking exercise and eating healthily, can affect your mental state and how you feel about yourself, too. If you have a poor diet, lack of exercise, and sleeping problems, you are more vulnerable to experiencing depression and other mental health problems.

TRADITIONAL AND MODERN MEDICINE IDEAS
—

Traditional Chinese, Ayurvedic, and complementary holistic medicine take a different approach from modern medicine to defining and treating disease and illness. Traditional approaches focus on looking at the person as a whole and not just their symptoms. They fully recognize that the mind and the body are connected. They acknowledge that an imbalance or illness affecting the mind can cause physical symptoms in the body, and vice versa.

A complementary practitioner works to find the underlying cause of the illness and then treats it on an individual basis – one person presenting with the symptoms of a cold will not necessarily receive the same treatment as another person.

On the other hand, modern or conventional medicine looks first at the symptoms of illness, then diagnoses the problem and provides treatment. Rather than focusing on the whole body, modern medicine often homes in on the specific part or organ of the body that is affected. Medical practitioners often specialize in particular areas, rather than covering the whole person, and standard treatments tend to be prescribed for certain ailments, such as ulcers.

Although the two approaches are inherently different, they can successfully be used alongside each other. Used well, they can balance each other and provide support and healing in different ways.

By seeing the link between mind and body, we can learn to unwind and to recognize the physical effects of mental stress.

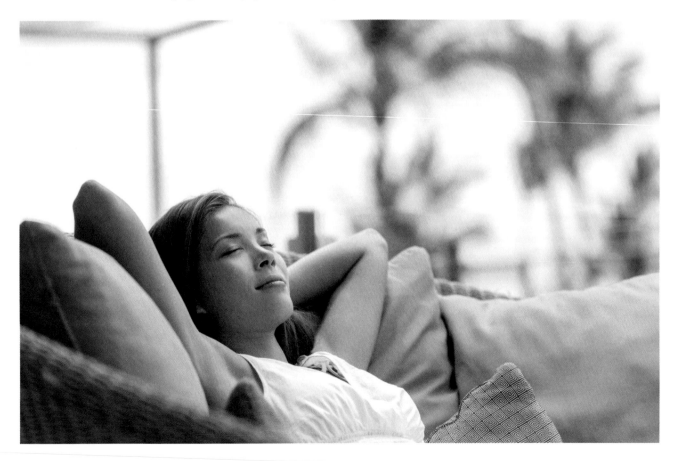

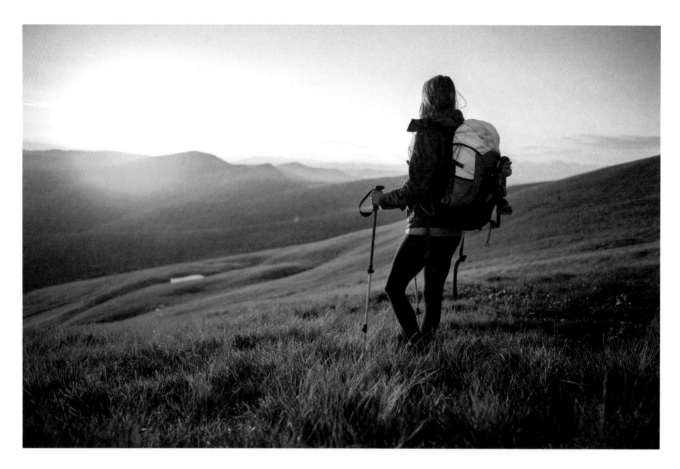

THE PLACEBO EFFECT

—

The term placebo comes from the Latin words "I will please" and refers to an inactive medication that is given in place of a working medication. The person receiving the placebo does not know it is inactive, but because they expect the drug or medication to work, sometimes they feel better after taking it. Clinical drug trials often include a placebo, so they can test the true effectiveness of actual treatments. In randomized double-blind research studies, neither the patients nor the researchers know which are the real treatments and which are the placebos, helping to rule out any element of bias.

The placebo effect highlights the true natural healing power of the body and especially the important part the mind plays in certain aspects of health, wellbeing, and healing.

THE EFFECT OF STRESS

—

Stress describes the feelings you have when the demands made on you, or that you feel

are being made, are more than you are able to fully cope with. Stress can affect all ages and is a normal reaction to pressure. It can be caused by external stressors, such as pressure from work, life experiences, family, or finances; or internal stressors, such as thoughts and feelings of inadequacy, uncertainty, or low self-esteem.

Sometimes the effect of stress can be positive, for example if it acts as encouragement or motivation to get on with the task in hand. This is because stress is a physical response, causing your body to move into the fight or flight mode. As it does so, the body releases a mix of hormones and chemicals, such as adrenaline, cortisol, and norepinephrine, that prepare your body for action. That is what causes physical symptoms such as a pounding heart, a rush of energy, and fast breathing, which can prove to be exhilarating and motivational for some.

However, stress is healthy and positive only when it is short-lived. Stress becomes a problem when you experience too much

Getting back in touch with your body, and with nature, can be the first step to both a healthy body and mind.

of it, causing it to become overwhelming and resulting in both physical and mental exhaustion. Too much cortisol can also affect your immune system, making it less efficient.

Stress can cause emotional and behavioral changes. You may be plagued by feelings of anxiety, fear, anger, depression, and frustration, and lack concentration, sleep, and the ability to make decisions. In turn, a build-up of all these feelings can produce physical symptoms, such as heart palpitations, headaches, and aches and pains.

Stress can be a highly unpleasant experience, and an important part of tackling stress is to accept you have a problem. As well as identifying the root causes and making lifestyle changes, exploring ways to release your stress, relax your mind, and rebalance your body are some of the key ways of combating it.

HEALING THE MIND

EXPLORING POSSIBILITIES
—

The first step to physical and emotional wellbeing is a clear, unstressed, and positive mindset. When it comes to healing the mind, there is a wealth of possibilities to explore, from meditation and mindfulness, to art and music, talking and ecotherapy. Some therapies can easily be practiced on your own, while others are best carried out in classes or on a one-to-one basis with a professional therapist, but they all share the common goal of helping to harness the healing power of your mind. Many of the therapies can be successfully combined, offering an even better boost to your mental and physical wellbeing. If troubling or negative thoughts and feelings are overwhelming or affecting your ability to live your daily life, consult with your healthcare provider about next steps.

PRAYER AND BREATHING
—

Sitting quietly to say a prayer can ease the mind. You may choose to pray for yourself or for others, or to focus on being thankful for all the good things in your life. You do not need to be religious to give thanks, and it is a technique that you can try at any time, on your own or in a group.

Controlled breathing techniques can help you relax and manage stress. Diaphragmatic breathing helps you learn how to breathe slowly and deeply from your abdomen and is particularly useful for dealing with panic attacks. Even if you think you breathe properly already, trying a specialist class can be an eye-opener into your normal breathing habits.

To get a taster of the technique, lie flat on your back, with your knees bent and your head on a pillow. Place a hand on your upper chest and the other just below your ribcage. Slowly breathe in through your nose so your stomach moves out against your lower hand. Now tighten your stomach muscles as you exhale through pursed lips. Throughout your inhalation and exhalation, the hand on your chest should remain as still as possible.

MEDITATION AND MINDFULNESS
—

Practicing meditation involves learning to clear your mind, so it becomes silent and you reach a sense of peace. Meditation helps the mind become free of random thoughts and feelings. Even a few minutes of meditation a day can be beneficial for relieving stress. Meditation is accessible to anyone and you can try it out at any time, anywhere, or join an organized group. If you find it hard to clear the chatter in your head, try focusing on the flame of a burning candle.

In contrast to meditation, where the emphasis is usually on clearing your mind, mindfulness focuses on giving full attention to the present moment. The idea is to focus on and be aware of "now," while acknowledging and accepting the feelings and thoughts in your body and mind. Doing so allows you to reconnect with sights, sounds, tastes, and smells, as well as how you feel, without

Pranayama is a yoga breathing technique. Shut your eyes. Close your right nostril with the right thumb and inhale through the left nostril. Remove your thumb. Use your fourth and middle fingers to close your left nostril. Exhale slowly and completely.

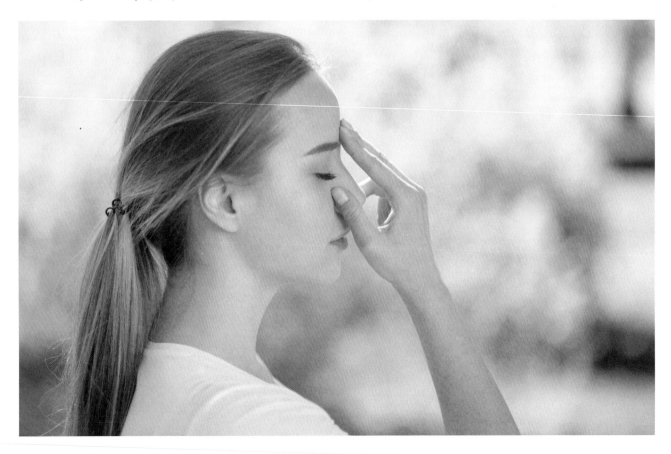

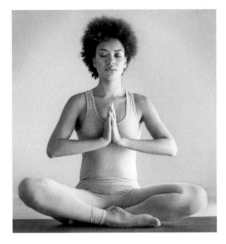

Meditation helps to calm mental chatter and may leave the body better able to cope with illness and physical stresses.

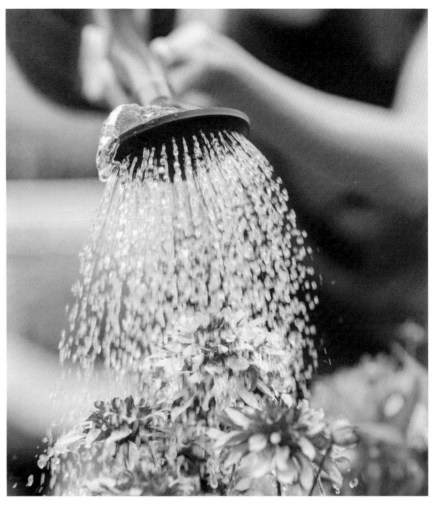

judging yourself. It encourages calm and awareness, so you can learn to manage negative thoughts and the effect they have on you. Research has found that mindfulness can help manage mild depression, anxiety, and other mental health problems.

BIOFEEDBACK

—

Biofeedback is a form of noninvasive therapy that helps to promote relaxation. A series of electrodes are attached to your skin and send signals to a monitor via a biofeedback device. Beeps, flashes, and images appear on the monitor, giving details on your heart rate, breathing, blood pressure, muscle activity, and temperature.

As your heart rate and other bodily functions change when you are under stress, you can see them as they happen and then get feedback to learn to control them better yourself. Other mind–body healing methods can be combined with biofeedback to help improve relaxation, such as mindfulness and deep breathing.

TALKING THERAPIES AND PSYCHOTHERAPY

—

There is a lot to be gained from talking to someone else and getting a different perspective on life and problems. A range of different talking therapies can be used to help you understand your behavior and feelings, and learn how to cope better with overwhelming emotions, difficult life events, and traumatic experiences.

Psychotherapy is one form of talking therapy that can be used to help you identify problems, habits, and worries, and devise ways to find solutions. As well as talking, psychotherapy sometimes combines the use of art, music, or drama too, all with the help of a professional therapist.

ART AND MUSIC THERAPIES

—

Art, music, dance, and drama therapies are often recommended or provided by psychotherapists and counselors. It can sometimes be hard to express your feelings, especially if you are confused about them yourself, so these therapies allow you to go beyond words to express how you feel and what you are going through.

One of the benefits of these therapies is that you do not need any prior experience or artistic skills. The key aim is to be guided to create something, such as a play, dance routine, piece of music, or

Gardening is an age-old form of ecotherapy.

painting, to express yourself in a way you feel comfortable with. Arts therapies can be physically relaxing and open up another outlet for mind–body healing.

ECOTHERAPY

—

Ecotherapy is a relatively new term in treatment programs, but the idea behind it is by no means new. Ecotherapy means using outdoor activities involving nature to help heal your mind and boost your mental and physical wellbeing. Ecotherapy can include activities like gardening, taking exercise outside, getting involved with a conservation project, helping with animals on a farm or refuge, or cycling through woodland. Research into ecotherapy shows that it can help with mild to moderate depression, and reduce anger and low self-esteem. It also offers the chance to connect with nature, other people, and improve your mood.

STARTING WITH THE BODY

EXERCISE
—

Looking after your body and your physical health is essential, both for reducing the risks of numerous health issues and for maintaining and improving your mental health. Ensuring you have regular sessions of physical activity is one crucial aspect of looking after your body. Exercise and activity is something that should be incorporated into your daily life and there are different benefits to be gained from different types of activity.

Health guidelines in the U.S.A. suggest that all adults should avoid inactivity: even some activity is far better than having none at all, and can trigger health benefits. To gain substantial benefits, aim for at least 150 minutes (2 hours and 30 minutes) of moderate-intensity exercise per week, or 75 minutes (1 hour and 15 minutes) of vigorous-intensity aerobic activity. Ideally, any aerobic exercise should be carried out in chunks of at least 10 minutes and spread throughout the week.

If you are looking to gain more extensive health benefits from exercise, then aim to increase your aerobic physical activity to 300 minutes (5 hours) a week of moderate-intensity exercise. Or aim for 150 minutes (2 hours 30 minutes) of vigorous-intensity exercise each week.

Good examples of moderate-intensity aerobic activity include brisk walking, skipping, cycling, or playing basketball. Good options for vigorous-intensity exercise include running, fast swimming, and doing jumping jacks.

In addition, bear in mind that a mix of different exercises is beneficial, to help look after different parts of your body. For example, combine digging in the gardening with cycling. Muscle-strengthening exercises, such as lifting weights, using resistance bands, yoga, or doing sit-ups are ideal and work well when performed at least two days per week.

EXERCISE THAT IS RIGHT FOR YOU
—

If it has been a while since you were last involved in regular exercise, or you are looking to try something new, find some beginners classes or exercise sessions to try out. There are numerous different types of exercise available, so there should be something that appeals to you, from dance classes or a tennis club to Sunday hiking groups. Sports centers and gyms often run taster classes, so you can see if you like an activity before you sign up. Even if finances are tight, exercising need not be expensive. Activities such as walking and running are easily accessible and relatively inexpensive, as long as you have supportive, good-quality footwear.

If you are nervous about exercising after a break away from it, try asking a friend to join you. Having a buddy to exercise with can help boost your motivation and staying power.

If you have been inactive for a while, or have existing health conditions, talk to your health practitioner first, before embarking on a new exercise regime. They will be able to tell you if it is suitable for your needs and advise on how much exercise to start with.

When you do start, take things slowly and gradually increase the amount of exercise you do over time. Do not push yourself to do more than you can manage, as you could end up straining your muscles and doing more harm than good. If you are attending an exercise class or going to the gym, follow the guidance of your trainer.

YOGA
—

Yoga is a great form of exercise for strengthening your muscles and improving flexibility. A series of yoga postures work on all the key areas of the body and, combined with breathing techniques, yoga can boost general physical and mental wellbeing. As a gentle form of exercise, yoga is suitable for all ages. Even if you are not currently feeling flexible, it can help loosen up your body and improve the range of your movements.

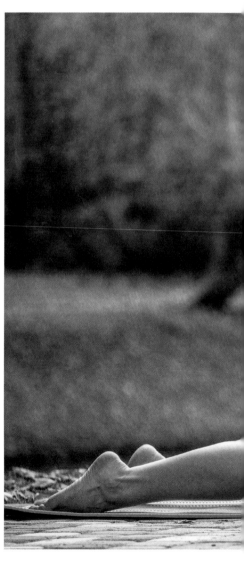

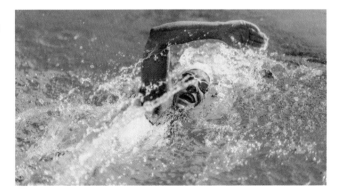

Swimming is a form of aerobic exercise, to improve the health of your heart and tone your muscles.

There are various different styles of yoga, such as Hatha, Ashtanga, Bikram, Iyengar and Vinyasa, and some are more vigorous and intense than others. Hatha yoga is a good starting point for learning the postural moves and breathing, as it is slow and gentle for beginners.

PILATES

—

Pilates exercise focuses on developing core strength to improve overall fitness and wellbeing and restore balance in the body. It is a low-impact, muscle-strengthening activity and, like yoga, it recognizes the connection between physical and mental health. Pilates is suitable for all ages and fitness abilities, making it a good form of exercise to try if you are getting back into more regular physical activity or want to improve movement and flexibility.

Unlike yoga, Pilates sometimes involves the use of apparatus or equipment, such as balls or elastic resistance bands. Exercises involve the whole body, targeting specific muscle groups, and performing the exercises can help correct issues such as poor posture that have previously led to pain and movement difficulties.

MASSAGE

—

Massage techniques have been used for thousands of years and can be very effective for easing stress, releasing pressure, boosting circulation, and generally improving physical and mental wellbeing. The skin is your body's largest sensory organ and as it is touched by the hands of a skilled masseuse, endorphins – the body's natural painkillers and "feel good" chemicals – are released (endorphins are also released when you exercise).

Massage should not be used as an alternative to exercise, but it is very effective used alongside it and especially after physical activity. Massage can help improve muscle flexibility and ease stiff joints.

There are various types of massage, including Swedish, Thai, deep tissue, hot stone, and special pregnancy massage. The standard type offered in most clinics, gyms, and spas is Swedish massage. Swedish massage is based on Western concepts of anatomy. Using lotion or oil, massage therapists typically begin with broad general strokes and then move on to address problem areas.

Yoga is a safe way to increase strength, flexibility, and balance. Regular yoga practice may be beneficial for people with high blood pressure, heart disease, lower back pain, depression, and stress.

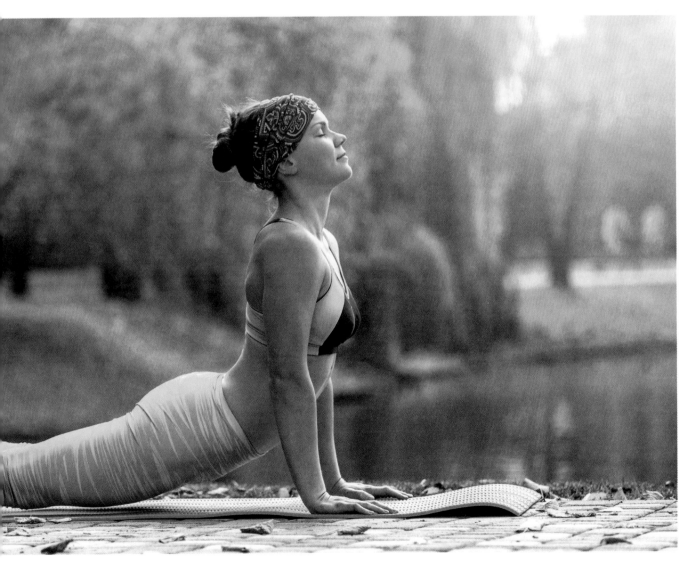

HEALING
REMEDIES

CHAPTER TWO

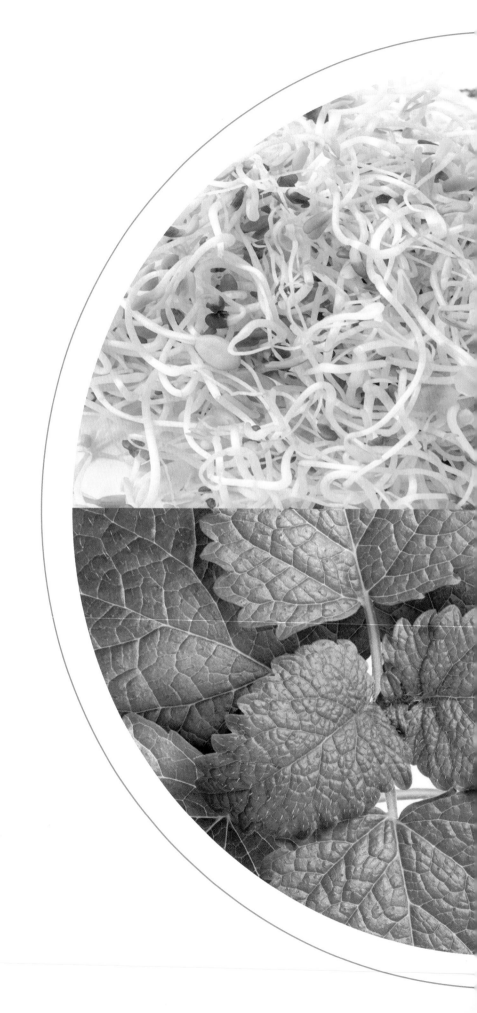

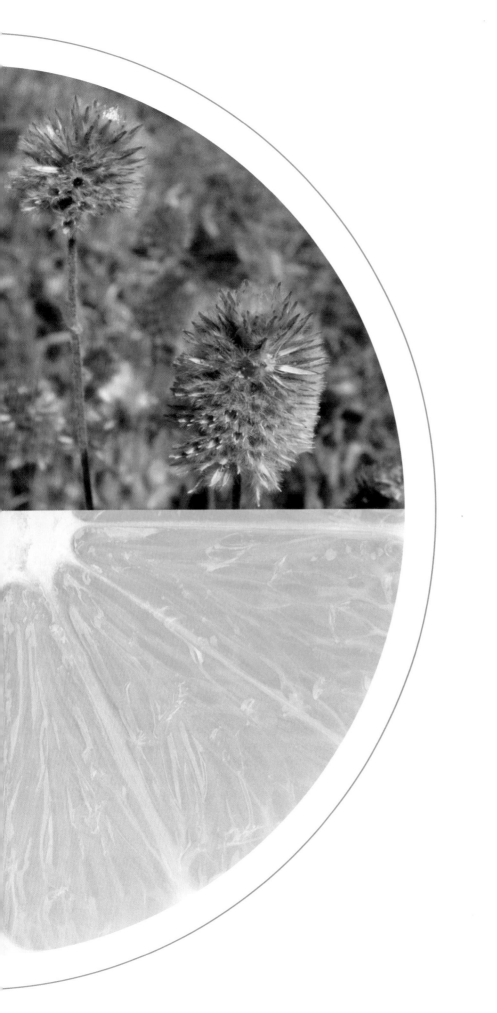

Acanthopanax gracilistylus
WU JIA PI

In Chinese herbal medicine, this herb is used to dispel wind dampness from the muscles, joints, and bones. Wind dampness causes rheumatic and arthritic ailments. Wu Jia Pi also treats damp cold conditions where the circulation is obstructed, as in the swelling of the legs or stiff knee joints.

DATA FILE

Properties
• Acrid • Warm

Uses
• Use for chronic wind cold damp painful obstruction (bi syndrome) when deficiency of the liver and kidneys causes weak sinews and bones.
• Helps to reduce water retention.

Notes and Dosages
Wu Jia Pi is a warm drying (acrid) herb that tonifies the liver and kidneys. These meridians decline as we get older, so the herb is especially helpful in treating rheumatism, arthritis, or stiffness in the elderly, as well as in those suffering from long-term illness. Wu Jia Pi is particularly helpful when the smooth flow of qi and blood is obstructed. It is also used for difficulties with urination and edema. The dried herb, or a decoction, can be taken in wine.

> **CAUTION**
> Use with caution in yin deficiency with heat signs, as it dries and heats further.

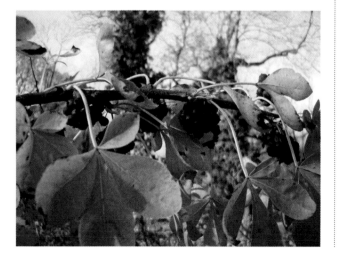

Achillea millefolium
YARROW

In Ayurveda, yarrow is called "gandana" and is believed to reduce pitta and kapha, and to increase vátha with its cooling, drying properties. It is used as a "heal-all" to balance emotional upsets and as an addition to treatments during the menopause.

DATA FILE

Properties
• Bitter • Pungent • Astringent • Cooling • Drying • Causes sweating
• Antispasmodic • Anti-inflammatory • Antiseptic • Tonic

Uses
• Use in the early stages of fevers, especially with hot, dry skin.
• Take for catarrh, sinusitis, hay fever, and dust allergies.
• For high blood pressure, take with hawthorn and linden.
• Take with a little ginger for cold feet.
• Supportive for people undergoing radiotherapy and intestinal infections.
• Use for diarrhea, colic, ulcers, and weak digestion.
• Take for irregular menstrual bleeding, cramps, and vaginal discharges.
• Take with sage and marigold for pelvic infections and pelvic congestion with menstrual cramps, and pain before menstruation.
• Wash the fresh root and chew for toothache.
• Press fresh leaves and flower tops into cuts to stop bleeding.
• Use as a cream or compress for bleeding piles.
• Apply the infused oil to inflammations associated with varicose veins.

Notes and Dosages
Yarrow is a common wild plant with feathery leaves and white or pink flowers. Gather yarrow in early summer, when it is in flower. The leaves, stalks, flowers, and fruits may all be used. It can be taken internally, as a tea, or externally, in the form of skin patches, lotion, in the bath, as a compress, or as massage oil. Use standard doses (see pages 39 and 41).

To make tea, steep 2 teaspoons of the dried herb in a cup of boiling water for about 10 minutes. Add honey to taste, and drink warm. The tea is excellent, on its own, for all feverish conditions, menstrual cramps, and hot flushes, and can be mixed with other herbs, such as elderflower and peppermint, to treat colds and flu.

RECIPE

Yarrow Soothing Bath
For a bath to ease aches and pains, simmer a handful of fresh leaves in 1pt. (500ml.) of water for 15 minutes. Strain and add to your bath water.

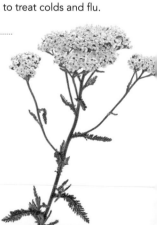

Acorus calamus

CALAMUS ROOT

Also known in the West as sweet flag or myrtle flag, this rhizome is a reddish, hairy root, used throughout Asia for its medicinal properties. Known in Ayurveda as "vacha," which means speech in Sanskrit, the root is used as a brain tonic and to improve the capacity for speech.

DATA FILE

Properties
• Pungent • Bitter • Astringent • Stimulant • Decongestant • Expectorant • Emetic • Bronchio-dilator • Increases circulation to the brain

Uses
• Use as a heating/drying agent to warm vátha and decrease kapha states.
• Take to strengthen the adrenals, improve muscle tissue, help arthritis and circulation, and in periods of weakness.
• Take for gingivitis (gum disease).
• Massage with calamus oil to stimulate lymphatic drainage.
• Use for coughs and nagging sinus headaches.

Notes and Dosages
As well as taking the root internally in powdered form (see Exam Rescue, below), it can be taken externally in a compress or as massage oil. Calamus mixes well with ginger, yarrow, lemon, orange, cinnamon, and also with cedar. Yarrow leaves can be used on a cut until you get the chance to clean it at home.

RECIPE

Exam Rescue
This simple formula is believed to boost your brain power, while reducing mental stress and overstimulation. It could be a great help at exam time! Mix ¼ of a teaspoon of the powdered root with a ½ teaspoon of honey. Take internally every morning and evening.

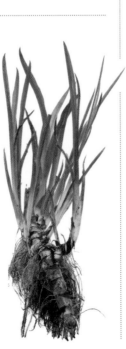

> **CAUTION**
> Calamus can cause bleeding disorders, such as nosebleeds and hemorrhoids, if used in excess. Use only the recommended dose. It can also have a very strong and long-lasting odor. It may be appropriate to use it in conjunction with rosemary, lavender, or a sweet-smelling herb.

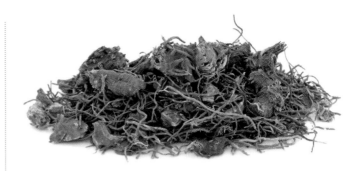

Actaea racemosa, Cimicifuga racemosa

CIMIC.

This homeopathic remedy is obtained from the root of black cohosh, also known as bugbane, black snakeroot, and rattleroot. Black cohosh was used by Native Americans to cure rattlesnake bites, and for rheumatism and gynecological problems.

DATA FILE

Properties
• Sedative • Soothing

Uses
• Eases intense emotions and fears.
• Helps cramps and backache when premenstrual.
• May help with depression after childbirth.
• May help with faints and flushes during menopause.

Notes and Dosages
In homeopathy, Cimic. is believed to be well-suited to many female complaints, and can be helpful for women who are restless and highly strung. It works well on the nerves and muscles of the uterus, making it useful for menstrual problems such as back cramps and headaches; and postnatal depression and menopausal problems, such as hot flushes. The upheaval in emotions associated with these problems, such as anxiety and irritability, can also be relieved.

> **CAUTION**
> Take advice from a qualified medical practitioner before taking black cohosh for an extended period.

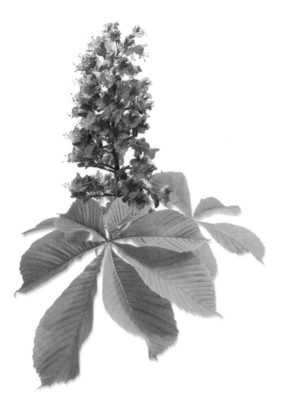

Aesculus carnea

RED CHESTNUT

This flower essence is extracted from the pink-flowered chestnut tree, which is frequently grown for ornamental decoration in parks.

DATA FILE

Properties
• Calming • Encourages rationality

Uses
• Useful for those who suffer intense and ceaseless fear and anxiety for loved-ones, often thinking that some unfortunate "worst case scenario" will occur.
• May help those whose level of anxiety is limiting the social interactions of both the sufferer and his or her loved-ones.
• Those who benefit from red chestnut may have forsaken worrying about themselves, but project their fear onto their loved-ones.
• Red chestnut brings the calm necessary to be sensitive to the real problems and concerns of our loved-ones, and to give empathetic support.

Notes and Dosages
Use the boiling method to prepare this flower remedy, as described on page 57. If harvesting for yourself, look for the red chestnut tree's distinctive bright pink flowers.

Aesculus hippocastanum

HORSE CHESTNUT

The common horse chestnut tree has distinctive, upright clusters of white flowers and divided spatulate leaves. It is used to make two flower remedies: white chestnut and chestnut bud.

DATA FILE

Properties
• Increases clarity • Calming

Uses
• White chestnut switches off unwanted thoughts and persistent mental chatter so that it is possible to find peace and clarity. It may help sleeplessness due to worry.
• Chestnut bud is for those who make the same mistake over and over again. It may help those who regretfully do not seem able to learn the lessons of past experience, events, and relationships. The sufferer may also have poor health, chronic conditions, or preventable illness. Chestnut bud helps focus the mind and enables us to see our path with greater objectivity.

Notes and Dosages
To make the white chestnut flower remedy, use the sun method (see page 56) to prepare the leaves and flowers of the horse chestnut.

For chestnut bud, pick the large leaf buds, called "sticky buds," when they are just about to open in early spring. Use the boiling method (see page 57) to prepare the essence.

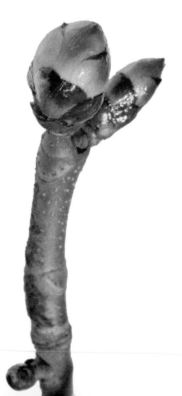

Agastache rugosa

HUO XIANG

Also known as wrinkled giant hyssop, in Chinese traditional medicine this herb transforms dampness, which creates stagnation in the middle burner (spleen and stomach), with digestive or fluid-retaining effects.

DATA FILE

Properties
• Acrid • Slightly warm

Uses
• Use for stuck digestion, leading to bloating either above or below the navel, nausea, fatigue, lack of appetite, and a moist white coating on the tongue.
• Harmonizes the middle burner and stops vomiting. May be useful for gastric flu.

Notes and Dosages
Huo Xiang comes from wrinkled giant hyssop, a summer-flowering perennial. The herb is the main herb in the patent formula Huo Xiang Zheng Qi Wan, which is used for gastric flu.

> **CAUTION**
> No herbs used for getting rid of damp (shown by a thick tongue coating or by the presence of phlegm) may be used in deficient yin with heat signs (shown by a peeled tongue): they will further dry the patient and make the condition worse.

Agrimonia eupatoria

AGRIMONY

A common wild plant with slender spikes of bright yellow flowers, agrimony is used both in herbalism and as a flower remedy. The seed vessels are covered in hooked hairs and cling to animals coming into contact with them.

DATA FILE

Properties
• Astringent • Tonic • Encourages self-acceptance

Uses
• Use as a tea or tincture for indigestion, heartburn, diarrhea, long-term food allergies and liverish feelings.
• Use with St. John's wort and horsetail for bedwetting and chronic cystitis.
• Apply as a lotion for the cleansing of wounds.
• Use as an eyewash for sore and inflamed eyes.
• The agrimony flower remedy may be useful for those who hide their problems behind a cheerful face and laughter. They may be reluctant to burden others and dread arguments, pursuing peace at all costs. This can lead to an inner anguish that is masked by alcohol or drugs.

Notes and Dosages
When preparing a herbal tea, tonic, tincture, lotion or eyewash, the whole herb is used. Follow the instructions and standard doses on pages 39 and 41.

To prepare the flower remedy, use the sun method (see page 56).

RECIPE

Agrimony Digestive Tonic
Combine equal parts of agrimony, raspberry leaf, and lemon balm. Store away from the light.
Make a tea from 1 teaspoon of the mixture to 1 cup of boiling water. Drink freely for colicky pains with looseness and nervous diarrhea.

> **CAUTION**
> If taken internally, agrimony may aggravate constipation.

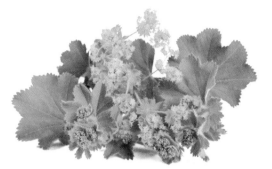

Alchemilla vulgaris
LADY'S MANTLE

A wild plant of wayside and meadows, lady's mantle also grows well in shady gardens, and bears sprays of greenish-yellow flowers.

DATA FILE

Properties
• Astringent • Tones and strengthens the womb

Uses
• Use for heavy menstrual bleeding, either alone or with an equal part of shepherd's purse or yarrow. Also for bleeding in the middle of the menstrual cycle and for irregular menstruation.
• To prevent menstrual cramps and for PMS, take during the second half of the menstrual cycle.
• For thrush and other vaginal discharges, take as a tea or douche.
• Traditional treatment for infertility in women with no obvious cause.
• For children's diarrhea.

> **CAUTION**
> Do not use in pregnancy except under professional guidance. Always seek medical advice for bleeding in mid-menstrual cycle.

Notes and Dosages
The whole herb should be gathered when the plant is in flower. Use standard herbalism doses (see page 39). Lady's mantle makes a pleasant drinking tea.

RECIPE

Lady's Mantle and Chamomile Wash
For a soothing wash for itchy genitals, in men and women, make a strong tea with 1 cup of boiling water to 1 teaspoon of lady's mantle and 2 teaspoons of chamomile flowers. Infuse in a covered vessel for 15 minutes.

Allium cepa
ONION

Onion is one of the oldest known medicinal plants. Ayurvedic practitioners, who call onion "dungri," believe that onion stimulates the production of saliva and digestive juices, as well as the flow of tears! Onions have also long been considered the mainstay of every household remedy chest.

DATA FILE

Properties
• Pungent • Heating • Drying • Stimulates circulation • Expectorant • Antispasmodic • Rejuvenating • Antibiotic • Diuretic

Uses
• Apply fresh onion to an abscessed tooth or a boil to draw out infection and encourage circulation to the area.
• Mix onion juice with honey to relieve the symptoms of a cold.
• Onion poultices are used to treat bronchitis.
• Onions are often recommended for gastric infections: onions will be effective cooked and raw.
• Place slices of raw onion on burned skin, bites, stings, bruises, and unbroken chilblains, or apply a homemade lotion of onion juice mixed with salt.
• Eat for joint problems, arthritis, and fluid retention.
• Cleanses the intestines and helps to maintain the balance of bacteria.
• For an antibiotic treatment, peel and eat (raw or cooked) one-quarter of one sweet white onion, two to four times a day.
• Eat daily if you are at risk of heart disease or circulatory disorders.
• In Ayurveda, onion reduces kapha and vátha, and increases pitta.

Notes and Dosages
If growing your own, ripe onions can be harvested 22 weeks after sowing. Onion is used both in its green stage as a scallion, or green onion, and in its mature stage as a bulb – the tightly packed globe of food-storage leaves containing the volatile oil that is the source of the onion's pungent flavor. The bulb can be used externally or peeled and eaten raw, cooked, powdered, juiced, taken as a tea, decoction, infusion, and as an oil. Onion combines well with ginger, black pepper, cumin, coriander, and eucalyptus. In homeopathy, the Allium remedy is often used to treat earache and toothache in children, as well as the acute symptoms of a cold and related headaches.

> **CAUTION**
> Nursing mothers beware: onion in your breast milk may cause colic in your infant. Some people have allergies to onion and may develop a skin rash. If one appears, discontinue use. Consult a physician before consuming large quantities of onion for medicinal purposes.

Allium sativum

GARLIC

Known as "lashuna" in Ayurveda, garlic belongs to the onion family and is one of the most-used medicinal plants. It has a strong odor, which many people find off-putting, but its health-giving and preventive properties make it well worth suffering the effects. Effective herbal preparations of garlic can be used at less cost and with fewer side-effects than most pharmaceutical drugs, and its use has been applauded by the conventional medical establishment.

DATA FILE

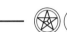

Properties
• Pungent • Heating • Drying • Stimulant • Expectorant • Antiseptic
• Antibiotic • Antifungal • Antispasmodic • Antioxidant
• Rejuvenating • Lowers blood pressure and cholesterol

Uses
• Garlic has been shown to lower total serum cholesterol as well as LDL cholesterol in human clinical trials. It may help to prevent high blood pressure and heart disease, and reduce the risk of atherosclerosis.
• Garlic juice can be used to treat infected wounds and infections of the stomach, as well as intestinal worms.
• Fresh garlic, eaten daily, can reduce chronic acidity of the stomach.
• Garlic syrup can be used to treat bronchitis, lung infections, asthma, flu, colds, and ear infections. Can be combined with echinacea.
• To obtain antibiotic effects, 6–12 cloves of garlic a day are recommended. Peel and chew three cloves of garlic at a time, two to four times a day.
• Garlic helps to boost the immune system.
• Helps to bring down fever.
• May be beneficial to diabetics and cancer patients.
• Garlic-infused oil can be used as a chest rub for respiratory ailments, or in the ear to reduce inflammation.
• Fresh garlic juice is antifungal, and can be applied neat to infections such as athlete's foot.
• In Ayurveda, garlic reduces kapha and vátha, and increases pitta.

CAUTION
Nursing mothers should be aware that garlic in breast milk may cause colic in your infant. Some people have allergies to garlic and may develop a skin rash. If one appears, discontinue garlic use. Consult a physician before consuming large quantities of garlic for medicinal purposes.

Notes and Dosages
Grow your own garlic by planting individual cloves in the fall. Garlic can be harvested about six to eight months after planting, in the summer. Bulbs not needed immediately can be dried in the sun and stored. Garlic cloves can be chewed, cooked, powdered, taken as a tea, decoction, infusion, in food, and as an infused oil. Garlic can be taken with other herbs, such as ginger, black pepper, cumin, coriander, eucalyptus. The smell of garlic on the breath can be reduced by eating an apple, drinking a little fresh lemon juice, or eating fresh parsley. Enteric-coated tablets are available. These are easier on the digestion.

RECIPES

Garlic Syrup
Garlic syrup boosts the immune system and relieves bronchitis and lung infections. Peel and chop 6–8 cloves of fresh garlic. Place the chopped garlic in a jar, and cover with 8 tablespoons of honey. Let it stand for several days, and then strain. The garlic-infused honey can be given by the teaspoonful (1 for children, 4 for adults).

Garlic or Onion Milk
Onion or garlic milk is an ideal respiratory disinfectant, and works well for fevers and croups, in infants and small children. Put 1 onion or 3 cloves of garlic, thinly sliced, into a pan with 2 cups of milk (cow's, goat's, sheep's, soy, or nut milk). Simmer over a very low heat for 20 minutes, then strain. The milk can be stored in a refrigerator for 2 or 3 days.

Infants can take 1 or 2 dessertspoons every four hours. Young children can drink freely if feverish and croupy.

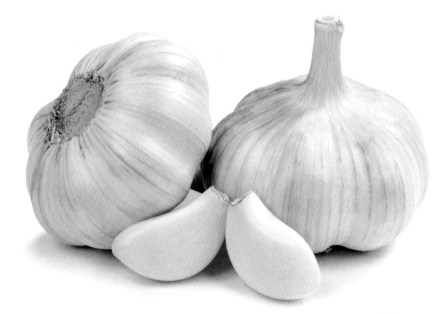

Aloe vera

ALOE VERA

Known as "kumara" in Ayurveda, aloe is a succulent, tropical plant that is often grown as a houseplant. Its fame as a treatment for burns and scalds goes back to Alexander the Great, who used an island off Somalia for the sole purpose of obtaining the "amazing wound-healing" plant. Another part of the aloe – the latex – is a powerful laxative, and is obtained in fresh aloe juice.

DATA FILE

Properties
• Soothing • Cooling • Antiseptic • Antifungal • Astringent

Uses
• Apply to burns and sunburn, ringworm, infected cuts, acne, shingles, eczema, wrinkles, and areas of dry, itchy skin.
• Use as a mouthwash for sore gums.
• Apply the gel directly to the outer eyelid for conjunctivitis.
• Can be used as an internal medicine for candidiasis (thrush).
• Aloe vera works on the thyroid, the pituitary gland, and the ovaries.
• For cosmetic purposes, the gel can give skin a healthy glow – but use only the fresh gel.
• In Ayurveda, aloe alleviates all three doshas, and specifically reduces pitta (cooling pitta rashes, burns, and ulcers).

Notes and Dosages
Aloes are easily grown as a houseplant, requiring sunlight and a minimum temperature of 50°F (10°C). The leaf, gel, and juice are used. Drink aloe juice for internal conditions, and apply the gel externally. Cut the leaf and apply the gel directly to the skin, or take 1 tablespoon, twice daily, as an internal medicine. The cut leaves will keep in the freezer and can be used again. There are many excellent preparations of aloe in the stores – follow the instructions on the packet. Barberry, cinnamon, cloves, licorice, and St. John's wort can all be used with aloe vera.

RECIPES

Aloe Gel
Wash the leaves. Cut into 2in. (5cm.) lengths. Slice each piece in half, to expose the largest amount of gel. Wrap each piece in plastic wrap and date.

To use, remove plastic and apply the gel side of the leaf to the skin: smear over the affected area, or hold in place with a bandage.

Aloe Oil
Cover the leaves with any vegetable oil. Allow the mixture to soak for 60 days, then strain. Keep the oil in a dark glass container. Label the container, as the scent is subtle and will not be easy to identify. The oil will keep indefinitely.

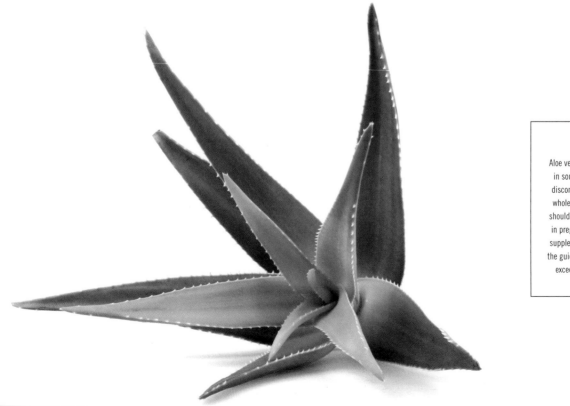

> **CAUTION**
> Aloe vera gel can cause skin irritation in some people. If irritation occurs, discontinue use. Preparations of the whole leaf are strongly laxative and should not be used for long periods or in pregnancy. If you use aloe juice or supplements as a laxative, use under the guidance of a physician, and never exceed the recommended dosage.

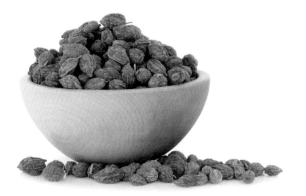

Alpinia oxyphylla
YI ZHI REN

In Chinese medicine, this herb warms internal cold. Yi Zhi Ren is a cardamom, and all cardamoms warm the middle area. It is good for urinary incontinence or frequency and enuresis (bed-wetting) from cold-deficient spleen and kidneys.

DATA FILE

Properties
• Acrid • Warm

Uses
• Warms the kidneys, firms the jing-essence and holds in urine: this herb is used when the yang aspect of the kidneys is deficient and cannot hold urine in place. It is also helpful in spermatorrhea, when men cannot hold the sperm or when it leaks out.
• Warms the spleen and helps stop diarrhea and other digestive symptoms.
• Helps to stop drooling.
• Warms the system, from infancy to old age.

Notes and Dosages
Yi Zhi Ren is the seed pod of *Alpinia oxyphylla*, an evergreen perennial.

> **CAUTION**
> Although useful for cases where symptoms are improved by warmth to the middle section, this herb is not to be used when spermatorrhea, frequent urination, or vaginal discharge are caused by heat.

Althea officinalis
MARSHMALLOW

Marshmallow is a wild plant easily grown in gardens. It reaches up to 4ft. (1.5m.) tall, with pale pink flowers. Its name comes from the Greek word *altho*, meaning "to cure."

DATA FILE

Properties
• Soothing • Mucilaginous

Uses
• Use for acid stomach, heartburn, ulcers, hiatus hernia, and irritable bowel.
• Helps nonproductive and dry coughs.
• Take for an irritable bladder.
• For cases of dry skin, take as a tea.
• For insect bites and weeping eczema, make a paste of powdered root mixed into a cream or added to water.

Notes and Dosages
Marshmallow leaves and root are used. Both have a high mucilage (a glutinous substance) content. This herb can be taken freely. To make a tea, for best results soak 1oz. (25g.) cut root or leaf in 1pt. (500ml.) cold water overnight. Strain and drink 3 cups daily.

RECIPE

Marshmallow Paste
This is an especially effective preparation for insect bites and stings. Take enough marshmallow root powder to cover the affected area, and add cold water to make a stiff paste.

Apply thickly and allow to dry. Wash off and replace the paste every 2 or 3 hours.

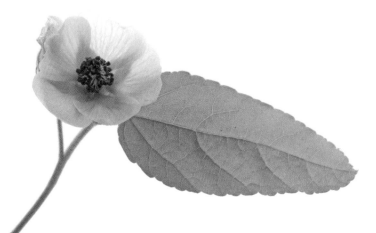

Angelica archangelica, A. glauca, A. sinensis

ANGELICA

Several angelica species are used in Ayurvedic and Chinese medicine, as well as in herbalism and aromatherapy. Ayurvedic practitioners prescribe *Angelica glauca*, also called "choraka," for menstrual problems, as well as arthritis, abdominal pains, and flu. In Chinese medicine, *Angelica sinensis*, known as Dang Gui, is used to treat patterns of blood deficiency.

DATA FILE

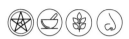

Properties
• Heating • Moisturizing • Stimulant • Expectorant
• Tonic • Antibacterial • May induce menstruation
• Diuretic • Strengthens digestion

Uses
• All these angelica species are used to treat painful menstrual cramps, PMS, and amenorrhea. Drink a cup of angelica decoction twice a day.
• These species are expectorants, which may help colds, flu, and bronchitis.
• Take as a digestive aid, helping cases of hiccups, heartburn, flatulence, and digestive problems caused by stress.
• For stomache ache, massage a few drops of blended angelica oil around the abdomen.
• In Chinese medicine, Dang Gui moistens the intestines and unblocks the bowels.
• Use Dang Gui for sores and abscesses.
• Also use these species for anemia, headaches, arthritis, rheumatism, poor circulation, adrenal excess, poor blood clotting, and poor liver function.

Notes and Dosages
The roots, leaves, and seeds may all be used, depending on the recipe. These herbs can be taken as an inhalant, as nose drops, in a vaporizer, or as a tea, tincture, or massage oil. In herbalism, the root alone is used. It should be dug up in the fall of the plant's first year, dried quickly, and stored in an airtight container. It will retain its medicinal properties for several years. Angelica root and the seeds are used to produce the essential oil, which has a musky, sweet, woody scent.

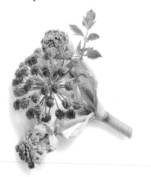

> **CAUTION**
> Do not use during pregnancy or if you are a diabetic. Do not use on skin exposed to sunlight. Fresh angelica roots are poisonous. Drying eliminates danger. Do not use with hypertension or heart disease.

Angelica dahurica

BAI ZHI

Bai Zhi belongs to a group of warm, acrid herbs that release exterior conditions: superficial illnesses caused by viruses, with symptoms in the skin or muscle layers. The herbs mainly affect the sweating mechanism, either causing the body to sweat, or if necessary stopping it from sweating.

DATA FILE

Properties
• Acrid • Warm

Uses
• A sudden headache (wind-caused), especially in the front of the head, will respond to treatment with Bai Zhi.
• Use for sinusitis and its symptoms.
• Reduces swelling and expels pus: use in the early stages of a sore in order to reduce swelling.
• Use for treating leukorrhea (vaginal discharge, especially for a white discharge) from damp cold in the lower abdominal area.
• Helps to open up the nasal passages.

Notes and Dosages
Bai Zhi works along the lung and stomach channels, expelling wind and alleviating pain. With the right combinations, this herb could be used to treat other types of headaches and discharges, in addition to those described above.

> **CAUTION**
> Contraindicated in deficient blood or deficient yin patterns because it is very drying. Use cautiously if sores have already burst.

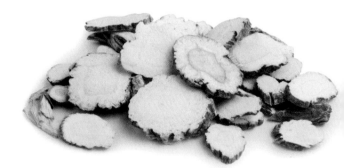

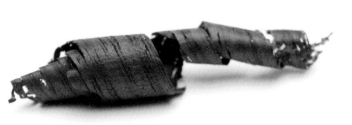

Aniba rosaeodora
ROSEWOOD

Most rosewood oil comes from Brazil. Distillation from wild trees contributes to the destruction of the rainforest, although cultivated trees are also used in the production of rosewood essential oil. For the sake of preserving the rainforests, it may be best to keep this oil for special occasions.

DATA FILE

Properties
• Tonic • Immune stimulant • Mild painkiller • Antidepressant
• Aphrodisiac • Tissue regenerator • Antiseptic • Antibacterial

Uses
• Diminishes scars, wrinkles, and stretch marks.
• Benefits sensitive or irritated skin, and suitable for acne and wounds.
• Helps coughs and headaches, especially when they are accompanied by nausea.
• Rebalances the nervous system in times of stress.

Notes and Dosages
Rosewood oil is distilled from the heartwood of the rosewood tree. It is extracted by steam distillation of the wood chippings. It has a subtle, woody, floral fragrance. It also blends well with lavender, sandalwood, frankincense, basil, patchouli, cedarwood, and most woody, citrus, and floral oils.

RECIPE

Replenishing Skin Care Oil
Pour 4 teaspoons sweet almond oil into a small, dark glass bottle. Add 4 drops rosewood, 3 drops sandalwood, and 3 drops frankincense. Seal and shake well. Smooth over face, neck, and dry skin patches, using gentle circular movements.

Anigozanthos manglesii
KANGAROO PAW

This large Australian perennial is one of the first plants to recolonize after bush fires. It is so named because the flowers at the end of the long stems resemble a kangaroo's front paw.

DATA FILE

Properties
• Encourages sensitivity and empathy • Gives courage

Uses
• Encourages sensitive and appropriate social interaction for people who have poor social skills and difficulties relating to and communicating with others.
• Gives courage to those who are so self-conscious that they feel "out of place" at work, at meetings, gatherings, or parties. This may be noticed by others and become a joke.
• Encourages kindness and empathy in those who find it impossible to find the space to think before acting, or to be aware of other people's feelings.

Notes and Dosages
Pick the whole cluster (or paw) of flowers. Use the sun method (see page 56) to prepare. The flowers of kangaroo paw are a more recent addition to the list of available flower remedies.

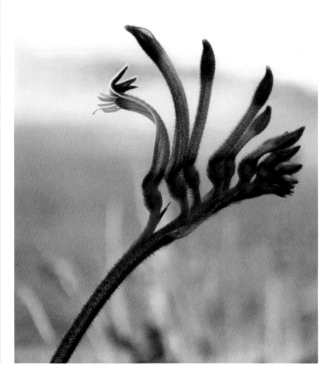

Apium graveolens
CELERY

Ayurvedic practitioners prescribe celery seed, called "ajwan," to reduce high vátha states: indigestion, nervous stomach, and ungrounded emotions. In aromatherapy, celery seed oil can be used to counteract jet lag and exposure to smog and toxic environments. Many folk remedies involve the whole plant.

DATA FILE

Properties
- Heating • Moisturizing • Diuretic • Encourages menstruation
- Sedative • Expectorant • Antispasmodic

Uses
- Take seeds as a diuretic to reduce fluid retention.
- Seeds may help with premenstrual syndrome and irregular menstruation.
- Drink celery seed tea before bed to lessen the risk of insomnia.
- Seeds help colds, coughs, sinus congestion, respiratory infections, bronchitis, and laryngitis.
- The seeds or stems can ease arthritis, gout, and rheumatic disorders.
- Grated, raw celery stems can be used as a poultice to apply to swollen glands.
- Raw, whole celery can be eaten regularly to reduce high blood pressure, and to act as a tonic for the liver.
- Celery juice or an infusion of celery seeds may be drunk to alleviate sciatica.
- Drink celery juice before meals to suppress the appetite.
- Chew celery seeds after a meal as a digestive.
- In Ayurveda, celery seed reduces kapha and vátha, and increases pitta.

Notes and Dosages
The juice, stems, leaves, and seeds of the plant may all be used, depending on the recipe. The seeds may be taken as a food, a tea or infusion, a steam, a powder, massage oil, or a gargle. Celery seeds combine with basil, black pepper, camphor, eucalyptus, and sandalwood. The seeds are rich in iron and many vitamins, including A, B, and C. Celery stems are best eaten raw, and the juice is particularly useful.

Celery seed aromatherapy oil blends well with lemon, peppermint, juniper, fennel, lavender, bergamot, pine, tea tree, cinnamon, and other spice oils. For a detoxifying massage blend, add 4 drops celery, 3 drops juniper, and 3 drops lemon to 4 teaspoons (20ml.) of grapeseed oil.

RECIPES

Celery Seed Infusion
For a mildly diuretic infusion, or to bring on menstruation, crush 1½ teaspoons of celery seeds. Add 1 cup of boiling water. Cover and let steep for 15–20 minutes. You may drink up to 3 cups of the infusion a day.

Celery Tonic
Celery seeds can be used to make a tonic that benefits the kidneys. Steep 2 tablespoons of bruised celery seeds in 1pt. (500ml.) of brandy. Take 1 tablespoon of the infused brandy, mixed with 2 tablespoons of water, three times daily.

CAUTION
Pregnant women should not use celery seed oil, take celery seed, or eat large quantities of celery. Do not give celery seed to children under two years old. If you are experiencing a stomach upset or diarrhea while taking celery seed, discontinue use. Drink extra water when taking this herb.

Arctium lappa, Arctium minus
BURDOCK

This common wayside plant has large wavy leaves and round beads of purple flowers. The root is commonly used.

DATA FILE

Properties
• Blood cleanser • Alterative • Diuretic • Lymphatic cleanser

Uses
• Take for "eruptive" and stubborn skin conditions, especially when hot and inflamed-looking: acne, spots, boils, rashes, and psoriasis.
• For eczema, combine with yellow dock and sarsaparilla.
• Take with dandelion root for skin and liver problems.
• Helps rheumatism and gout.
• Alleviates chronic cystitis.
• May help with loss of appetite.

Notes and Dosages
Take 2 teaspoons of dried root, decocted, daily, or 1 teaspoon of the tincture twice daily for some months. For lack of appetite, take the tincture 3 times daily, before meals, in a little water or fruit juice, 5–10 drops for children and 20 drops for adults.

RECIPE

Pickled Burdock Root
Pickled burdock root makes a good daily tonic, digestive, and blood strengthener. It is a useful way to use the roots after weeding. Wash the root and cut into small rounds. Simmer in water until soft. Strain and put into a clean jar. Pour hot cider vinegar over the root. Label and date.

As a tonic, chew a piece first thing every morning. As a digestive, chew a piece 20 minutes before your meals.

> **CAUTION**
> Avoid in early pregnancy. Large doses may cause a cleansing rash, so it is best to start with small doses and then slowly increase them.

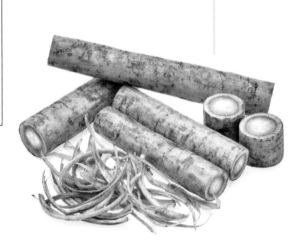

Arctostaphylos uva-ursi
UVA URSI LEAVES

This small evergreen shrub of moors and mountains is also known as bearberry. The leaves are astringent and have a high tannin content.

DATA FILE

Properties
• Diuretic • Urinary antiseptic • Astringent

Uses
• For cystitis, take with soothing herbal remedies such as marshmallow.
• For irritable bladder with persistent frequency, take with horsetail or nettle.
• For thick, white vaginal discharges, take with lady's mantle or shepherd's purse.
• For diarrhea, take along with agrimony.

Notes and Dosages
The best time to collect the leaves is in spring and summer. Hang them to dry before storing. Take as a tea or tincture. For a tea, use 1 teaspoon dried leaves to 1 cup water and infuse for 10 minutes.

For acute cystitis, take 1 cup of tea, or 1 teaspoon of tincture, 2 or 3 times daily for up to a week. Take in combination with the suggested herbs for long-term use.

> **CAUTION**
> Do not use during pregnancy or breastfeeding, or during kidney disease. Do not use for more than two weeks without consulting a professional herbalist.

Armoracia rusticana

HORSERADISH

Horseradish is a member of the mustard family, and is widely cultivated for its pungent, fleshy root. Japanese horseradish, or wasabi (*Wasabia japonica*), is used both for cooking and for therapeutic purposes, and the grated rhizomes are often sold as a dry, green-colored powder.

DATA FILE

Properties
• Diuretic • Stimulant • Clears nasal passages • Warming
• Antiseptic • Stimulates blood flow • Aids digestion

Uses
• Apply tincture of horseradish root to skin eruptions, including those associated with acne, to draw out the infection and encourage healing.
• Add some horseradish root to your toothpaste to clean teeth effectively, kill bacteria, and control mouth ulcers.
• Eat fresh horseradish, mixed with a little lemon juice, for the relief of sinus infections and nasal blockages.
• Eat freshly grated horseradish root for the swelling associated with premenstrual symdrome.
• A horseradish poultice can be applied to chilblains and hemorrhoids to encourage healing and improve the circulation of the blood.
• Chronic rheumatism may respond to eating tiny pieces of horseradish root without chewing, continuing for several weeks.

Notes and Dosages
Horseradish is rich in sulfur, which may contribute to its antibacterial action and its many beneficial effects on the body.

CAUTION
Too much horseradish taken internally can cause night sweats, and occasionally diarrhea and abdominal cramping.

Arnica montana

ARNICA

Arnica has been used for its healing properties for centuries. It grows in the mountain regions of Europe and Siberia. In folk remedies it is used externally for aches and bruises. Homeopathically, it is also taken internally for shock.

DATA FILE

Properties
• Soothing • Reduces bruising

Uses
• Applied externally, arnica cream is used for sprains, strains, and bruising.
• Taken internally, arnica may be useful for shock, after either an injury or emotional trauma.
• It can be used for long-term joint and muscle complaints such as osteoarthritis.
• Internal treatment can possibly aid external conditions such as eczema and boils.

Notes and Dosages
To make the homeopathic remedy, the whole fresh plant is used when in flower.

CAUTION
Do not use arnica cream on broken skin. Arnica is toxic if taken in large quantities. Contact with the plant can cause skin irritation.

Asparagus officinalis
ASPARAGUS

A herbaceous perennial of the Liliaceae family, asparagus is cultivated for its tender shoots, which appear in early spring. In 1806 the French chemist Louis Nicolas Vauquelin isolated asparagine, the first amino acid to be discovered, from the asparagus plant.

DATA FILE

Properties
• Diuretic • Liver tonic • Aids digestion

Uses
• For urinary complaints, arthritis, and rheumatism, drink asparagus water (the water remaining after steaming asparagus spears).
• Freshly cooked asparagus will tonify the liver, and may be used in cases of liver congestion and conditions such as hepatitis. It promotes elimination through the urine.
• Asparagus tincture can be added to food and drinks to encourage the elimination of urine.
• May help control the symptoms of premenstrual syndrome, including breast tenderness and abdominal bloating

Notes and Dosages
Asparagus is taken internally: it may be eaten as a food or prepared as a tincture.

CAUTION
Asparagus is high in purines, so anyone suffering from gout should avoid it.

Astragalus membranaceus
ASTRAGALUS

This herbaceous perennial plant belongs to the pea family. The root is used for therapeutic purposes, both in Western and Chinese herbalism. To Chinese herbalists, it is known as Huang Qi.

DATA FILE

Properties
• Tonic • Strengthens the immune system

Uses
• Take as a decoction or tincture for chronic fatigue, persistent infections, multiple allergies, and glandular fever.
• Use as a soup stock with other nourishing herbs for people with severe immune deficiencies.
• May help to counteract tiredness and lack of appetite in patients undergoing chemotherapy and radiotherapy for cancer.
• Soothing and healing for stomach ulcers.
• May help night sweats.
• Good for edema and pus-filled sores that have not yet discharged.

Notes and Dosages
If preparing your own remedy, use standard doses of the root (see pages 39 and 41). The root can also be bought in Chinese herb stores as Huang Qi. In Chinese medicine, this herb treats qi deficiency and spleen-deficient symptoms such as lack of appetite, fatigue, and diarrhea.

CAUTION
Always tell the hospital if you are taking herbal medicine in conjunction with their treatment. Severely debilitated patients should always be seen by a professional herbalist, who will prescribe according to the individual's condition and circumstances.

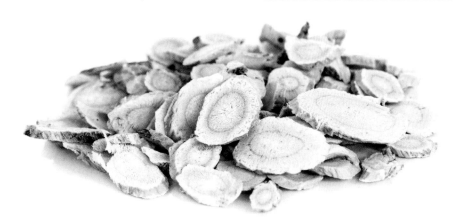

Atractylodes macrocephala
BAI ZHU

This herb is one of a group that is used in traditional Chinese medicine to treat qi deficiency. As we replenish our day-to-day energy from air and food, the two main organs involved are lungs and spleen.

DATA FILE

Properties
• Sweet • Bitter • Warm • Tonic • Dries dampness

Uses
• Use for digestive disorders, diarrhea, and vomiting.
• May help rheumatic ailments, or damp painful obstruction.
• Helps with excessive sweating due to qi deficiency.
• Helps damp disorders such as water retention and reduced urination.
• Gives a boost when fatigue is experienced, and helps with lack of appetite.

Notes and Dosages
Bai Zhu is one of the herbs in the seminal tonifying prescription of the "Four Gentlemen" (Si Jun Zi Wan). It is also used in the "Jade Screen" prescription for spontaneous sweating.

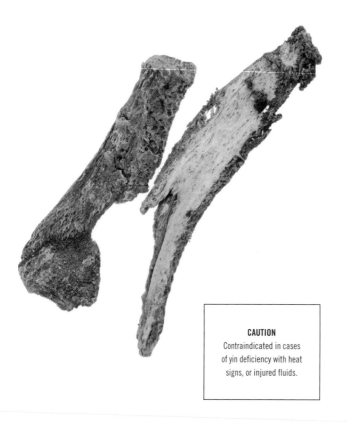

> **CAUTION**
> Contraindicated in cases of yin deficiency with heat signs, or injured fluids.

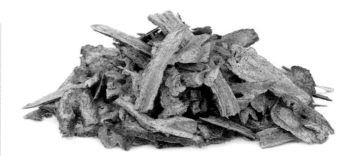

Aucklandia lappa
MU XIANG

The traditional Chinese herb Mu Xiang regulates and invigorates the qi when it becomes stuck or "stagnant," optimizing the function of the gastrointestinal tract and helping stop pain. In the West, it is known as costus root or saussurea.

DATA FILE

Properties
• Acrid • Slightly bitter • Warm • Prevents stagnation

Uses
• Promotes the movement of qi and alleviates pain, swelling, and soreness in the spleen, stomach, liver, or gall bladder.
• Helps digestive difficulties and pain: lack of appetite, epigastric (above the navel) or abdominal pain or swelling, nausea, diarrhea, vomiting, and tenesmus (a spasm of the rectum where one feels the need to defecate without being able to).
• Strengthens the spleen.

Notes and Dosages
Mu Xiang is part of the ginger family, and is a rhizomatus perennial. Use with tonifying herbs to prevent their cloying side-effects.

> **CAUTION**
> Contraindicated in cases of yin deficiency or depleted fluids.

Avena fatua

WILD OATS

This wild grass is the origin of cultivated oats (*Avena sativa*). The whole plant (called oat straw) is used, picked while still green. Cultivated oats may be substituted. Groats, or oat grains, may be substituted, although they are not quite as good.

DATA FILE

Properties
• Restorative • Antidepressant • Strengthening

Uses
• Use for weakness and nervous exhaustion; take with vervain for weakness following illness.
• Alleviates restless sleep from overexcitement.
• Take with valerian to ease the symptoms of withdrawal from tranquilizers.
• Helps premenstrual syndrome with scanty menstruation and cramps.
• Take for exhaustion after childbirth and during breastfeeding.
• Addresses loss of libido in both sexes.
• Take with horsetail to strengthen the bones of children and the elderly.
• For eczema, use in baths and lotions.

Notes and Dosages
For oat straw, make a tea with 2 teaspoons to 1 cup of water. Infuse for 15 minutes. For oats in general, buy the tincture. Use 20 drops every 2 hours when you need to keep going or 1 teaspoon 3 times daily for weakened states.

For a bath, fill a muslin bag with porridge oats and hang it under the hot faucet, so that the water flows through it. Preparations of oats for making baths can also be bought at general and herbal pharmacies.

Avena sativa

CULTIVATED OATS

Oats are a cereal plant, and are both extremely nutritious and useful therapeutically. Oats are one of the best sources of inositol, which is important for maintaining optimum blood cholesterol levels. Eaten daily, they provide a wealth of excellent effects.

DATA FILE

Properties
• Tonic • Lowers cholesterol • Antidepressant • Cleansing
• Rich in B vitamins and minerals

Uses
• Eat porridge daily to reduce fatigue, strengthen the nervous system, and lower cholesterol.
• Eat raw oats as a source of fiber to ease constipation.
• Oatmeal (unrefined) can be eaten regularly to reduce the effects of stress and nervous disorders.
• Eat daily to control hormonal activity.
• Use the tincture for stress, addictions, eating disorders, and depression.
• For eczema and other skin conditions, use a compress of oatmeal or an oatmeal bath.

Notes and Dosages
To prepare a nourishing nerve tonic, boil a tablespoon of oats in ½pt. (250ml.) of water for several minutes and drain.

RECIPE

Oat Water
Prepare oat water as a soothing drink for diarrhea, cystitis, and stomach upsets caused by antibiotics. Take 1 dessertspoon of porridge oats and rub well between your fingers. Add to 1 cup of cold water. Stir well and leave for 20 minutes. Stir again and pass through a tea strainer.

CAUTION
Oats contain gluten, which causes an allergic reaction in some individuals.

Berberis vulgaris

BARBERRY

Barberry has been in use as a healing herb for thousands of years. The Egyptians used it to prevent plagues – a testimony to its antibiotic properties. Ayurvedics are more likely to prescribe it for dysentery, mouth ulcers, sore throats, and skin infections.

DATA FILE

Properties
• Antibiotic • Antibacterial • Antifungal • Stimulant • Respiratory aid

Uses
• Use for skin infections, urinary tract infections, conjunctivitis, throat infections, and mouth ulcers.
• Helps with diarrhea and dysentery.
• May be useful for arthritis and high blood pressure.

Notes and Dosages
The plant's berries, roots, and ground bark are used. May be taken as a tea or infusion, gargle, eyewash, douche, compress, or powder. Can be taken with garlic, ginger, saffron, and wild sunflower.

RECIPE

Barberry Decoction
Barberry can be used to treat a variety of symptoms in its decoction form. Put 1 teaspoon of powdered root bark in a small enamel pan. Add 2 cups of water. Cover and boil for 15–30 minutes, with as little liquid loss as possible. Allow to cool. The taste will be quite bitter. Sweeten with honey as required. Drink up to one cup a day.

For a compress to treat conjunctivitis, soak a clean cloth in the decoction (before you add any honey). Place over the eye.

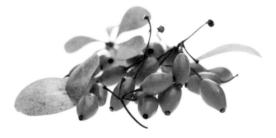

CAUTION
Barberry may stimulate the uterus and should not be taken by pregnant women. Barberry is a very powerful herb, and should be used in small doses and under the supervision of a physician or alternative healthcare practitioner. If the dosage is too high, barberry can cause nausea, vomiting, hazardous drops in blood pressure, and dizziness.

Boswellia carteri

FRANKINCENSE

Frankincense essential oil, also known as olibanum, is distilled from the resin produced by the bark of a small North African tree. Wonderfully calming and richly fragrant, it is considered a spiritual oil, used by many to encourage meditation.

DATA FILE

Properties
• Immune stimulant • Expectorant • Antiseptic
• Anti-inflammatory • Calming

Uses
• Slows the breathing and calms the nervous and digestive systems, relieving anxiety, depression, nervous tension, emotional upsets, and stress-related digestive problems.
• Helps respiratory and catarrhal conditions such as asthma, colds, chest infections, and chronic bronchitis.
• Its wound-healing properties make the oil ideal for treating cuts, scars, blemishes, and inflammation, and it is recommended for firming aging skin.
• Helpful for cystitis.
• Irregular or heavy menstrual bleeding and nosebleeds may be improved.

Notes and Dosages
The gum resin used to make frankincense essential oil oozes out from the tree as a milky-white liquid and then solidifies into tear-shaped, amber to orange-brown lumps. Frankincense blends well with rose, lavender, geranium, neroli, orange, bergamot, mandarin, sandalwood, pine, black pepper, cinnamon, and other spice oils.

RECIPE

Inhalation for Dry Coughs
Add 2 drops frankincense, 2 drops lavender, 2 drops cypress to a bowl of steaming hot water. Lean over the bowl, cover your head with a towel, and inhale the aroma for 5–10 minutes.

CAUTION
Do not take frankincense internally and keep it out of children's reach.

Brassica nigra, Sinapis alba

MUSTARD

Mustard is an annual plant cultivated as a spice all over the world. It has been used for centuries as a pungent condiment and healing herb, by the Greeks, Ayurvedics, and folk practitioners. Mustard's strong taste develops only after the seeds are crushed and come into contact with water or saliva.

DATA FILE

Properties
- Antiseptic • Warming • Antibacterial • Antiseptic • Antiviral
- Aids digestion • Emetic • Laxative • Irritant • Expectorant

Uses
- Use mustard poultices to treat chest colds and coughs.
- Eases constipation, acting as a laxative, and improves digestive upsets and hiccups.
- Use diluted mustard oil as a lotion, or a poultice of mustard seeds, for backache, joint pain, muscle stiffness, rheumatism, neuralgia, and sciatica.
- Use mustard flour as an antiseptic and deodorizer.
- Eat fresh mustard leaves when convalescing to encourage healing: they are rich in vitamin A, iron, and zinc.
- In Ayurveda, mustard reduces pitta and kapha, and has a neutral effect on vátha.

Notes and Dosages
The leaves, flowers, seeds, and oils of the black mustard are used, while only the seeds of the white mustard are useful. Take as a spice or oil, in compresses and poultices. Mustard oil can be rectified with alcohol (1 part oil to 40 parts alcohol). To make a poultice, mix ready-powdered mustard seeds with warm water to form a thick paste. Spread on a piece of cloth. In Ayurvedic practice, black mustard can be taken with aloe vera, ginger, garlic, and onion.

RECIPE

Mustard Foot Bath
A mustard foot bath will clear blood congestion in the head, warm up cold feet, and lower a fever in the early stages of illness. Put one-quarter of a cup of mustard seed in a small cloth bag or a large tea strainer. Steep in hot water for 5 minutes. Soak the feet until the water cools.

CAUTION

Large amounts of mustard can cause irritation and inflammation. Avoid contact with the mucous membranes, and with sensitive skin. Do not let undiluted mustard oil come in contact with the skin. Do not use mustard poultices for more than 10–15 minutes at a time, or blistering and irritation can occur.

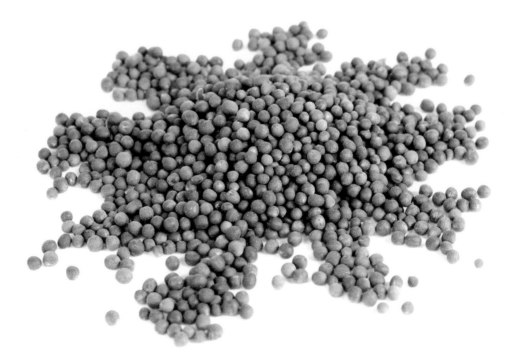

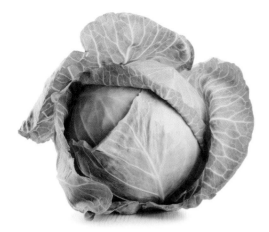

Brassica oleracea
CABBAGE

The ancient Greeks used fresh white cabbage juice to relieve sore or infected eyes. The Romans and Egyptians would drink cabbage juice before big dinners to prevent intoxication.

DATA FILE

Properties
• Anti-inflammatory • Reduces pain • Soothing • Anti-cancer
• Expectorant

Uses
• Make cabbage a regular part of your diet to reduce the risk of cancer.
• A cabbage poultice can be applied to boils and infected cuts to draw out the infection and disperse pus.
• Applied to bruises and swelling, macerated cabbage leaves will encourage healing.
• Dab white cabbage juice on mouth ulcers, and gargle for sore throats.
• A warm cabbage compress, on the affected area, reduces the pain of headaches and some kinds of neuralgia.
• Drink fresh cabbage juice daily to reduce the discomfort of gastric ulcers, bronchial infections, psoriasis, chronic headaches, asthma, and cystitis.
• For mastitis, place a cabbage leaf, lightly pounded, directly on the breast.
• Cabbage seeds are said to prevent hangovers.

Notes and Dosages
When consuming raw cabbage juice, drink l–2fl.oz. (25–50ml.) daily for best effects.

> **CAUTION**
> Do not eat red cabbage raw, and beware eating large quantities cooked, because the high levels of iron can interfere with gut absorption, causing constipation. Avoid cabbage if you suffer from goiter or take MAOI antidepressants.

Bromus ramosus
WILD OAT

Although called "wild oat," this flower remedy is actually made from hairy or wood brome grass, named for its soft, hairy leaves. An elegant woodland grass, it stands between 2 and 5ft. (½–1½m.) high.

DATA FILE

Properties
• Helps to find purpose • Aids decision-making

Uses
• For capable people who have ambition to do something meaningful in their lives but have not yet found their true calling. They may be aimless and frustrated. Wild oat helps them to find true meaning and purpose.
• Helps us to make choices, sometimes difficult, and to balance the needs of spirituality and making a living.

Notes and Dosages
"Wild oat" is made from a hairy woodland grass, not to be confused with the common wild oat of open pastures (see page 89). Use the sun method (see page 56) to prepare this flower remedy.

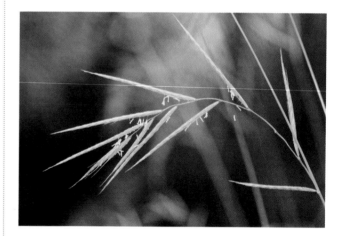

Calendula officinalis

MARIGOLD

Marigold is a popular garden plant with orange or yellow flowers. Do not confuse it with French and African marigolds (*Tagetes* species), which must not be taken internally. Marigold is used in herbalism, aromatherapy and homeopathy.

DATA FILE

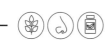

Properties
• Lifts the spirits • Antispasmodic • Antiseptic • Antifungal
• Healing • Anti-inflammatory

Uses
• Take marigold tea for digestive colic, stomach, and duodenal ulcers, as well as for children's infections and fevers.
• Use marigold tea as a gargle for sore throats and tonsillitis.
• Use marigold as a wash, cream, or compress for boils, spots, inflamed wounds, painful varicose veins, leg ulcers, sore nipples in nursing mothers, and sore eyes.
• Use as a lotion for itchy skin rashes, grazes, cuts, broken chilblains, eczema, and fungal infections.
• Put in a douche or bath for thrush and vaginal infections.
• Calendula-infused oil helps cradle cap.
• For dry skin, add a few teaspoons of calendula oil to the bath.
• Calendula-infused oil has valuable wound-healing properties, so it is a first-aid kit essential for cuts, grazes, wounds, and insect bites.
• After childbirth, calendula is used by midwives in baths or lotions to aid perineal tears.

Notes and Dosages
Marigold preparations are also sold as calendula lotion. For compresses and fomentations, use 1 dessertspoon of marigold tincture to 1 cup water. Dip cloth into the cooled water, then wring out. Use cold water to soothe and draw heat, for sprains, congestive pain, and hot joints. Use hot water to relax and encourage circulation for spasm, stiffness, and cold joints. Wrap around the affected part, then cover.

Calendula essential oil is not widely available, as the bright orange flowers of the common pot marigold yield only small amounts of oil. More common is infused oil of calendula, where the flowers are infused in warm oil, macerated, and strained.

Homeopathically, the fresh leaves and flowers of the plant are used to make a healing remedy, and a cream for external use.

RECIPES

Marigold Tea
Add 2 or 3 flowers to 1 cup of boiling water. Infuse for 10 minutes. Drink 3 cups a day, or 1 cup every 3 hours for acute complaints. Give a half dose for children over five years old. Give infants 3 or 4 teaspoons of a weak tea in fruit juice.

Calendula Cream
To make a soothing skin cream, add calendula oil drop by drop to any ready-made unperfumed pure plant cream, and blend thoroughly. Stop adding the oil when the cream reaches a soft, usable consistency. Do not worry about adding too much calendula oil. Pure plant creams are often available from the suppliers of essential oils.

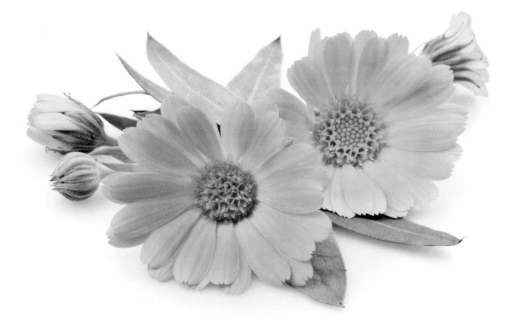

Calluna vulgaris
HEATHER

This common plant is often found in alpine areas, on heaths, and waste ground. Calluna prefers acid soil. According to variety, flowers are produced from summer to fall.

DATA FILE

Properties
• Encourages listening • Discourages self-obsession

Uses
• For people who are caught up with themselves and their own interests, are poor listeners, find it hard to share, and do not like to be alone, heather helps us to look after ourselves without being obsessed with our own personal needs, gives us the space to listen to others, and experience genuine love and companionship.
• People who need heather often become isolated from others, as friends may avoid them because they demand too much. Heather encourages them to nurture themselves and give others space.
• Discourages clinginess, hyponchondria, and tearfulness.

Notes and Dosages
Gather wild heather on acid heathland. Prepare the flower remedy using the sun method (see page 56).

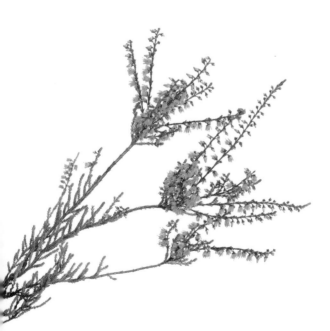

Camellia sinensis
TEA

Native to Southeast Asia, the tea plant is a small, shrub-like, evergreen tree that belongs to the family Theaceae. Its seeds contain a volatile oil, and its leaves contain the chemicals caffeine and tannin.

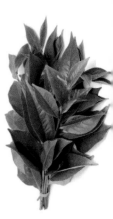

DATA FILE

Properties
• Diuretic • Astringent • Antioxidant • Boosts immune system
• Stimulant

Uses
• The fluoride in tea may be beneficial in preventing dental caries.
• Tea may help in the treatment of diarrhea, dysentery, hepatitis, and gastroenteritis.
• The flavonoids contained in tea may destroy harmful bacteria and viruses, and act on the immune system.
• Cold, steeped tea bags placed over the eyes will soothe soreness and irritation; they are also useful for treating minor injuries and insect bites.
• Tannins in the leaves of green and black tea may be beneficial in the prevention of heart disease and stroke.
• Green tea may help to prevent cancer if it is drunk on a regular basis.
• Provides folic acid (vitamin B9), some potassium, and also magnesium.

Notes and Dosages
Green tea is made from the tips, or shoots, of the shrub *Camellia sinensis*; black tea is made from the fermented dried leaves. An essential oil, called tea absolute, is distilled from black tea. Both the leaves and the oil are used for medicinal purposes. Fruit teas do not actually contain tea but can also be beneficial to the health.

CAUTION
Tea can interfere with the effectiveness of drugs such as allopurinol (for the treatment of gout), antibiotics, antiulcer drugs, and the drug theophylkline, prescribed for asthma. It can prevent the absorption of iron and interfere with the effectiveness of sedative drugs. Drinking tea to excess can cause constipation, indigestion, dizziness, palpitations, irritability, and insomnia.

Cananga odorata var. genuina

YLANG YLANG

This essential oil is extracted from a tropical tree that grows in the Philippines, Indonesia, the Comoros, and Madagascar. Ylang ylang means "flower of flowers." The name suits the heady floral fragrance of this oil, distilled from the freshly picked flowers.

DATA FILE

Properties

- Sedative • Antidepressant • Tonic • Aphrodisiac • Rebalancing

Uses

- Depression, anxiety, tension, irritability, and stress-related insomnia can all benefit from ylang ylang's soothing properties.
- It helps to rebalance sebum production in oily skin, acne, and both dry and greasy scalps.
- Calms irritated skin, bites, and stings, and is a traditional topical remedy for infections and skin diseases.
- Ylang ylang is reputed to be an aphrodisiac and can be used to treat sexual problems.
- Helps to reduce blood pressure, and slows down breathing and heart rate in cases of shock, panic, or rage.

Notes and Dosages

Ylang ylang essential oil blends well with rosewood, rose, bergamot, vetiver, frankincense, chamomile, lavender, and cedarwood.

RECIPE

Bath Blend for Nervous Tension

Add 3 drops ylang ylang, 2 drops rosewood, 3 drops lavender to 1½ teaspoons (8ml.) of a dispersible bath oil such as red turkey oil, and add to a warm bath. Alternatively, drip the oils directly into the bath water and disperse with your hand. Relax in the bath for 10 minutes.

> **CAUTION**
> Ylang ylang can cause nausea or headaches in high concentrations. It may irritate the skin of some hypersensitive people.

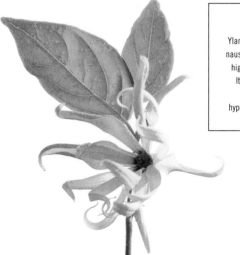

Cannabis sativa

HUO MA REN

Huo Ma Ren is ungerminated cannabis seeds, but does not have the effects that smoking cannabis leaves or resin has. Huo Ma Ren comes into the category of descending downward: it facilitates the expulsion of the stool in cases of constipation.

DATA FILE

Properties

- Sweet • Neutral

Uses

- Nourishes and moistens the intestines, but does not have a harsh effect so is most suitable for constipation in the weak and elderly.
- Mildly tonifies the yin, which is often depleted during a long illness like ME (or post-viral syndrome) and in the elderly.
- Taken orally or applied topically (locally), it clears heat and promotes healing of sores and ulcerations.

Notes and Dosages

These seeds have been processed and therefore cannot germinate, so they cannot be considered an illegal drug.

> **CAUTION**
> Long-term use may possibly result in vaginal discharge. Overdose may lead to nausea, vomiting, and diarrhea.

Cephaelis ipecacuanha

IPECAC.

Ipecacuanha is a small, perennial shrub grown in the tropical rainforests of South and Central America. It is used in conventional medicine to induce vomiting in cases of drug overdoses or poisoning, and as an expectorant. Homeopathically, the root is used to treat nausea and vomiting.

DATA FILE

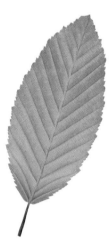

Properties
• Relieves nausea • Helps breathing difficulties

Uses
• Commonly used for nausea and vomiting, and accompanying sweats and clamminess.
• May be good for stomach complaints accompanied by salivating, lack of thirst, weak pulse, and fainting.
• May help conditions causing breathing difficulties and coughing.

Notes and Dosages
The homeopathic remedy is obtained from the dried root of the ipecacuanha plant, collected when the plant is in flower.

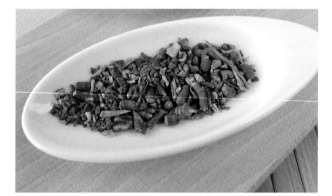

Carpinus betulus

HORNBEAM

This flower remedy is obtained from the hornbeam, a medium-sized, deciduous tree common in woods. It grows well in a sunny or lightly shaded position, and its leaves turn a rich yellow-orange in fall.

DATA FILE

Properties
• Restores confidence • Encourages optimism

Uses
• Hornbeam helps those who feel they do not possess enough strength to fulfill the responsibilities of daily life, for the "Monday morning blues." This feeling often comes from boredom, frustration, or pessimism.
• Gives strength, confidence, and optimism, and helps us find satisfaction in the mundane "nine-to-five" aspects of our lives.
• Prevents procrastination.

Notes and Dosages
Prepare using the boiling method (see page 57). Hornbeam is the right remedy if the feelings of weakness are temporary: if they are a regular occurrence, the person may be exhausting himself or herself in the wrong direction, and other remedies may be needed.

Carthamus tinctorius
HONG HUA

In traditional Chinese medicine, this herb invigorates (or "regulates") the blood, treating problems associated with blood stasis. These problems include pain and internal masses or growths.

DATA FILE

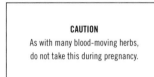

Properties
• Acrid • Warm • Invigorates the blood • Alleviates pain

Uses
• May be useful for gynecological problems such as amenorrhea, postpartum dizziness, or fibroids.
• Helps many skin diseases, such as Kaposi's sarcoma and scarlet fever.
• Useful for pain in the limbs and joint pain such as arthritis.
• May help tumors if they are caused by congealed blood.
• Good for wounds or painful sores.

Notes and Dosages
This Chinese remedy is prepared from the flowers of the safflower plant.

> **CAUTION**
> As with many blood-moving herbs, do not take this during pregnancy.

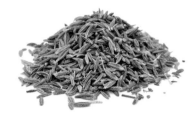

Carum carvi
CARAWAY SEED

This perennial plant, known as "sushavi" in Ayurveda, is found in the wild in North America, Europe, and Asia. Caraway is best known in Europe in the making of rye bread, where the addition of caraway seeds aids in the digestion of starch.

DATA FILE

Properties
• Pungent • Heating • Drying agent • Stimulant • Carminative
• Antispasmodic • Muscle relaxant

Uses
• Relaxes uterine tissue and is therefore beneficial for menstrual cramps.
• Chewing a teaspoonful of seeds aids the digestive process, soothing indigestion, gas, colic, flatulence, and accumulation of toxins and fluids.
• A cool caraway infusion soothes colicky children.
• Caraway oil is beneficial as a scalp treatment.
• Caraway oil can be used as an enema for intestinal parasites.
• Massage the stomach with a very small amount of oil to reduce flatulence.
• Seeds can be added to any laxative to temper its strength and to soothe the colon.
• Caraway reduces vátha and kapha, and increases pitta.

Notes and Dosages
The seeds can be used to make teas, an oil for stomach massage, used in an inhaler, and as a spice to aid the digestion of starches. Caraway blends well with dill, fennel, anise, basil, cardamom, and jasmine.

RECIPE

Caraway Infusion
Finely crush 9 teaspoonfuls of seeds using a pestle and mortar. Place the seeds in a pot and add boiling water. Allow the infusion to stand for 20 minutes, then strain and drink as needed, up to 3 cups a day.

Capsicum annuum

CAYENNE

This fiery red pepper, used the world over in cooking, is known to many Westerners by its Caribbean name, cayenne, or as "chilli pepper." In Ayurvedic practice, it is known as "merchi." Cayenne pepper is one of several different cultivars of *Capsicum annuum*, a milder cultivar being red pepper (see opposite).

DATA FILE

Properties

- Assists digestion • Analgesic • Warms circulation • Carminative
- Emetic • Decongestant • Expectorant • Antispasmodic

Uses

- Taken internally, cayenne helps colds, fevers, and toothache.
- Taken internally, it can help catarrh and sinus problems.
- Internally, cayenne soothes gastrointestinal and bowel problems, including diarrhea and constipation, and is used as a digestive aid.
- Externally, cayenne oil can treat arthritis, cold joints, muscle soreness, cramps, aches and pains, and unbroken chilblains.
- For shingles, creams containing cayenne may be used.
- For the elderly, cayenne infusions help poor circulation, chills, and inefficient digestion.
- In winter, sprinkle cayenne into your socks to heat your feet.
- For poor circulation, add cayenne to any herbal medicines.
- In Ayurveda, cayenne increases pitta and reduces kapha and vátha.

Notes and Dosages

The pod is used for all remedies. It can be taken raw, powdered, as a spice, oil, tea, or poultice. It mixes well with garlic, onion, coriander, lemon, and ginger. Use only in very small quantities. A small pinch of the powder or 5–10 drops of the tincture is sufficient for a single dose. For a pain-relieving muscle rub, mix a half-teaspoon of cayenne powder or puréed fresh cayenne to 1 cup of warm vegetable oil.

RECIPE

Cayenne Oil

Make an infused oil using 1 dessertspoon cayenne pepper, 2 dessertspoons powdered mustard seed, 2 teaspoons powdered ginger root, and 1 cup unblended vegetable oil, sunflower, or grapeseed oil. Use as a rub for cold joints and muscle spasm.

CAUTION

Do not give to children under two years old. Use rubber gloves when chopping cayenne peppers, as they may burn. If burning does occur, wash with vinegar several times, rinsing carefully. Pepper oil will cause severe pain on contact with sensitive tissues, such as eyes or genitals. Cayenne-based creams, liniments, and infused oils should only be used on small areas and rubbed in well.
Cayenne can aggravate acidity and heartburn.

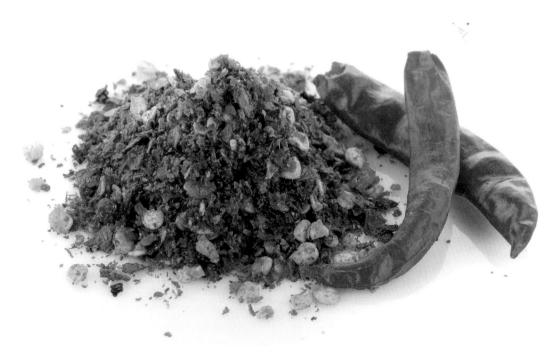

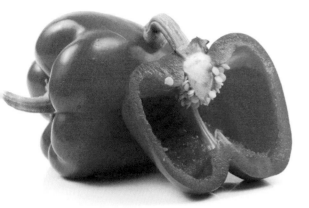

Capsicum annuum
RED PEPPER

The red pepper is also known variously as bell pepper, sweet pepper, and capsicum. It is a milder cultivar than cayenne (see opposite). Red peppers are the ripened fruit (some varieties ripen to yellow or purple), while green peppers are immature.

DATA FILE

Properties
• Tonic • Stimulates digestion • Warms circulation

Uses
• Helps in the treatment of varicose veins, asthma, and digestive complaints.
• Acts as a tonic for those suffering from tiredness and cold.
• Encourages the elimination of toxins from the body.

Notes and Dosages
Peppers are an excellent source of vitamin A and C (a fresh green pepper contains 10 percent vitamin C) and also contribute small amounts of iron and vitamin A: the largest amounts of vitamin A are found in fresh red peppers. Peppers are also a good source of potassium. The best way to consume red peppers is raw, in salads.

Cassia angustifolia
SENNA

Senna has a very strong laxative effect on the body. Indian senna, used by Ayurvedic practitioners, is a close relative of North African and American senna, but its properties are much milder. Still a powerful laxative, it is gentler on the body.

DATA FILE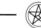

Properties
• Laxative • Cooling • Antispasmodic • Cleansing

Uses
• Senna is the most powerful herbal treatment for constipation, especially when it is chronic.
• Senna reduces kapha and vátha, and increases pitta.

Notes and Dosages
The leaves and the whole seed pods may be used, with the seed pods having a milder effect. Senna may be taken as a powder, a tea, or supplement. Only use North American and African senna with other herbs. Senna may be combined with anise, cardamom, cinnamon, coriander, fennel, ginger, nutmeg, and orange.

RECIPE

Senna Infusion
A senna infusion will give you the benefits of senna's laxative power. Steep 3½oz. (80g.) of senna leaves, ½ teaspoon of coriander, and ½ teaspoon of ginger in 1 quart (1l.) of hot water for 15 minutes. Take 1–4 tablespoons at a time. The infusion is more palatable cold than hot.

For children or the elderly, senna pods have a more gentle laxative effect. Steep 3–4 pods in 4–5 tablespoons of cold water. Take 1 or 2 tablespoons at a time. For healthy adults, use 6–12 pods for the same amount of water.

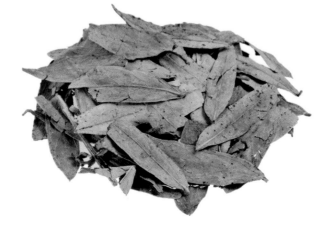

CAUTION
Senna has a powerful laxative effect. Do not use if you suffer from hemorrhoids.

Castanea sativa

SWEET CHESTNUT

This chestnut tree produces edible fruits after its creamy flowers. The tree grows to 100ft. (30m.) and is deciduous. The flower remedy is used for moments of great anguish.

DATA FILE

Properties
• Brings out reserves of strength • Expands limits

Uses
• Sweet chestnut is for times when anguish is so great it seems unbearable, when people feel stretched beyond endurance. The sufferer may feel hopeless, despairing, and unable to sleep.
• Sweet chestnut helps to bring out hidden reserves of strength, opening boundaries and transforming the sufferer in the "dark night of the soul."

Notes and Dosages
Prepare the leaves and fruits using the boiling method (see page 57).

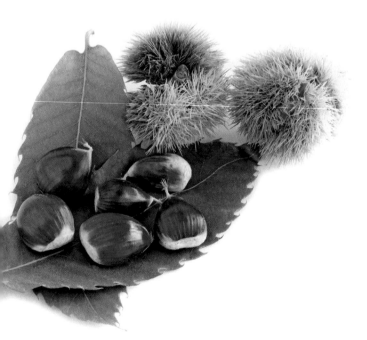

Cedrus atlantica, Cedrus deodara

CEDAR

The wood we know of for its insect-repellent qualities is also, according to the Ayurvedics, an excellent treatment for dandruff. The Ayurvedics use the Himalayan cedar (*Cedrus deodara*). In aromatherapy, the oil of the *Cedrus atlantica* species is used, sold as "cedarwood." It has a rich, woody, masculine scent.

DATA FILE

Properties
• Pungent • Antiseptic • Diuretic • Expectorant • Astringent
• Tonic • Grounding

Uses
• Used as a massage oil, cedar is an excellent antidote to oily skin, oily scalp, and dandruff.
• For an air freshener, deodorizer, and insect repellent, add oil of cedar to water in an atomizer and spray the room, or add 10 drops to a tablespoon of vegetable oil and rub it onto skin.
• Taken internally, cedar may help urinary infections and provoke sluggish menstrual cycles.
• Used in massage and inhaled, the aromatherapy oil is warming, physically cleansing, and emotionally grounding. It helps to relieve nervous tension and stress-related conditions.
• Inhale cedarwood oil for treatment of catarrhal problems, especially bronchial congestion and infections.
• In Ayurveda, cedar reduces pitta and kapha, while increasing vátha.

Notes and Dosages
The wood and bark are used to produce oil for massage and inhalation; or made into a tea or an infusion. The aromatherapy oil is extracted by steam distillation from the wood chips. However, note that several varieties of cedar trees are used to produce oil that is sold as cedarwood. Some of this oil is very different from *Cedrus atlantica*: always make sure you buy Atlas cedarwood oil. It blends well with camphor, sandalwood, and vetiver.

RECIPE

Antidandruff Treatment
Add 6 drops cedarwood, 6 drops rosemary, and 4 drops cypress oil to 1½fl.oz. (50ml.) olive oil. Massage into the scalp with your fingertips, cover, and leave overnight, if possible. Shampoo thoroughly. Use half the recipe for children.

> **CAUTION**
> Cedar should not be used by pregnant women, as it stimulates the menstrual cycle, and acts as a possible abortifacient.

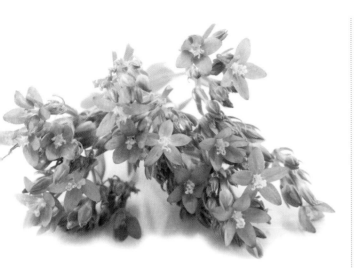

Centella asiatica
GOTU KOLA

According to tradition, the natives of Sri Lanka were the first people to use gotu kola. They noticed that elephants, animals renowned for their longevity, loved to eat the rounded gotu kola leaves. Known as "brahmi," gotu kola is used widely in Ayurvedic practice.

DATA FILE

Properties
• Bitter • Stimulating • Cooling • Tonic • Diuretic • Rejuvenating
• Encourages hair growth

Uses
• Used as a shampoo, gotu kola benefits the head and scalp and is used by some as a treatment for baldness.
• Drunk as an infusion, gotu kola will act as a soporific in cases of insomnia.
• Infusions improve circulation in the legs and treat varicose veins.
• Gotu kola decreases depression and stress, and stimulates sexual appetite.
• Aids in the elimination of fluids.
• Used as a compress, the infusion will relieve psoriasis.
• May help infections such as a sore throat, tonsillitis, and cystitis.
• May aid treatment of rheumatism and high blood pressure.
• Gotu kola has a balancing effect on all three doshas.

Notes and Dosages
The seeds, nuts, and roots can be used to prepare massage oil, shampoo, poultices, tea, and skin cream. Gotu kola can be taken with sandalwood and lemon.

RECIPE

Gotu Kola Infusion
To make an infusion, pour 2 cups of boiling water over 1 teaspoon of the herb. Let steep for 10 minutes. Drink up to 2 cups a day, adding lemon or honey to taste if desired. If the results of a compress are disappointing, try strengthening the infusion used.

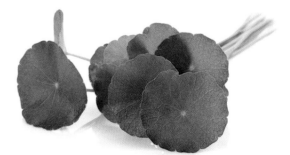

Centaurium erythraea
CENTAURY

A small pink flower of chalky soil, centaury is named after a centaur in Greek mythology, who used it to cure himself from a poisoned arrow wound.

DATA FILE

Properties
• Strengthens willpower • Aids decision-making

Uses
• Centaury is for people who have an excessive desire to please and a willingness to serve. They can be taken for granted and exploited. This leads to frustration, loss of self-confidence, drudgery or self-martyrdom.
• Centaury helps balance the desire to serve by strengthening our willpower and appreciation of ourselves. It may help the "weaker" partner in a co-dependent relationship.

Notes and Dosages
Centaury grows more readily in the wild than in cultivation. Prepare the flowers using the sun method (see page 56).

Ceratostigma willmottiana
CERATO

A small shrub with bright blue flowers that is often grown in gardens, cerato originated in China and the Himalayas. Cerato is the only Bach Flower Remedy to be made from a cultivated plant.

DATA FILE

Properties
• Gives confidence • Encourages trust in intuition

Uses
• Cerato is for those who lack trust in their own abilities and judgment. People who need cerato are intelligent and curious, but constantly seek the advice and approval of other people. They may join cults or take up fads.
• Cerato helps us to listen to advice from within, restores confidence, and strengthens our trust in ourselves to follow our path even if it runs contrary to the expectations of others.

Notes and Dosages
Blue cerato flowers grow on a species of hardy Chinese shrub cultivated as a garden plant. Use the sun method (see page 56) to prepare.

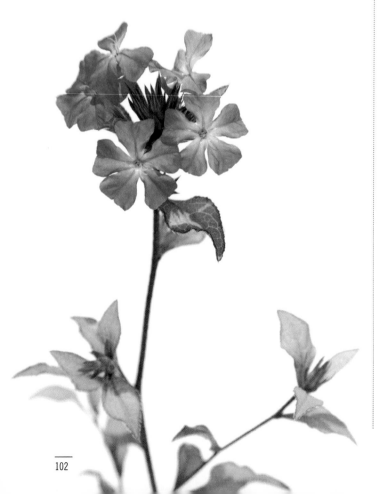

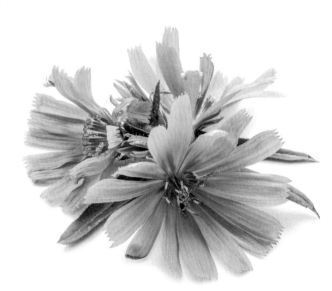

Chicorium intybus
CHICORY

A wayside plant with bright blue flowers, chicory is cultivated as a vegetable and blanched to add to salads. The flowers close in the afternoon and open again in the morning. They may be used to prepare a flower remedy.

DATA FILE

Properties
• Encourages selfless love

Uses
• Chicory flower remedy is for those who see love as a method of control, giving love in order to receive it. They love and care publicly, even melodramatically, building up a stock of good works which they expect to be reciprocated, but love still does not flow their way. They may be prone to illness if not "loved," or to hypochondria.
• Chicory helps us to see love as a universal force, to give love selflessly and freely so that it may freely return to us.

Notes and Dosages
Prepare the chicory remedy from the pretty sky-blue flowers, using the sun method (see page 56).

Cinchona officinalis

CHINA

The China homeopathic remedy is made from Peruvian bark, grown in the tropical rainforests of South America, in India, and Southeast Asia. Quinine, an extract of the bark, is used in conventional medicine as part of the treatment for malaria. Homeopathically, China is used for exhaustion.

DATA FILE

Properties
• Relieves nervous exhaustion • Improves weakness after illness

Uses
• May aid recovery from nervous exhaustion after illness and as a result of loss of fluids from vomiting, diarrhea, or sweating.
• May help digestive conditions such as gastroenteritis, flatulence, and gall bladder problems.
• Works against mental upsets such as lack of concentration, indifference, and outbursts that are out of character.

Notes and Dosages
To prepare the homeopathic remedy, the bark of the tree is stripped and dried.

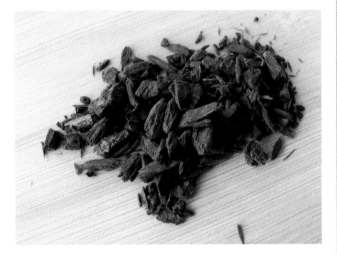

Cinnamomum camphora

CAMPHOR

When camphor is steam-distilled, it is fractionalized into blue, brown, and white camphors. Blue camphor is the heaviest and weakest, and it is used mostly in perfume distillation. Brown camphor contains strong carcinogens and should be avoided. White camphor has medicinal qualities and is called "karpura" by Ayurvedic practitioners.

DATA FILE

Properties
• Heating • Expectorant • Decongestant • Bronchio-dilator
• Analgesic • Antiseptic

Uses
• Camphor clears the mind and eases headaches.
• It alleviates joint and muscle pain, as well as helping arthritis, rheumatism, and gout.
• Useful for bronchitis, asthma, coughs, and nasal and sinus congestion.
• Camphor reduces kapha and vátha, and it increases pitta when used in excess.

Notes and Dosages
The camphor tree is a large evergreen grown in warm regions. The twigs and the leaves are used. Both have a strong camphor smell. Make sure that you purchase camphor that has been steam-distilled from natural sources. Use as a massage oil, compress, salve, steam inhalation, and in lotions. Camphor blends with rosemary, eucalyptus, and juniper.

RECIPE

Camphor Inhalation
For bronchitis and colds, try a camphor inhalation. Half-fill an enamel pan or heatproof dish with just-boiled water. Add 7 drops of oil of camphor. Use a towel to form a "tent" over the bowl. Inhale deeply for several minutes. Stop if you feel dizzy or if the steam is too hot for your skin.

CAUTION
Use camphor in small doses only.

Cinnamomum cassia
GUI ZHI

Gui Zhi belongs to a group of warm, acrid herbs that are used in traditional Chinese medicine to help illnesses caused by viruses, with symptoms in the skin or muscle layers. These herbs mainly cause sweating, or stop sweating where necessary.

DATA FILE

Properties
• Sweet • Warm

Uses
• Use for colds and flu, commonly in combination with Bai Shao, when there is too much sweating and the patient is becoming weak.
• Warms the meridians, helping conditions such as rheumatism and gynecological problems such as menstrual cramps or irregular menstruation caused by cold obstructing the blood.
• Use for water retention (edema) from cold, where poor circulation of yang qi has failed to move the fluids in the body.
• Use with licorice (Gan Cao) to strengthen the heart yang in cases of palpitations and shortness of breath.

Notes and Dosages
Gui Zhi is prepared from the twigs of the evergreen Chinese cinnamon tree.

> **CAUTION**
> Contraindicated in warm diseases, either from fever, deficient yin with heat signs or heat in the blood with vomiting.

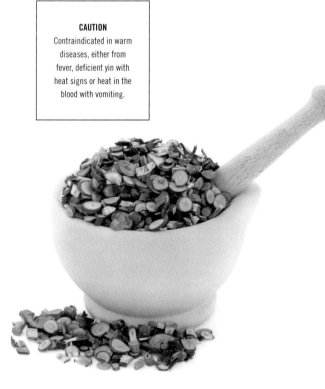

Cinnamomum zeylanicum
CINNAMON

Ancient Ayurvedic practitioners used cinnamon as a treatment for fevers, diarrhea, and to mask unpleasant flavors in other healing herbs. The Greeks used cinnamon to treat bronchitis, but the Europeans championed the use of cinnamon in baking. Oil made from cinnamon leaves is used in aromatherapy.

DATA FILE

Properties
• Pungent • Sweet • Astringent • Stimulating • Heating
• Antispasmodic • Aphrodisiac • Analgesic • Diuretic • Antiseptic
• Antibacterial • Antifungal • Parasiticide

Uses
• Take for respiratory ailments such as colds, sinus congestion, and bronchitis.
• As a digestive aid, it relieves dyspepsia, intestinal infections, and parasites.
• Aids circulation and helps to alleviate anemia, particularly during the menopause.
• Helps in the treatment of scabies and lice.
• Increases the appetite – both sexual and gastronomic.
• Powdered cinnamon can be used for its antibacterial effect on minor scrapes and cuts.
• Cinnamon leaf oil can relieve mental fatigue, improve poor concentration and nervous exhaustion, and help to lift depression.
• In Ayurveda, cinnamon reduces vátha and kapha, and increases pitta.

Notes and Dosages
Cinnamon can be taken as a tea, spice, inhalant, massage oil, or powder. The bark and leaf are used for Ayurvedic remedies, but only the leaf should be used for the aromatherapy oil. Use cinnamon leaf oil only in a 1 percent dilution, and in moderation.

RECIPE

Cinnamon Room Freshener
Sprinkle a few drops of cinnamon leaf oil on rolled cinnamon sticks and add to potpourri made from dried orange peel, orange oil, and basil for a room freshener that stimulates and refreshes the mind, relieves tension, and soothes the nerves.

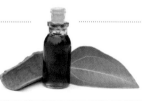

> **CAUTION**
> Cinnamon bark oil is irritant and should not be used on the skin: only use cinnamon leaf for aromatherapy. However, cinnamon leaf may also cause skin irritation. Cinnamon will aggravate bleeding, and can be a convulsive in high doses. Cinnamon infusions should not be given to children under two.

Citrullus colocynthis

COLOCYNTHIS

In the past, the bitter apple, as it is also known, was used by Arab and ancient Greek physicians to induce abortion, and to treat derangement, lethargy, and dropsy. When the whole fruit is eaten, it causes bowel inflammation and cramping pains. Homeopathically, the fruit is dried and powdered, without the seeds.

DATA FILE

Properties
• Aids digestion • Analgesic

Uses
• May treat digestive complaints and colic.
• May treat symptoms brought on by suppressed anger, such as neuralgia, abdominal pain, and headaches.
• May help gout, sciatica, and rheumatism.

Notes and Dosages
Coloc. may be suitable for those whose symptoms improve in the warmth, after flatulence, or drinking coffee, but worsen after eating, when indignant or angry, and in damp, cold weather.

Citrus aurantifolia

LIME

Limes were traditionally used as a digestive remedy and to prevent scurvy among sailors. Lime has a fairly wide application in modern aromatherapy. It has properties similar to those of lemon, and the two oils are often used interchangeably.

DATA FILE

Properties
• Digestive stimulant • Tonic • Boosts immunity • Fever-reducing • Antiseptic • Antiviral • Antibacterial

Uses
• Valuable in fighting colds, flu, fever, and chest and throat infections.
• Boosts the immune system.
• Stimulates the appetite and helps to treat the symptoms of dyspepsia.
• Helps oily skin and conditions such as acne, boils, and warts.
• May help in the treatment of rheumatism.
• Restores and increases mental alertness and assertiveness.

Notes and Dosages
Lime is a small evergreen tree, up to 15ft. (4.5m.) tall, with stiff, sharp spines, smooth ovate leaves, and small white flowers. The pale green fruit is the size of a small lemon. Lime essential oil is expressed from the peel of the fruit, or steam-distilled from the whole fruit. Lime blends well with lavender, rosemary, clary sage, black pepper, bergamot, and other citrus oils.

RECIPE

Stay-Alert Diffuser Blend
Fill the dish of a pottery burner with water and add 4 drops lime, 2 drops black pepper, and 2 drops peppermint. Light the nightlight and let the heat diffuse the oil into the air.

CAUTION
Lime increases the skin's sensitivity to sunlight. Do not apply to the skin within two days of exposure to sunlight.

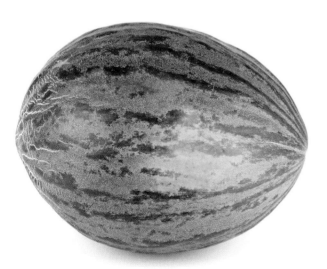

Citrus aurantium var. amara, Citrus sinensis

ORANGE

Originally from China, oranges have a history of use in traditional Chinese medicine. Dried sweet orange is used to treat coughs and colds, while bitter orange is used to treat diarrhea. The outer peel of both bitter (*Citrus aurantium var. amara*) and sweet oranges (*Citrus sinensis*) is pressed to produce the sweet, fruity orange essential oil.

DATA FILE

Properties
• Cheering • Stimulating • Warming

Uses
• Good for nervous tension and related insomnia, either blended with lavender, or alternated with lavender or sandalwood.
• Enlivens the mind and dispels depression.
• Beneficial for painful spasms, constipation, and diarrhea.
• Fights chills, bronchitis, colds, and flu, especially when mixed with complementary winter spice oils such as cinnamon and clove.

Notes and Dosages
Both bitter and sweet orange trees are evergreen, but the sweet variety is more hardy. Sweet oranges are larger and lighter in color than bitter oranges. Orange essential oil blends well with lavender, ylang ylang, neroli, cinnamon, black pepper, clary sage, lemon, myrrh, cinnamon, and clove

RECIPE

Massage Blend for Constipation
Mix 3 drops orange, 3 drops black pepper, 4 drops rosemary, and 3 teaspoons (15ml.) sweet almond or grapeseed oil. Warm a little oil in the hands, then massage into the abdomen clockwise.

CAUTION
Orange oil can increase skin sensitivity to the sun and may cause contact dermatitis in some people. Do not use more than four drops in the bath.

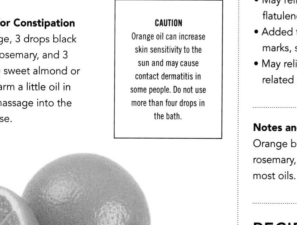

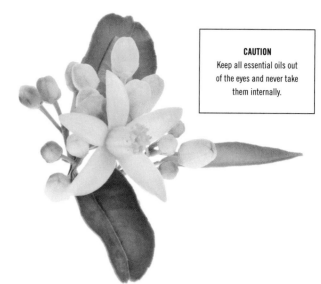

CAUTION
Keep all essential oils out of the eyes and never take them internally.

Citrus aurantium var. amara

NEROLI

The blossoms of the bitter orange tree yield this oil, also called orange blossom, which has an exquisite fragrance. Neroli is named after an Italian princess, Anne-Marie of Nerola, who used it as a perfume. In folk traditions, orange flowers were included in bridal bouquets as a symbol of innocence and fertility, and to calm nervous couples on their wedding night.

DATA FILE

Properties
• Tonic • Carminative • Antispasmodic • Soothing

Uses
• May relieve digestive problems such as indigestion, diarrhea, flatulence, and stomach cramps.
• Added to cream or diluted in oil, neroli is used to prevent stretch marks, scarring, and wrinkles, and to soothe sensitive skin.
• May relieve anxiety, depression, nervous tension, and stress-related problems.

Notes and Dosages
Orange blossom oil blends well with lavender, lemon, bergamot, rosemary, rose, ylang ylang, chamomile, geranium, benzoin, and most oils.

RECIPE

Massage Blend for High Blood Pressure
Add 3 drops neroli, 3 drops celery, 4 drops rose to 1fl.oz. (25ml.) or 5 teaspoons grapeseed or other vegetable oil. Use for gentle massage.

Citrus aurantium var. amara

PETITGRAIN

Petitgrain is often regarded as a cheaper alternative to neroli. It is distilled from the leaves and twigs of the bitter orange tree, whereas neroli comes from the blossom. Both oils have similar properties and fragrances, but petitgrain is also a valuable oil in its own right.

DATA FILE

Properties
• Revitalizing • Restorative • Antispasmodic • Antiseptic

Uses
• Petitgrain can refresh or relax, depending on which oils it is blended with.
• Soothes many stress-related problems, such as anxiety, nervous exhaustion, and insomnia.
• Feelings of being "rundown," apathy, mild depression, loneliness, and pessimism can all get a lift from petitgrain's antidepressant properties.
• Helps to tone the digestive system, relieving flatulence and indigestion.
• Acts as a deodorant, and is sometimes used to control excessive perspiration.
• Controls the overproduction of sebum in the skin and has gentle antiseptic properties, making it ideal for acne and greasy hair.

Notes and Dosages
Petitgrain blends well with lavender, geranium, bergamot, jasmine, clove, palmarosa, clary sage, and other orange oils.

RECIPE

Invigorating Room Fragrancer
Add 3 drops petitgrain, 3 drops lime, and 2 drops cypress to a vaporizer dish filled with water. Light and burn for 10–15 minutes.

> **CAUTION**
> Keep out of the reach of children.

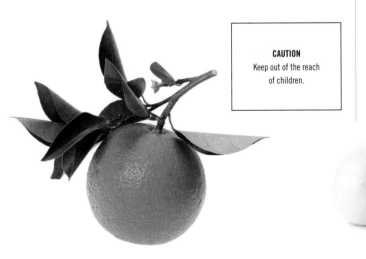

Citrus bergamia

BERGAMOT

The bergamot tree was originally cultivated in Italy, where the fruit has a history of use in folk medicine. The refreshing essential oil is expressed from the peel of the fruit, which resembles a small yellow orange when it is ripe. Outside Italy, bergamot is perhaps best known as an ingredient in Earl Grey tea and eau de Cologne.

DATA FILE

Properties
• Antidepressant • Antiseptic • Antiviral • Repels insects

Uses
• Joyous and uplifting, bergamot is a powerful antidepressant.
• Use for acne, boils, oily skin, eczema, psoriasis, cuts, and insect bites.
• Dilute in alcohol then dab on cold sores, chicken pox, and shingles.
• The fragrance repels insects and the oil can be used to expel worms.
• Use as a wash for cystitis, thrush, and other types of vaginal itching and discharge.

Notes and Dosages
Bergamot blends well with chamomile, geranium, lemon, sandalwood, myrrh, juniper, lavender, neroli, cypress, jasmine, and tea tree.

RECIPE

Bergamot Wash for Cystitis Relief
Cystitis is a bacterial infection causing inflammation of the bladder. This soothing wash will ease the characteristic burning sensation that occurs while urinating. You can also use absorbent cotton soaked in the solution to swab the opening of the urethra after passing urine.

Add 3 drops bergamot, 3 drops lavender, 3 drops niaouli to a warm bath and soak for at least 10 minutes, or fill a bowl that is big enough to sit in with lukewarm water and add 1 drop of each oil. Agitate the water thoroughly with your hand to disperse the oil.

> **CAUTION**
> Bergamot increases the skin's sensitivity to sunlight. Never use undiluted on the skin, and avoid it if you have sensitive skin. Mix with a carrier oil before adding to bath water to ensure it disperses well in the water.

Citrus limon

LEMON

The ancient Greeks and Romans included lemon in their medicine chest and it has a history of use in European folk medicine. The essential oil, which is expressed from the fresh peel, has many applications, making it invaluable in the home aromatherapy kit.

DATA FILE

Properties
• Refreshing • Boosts immune system • Tonic • Diuretic • Laxative • Astringent • Antacid • Antifungal

Uses
• Lemon can stimulate the body's defenses to fight all kinds of infection, to remove warts and verrucas, and to clear herpes blisters.
• Use on cuts and grazes to stop bleeding.
• Apply pure lemon juice to a wasp sting to relieve the pain.
• Have a lemon drink before going to bed to relieve cramp and "restless legs" syndrome.
• A drop of lemon juice several times a day will benefit cold sores, ulcers on the tongue and in the mouth.
• Lemon juice taken in hot water will ease stomach acidity.
• Lemon may help with the symptoms of colds, flu, and bronchitis.
• Drinking lemon juice mixed with olive oil may help to dissolve gallstones.
• Regular intake of fresh lemons may be useful in the treatment of hemorrhoids, kidney stones, and varicose veins.
• Massaging with lemon oil benefits circulation and is often used to treat varicose veins, high blood pressure, and fluid retention.
• Lemon oil may benefit greasy skin.
• The scent of lemon essential oil dispels depression and indecision.

Notes and Dosages
For a lemon drink, boil 3 sliced lemons in 1pt. (600ml.) water, until the liquid is reduced by half. Add honey to taste.

Lemon essential oil is expressed from the peel of the fresh fruit. It blends well with geranium, fennel, juniper, eucalyptus, sandalwood, frankincense, chamomile, lavender, ylang ylang, rose, neroli, and other citrus oils.

RECIPE

Hangover Bath Oil
Add 4 drops lemon oil, 2 drops fennel, and 2 drops lavender to a warm bath and agitate the water with your hand. Relax for 10 minutes and inhale deeply.

CAUTION

Lemon essential oil can irritate sensitive skin. Do not use before sunbathing. Dilute well for massage and bath blends, and do not use for more than a few days at a time.

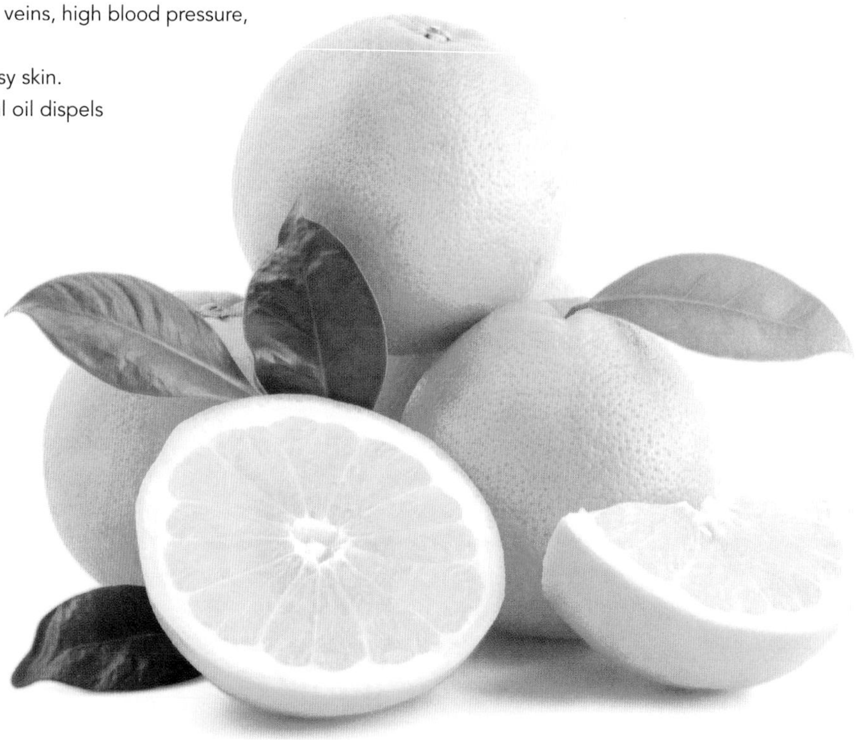

Citrus reticulata
MANDARIN

The mandarin tree was brought to Europe in 1805 and to the U.S. 40 years later, where it was renamed tangerine. The essential oil is expressed from the peel. It has a delicate, fruity, floral aroma and a gentle healing action. In traditional Chinese medicine, Chen Pi, or "tangerine peel," regulates and invigorates the qi when it becomes stagnant.

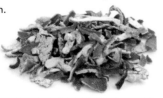

DATA FILE

Properties
• Antispasmodic • Soothes indigestion • Mildly laxative
• Mildly diuretic • Soothing

Uses
• Chen Pi is given for symptoms like abdominal bloating, belching, nausea, and vomiting.
• Tones the liver, the body's main chemical processing and elimination organ.
• Relieves fluid retention and stored toxins.
• Mandarin oil can be used as a skin toner for oily skin, acne, or congested pores.
• The oil's scent relieves nervous tension and insomnia during pregnancy, and can help to settle restless children.

Notes and Dosages
Chen Pi is a very important herb as it "awakens the spleen." It is for stagnant qi patterns and is used for disorders affecting both the spleen and the lungs. It is particularly important for putting into tonifying prescriptions to make them more digestible.

Mandarin oil blends well with frankincense, chamomile, lavender, rosewood, neroli, and other citrus oils and spice oils, such as clove and cinnamon.

RECIPE

Oil to Prevent Stretch Marks
Add 4 drops mandarin, 3 drops neroli, and 3 drops lavender to a bottle containing 1fl.oz. (25ml.) or 5 teaspoonfuls of sweet almond oil and 1 teaspoonful of wheat germ oil. Massage into the abdomen twice a day from the fifth month of pregnancy.

> **CAUTION**
> Mandarin oil may increase the skin's sensitivity to the sun. Chen Pi is contraindicated in dry coughs due to yin or qi deficiency, as it is drying (fragrant) and warm. Use with caution with a red tongue or yellow phlegm (symptoms of heat).

Citrus x paradisi
GRAPEFRUIT

Like all citrus fruit, grapefruit is rich in vitamin C and potassium. Pink grapefruit is rich in vitamin A, and acts as a natural antioxidant. Grapefruit is an excellent cleanser for the digestive and urinary systems. Refreshing grapefruit oil is expressed from the peel of the fruit. It has a fresh, tangy citrus scent that disperses feelings of gloom. Unlike many citrus oils, grapefruit does not increase the skin's sensitivity to sunlight.

DATA FILE

Properties
• Diuretic • Detoxifying • Tonic • Stimulates digestion
• Boosts the immune system • Antidepressant

Uses
• Fresh grapefruit relieves symptoms of colds and flu.
• Eat grapefruit seeds to rid the body of worms.
• Grapefruit pith and membranes lower cholesterol in the blood.
• Drinking grapefruit juice can encourage healthy skin, cleanse the kidneys, and eliminate toxins.
• Drinking grapefruit juice with iron supplements or foods rich in iron increases the absorption of iron in the body.
• Massage with grapefruit oil is invigorating and uplifting, and may help to treat depression. It also stimulates the immune system, which is particularly useful when suffering from infections.
• After exercise, massage with grapefruit oil to ease stiff muscles.
• Local massage, with a few drops of essential oil blended in a carrier oil, will relieve the severity of a headache.
• Used in steam inhalation or burnt in a room, grapefruit oil is beneficial in the treatment of colds, flu, and respiratory problems.

Notes and Dosages
Grapefruit oil blends well with orange, lemon, sandalwood, bergamot, neroli, lavender, cypress, rosemary, geranium, juniper, cardamom, coriander, and other spice oils.

RECIPE

Wake-Up Shower Gel
Mix 2 drops grapefruit essential oil, 2 drops petitgrain, and 1 drop rosemary with a dollop of unscented shower gel and work to a lather with a sponge.

> **CAUTION**
> Do not take grapefruit essential oil internally. Keep out of the eyes.

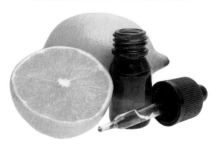

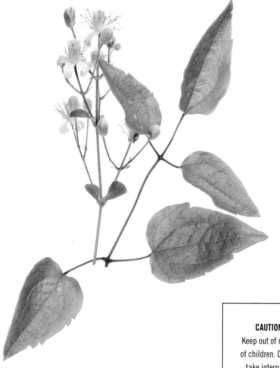

Codonopsis pilosula
CODONOPSIS

This sprawling herb with yellow, bell-shaped flowers is called codonopsis root in Western medicine and Dang Shen in traditional Chinese medicine. It is similar to Ren Shen: it treats qi deficiency, affecting primarily the lungs and spleen (the main digestive organ in TCM).

DATA FILE

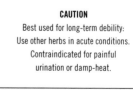

Properties
• Sweet • Neutral • Soothing • Strengthening
• Boosts the immune system

Uses
• Use for general debility, exhaustion, weakness, and lack of appetite.
• May be useful for digestive difficulties and chronic diarrhea.
• Take for chronic coughs, asthma, and shortness of breath.
• May alleviate excessive perspiration.

Notes and Dosages
Take 1oz. (25g.) of the powder daily, sprinkled onto soups or made into a decoction. In traditional Chinese medicine, Dang Shen does basically the same work as Ren Shen, but is not as strong. In prescriptions it is used in place of ginseng to tonify the qi of the spleen and lungs, while ginseng is preferred for more serious situations, such as a patient who is barely conscious.

RECIPE

Soup of the "Four Gentlemen"
This is a famous traditional Chinese digestive and energy tonic. It is made from codonopsis, white atractylodes (Bai Zhu), Chinese angelica (Dang Gui), poria (Fu Ling), and licorice. Add 1oz. (25g.) of the herb mixture to 1pt. (500ml.) of water. Simmer for 15 minutes, strain, and drink daily.

> **CAUTION**
> Best used for long-term debility:
> Use other herbs in acute conditions.
> Contraindicated for painful
> urination or damp-heat.

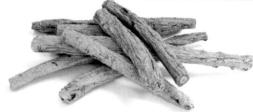

> **CAUTION**
> Keep out of reach
> of children. Do not
> take internally.

Clematis vitalba
CLEMATIS

The wild clematis is a rambling, perennial climber of woods and country hedges. Its common name is travelers' joy, and it bursts forth with a mass of beautiful flowers.

DATA FILE

Properties
• Grounding • Wakening

Uses
• For those who are dreamy and prefer to live in the mind or the spirit, rather than deal with contemporary issues and the mundane functions of everyday life. They tend to be airy and impractical individuals, the typical "mad professor." They may forget to eat, and experience faintness and tiredness.
• Clematis encourages feeling grounded in the body and in the present.
• If children resort to daydreaming as an escape, clematis may be useful, but the child should be questioned to find the underlying cause.

Notes and Dosages
Wild clematis, also called travelers' joy or old man's beard, is a poisonous plant and must be used carefully. Use the sun method (see page 56) to prepare the flowers.

Coffea arabica
COFFEA

Coffee has been used widely for medicinal purposes as a diuretic, painkiller, and to ease indigestion. It is also a well-known stimulant. Homeopathically, coffea is made from the raw berries of the coffee tree and is mainly used to treat those who are excitable and mentally overstimulated.

DATA FILE

Properties
• Calming

Uses
• May be useful for irritability and anxiety leading to restlessness.
• Eases heightened senses and a mind buzzing with ideas.
• For physical symptoms caused by anger and irritability, such as trembling limbs, palpitations, and headaches.
• May ease acute premenstrual symptoms.

Notes and Dosages
Symptoms that might be treated by coffea may appear after a failed relationship, and with exhaustion or after a trauma.

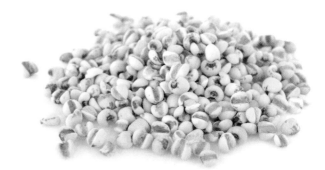

> **CAUTION**
> Use with caution during pregnancy.

Coix lachryma-jobi
YI YI REN

Also known as seeds of Job's tears, this is one of the Chinese herbs that transforms dampness, but it is more active on the lower burner than the middle burner.

DATA FILE

Properties
• Sweet • Bland • Slightly cold

Uses
• Promotes urination and leeches out dampness, so is helpful for edema or water retention in the legs.
• Clears wind dampness, making it useful for arthritic conditions.
• Pushes pus out when sores have become full.
• Strengthens the spleen and stops diarrhea.

Notes and Dosages
Like Fu Ling, Yi Yi Ren clears dampness by promoting urination, but its spleen-strengthening function is not as strong, and it works more on the lower burner (kidneys) than on the middle burner (spleen and stomach).

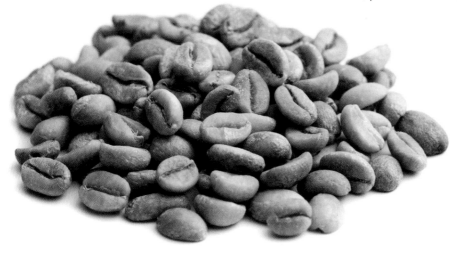

Commiphora myrrha
MYRRH

Known as "bola" in Ayurvedic practice, myrrh is the gum from a shrub native to northeast Africa and southwest Asia. It has been used for thousands of years for its healing properties. In the Bible, myrrh was one of the gifts the wise men brought to the Christ child. Essential oil of myrrh has a musty, balsamic odor and is closely related to frankincense, with which it is often linked.

DATA FILE

Properties
- Alterative • Analgesic • Rejuvenating • Astringent • Expectorant
- Antispasmodic •Antiseptic • Tonic

Uses
- Myrrh is a treatment for amenorrhea, menstrual cramps, and menopause.
- It helps sore throat, coughs, asthma, and bronchitis.
- Use a gargle for halitosis, gum disease, and mouth ulcers. Myrrh oil can also be used directly on sore gums.
- Massage with myrrh for arthritis and rheumatism.
- Its antiseptic and antifungal qualities suit myrrh to cleaning wounds, being used as a vaginal wash for thrush, or in a foot bath for athlete's foot.
- It can speed the healing of weepy eczema.
- In Ayurveda, myrrh reduces kapha and vátha, while increasing pitta.
- The essential oil relieves agitation, calms fears, and has a positive, balancing effect on the emotions.

Notes and Dosages
The sap or gum is used. Myrrh exudes from natural cracks or man-made incisions in the bark of *Commiphora myrrha*. It leaves the tree as a pale yellow liquid, which hardens into a yellowish-red or reddish-brown substance, which is collected for use. Myrrh can be used as a lotion or salve, a massage oil, an incense, poultice, gargle, or infusion. In Ayurvedic treatment, myrrh can be mixed with frankincense, juniper, cypress, geranium, aloe, and pine.

The essential oil blends well with frankincense, sandalwood, mandarin, lavender, lemon, rose, eucalyptus, thyme, benzoin, geranium, peppermint, cypress, pine, and spice oils.

RECIPES

Myrrh Gargle
Mix 1 teaspoon of myrrh and 1 teaspoon of boric acid in 1pt. (500ml.) of boiling water. Stand for 30 minutes, then strain. Reheat and gargle. Do not swallow. Add 1 teaspoon of golden seal to cure bad breath.

Chapped Skin Cream
Add 5 drops myrrh, 5 drops benzoin, and 4 drops geranium to 1oz. (30g.) of good unperfumed, lanolin-free cream. Mix well and apply to the skin.

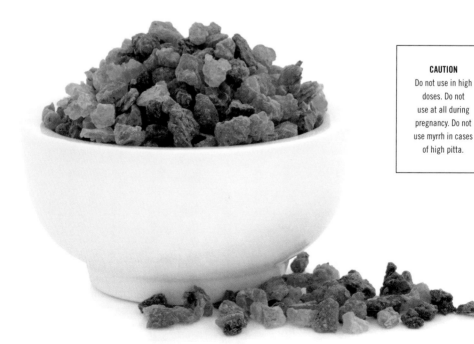

CAUTION
Do not use in high doses. Do not use at all during pregnancy. Do not use myrrh in cases of high pitta.

Coptis chinensis

HUANG LIAN

In traditional Chinese medicine, this herb clears heat, including febrile conditions and illnesses with heat signs. It is one of the "Three Yellows," which are used together for severe infections.

DATA FILE

Properties
• Bitter • Cold

Uses
• Helps sore throats.
• A decoction may be placed on sore, red eyes, boils, and anal fissures, and used locally it is very good for treating trichomoniasis, a protozoan infection of the vagina.
• Clears heat and drains dampness, especially in the stomach and intestines, including diarrhea, acid regurgitation, vomiting, and digestive dysfunction leading to bad breath and belching.
• Clears heart fire causing symptoms such as irritability and insomnia.
• Use topically for red mouth ulcers, boils, and abscesses.

Notes and Dosages
Huang Lian works in the heart, liver, stomach and large intestine channels.

> **CAUTION**
> Do not use for deficient yin patterns, where the fluid may be deficient anyway, as Huang Lian would dry it out more. Like all the clearing heat herbs, it is cold in energy, so it is contraindicated in any diseases caused by cold.

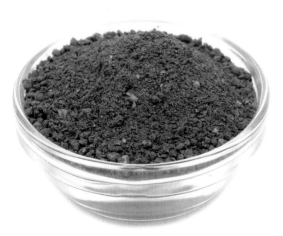

Coriandrum sativum

CORIANDER

Known as "dhanyaka" or "dhania" to the Ayurvedics, coriander is a highly aromatic annual herb. The seeds and leaves are both used in cooking, and the Ayurvedics use the whole herb for medicinal purposes. The essential oil, distilled from the crushed seeds, has a sweet and slightly musky, spicy, and woody aroma.

DATA FILE

Properties
• Pungent • Cooling • Moisturizing • Stimulant • Alterative
• Diuretic • Aphrodisiac

Uses
• Coriander is beneficial for respiratory problems and eases allergies and hay fever.
• Alleviates urinary infections, cystitis, rashes, hives, burns.
• Helps digestive disorders such as gas pains, vomiting, and indigestion.
• Purifies the blood, decongests the liver, and reduces heat and fever in the body.
• As an anti-inflammatory, coriander benefits arthritis.
• Coriander powder can be sprinkled on cuts and scrapes to prevent infection.
• Coriander essential oil is an aphrodisiac which has a warming, stimulatory effect on the emotions.
• For a rub for tired muscles, blend with juniper and black pepper.
• In Ayurveda, coriander reduces all three doshas.

Notes and Dosages
Coriander can be used as a spice, a tea or infusion, a compress, douche, shampoo, and massage oil. In Ayurveda it can be used with lemon, cajeput, lavender, cardamom, clove, nutmeg, jasmine, sandalwood, and cypress.

RECIPE

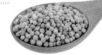

Coriander Infusion
The infusion makes an excellent digestive aid. Bruise 1 teaspoon of the seeds (or use ½ teaspoon of the powder). Place in a cup, and add 1 cup of boiling water. Let steep for 5 minutes. Drink up to 3 cups a day after meals. This same infusion, at half-strength, may be given, with caution, to children under two years of age for colic.

> **CAUTION**
> During pregnancy, use only under recommendation from your physician. In high doses, coriander may cause kidney irritation. Keep all essential oils out of the reach of children.

Cornus officinalis

SHAN ZHU YU

In traditional Chinese medicine, Shan Zhu Yu stabilizes and binds. It is sour and astringent, and helps keep in bodily substances that may leak, such as urine.

DATA FILE

Properties
• Sour • Slightly warm

Uses
• Use for leakage of fluids due to weak jing-essence, with symptoms such as excessive urination, incontinence, spermatorrhea, and premature ejaculation.
• Firms, tonifies and builds the liver and kidneys.
• Absorbs sweating.
• Use for devastated yang and qi, as in cases of shock.
• Stabilizes the menses and stops excessive bleeding, if the cause is deficiency.

Notes and Dosages
Shan Zhu Yu is the fruit of the dogwood, also called the cornelian cherry. It enters the kidneys, where jing is stored. It is one of the six herbs in the basic yin-tonifying prescription Liu Wei di Huang Wan ("Six Flavor"), so if carefully combined it may tonify yin or yang.

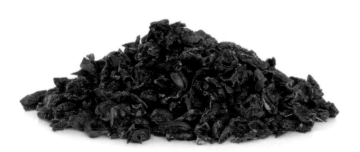

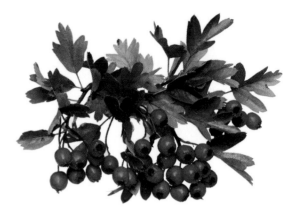

Crataegus monogyna

HAWTHORN

In herbalism, the berries and flowering tops of the common hawthorn tree are used to strengthen the heart. Hawthorn's genus name, *Cretaegus*, comes from Greek words meaning hard and sharp.

DATA FILE

Properties
• Strengthens the heart • Lowers blood pressure • Relaxes arteries

Uses
• May be useful for heart failure or an irregular heartbeat.
• May be helpful for angina and high blood pressure, as part of an overall strategy.
• Take with nervine herbs, such as valerian and linden, for anxiety with palpitations.
• Hawthorn berries can be used in a decoction for a sore throat.

Notes and Dosages
Take standard doses (see pages 39 and 41). Make a tea of the flowering tops or a decoction of the berries. For a tincture, take 1 teaspoon in a little water twice daily. For heart disease, take this dosage for at least 6 months.

RECIPE

Hawthorn Brandy
This is the nicest way of taking hawthorn as a heart-strengthening tonic. Pick the flowering shoots (with flowers and leaves), wash, dry, and pack into a large jar. Cover with brandy and leave in a cool place for two weeks. Strain off the liquid, bottle, and label. Take 2 dessertspoons daily.

CAUTION
Always seek advice from a qualified medical practitioner. If you are taking drugs for heart problems, seek professional advice before taking any herbal medicine.

Crataegus pinnatifida

SHAN ZHA

The mountain or Chinese hawthorn is used in traditional Chinese medicine to relieve digestive problems resulting from over-indulgence in greasy foods, and helps to promote efficient digestion by increasing gastrointestinal secretions and enzymatic functions.

DATA FILE

Properties
• Sour • Sweet • Slightly warm • Astringent • Unblocking

Uses
• Reduces digestive stagnation and obstruction brought on by meat or greasy foods, causing abdominal distension, belching, pain, and reduced appetite.
• Indicated for postnatal abdominal pain and menstrual pain when the cause is congealed blood.
• May help hernias with testicular pain and swelling.
• When the herb is slightly charred, helps to stop diarrhea.
• May help hypertension (high blood pressure), coronary artery disease, and high cholesterol.
• May be used for children who fail to thrive.

Notes and Dosages
This herb works through the liver, spleen, and stomach channels.

> **CAUTION**
> Use with caution in cases of spleen and stomach deficiency without food stagnation, and in diseases with acid regurgitation.

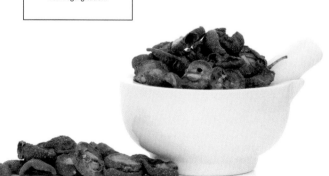

Crocus sativus

SAFFRON

Known as "kesar" or "nagakeshara" in Ayurveda, saffron is a small, perennial crocus with purple flowers. When the plant matures, it produces flowers with golden stigmas, which are quite expensive to harvest. The stigmas, or threads, are highly valued for their medicinal and aphrodisiac properties, as well as their delicious flavor.

DATA FILE

Properties
• Balancing • Warming • Digestive • Aphrodisiac • Stimulant
• Rejuvenating • Antispasmodic • Expectorant • Emmenagogue

Uses
• Aids digestion and improves appetite, helping gastrointestinal complaints such as colic and chronic diarrhea.
• Use for menstrual pain and irregularity, menopause, impotence, and infertility.
• Calms hysteria, depression, and insomnia.
• Take for coughs and asthma.
• Soothes neuralgia, lumbago, and rheumatism.
• May help cases of anemia and enlarged liver.

Notes and Dosages
Whole threads can be taken as a spice, in oils, infusions, and food. When taking internally, do not exceed the amounts recommended below. The oil can be used as a massage oil, a perfume, or a bath. Saffron can be used to balance all three doshas. It can be taken with cedarwood, champa, lavender, rosewood, and sandalwood.

RECIPE

Saffron Infusion
A saffron infusion can be helpful for irregular menstruation and menstrual pains, and may also be taken as an aphrodisiac. Steep 6–10 stigmas in ½ cup of boiling water. Take 1 cup a day, unsweetened.

> **CAUTION**
> Do not use saffron during pregnancy, as it can promote miscarriage. Saffron can be narcotic in large doses: Do not exceed the medicinal amount indicated. A dose of ½oz. (10–12g.) can be fatal.

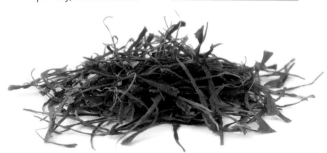

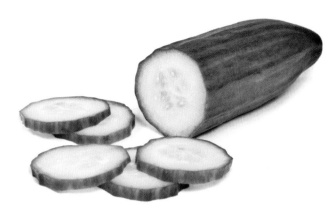

Cucumis sativis
CUCUMBER

The cucumber is a vine fruit that can be eaten fresh or pickled. Cucumbers originated in northwestern India but have long been distributed throughout Asia, Europe, and Africa. Cucumber has been widely used in folk medicine to reduce heat and inflammation.

DATA FILE

Properties
• Diuretic • Cooling • Cleansing • Soothing • Anti-inflammatory

Uses
• To soothe the eyes, lie down for half an hour with a slice of cucumber on each eye.
• Drink cucumber juice or eat fresh cucumber to soothe heartburn or to improve an acid stomach.
• Drink 3–5fl.oz. (100–150ml.) of cucumber juice every two hours for a gastric or duodenal ulcer.
• Apply fresh cucumber or cucumber juice to sunburned skin to cool it down.
• Ground dried cucumber seeds can treat tapeworm.
• Cucumber juice, drunk daily, may help to control eczema, arthritis, and gout.
• Eat fresh cucumber regularly to help skin conditions.
• Use cucumber ointment externally on inflammatory skin conditions.
• Drink cucumber juice to treat lung and chest infections, and to bring down fever.

Notes and Dosages
Taken internally, cucumber is a rich source of vitamin C. Externally, it can be used to cool and cleanse.

Cuminum cyminum
CUMIN

Known as "jeera" in Ayurvedic medicine, cumin seeds are pungent and savory brown seeds with a flavor common to Indian and Middle Eastern cooking. Heating the seeds, by cooking or infusing, aids the digestive power of the cumin. Cumin is very rich in vitamins and minerals, and is an antidote to weakness and fatigue.

DATA FILE

Properties
• Pungent • Bitter • Carminative • Stimulant • Antispasmodic
• Alterative • Lactagogue • Boosts immune system

Uses
• To relieve abdominal pain caused by gas, add the seeds to food.
• Builds up the immune system of people who suffer from severe allergies.
• Helpful for anemia, migraine, and nervous conditions.
• Take for low breast milk.
• Helps with lack of sexual drive.
• Cumin reduces kapha and pitta, and increases vátha.

Notes and Dosages
The seeds may be used in a compress, as a spice and infusion, in massage oil, and as an inhalation. Because of its overpowering smell, use cumin in small amounts when mixing with other herbs. Cumin is frequently used with lemon, black pepper, coriander, lavender, and rosemary.

RECIPE

Cumin Seed Poultice
This poultice is helpful for relieving liver, stomach, and gall bladder pains. First, soak 2 tablespoons of cumin seeds in hot water for 2 hours. Strain, dry, then crush the seeds with a heavy object or pestle and mortar. Add several drops of peppermint oil, a little flour, and some hot water – just enough to make a paste. Mix well. Spread this mixture on a piece of muslin or thin cloth, and apply over the abdomen.

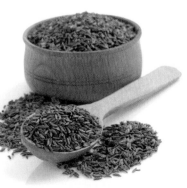

CAUTION
An excess of cumin may cause nausea.

Cupressus sempervirens
CYPRESS

Ancient civilizations used the tall evergreen cypress tree as a source of incense for religious ceremonies and medicinal purposes. The oil, which is distilled from the twigs and needles of the cypress, has a pleasant, smoky, wood aroma, and a number of therapeutic uses in aromatherapy.

DATA FILE

Properties
• Antispasmodic • Astringent • Stops bleeding • Tonic

Uses
• Use in a vaporizer for respiratory problems such as bronchitis or asthma, or to prevent coughing attacks.
• Use in a wash for hemorrhoids and for excessively oily skin.
• Apply to cuts to stop bleeding and use as a mouthwash for bleeding gums.
• Cypress is a circulatory tonic, which can improve poor circulation, relieve fluid retention, and soothe muscular cramp, and can be applied gently to varicose veins.
• Put in a foot bath to counteract excessively sweating and smelly feet.
• Use for premenstrual syndrome, to regulate the menstrual cycle, and to counteract heavy bleeding.
• Alleviates menopausal symptoms such as hot flushes and irritability.

Notes and Dosages
The oil is for external use. It blends well with juniper, pine, lavender, sandalwood, lemon, mandarin, orange, bergamot, and clary sage.

RECIPE

Varicose Vein Toner
Add 5 drops cypress and 10 drops geranium oil to 5 teaspoons (25ml.) of vegetable oil. Starting at the ankle, gently stroke up the legs toward the heart.

> **CAUTION**
> Do not use undiluted on the skin. Do not take internally.

Curcuma longa
TURMERIC

Turmeric, known as "haridra" or "haldi," holds a place of honor in Ayurvedic medicine. It is believed to be a cleanser for all the systems in the body. Turmeric is prescribed as a digestive aid, and a treatment for fever, infections, dysentery, arthritis, and jaundice.

DATA FILE

Properties
• Warming • Pungent • Bitter • Astringent • Stimulant • Alterative
• Carminative • Vulnerary • Antiseptic • Antibacterial

Uses
• Use externally for skin disorders, wounds, and bruises.
• Apply turmeric face cream to spot-prone areas of the skin.
• Take internally for indigestion, poor circulation, coughs, amenorrhea, pharyngitis, diabetes, arthritis, and anemia.
• Because of its energizing effect on the immune system, turmeric is being studied for use in the treatment of HIV and AIDS.
• Reduces kapha and vátha, and increases pitta.

Notes and Dosages
Turmeric roots are used to make these remedies. They have a bright yellow color, and are sometimes used as a dye and a food coloring. The roots may be used in a massage oil, in facial creams and lotions, in compresses, or as a food or spice. Take with ginger, musk, and wild sunflower.

RECIPE

Turmeric Infusion
This infusion benefits digestion, and can help rid the body of intestinal parasites. It also reduces arthritis pain, reduces fat, purifies blood, and aids circulation. Warm 1 cup of milk and remove it from the heat before it boils. Stir in 1 teaspoon of turmeric powder. Drink up to 3 cups a day.

> **CAUTION**
> Do not use in cases of hepatitis, extremely high pitta, or pregnancy. Turmeric is said to reduce fertility, so it would not be recommended for someone trying to conceive.

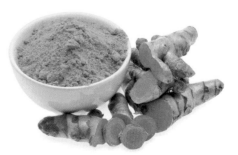

Cuscuta chinensis
TU SU ZI

Also known as Chinese dodder seed, in traditional Chinese medicine this herb tonifies the yang, mainly affecting the kidneys and liver. Kidneys are believed to house the body's reserves, and kidney yang is responsible for sexual and endocrine disorders.

DATA FILE

Properties
• Acrid • Sweet • Neutral • Moistening

Uses
• Stops persistent diarrhea.
• Good for impotence, for nocturnal emissions, and for premature ejaculation.
• Take for frequent urination, incontinence, and vaginal discharge.
• Use for sore lower back and knees.
• May help liver and kidney deficient symptoms as tinnitus (ringing in the ears), dizziness, blurred vision, or spots in front of the eyes, although the advice of a qualified medical practitioner should also be sought for these conditions.

Notes and Dosages
Unlike most kidney yang herbs, which are heating and therefore drying, Tu Su Zi is also moistening, so helps preserve the yin fluid. Use for patterns of deficient liver and kidney yin and yang.

> **CAUTION**
> Although this is a neutral herb, it leans more toward tonifying the yang and should therefore not be used for fire from yin deficiency.

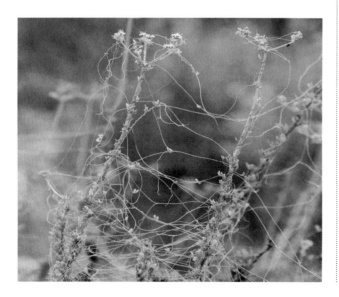

Cymbopogon citratus
LEMONGRASS

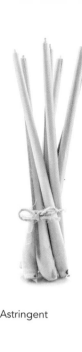

Lemongrass is a tall, aromatic grass. It is used as a flavoring in Thai cuisine and has been used in Ayurvedic medicine for centuries. The essential oil is distilled from the grass leaves. It has a strong, refreshing citrus smell that has many aromatherapy and domestic uses.

DATA FILE

Properties
• Tonic • Painkilling • Antidepressant • Deodorant • Astringent
• Insect repellent • Boosts immune system

Uses
• Use for depression, headaches, lethargy, and symptoms of stress.
• Relieves muscular pain and poor muscle tone.
• Reduces fevers and helps the immune system to fight infections.
• Use as a deodorant for excessive perspiration and sweaty feet.
• Apply as a skin toner to close open pores.
• The oil is an effective flea, lice, and tick repellent.
• Use in a vaporizer to keep flies out of the kitchen in summer and to get rid of pet smells.

Notes and Dosages
The long, thin leaves of lemongrass are the source of its essential oil. This aromatherapy oil blends well with lavender, orange, geranium, jasmine, rosemary, neroli, basil, sandalwood, and eucalyptus.

RECIPE

Greasy Hair Shampoo
Add 2 drops of lemongrass to a dollop of mild, unscented shampoo, rub between your palms, and wash your hair as normal.

> **CAUTION**
> Dilute well, as lemongrass may cause skin irritation in some people. Do not use on babies or children. Do not use around the eyes.

Cymbopogon martinii
PALMAROSA

In Ayurvedic medicine, palmarosa has long been used to combat infectious diseases. Distilled from a fresh scented grass, in the same genus as lemongrass, palmarosa has a gentle floral fragrance like a mix of rose and geranium. In the past it was also known as Indian or Turkish geranium.

DATA FILE

Properties
• Healing • Antiseptic • Antibacterial • Balancing
• Stimulates circulation and digestion

Uses
• Diluted oil applied to the skin rebalances sebum production, hydrating dry skin conditions.
• Rejuvenates wrinkled or aging skin by promoting cellular regeneration.
• Dab diluted oil onto wounds to aid healing.
• Benefits acne, dermatitis, and skin infections.
• Helps to increase appetite and activate a sluggish digestion.
• Prevents and treats intestinal infections.
• Used in a massage blend, palmarosa is good for nervous exhaustion and stress-related problems.

Notes and Dosages
Palmarosa is a perennial plant with long stems and terminal flowering tops. Its essential oil blends well with sandalwood, lavender, geranium, rosewood, cedarwood, frankincense, lemon, floral, citrus oils, and woody oils.

RECIPE

Skin Rejuvenator
Add 6 drops palmarosa, 3 drops rose, and 3 drops frankincense to a small bottle containing 5 drops evening primrose and 3 teaspoons (15ml.) apricot kernel oil. Shake well. Gently massage into the face at night.

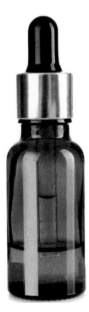

Cymbopogon nardus
CITRONELLA

The leaves of this tropical scented grass are valued in many countries for their medicinal properties. The essential oil, which is distilled from the dried leaves, has a strong, fresh, lemony scent. Although it is not widely used in aromatherapy, it is highly valued as a household disinfectant and insecticide.

DATA FILE

Properties
• Deodorant • Refreshing • Uplifting • Antifungal • Insect repellent
• Digestive

Uses
• Helps to combat headaches, fatigue, and feelings of depression.
• Refreshes tired or sweaty feet, while treating fungal infections such as athlete's foot.
• Use as a rub for rheumatic pain.
• May be used to settle digestion and menstrual problems.
• Makes an excellent insect repellent, used in a room spray, vaporizer, or dropped onto a square of cotton and added to a linen cupboard to keep clothes free from moths.
• Cats dislike the smell of citronella, so it can be used to keep them away from areas of the garden.

Notes and Dosages
This essential oil blends well with geranium, lemon, orange, cedarwood, cypress, tea tree, bergamot, eucalyptus, and pine.

RECIPE

Refreshing Foot Soak
Add 4 drops citronella, 2 drops tea tree, and 3 drops cypress to a foot bath to refresh hot and sweaty feet.

> **CAUTION**
> Do not use during pregnancy. Dilute well, as it may cause irritation to some people with sensitive skin.

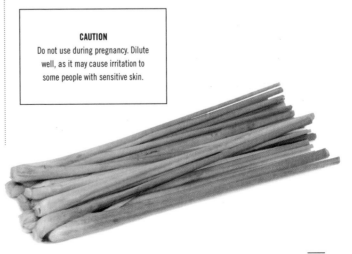

Cyperus rotundus
XIANG FU

In traditional Chinese medicine, the nut-grass rhizome regulates and invigorates the qi when it becomes stuck or "stagnant," optimizing the function of the gastrointestinal tract and helping stop pain in various parts of the body, particularly menstrual and digestive pain.

DATA FILE

Properties
• Acrid • Slightly bitter • Slightly sweet • Neutral • Relieves pain

Uses
• Suitable for pain in the sides, fullness in the epigastrium (above the navel), pain and stuffiness in the chest, lack of appetite, wind and indigestion, as well as vomiting and diarrhea due to liver qi invading the spleen.
• Take for swollen, tender breasts due to premenstrual syndrome.
• Essential in prescriptions for dysmenorrhea (menstrual cramps) or irregular menstruation, by treating liver qi stagnation.

Notes and Dosages
Xiang Fu is a very widely used herb, as it has the ability to disperse stuck liver qi and to harmonize energy, both in digestive and in gynecological disorders.

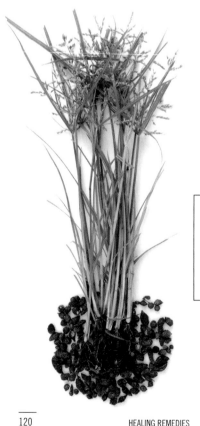

CAUTION
Contraindicated in qi deficiency without stagnation, and in yin deficiency or heat in the blood.

Daucus carota
CARROT

Carrots were first used as medicinal herbs rather than as vegetables, and they have the dual purpose of acting as therapeutic agents, and providing the best source of beta carotene (a form of vitamin A) in the human diet. They are rich in vitamins A, B, C, and E, and the minerals phosphorus, potassium, and calcium. Chinese medical practitioners suggest eating carrots for liver energy.

DATA FILE

Properties
• Energizing • Cleansing • Anti-inflammatory • Antiseptic
• Antibacterial

Uses
• Drink fresh, raw carrot juice daily to energize and cleanse the body. It will help to relieve the effects of stress and fatigue, and boost the body after illness.
• Eating plenty of raw carrots may help in the treatment of eye problems.
• Carrot soup may help infant diarrhea as it soothes the bowel and slows down bacterial growth.
• Raw, grated carrots or cooked, mashed carrots can be applied to wounds, cuts, inflammations, and abscesses to discourage infection and encourage healing.
• Dried carrot powder will restore energy, and can help to treat infections, glandular problems, headaches, or joint problems.
• Taken daily, carrots may help to regulate the menstrual cycle.
• Carrots may help to relieve skin disorders.
• Carrots contain beta carotene, an antioxidant which protects the body against cancer and may help to prevent some of the damage caused by smoking.

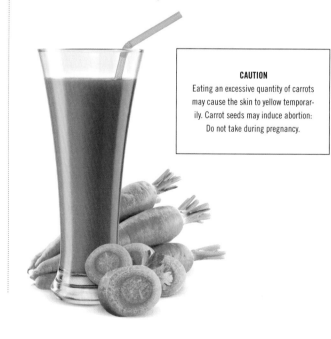

CAUTION
Eating an excessive quantity of carrots may cause the skin to yellow temporarily. Carrot seeds may induce abortion: Do not take during pregnancy.

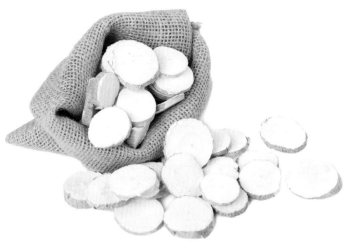

Dioscorea villosa
WILD YAM

The rhizome of the Mexican wild yam is used in Western herbalism as an anti-inflammatory. In addition, wild yams are a key source of dehydroepiandrosterone (DHEA), a hormone that we produce in our adrenal glands.

DATA FILE

Properties
• Anti-inflammatory • Antispasmodic • Tonic

Uses
• Take for stomach cramps, nausea, vomiting, hiccups, recurrent colicky pains, pain of diverticulitis, and gall bladder pains. Add a little ginger for a quicker action.
• Use for menstrual cramps, pain on ovulation, menopausal symptoms, and vaginal dryness.
• Use for the treatment of rheumatoid arthritis.

Notes and Dosages
The plant is dug up in the fall to harvest the root. The dried root retains its medicinal value for up to a year. Wild yam is the starting point for synthesization of hormones for the contraceptive pill and for "natural progesterone," used in a prescription cream for the menopause. When using as a herbal medicine, take standard doses (see page 39).

RECIPE

Decoction for Arthritic Pains
Add 1oz. (25g.) each of wild yam root and willow bark to 3pt. (1.5l.) water. Simmer together for 20 minutes. Strain. The decoction will keep in the refrigerator for two or three days. Take ½ cup 3 times daily, adding honey to taste.

Drosera rotundifolia
DROSERA

The sundew is a carnivorous plant that grows widely in the heaths and boggy areas of Europe, South America, the U.S.A, China, and India. Insects are attracted by the long, red hairs on the leaves of the plant. Glands on the surface of the leaves then secrete a fluid which traps and breaks down the insect, digesting it. The juice of the plant is caustic, affecting the respiratory system, and when eaten by sheep, leads to a harsh, spasmodic cough. Homeopathically, the whole fresh plant is used, mainly to treat coughs.

DATA FILE

Properties
• Relieves coughs

Uses
• Take for coughs characterized by a violent, spasmodic, hollow-sounding cough, triggered by a tickling sensation in the throat.
• May help the uncomfortable tingling sensation associated with growing pains.
• May help with difficulty in concentrating.

Notes and Dosages
May help coughs that worsen after midnight, after cold food and drinking, when lying down, and if the bed is too warm.

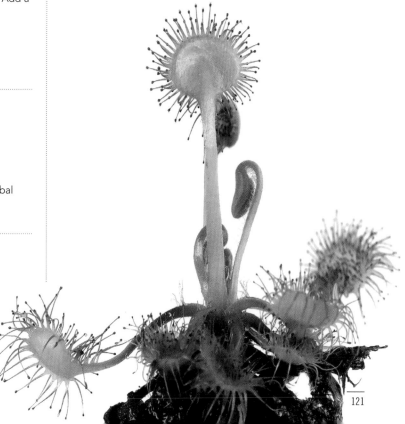

Echinacea angustifolia, Echinacea purpurea

ECHINACEA

Echinacea is a summer-flowering perennial which grows best in the sun. The root of the plant is used in Western herbalism to rid the body of microbial infections and is effective against both bacteria and viruses.

DATA FILE

Properties
• Antiseptic • Stimulates the immune system • Antimicrobial

Uses
• Take regularly for a weak immune system if the patient suffers chronic tiredness and is susceptible to minor infections.
• Take for boils, acne, duodenal ulcers, flu, herpes, and persistent infections.
• Use as a gargle and mouthwash for sore throats, tonsillitis, mouth ulcers, and gum infections.

Notes and Dosages
For acute conditions, take large doses, 1 cup of the decoction or 1 teaspoon of the tincture every 2 hours for 10 days. For chronic conditions, use in combinations and take ½ cup of the combined decoction or 1 teaspoon of the combined tincture, 3 times daily.

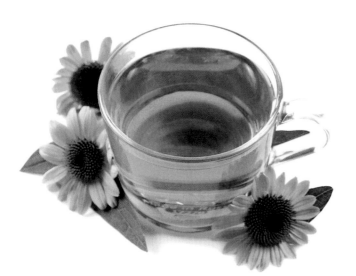

Elettaria cardamonum

CARDAMOM

Known as "elaichi" in Ayurvedic practice, cardamom is a stimulating plant that eases the brain, and the respiratory and digestive systems. Its sweet, warming energy brings joy and clarity to the mind, and is particularly good for opening the flow of prana, or vital energy, through the body. In aromatherapy, the essential oil has a warm, sweet, spicy aroma and a warming quality similar to ginger.

DATA FILE

Properties
• Pungent • Sweet • Heating • Stimulant • Expectorant
• Diaphoretic • Aphrodisiac • Diuretic

Uses
• Aids respiratory problems such as coughs, colds, bronchitis, asthma, and loss of voice.
• Benefits the digestive system in cases of belching, acid regurgitation, and indigestion.
• Suppresses vomiting when eaten with a banana.
• Cardamom's stimulating effects bring mental clarity and good humor.
• Added to milk, cardamom will neutralize mucus-forming properties; added to coffee, it neutralizes the caffeine.
• The essential oil makes a refreshing bath which can relieve fatigue and soothe strained nerves.
• For a massage oil for stomach cramps, add 1 drop cardamom, 1 drop basil, 2 drops marjoram to 2 teaspoons (10ml.) vegetable oil and massage in a clockwise direction.
• In Ayurveda, cardamom reduces kapha and vátha, and stimulates pitta.

Notes and Dosages
Cardamom is a reedlike herb with long, blade-shaped leaves and yellowish flowers with purple tips, ripening into oblong seed pods. The seeds and root are used in Ayurvedic practice, while the aromatherapy essential oil is distilled from the seeds. Cardamom can be taken as a tea, as an additive to milk and food, as a bath, inhalation, or massage oil. The essential oil should not be taken internally. In Ayurveda, cardamom blends well with orange, anise, caraway, ginger, and coriander. In aromatherapy, the essential oil blends well with bergamot, rose, frankincense, clove, ylang ylang, neroli, basil, cedarwood, fennel, lemon, and ginger.

> **CAUTION**
> Do not take the essential oil internally. Use it sparingly, as spicy oils may cause irritation in some people. Do not take cardamom internally if you have ulcers, or in high pitta states.

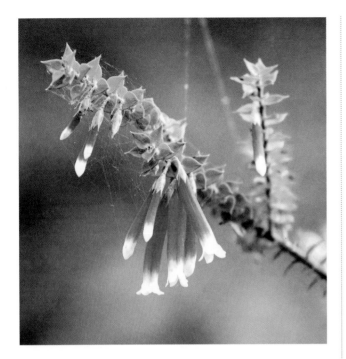

Epacris longiflora
BUSH FUCHSIA

A low, straggly shrub, bush fuchsia flowers throughout the year with bright red, elongated, bell-like flowers hanging in a row from the stem. The leaves are small and heart-shaped. The plant needs full sun.

DATA FILE

Properties
• Balances the left and right sides of the brain • Boosts confidence

Uses
• Balances the rational left side and creative right side of the brain so they can be expressed with confidence.
• Useful for children with dyslexia and learning difficulties, or difficulties translating marks from the page (words, symbols, music) into physical action. Advice from qualified practitioners should also be sought.
• Boosts confidence when performing or speaking in public.
• Aids concentration.
• Helps nervousness and stammering.

Notes and Dosages
Prepare this flower remedy using the sun method (see page 56).

Equisetium arvense
HORSETAIL

A weed that is common on damp ground, horsetail reproduces by spores, like ferns. Galen, a physician of ancient Greece, used horsetail to heal sinews.

DATA FILE

Properties
• Styptic • Diuretic • Strengthens the bladder • Antifungal

Uses
• Take for irritable bladder with urgency and frequency.
• For bedwetting problems, take with cramp bark or St. John's wort.
• Use for arthritis.
• Strengthens nails and hair.
• Speeds healing after surgery.
• Apply in a compress for infected, weepy skin conditions.

Notes and Dosages
Collect horsetail in early summer. Hang in large bunches and leave it to dry. The healing properties of horsetail are due to its high content of silica and zinc.

RECIPE

Horsetail Decoction
Simmer 1 teaspoon in 2 cups of water for half an hour. Make up a pitcher and keep it in the refrigerator. Drink twice daily for one month.

> **CAUTION**
> Avoid large doses in early pregnancy.

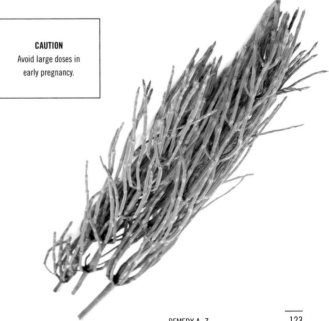

Eucalyptus globulus

BLUE GUM EUCALYPTUS

Several of the 700 species of eucalyptus are used to distill medicinal-quality essential oil, but the Australian "blue gum" is by far the most widely used. Eucalyptus is a traditional remedy in Australia and a familiar ingredient in chest rubs and decongestants.

DATA FILE

Properties
• Decongestant • Anti-inflammatory • Deodorant • Antiseptic
• Antiviral • Boosts immune system • Insect repellent • Painkiller

Uses
• Use for coughs, colds, chest infections, and sinusitis.
• The oil eradicates lice and fleas.
• Alleviates inflammation and is helpful in treating rheumatism, muscular aches and pains, and fibrositis.
• Use for urinary tract problems, such as cystitis.
• Reduces fevers.
• Treat skin infections, cuts, and blisters, genital and oral herpes, chicken pox, and shingles.
• Eases the pain of burns and helps new tissue to form.
• Prevents and relieves insect bites.

Notes and Dosages
This evergreen tree bears long, narrow, yellowish leaves. Eucalyptus oil is extracted from the leaves and young twigs. It blends well with peppermint, tea tree, rosemary, thyme, lavender, cedarwood, lemon, and pine.

RECIPE

Disinfectant Wash for Insect Bites
Add 3 drops eucalyptus, 3 drops thyme, 3 drops lavender to a bowl of clean water. Use cotton wool or a clean cotton cloth to dab repeatedly on the affected area.

> **CAUTION**
> Do not take when using homeopathic remedies.
> Do not use for more than a few days at a time because of the risk of toxicity.
> Do not use on babies or very young children.

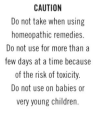

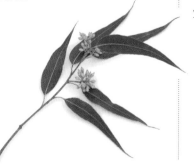

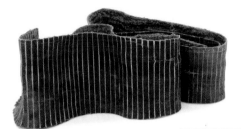

> **CAUTION**
> Contraindicated for heat from yin deficiency.

Eucommia ulmoides

DU ZHONG

This herb, made from eucommia bark, belongs to a group that in traditional Chinese medicine is believed to tonify the yang, mainly affecting the kidneys. In TCM the kidneys house the body's reserves, and the kidney yang is responsible for sexual and endocrine disorders.

DATA FILE

Properties
• Sweet • Slightly acrid • Warm • Tonic • Strengthening

Uses
• Use for lower back pain and knee problems caused by qi and blood stagnation.
• Strengthens the tendons and bones, which makes it useful for sports injuries.
• Promotes circulation.
• Helps with spermatorrhea (leaking of sperm) and frequent urination.
• Use for dizziness and lightheadedness due to hypertension from rising liver yang.

Notes and Dosages
Du Zhong is an expensive herb as it is necessary to kill the *Eucommia ulmoides* tree in order to get the bark. The liver rules the sinews, the kidneys rule the bones, so Du Zhong is used for weak, sore, or painful lower back and knees, chronic fatigue, and yang deficient symptoms, which are always accompanied by cold.

Eugenia caryophyllata

CLOVES

Cloves are the dried buds of a tree of the myrtle family. Almost 20 percent of the clove's weight is essential oil, obtained by distilling, and used in perfumes, blends of spices, medications, and candies. Cloves' deodorizing properties have long been used externally, but they may also be used as an internal deodorizer, freshening the breath and reducing body odor.

DATA FILE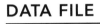

Properties
• Warming • Antiseptic • Analgesic • Anti-inflammatory
• Digestive • Antiparasitic • Antifungal • Mildly sedative
• Deodorant • Expectorant • Carminative

Uses
• Oil of cloves can be placed directly on a sore tooth or mouth abscess to draw out the infection and ease the pain before visiting the dentist. Chew cloves for the same effect.
• Use locally to reduce swellings.
• Dab a tiny amount of neat oil on insect bites.
• Drink clove tea to encourage sweating, which is helpful for high fever or vomiting.
• Oil of cloves may be used during a long labor to hasten birth.
• Clove tea soothes wind and eases nausea, particularly the nausea of travel sickness.
• Inhale an infusion of cloves to clear the lungs and refresh the airways.
• A clove and orange pomander can be hung in cupboards as an insect repellent.
• Use clove oil for treating athlete's foot.
• Drink a cup of clove tea a day to ease depression.
• In Ayurveda, cloves reduce kapha and vátha, and increase pitta.

Notes and Dosages
The clove tree, which may reach a height of 40ft. (12m.), produces abundant clusters of small red flower buds that are gathered before opening and dried to produce the dark brown, nail-shaped spice, clove. Cloves can be used as an oil, a compress, inhalation, massage oil, lotion, spice, and tea.

To make tea, steep cloves in boiling water and then simmer. Strain and use the remaining liquid. In Ayurvedic practice, cloves combine well with cardamom, cinnamon, lavender, ginger, orange, and bay leaf.

> **CAUTION**
> Cloves can cause uterine contractions, and should not be used in pregnancy. Cloves should also not be given to children under two or to nursing mothers. External use of the oil may cause a rash.

Euphrasia officinalis, Euphrasia stricta

EUPHRASIA

Grown in Europe and America, eyebright – as its name suggests – has been used for centuries to treat eye problems. It is commonly used in herbal medicine. Homeopathically, the whole fresh plant is used when in flower to make a remedy for sore, irritated eyes.

DATA FILE

Properties
• Relieves sore eyes

Uses
• Use for any eye irritation or inflammation, such as conjunctivitis, inflammation of the eyelid or iris, small blisters on the cornea, or running eyes associated with hay fever.
• May also help dry eyes associated with the menopause.

Notes and Dosages
May be useful for symptoms that improve after lying down in a darkened room and worsen in bright light, in the evening, in enclosed spaces, and during warm, windy weather.

> **CAUTION**
> See a qualified medical practitioner in the case of eye injury, vision disturbances, or if symptoms persist or worsen.

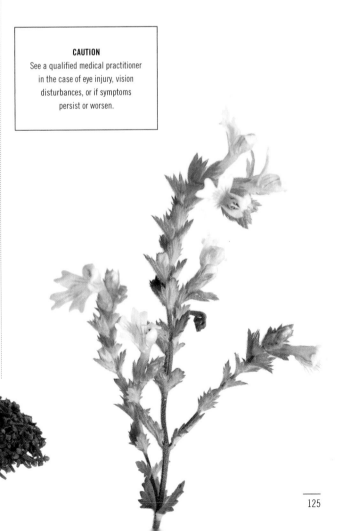

Fagus sylvatica

BEECH

This flower remedy is obtained from the leaves and twigs of the common beech tree, which grows to a majestic 100ft. (30m.) and has a spread of 80ft. (25m.). The leaves take on rich yellow and orange hues in the fall.

DATA FILE

Properties
• Encourages tolerance • Fills hearts with empathy

Uses
• Beech is for those who are being overcritical and intolerant, who think problems can be solved only in their way, and are irritable and short-tempered with those who cannot do this. They do not understand that everyone has different strengths and experiences. Their lack of understanding may lead to loneliness.
• Beech encourages empathy and opens eyes to see beauty without judgment. It shows that we are individuals, with different ways of dealing with the world.

Notes and Dosages
To make this flower remedy, the leaves and twigs of the common beech tree are prepared using the boiling method (see page 57).

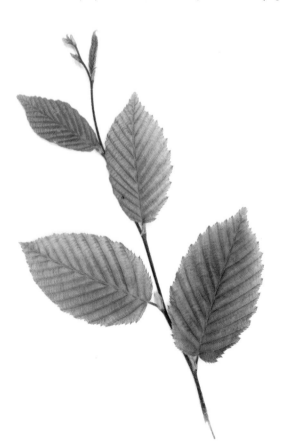

Ficus carica

FIG

Figs comprise a large family of deciduous and evergreen tropical and subtropical trees, shrubs, and vines belonging to the mulberry family, Moraceae. The *Ficus carica* tree produces the edible fig fruit. Figs are a nutritious and sustaining food, with a long history of medicinal use.

DATA FILE

Properties
• Highly alkaline • Healing agent • Antifungal • Antibacterial
• Digestive • Anti-inflammatory • Laxative

Uses
• For warts, use a preparation of the stem of the fresh fruit, which is antifungal.
• Eat dried figs to ease constipation.
• To bring a boil to a head, or to treat mouth ulcers or hemorrhoids, split a fig, heat it, and place it directly on the boil.
• Drunk daily, fig juice may act as a cancer preventive.
• Digestive troubles can be eased by eating fresh figs after light meals or just prior to heavy meals.
• Fresh figs can soothe respiratory ailments by acting as an anti-inflammatory agent.

Notes and Dosages
For sore throats, boil four or five fresh figs in about 1pt. (500ml.) of water. Bring to the boil, strain, cool, and drink the liquid.

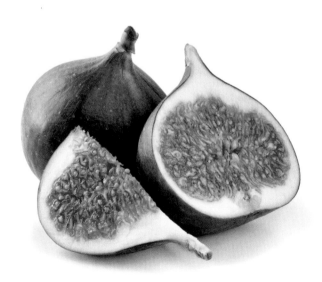

Filipendula ulmaria
MEADOWSWEET

This wild plant is common in damp meadows. The leaves, stalks, and flowers are used in Western herbalism. The flowers are very fragrant, and the plant was a medieval strewing herb. Culpeper described it as a help to acquiring a "merry heart."

DATA FILE

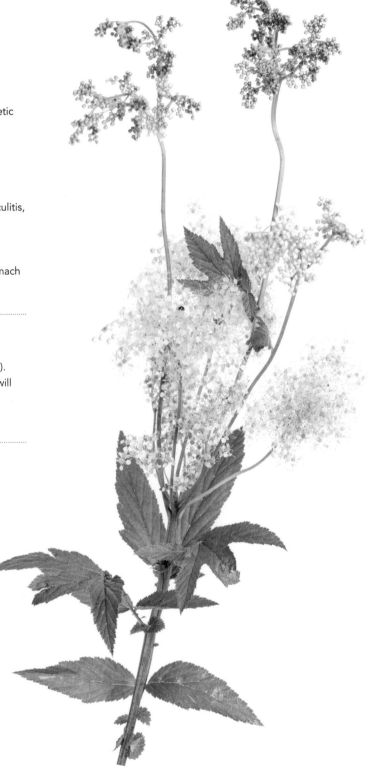

Properties
• Antacid • Digestive • Astringent • Anti-inflammatory • Diuretic

Uses
• For acid stomach, heartburn, ulcers, and hiatus hernia, meadowsweet combines well with comfrey, marshmallow, and chamomile.
• Take with peppermint or chamomile for indigestion, diverticulitis, and wind.
• Helpful for rheumatism and arthritis.
• Clears sandy deposits in the urine.
• Excellent for summer diarrhea and fevers with an upset stomach in children.

Notes and Dosages
Meadowsweet bears cream flowers in summer and should be picked at this time. Use standard doses (see pages 39 and 41). Give half dosages for children and elderly people. This herb will give quick relief for stomach pains, but the best results come from long-term use.

RECIPE

Tea for Acid Stomachs
Take equal parts of meadowsweet, chamomile flowers, and comfrey leaves, dried. Mix together and store in a clean jar. Use 1 teaspoon of the mixture to 1 cup of boiling water. Allow the tea to draw for 10 minutes. Drink 3–6 cups daily.

Foeniculum vulgare

FENNEL

The leaves and seeds of this familiar cooking herb are used in both Western herbalism and aromatherapy. Fennel has feathery leaves and grows to about 6ft. (2m.). It was traditionally reputed to give strength and courage. The essential oil, distilled from the crushed seeds, is still valued for its detoxifying properties.

DATA FILE

Properties
• Warming • Carminative • Antispasmodic • Antidepressant • Lactagogue • Balances hormones • Diuretic • Antimicrobial

Uses
• Take for wind, nausea, stomach cramps, and irritable bowel.
• For colic in infants, give the tea in teaspoon doses, as much as they will take, or add 2 teaspoons to milk formulas.
• Drink fennel tea while breastfeeding to help milk flow and reduce colic.
• Take for anxiety, depression, and disturbed spirits.
• Use for arthritis and water retention or edema.
• Use in mouthwashes to treat gum diseases and infections.
• Drink fennel tea during fasts to reduce hunger.
• Helps to stabilize hormone activity during the menopause.
• Fennel is a good diuretic and antiseptic, which can help with premenstrual water retention and urinary tract infections.

Notes and Dosages
For herbal remedies, use standard doses (see pages 39 and 41). Fennel seed tea bags are also available from health food stores. Remember to cover the cup to avoid losing any goodness. The essential oil is distilled from the crushed seeds. It blends well with lavender, lemon, orange, peppermint, rose, geranium, juniper, sandalwood, rosemary, cypress, and clary sage.

RECIPES

Fennel Eye Bath
Fennel tea that is diluted 1:1 with water and with the addition of a pinch of salt helps ease tired, dry eyes and maintain clear vision. As with any liquid used for the eyes, absolute cleanliness must be observed. Strain the tea through a very fine strainer before use, and make fresh every day.

Anticellulite Massage Oil
Add 8 drops fennel oil, 8 drops juniper, and 10 drops grapefruit oil to 5 teaspoons (25ml.) sweet almond oil and 5 drops jojoba oil. Store in a dark glass bottle and massage into the affected area every day after your bath or shower.

> **CAUTION**
> Do not use during pregnancy. Not suitable for epileptics or children under six years old. Fennel is narcotic in large doses. When making the essential oil, use only sweet fennel (also known as Roman or French fennel), as bitter fennel should not be used on the skin.

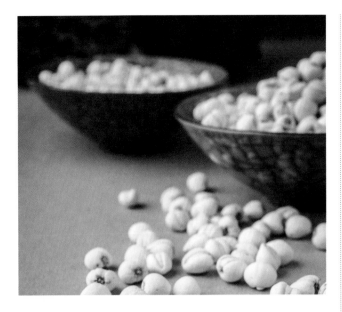

Fritillaria thunbergii
ZHE BEI MU

Like Ban Xia, this herb transforms phlegm, which in traditional Chinese medicine is the accumulation of thick fluid mainly in the respiratory and digestive tracts, but which may occur in the muscles and other body tissues.

DATA FILE

Properties
• Bitter • Cold

Uses
• Clears and transforms phlegm heat: use for acute lung heat patterns with productive yellow sputum (often caused by a heavy cold).
• Use for phlegm fire which congeals and causes neck swellings or lung abscesses.

Notes and Dosages
This herb is obtained from the bulb of *Fritillaria thunbergii*. Zhe Bei Mu is a cold herb which treats phlegm heat (as opposed to Ban Xia, which is warming), characterized by yellow sputum or sputum which is difficult to bring up. Chuan Bei Mu is another form of this herb which is milder and not so cooling, and may be used for many types of cough, including dry yin-deficient ones.

> **CAUTION**
> Ineffective in coughs due to phlegm cold.

Fucus vesiculosus
BLADDERWRACK

This common dark brown seaweed, also called kelp, is found on the coasts of the U.S.A. and Europe. It is used in herbalism as a tonic.

DATA FILE

Properties
• Nourishing • Soothing • Stimulates the thyroid gland

Uses
• Take as a tonic for old age.
• May help obesity with tiredness.
• Take for cellulite and chronic dry skin.
• Eases stubborn constipation.
• Regular use may delay the progress of arthritis and hardening of the arteries.
• May help children with slow mental and physical development.

Notes and Dosages
Gather bladderwrack from clean beaches, keeping away from sewage outlets. Alternatively, take 1 tablet 3 times a day, or follow the instructions on the packet. When using powder, 1 or 2 teaspoons may be sprinkled onto cooked meals or soups. Give half doses to children aged over five.

RECIPE

Bladderwrack Liniment
To make an excellent liniment for rheumatism and arthritis, add 1oz. (25g.) of dried bladderwrack to 1pt. (500ml.) of water. Simmer for half an hour. Strain and add to an equal amount of comfrey infused oil (see page 186). Shake before use and rub in well twice daily.

> **CAUTION**
> Avoid in overactive thyroid conditions, except with professional guidance. Not recommended for children under five. It is best to seek advice before using herbs for weight loss.

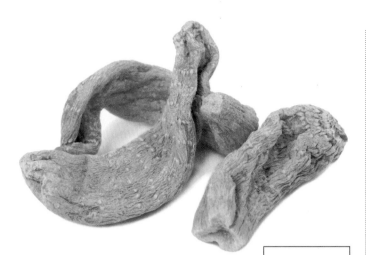

CAUTION
May be toxic in large doses.

Gastrodia elata

TIAN MA

In traditional Chinese medicine, this rhizome has a sinking action, which means that it takes qi down strongly, working through the liver channel.

DATA FILE

Properties
• Sweet • Neutral • Tonifies qi • Treats the liver

Uses
• Treats internal liver wind, with symptoms such as childhood convulsions or tantrums, epilepsy, spasms, or seizures.
• Use for headaches, dizziness, and migraines caused by wind phlegm patterns.
• May help in cases of wind stroke (stroke) with hemiplegia and numbness in the extremities.
• Good for rheumatic ailments in the lower back and limbs.
• Alleviates pain: especially wind mucus head pain.

Notes and Dosages
There are two kinds of wind in TCM: external (which brings in cold or flu, or arthritic symptoms) and internal, which is generated by dysfunction of the liver. This herb treats the second.

Gentianella amarella

GENTIAN

Gentianella amarella flowers from late summer onward, with rich blue, violet to purple flowers. It likes dry, well-drained conditions, and sandy or chalky soils. The flowers are used to make a flower remedy for alleviating mild depression.

DATA FILE

Properties
• Restores courage • Encourages positivity

Uses
• Gentian is used to treat despondency and mild depression due to circumstances. People who benefit from gentian are easily discouraged and lack faith.
• Gentian gives the courage to recognize that there is no failure when trying our best. It helps us to put disappointments into perspective, and to once again display a positive attitude.

Notes and Dosages
The purple flowers of this *Gentianella* species are similar to those of the honeysuckle. Prepare them using the sun method (see page 56).

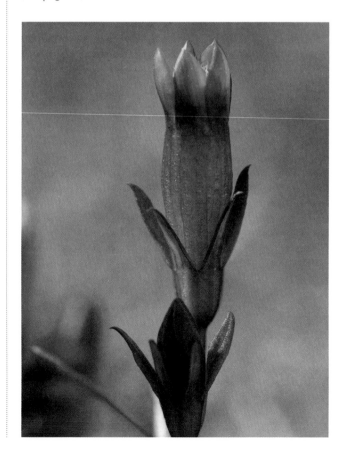

Ginkgo biloba

GINKGO

The leaves of the maidenhair or ginkgo tree, originally from China and often grown in parks, are used to make herbal remedies to treat poor circulation, thrombosis, and varicose veins. The tree grows to almost 100ft. (30m.) and is a deciduous conifer.

DATA FILE

Properties
• Improves blood flow • Strengthens blood vessels
• Anti-inflammatory • Relaxes the lungs

Uses
• Use for poor circulation, white finger, thrombosis, varicose veins, cramp that comes on when walking, and spontaneous bruising.
• Helpful for failing circulation to the brain in elderly people.
• Strengthens memory.
• Often improves deafness, tinnitus, vertigo, and early senile dementia.
• Helpful in asthma.

Notes and Dosages
Ginkgo may be taken as tea, tincture, or tablets. The tea is best taken in large doses: at least 3 cups a day for some months. It is a pleasant drinking tea. Follow the dose on the packet of any tablets.

RECIPES

Ginkgo Tincture
A good way to take ginkgo leaf over the medium term is by making it into a tincture. Place around 5oz. (150g.) of dried ginkgo leaf in a jar, then add 2 cups (500ml.) of vodka. Store in a dark place for a month, shaking daily. Finally, strain the leaves, pressing all the liquid from them. Keep in a labeled glass container. Take one teaspoon a day.

Ginkgo and Ginger Tea
Taken regularly, this tea is a good circulation-booster. Peel and thinly slice 2in. (5cm.) of fresh ginger. Boil the ginger in 1½ cups (350ml.) of water for at least 10 minutes. Strain out the ginger. Bring the water back to boiling point, then pour over 1 teaspoon of ginkgo leaves. Let steep for 5 minutes. Strain, then serve with lemon juice or honey to taste.

> **CAUTION**
> Exercise caution when using ginkgo with anticoagulant or antiplatelet medication such as warfarin and aspirin. It may also interact with MAOIs and NSAIDs. Avoid before surgery. When taking ginkgo regularly, take a break for 6 weeks every 6 months.

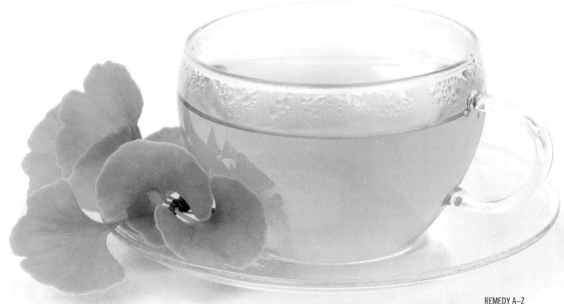

Glycyrrhiza glabra
LICORICE

Licorice has been used for ulcers and malaria, to treat throat and respiratory problems, and to soothe rashes and infections. Due to its strong, sweet taste, the herb is sometimes used in recipes to mask the unpleasant taste of another herb.

DATA FILE

Properties
- Sweet • Astringent • Demulcent • Expectorant • Antibacterial
- Antiviral • Mildly laxative • Alterative • Anti-inflammatory
- Adrenal tonic • Detoxifying • Raises blood pressure • Strengthening

Uses
- Take licorice syrup for colds, stubborn coughs, and to reduce the incidence of asthma attacks.
- For bronchitis, take ¼oz. (5g.) of the powdered root 3 times daily with honey or in capsules, for up to 2 weeks.
- A strong infusion drunk three times a day can protect against and heal ulcers, as it inhibits gastric secretions.
- Steep licorice root with a blend of other soothing herb teas to treat gastric disorders, such as constipation and gastritis, and to stimulate kidneys and bowel.
- For exhaustion, use with other strengthening herbs, such as ginseng.
- Mix in creams or pastes for the relief of inflamed psoriasis and hot and weepy skin conditions.
- Helps in the treatment of low blood pressure.
- Apply licorice powder externally to treat genital herpes and cold sores.
- May help disorders of the spleen, liver disease, Addison's disease, and inflamed gall bladder.

Notes and Dosages
The root and bark of the plant are used. Licorice can be chewed, taken as a powder, a tea or infusion, or as an oil. To make a decoction, use ½ teaspoon to 1 cup of water. Take 3 cups daily, or half this for long-term use. Boiling the decoction for an hour and drying it in a low oven produces an extract that is easy to take.

> **CAUTION**
> In large doses, licorice can exacerbate high blood pressure, cause mild adrenal stimulation, and water retention. Avoid in pregnancy. In nursing women, cases of high blood pressure or high adrenal function, it should be used only on the advice of a physician.

Glycyrrhiza uralensis
GAN CAO

This herb, also known as Chinese licorice, is one of a group that is used in traditional Chinese medicine to treat qi deficiency and tonify the spleen.

DATA FILE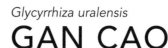

Properties
- Sweet • Neutral (raw) • Warm (toasted) • Moistening

Uses
- Moistens the lungs and stops coughing: because it is neutral it can be used to treat either heat or cold in the lungs.
- Use for sores or sore throats with pus, particularly strep throat, as it clears heat and detoxifies fire-poison.
- Take for spleen deficiency with shortness of breath, tiredness, and loose stools.
- Take for blood deficiency with an irregular pulse and palpitations.
- Moderates spasms or cramps in the abdomen and legs.
- Moderates and harmonizes the effects of other herbs.

Notes and Dosages
Can Cao is a very useful herb, primarily because it is sweet and mild, so that it moderates the violent properties of other herbs in a prescription and makes them more digestible. Furthermore, it enters all 12 channels, so it can lead other herbs into those channels.

> **CAUTION**
> Contraindicated for cases of excess dampness, nausea, or vomiting. May cause high blood pressure or edema if taken for an extended period of time.

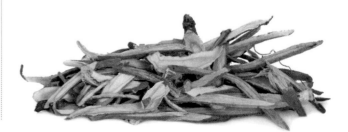

Gossypium sturtianum

STURT'S DESERT ROSE

Sturt's desert rose is a small shrub with mauve, hibiscus-like flowers. It likes dry, stony ground. The flower remedy is good for feelings of worthlessness.

DATA FILE

Properties
• Enables self-acceptance • Encourages reconciliation

Uses
• People who need Sturt's desert rose are always apologizing for themselves, blaming themselves, and feeling guilt. They have low self-esteem and a sense of shame. They may have an acute sense of obligation that is hard to live up to. Associated symptoms include anxiety dreams and depression.
• Sturt's desert rose enables self-acceptance, the understanding that we do what we can and must take responsibility (not blame) for the consequences. It enables reconciliation, allowing us to accept, forgive, and move on to pastures new.

Notes and Dosages
Sturt's desert rose is a delicate-looking, sun-loving plant that thrives in poor, dry soil and is a tough survivor. Use the sun method (see page 56) to prepare this flower remedy.

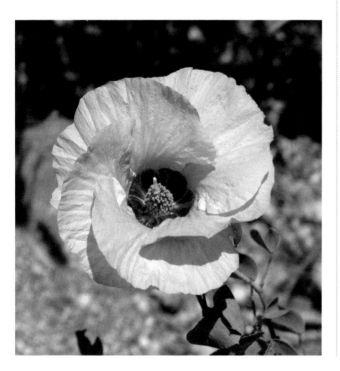

Grevillea buxifolia

GRAY SPIDER FLOWER

A common Australian evergreen, this shrub flowers for most of the year. It prefers acid soil and full sun.

DATA FILE

Properties
• Calms bad dreams • Gives courage • Frees from panic

Uses
• Gray spider flower is for extreme and intense feelings of terror, a blind panic that is immobilizing. The fear may be known or unknown, and may strike during the day or night.
• This remedy frees the body and the mind to move, bringing courage and the faith that the terror will pass.
• Gray spider flower eases nightmares, disturbed sleep, or fear of sleep. It is ideal for children terrorized by bad dreams.
• Eases the symptoms associated with terror, including shivering, pallor, palpitations, depression, and feelings of being psychically drained and exhausted.
• Take with fringed violet flower for protection from fear of the supernatural and of psychic attack.

Notes and Dosages
The plant that yields the gray spider flower remedy is a tender evergreen that can be grown in sheltered areas outdoors in milder regions. Pick the whole flower head at the end of the branch. Use the sun method (see page 56) to prepare.

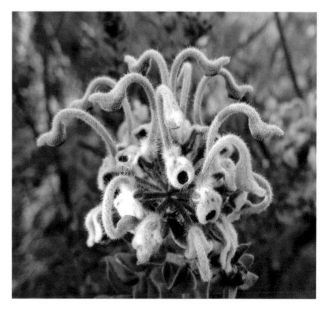

Hamamelis virginiana

WITCH HAZEL

This witch hazel species is a common tree of the U.S.A. Its leaves, bark, or roots are used in folk medicine, Western herbalism and homeopathy. The common name arose as a result of the remarkable medicinal properties of the alcoholic extract from the leaves and bark of the plant, which is used on bruises and inflammations, and as a rubbing lotion. The homeopathic remedy Hamamelis is used to treat piles and varicose veins.

DATA FILE

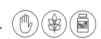

Properties
• Analgesic • Antiseptic • Astringent • Anti-inflammatory • Styptic

Uses
• Use diluted to wash cuts and grazes.
• Use a facial wash for oily skin and spots.
• Drink as an infusion two or three times daily when there is inflammation (such as that of arthritis or rheumatism, sprains, or bruising) and for internal bleeding.
• Apply externally (as a decoction, tincture, or cream) for the treatment of bruising, hemorrhoids, or varicose veins.
• Use as a compress for sprains, strains, and sunburn.
• Dilute one part witch hazel to 20 parts boiled, cooled water, and use as an eyewash for sore and inflamed eyes.
• Add to the bath to reduce the aches and pains of rheumatic conditions.
• Helps to control diarrhea when taken internally, and can encourage the health of the digestive tract.
• In homeopathy, the remedy is also used to treat inflammation of the ovaries or uterus, heavy menstrual bleeding, and pain at the time of ovulation.

Notes and Dosages
The small tree or shrub is often grown in gardens for its fragrant yellow spring flowers. Witch hazel's oval leaves turn yellow in the fall. It grows to 12ft. (3.6m.). Distilled witch hazel and other preparations are also easily available to buy. The decoction and tincture are stronger but tend to stain clothes. Dilute the tincture with 3 parts of water to use as a compress or lotion.

RECIPE

Witch Hazel Compress
For sunburn, swollen and inflamed joints, and aching varicose veins, make a compress. Take 1oz. (25g.) cut bark and 1pt. (500ml.) water. Simmer together for 10 minutes. Strain and allow to cool. Dip a cloth into the decoction, wring, and apply for a half-hour, wetting it again as needed.

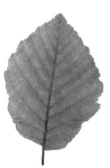

Harpagophytum procumbens
DEVIL'S CLAW

This remedy is made from the tuber of a South African plant that survives in very arid conditions. Devil's claw contains a glycoside called harpagoside that helps to reduce inflammation in the joints.

DATA FILE

Properties
• Bitter • Tonic • Anti-inflammatory

Uses
• Take the decoction or tincture for all types of arthritis, especially for inflamed joints and arthritis affecting a number of joints.
• Take for gout, lumbago, sciatica, rheumatism, gallbladder inflammation, piles, and phlebitis.
• May help itchy skin with no obvious cause.

Notes and Dosages
Devil's claw tubers are dug up at the end of the rainy season and dried. For a decoction, add ½ teaspoon powdered devil's claw to 1 cup of water, twice daily. For a tincture, use 1 teaspoon to 1 cup twice daily. Tablets are available in most health food stores: follow the dosage on the box. For acute flare-ups, double the dosage for a week or two.

RECIPE

Devil's Claw Capsules
Capsules are a good way of producing a customized remedy, and useful if you do not want to take a lot of liquid decoctions. Buy 120 empty gelatin capsules from a herb store. Get out a flat dish and a coffee grinder. Powder 1oz. (25g.) chopped devil's claw in the coffee grinder (some stores sell it pre-ground). Put the powder in the dish. Fill each capsule by pushing the halves through the powder. Take two capsules three times daily.

> **CAUTION**
> Avoid in pregnancy. Devil's claw may aggravate stomach acidity, so do not use in gastritis and with ulcers.

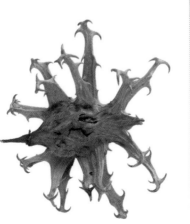

Helianthemum nummularium
ROCK ROSE

The yellow flowers of this low-growing plant, found on chalky or gravelly soils, are used to make a flower remedy. Some varieties of rock rose are cultivated in rock gardens, but these are not suitable for use as flower remedies. Rock rose is one of the main ingredients of Rescue Remedy (see page 158).

DATA FILE

Properties
• Gives courage • Brings faith

Uses
• Rock rose is to be taken in all cases of extreme fear, panic, urgency, or danger. Fear may cause palpitations, heart jitters, or panic attacks.
• This remedy gives the courage to face life and death, frees the mind to act, and brings faith that the terror or panic will soon pass.
• May be taken for any perceived threat to the person, self-image, or personal integrity.

Notes and Dosages
The rock rose thrives in a dry, stony, sunny spot and bears an endless succession of short-lived, fragile flowers. Prepare them using the sun method (see page 56).

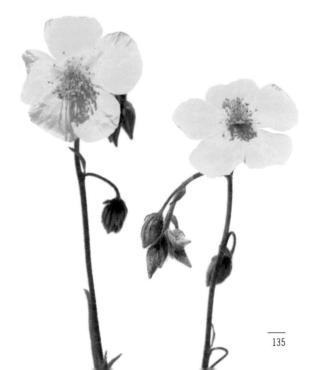

Hibbertia pedunculata

HIBBERTIA

This flower remedy is good for studious young people who may neglect the physical side of themselves. It is made from the flowers of hibbertia, commonly known as stalked Guinea-flower, a low, trailing plant of the open bush. Its large, bright, and gleaming yellow flowers bloom in spring.

DATA FILE

Properties

• Encourages contentment • Opens the mind to true wisdom

Uses

• People who need hibbertia love ideas and pursue knowledge at all costs. They may repress or deny their body and its needs, or have a rigid or dogmatic lifestyle. They continually read, attend lectures, courses, and workshops to improve themselves. Such people may be fanatical or cult followers. They look deep within books, but never around at their surroundings. Their head is in the air and they are ungrounded. Their search may be ultimately unsatisfactory. They may suffer sedentary and stress-related illnesses, indigestion, skin rashes, and wasting or stiffness of muscles and joints.
• Hibbertia encourages the user to understand that real knowledge grows from within and they must find themselves before they can gain true wisdom.

Notes and Dosages

Prepare the flowers using the sun method (see page 56).

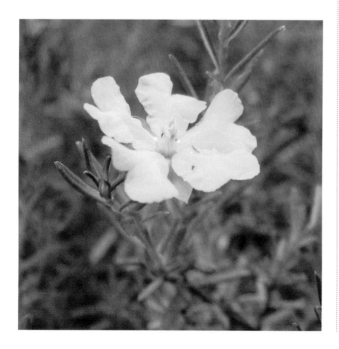

Hordeum sativum vulgare

BARLEY

Barley is rich in minerals (calcium, potassium, and B-complex vitamins), which makes it useful for convalescents or people suffering from stress. Barley has been used for its restorative qualities, in medicine and in cooking, for thousands of years. Malt is produced from barley.

DATA FILE

Properties

• Nutritious • Anti-inflammatory • Digestive
• May lower cholesterol levels

Uses

• Barley water can be used in the treatment of respiratory disorders, and eases dry, tickling coughs.
• Drink barley water for urinary tract infections and cystitis, and for flatulence and colic.
• Cooked barley is a traditional remedy for constipation and diarrhea.
• Barley water reduces acid in the spleen if drunk twice a day for a month.
• Make a poultice of barley flour to reduce inflammation of the skin.
• Barley may help to prevent heart disease, as it promotes the normal functioning of the heart and may stabilize blood pressure.
• Eat barley in soups and stews when convalescing.

Notes and Dosages

Barley is a cereal crop cultivated for humans and animals. It may be cooked and eaten, drunk as barley water, or used in a poultice.

RECIPE

Barley Water

Add 2 tablespoons of pearl barley to 1pt. (500ml.) of water and boil for 10 minutes. Strain, then add the barley to a fresh pint of water. Boil this water and barley for another 10 minutes. Strain out the barley and serve the water warm or cold, with lemon and honey.

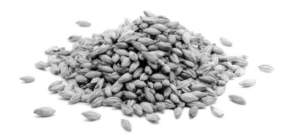

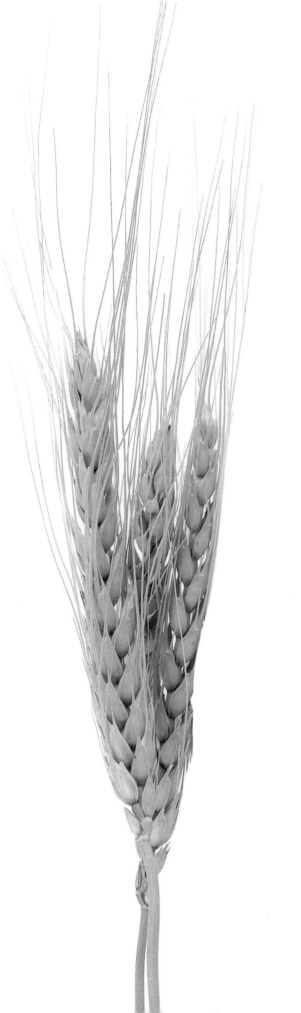

Hottonia palustris

WATER VIOLET

This is a delicate perennial plant with pale violet flowers and feathery leaves. Water violet is often found in ditches, as it grows submerged in water. The flowers appear above the water in summer.

DATA FILE

Properties
- Gives confidence to share

Uses
- Water violet is for self-reliant people with an aloof, "live-and-let-live" attitude. They are quiet and spend much time alone, keeping others at a distance. When ill they keep to themselves and do not wish to be any "trouble" to those around them. They find it hard to share. In their isolation they may feel special, or chosen, a sensation which can distort their sense of belonging and self-worth.
- Water violet gives the confidence to share one's strengths and weaknesses, the ups and downs, all of life's rich tapestry. Water violet allows us to acknowledge the inner self as a starting point from which to expand and communicate with the world.

Notes and Dosages
Water violets issue forth delicate lilac-colored flowers in early spring. Use the sun method (see page 56) to prepare them.

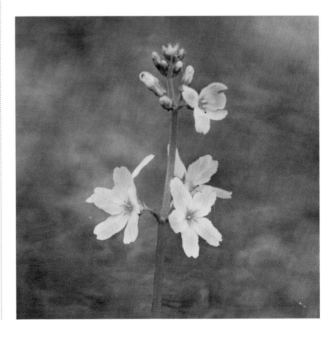

Hypericum perforatum
ST. JOHN'S WORT

This common wild plant is easy to grow, but make sure you get the right species: *perforatum* has oil glands in the leaves which show up as transparent dots against the light. The leaves and flowers are used as a remedy for mild depression in Ayurvedic practice, Western herbalism, and homeopathy.

DATA FILE

Properties

- Antidepressant • Diuretic • Emmenagogic • Expectorant
- Analgesic • Antiviral • Anti-inflammatory • Antispasmodic
- Moisturizing • Vulnerary • Strengthens the nervous system
- Speeds healing

Uses

- Take regularly for mild depression, not for severe depression.
- Eases the pain of neuralgia, sciatica, back pain, and deep wounds.
- Use as a tincture for shingles, cold sores, and herpes.
- Apply as a cream for sore skin, inflamed rashes, burns, and cuts.
- The infused oil may be used for massage, with the addition of lavender essential oil for neuralgia.
- May ease uterine cramping and menstrual problems.
- An oil extract of St. John's wort can be used internally for stomach ache, colic, or intestinal disorders.
- In Ayurveda, St. John's wort reduces pitta and kapha, and increases vátha.
- In homeopathy, Hypericum is most often given to treat nerve pain following injury.

Notes and Dosages

The tops of the plant are picked in full flower. Use standard herbalism doses (see pages 39 and 41). Take internally as a tea, tincture, or infusion. In cases of depression, it may be a week before depression begins to lift. The best preparations for external use are the infused oil and creams based on the infused oil (see recipe, below). For nerve damage, you may need to use regularly for some months. In Ayurvedic practice, St. John's wort combines well with angelica, chamomile, rosewood, and yarrow.

RECIPE

St. John's Wort Oil

Use this oil on the skin, healing nerve damage, as a base for massage oils, or as a salve. Pick the flowering tops. Put into a pestle, then add a small amount, just enough to cover, of a pure, light vegetable oil such as sunflower oil. Pound together to crush and bruise. Put into a large, clear glass jar. Cover with more oil so that all of the herb is well covered. Shake well. Then add another inch of oil. Leave outside in direct sunlight for 20 days. The oil will turn red when it is ready. Stored in a dark container, the oil will keep for up to two years. Use the oil externally or take internally, 10–15 drops in water.

CAUTION
St. John's wort can cause photosensitivity in direct sunlight.

Hyssopus officinalis
HYSSOP

Revered as a sacred cleansing herb by the Hebrews and the ancient Greeks, hyssop has also long been valued by herbalists for its medicinal properties. Both the leaves and the small blue or mauve flowers are distilled for their essential oil, which has a strong, spicy, herbaceous scent.

DATA FILE

Properties
- Expectorant • Antispasmodic • Bactericidal • Antiseptic
- Hypertensive • Emmenagogue • Digestive • Tonic • Sedative

Uses
- Helpful for coughs, catarrh, sore throats, and chest infections.
- Use in skin care for cuts, bruises, and inflammation.
- May be useful in the treatment of low blood pressure, and has a general tonic effect on circulation.
- Can be used for scanty or no menstrual bleeding.
- Soothes indigestion and relieves colicky cramps.
- Can benefit stress- or anxiety-related problems, relieving fatigue and increasing alertness.

Notes and Dosages
Hyssop is a perennial, almost evergreen shrub, with woody stems and small, lance-shaped leaves. The oil blends well with sandalwood, lavender, ylang ylang, rosemary, clary sage, cypress, geranium, lemon, and other citrus oils.

RECIPE

Inhalation for Chest Infections
Add 2 drops hyssop, 2 drops lavender, and 2 drops benzoin to a bowl of steaming water. Cover your head with a towel, bend over the bowl, and inhale.

CAUTION

Dilute well and use for no more than a few days at a time because there is some risk of toxicity. Do not use during pregnancy. Do not use if you are epileptic. For people with high blood pressure, hyssop should be used only as directed by a qualified aromatherapist.

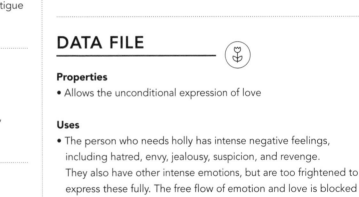

Ilex aquifolium
HOLLY

Holly is a common evergreen tree, with spiky leaves and red berries. It is a powerful symbol of winter and is used in Christmas decorations. To produce berries on a female plant, a male plant needs to be grown nearby. The holly is not noted for its flowers, but these have an unmistakable and pervasive scent.

DATA FILE

Properties
- Allows the unconditional expression of love

Uses
- The person who needs holly has intense negative feelings, including hatred, envy, jealousy, suspicion, and revenge. They also have other intense emotions, but are too frightened to express these fully. The free flow of emotion and love is blocked or expressed unclearly, leading to tension, unclear communication, frustration, anger, and emotional outbursts.
- Holly allows us to recognize these negative feelings and gives us the strength to open our hearts to the full flow of love.
- May also be useful for the "No!" negative states and temper tantrums of toddlers.

Notes and Dosages
Prepare this flower remedy using the boiling method (see page 57).

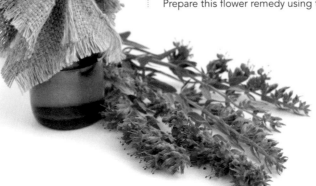

Impatiens glandulifera
IMPATIENS

A tall annual with large mauve flowers, impatiens is common in damp places. It is sometimes called "touch me not," as the tightly coiled seed pods are apt to explode at the slightest touch. The flowers are used to prepare a flower remedy.

DATA FILE

Properties
• Encourages patience

Uses
• Impatiens is for those who are quick in thought and action, and want things to be done at speed. They become irritable at hindrance, hesitation, and delay, and impatiently blame others. They can alienate people by being brusque and unsympathetic, speaking their mind quickly and without thought. They refuse to slow down even when illness overtakes them. People who need impatiens may find it hard to sit still, and therefore suffer from indigestion and nervous tension.
• Impatiens restores acceptance of the natural pace of life, rather than fighting against it. People who have learned the lesson of impatiens have patience, are capable and decisive, and know how to turn the pace of life to advantage.

Notes and Dosages
Impatiens grows on the banks of streams and ditches, and its flowers nod gently in the breeze. Prepare the flower remedy using the sun method (see page 56).

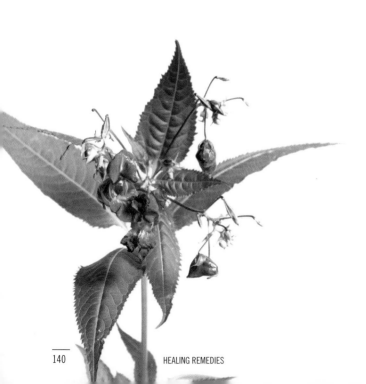

Inula helenium
WILD SUNFLOWER

Ayurvedic herbalists have long used the dried root of the wild sunflower, or elecampane, to treat bronchial infections, asthma, and whooping cough. The Greeks were convinced of the healing properties of the herb for intestinal disorders such as dysentery, pinworm, and parasites.

DATA FILE

Properties
• Sweet • Bitter • Pungent • Warming • Drying • Expectorant
• Tonic • Rejuvenative • Lactagogue • Antibacterial • Antifungal
• Antiparasitic

Uses
• Helps colds, bronchial infections, coughs, lung congestion and infection.
• Aids digestive infections such as amebic dysentery, pinworms, hookworms, and giardiasis.
• It stimulates the brain, kidneys, stomach, and uterus, and eases sciatica.
• Can treat menstrual cramps.
• Increases pitta, and reduces kapha and vátha.

Notes and Dosages
The root of the wild sunflower is dug up in the fall and dried. It can be used for inhalations, massage oils, and lotions, or taken as a decoction. It mixes well with cedarwood, cinnamon, lavender, frankincense, musk, and tuberose.

RECIPE

Wild Sunflower Decoction
A decoction treats both respiratory and digestive upsets. Put 3 cups of water and 2 teaspoons of powdered root into an enamel pan. Cover and boil gently for 30 minutes. Allow to cool. The taste will be bitter, so sweeten with honey if desired. Take 2 tablespoons at a time, up to 2 cups a day. Store the mixture in a refrigerator.

> **CAUTION**
> Wild sunflower should not be taken by pregnant women as it stimulates the uterus. Some people develop a rash when in contact with the herb or its oil. Do not give wild sunflower to children under two years of age.

Jasminum officinale

JASMINE

It takes huge quantities of jasmine flowers to produce a small amount of this very expensive essential oil. However, very little is needed to produce an effect, and the sensual floral perfume makes it a highly prized oil.

DATA FILE

Properties
• Aphrodisiac • Uterine tonic • Strengthens male sex organs • Antidepressant • Antiseptic • Expectorant • Anti-inflammatory • Analgesic

Uses
• Massage with jasmine oil benefits impotence in men and acts as an aphrodisiac in women.
• Helps with menstrual cramp and disorders of the uterus.
• Its pain-relieving properties and ability to strengthen contractions make it one of the best oils to use during childbirth.
• May help prostate problems.
• May help postnatal depression, stress, and lethargy.
• Soothes and warms joints.
• Rejuvenates dry, wrinkled, or aging skin.
• May help catarrh, and infections of the chest and throat.

Notes and Dosages
Jasmine is an evergreen shrub or vine, up to 33ft. (10m.) high, with delicate leaves and highly fragrant flowers. Jasmine oil blends well with lavender, geranium, chamomile, clary sage, sandalwood, rose, neroli, and other citrus oils.

RECIPE

Jasmine Massage for Menstrual Cramps
Add 4 drops jasmine, 4 drops clary sage, and 2 drops lavender to 5 teaspoons (25ml.) sweet almond oil. Start the massage by sliding your hands from your hips across your abdomen. Gently stroke around the abdomen in a clockwise direction, sliding one hand after the other. Stroke your hands back up and around your hips, and around to the small of your back. Repeat.

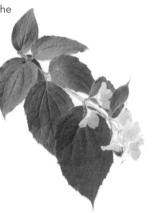

> **CAUTION**
> Jasmine may cause an allergic reaction in rare cases.

Juglans regia

WALNUT

A large, handsome, deciduous tree that is easily recognized by its popular edible nuts, walnut grows to about 50ft. (15m.) tall and is wide-spreading. Walnut bark and nuts are used in folk remedies, while the flowers can be made into a remedy to protect and strengthen the mind.

DATA FILE

Properties
• Astringent • Cleansing • Anti-inflammatory • Discourages milk flow • Aphrodisiac • Mildly laxative • Antiparasitic • Digestive • Protective

Uses
• Eat nuts daily while convalescing to relieve fatigue and strengthen the body.
• Walnut bark strengthens the gums and acts as an anti-inflammatory.
• The bark discourages milk flow in nursing mothers.
• Fresh walnuts and walnut oil can encourage circulation, and because they are rich in potassium, will keep the heart healthy.
• Add walnut bark to the bath for rheumatism, and sore and aching muscles and joints.
• Apply walnut bark tincture, in a little carrier oil, to swellings and skin problems, to encourage healing.
• Eat walnuts for heartburn, diarrhea, gas, and intestinal worms.
• Walnut oil, added to salads and vegetables, will help to ease the discomfort of irritable bowel syndrome and act as a mild laxative.
• Walnut leaves can be rubbed on a pet's coat to repel fleas.
• The walnut flower remedy is for people who need to move on and break links and old patterns with people and things. Walnut gives protection and freedom when on the brink of some major decision or change, for example puberty, leaving home, the menopause, marriage, or having a baby.

Notes and Dosages
Make the flower remedy using the boiling method (see page 57).

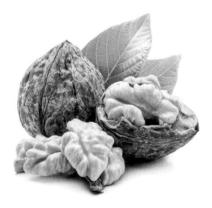

Juniperus communis

JUNIPER

Used in ancient Greece and Egypt to combat the spread of disease, juniper was still being used in French hospitals during World War II. A warm woody-scented aromatherapy oil can be distilled from juniper berries and twigs, but the best oil is produced by distilling the ripe berries only.

DATA FILE

Properties
• Cleansing • Diuretic • Tonic • Astringent • Antiseptic • Healing
• Stimulates appetite • Soothing

Uses
• Helps to detoxify the body of harmful waste products that contribute to problems such as rheumatoid arthritis and cellulite, and clears the mind of confusion and exhaustion.
• Excellent for treating cystitis.
• Helps skin problems, especially weepy eczema and acne.
• Apply to cuts and scrapes to aid healing.
• May help hemorrhoids and hair loss.
• Relieves nervous tension.

Notes and Dosages
Juniper is an evergreen shrub with bluish-green stiff needles. Juniper essential oil blends well with pine, lavender, cypress, clary sage, sandalwood, vetiver, benzoin, rosemary, fennel, geranium, bergamot, and other citrus oils.

RECIPE

Hair and Scalp Tonic
Add 10 drops juniper, 8 drops rosemary, and 7 drops cedarwood to 1½fl.oz. (50ml.) or 10 teaspoons olive oil and massage into your hair and scalp before you wash it. Wrap your hair in a warm towel and leave for about 2 hours. Wash out with a mild shampoo, massaging the shampoo into the hair before you wet it to remove all the oil.

> **CAUTION**
> Do not use in pregnancy. Not suitable for people with kidney disease.

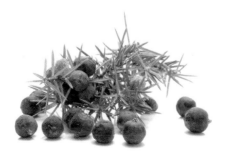

Lactobacillus acidophilus, Lactobacillus bulgaricus

LIVE YOGURT

Yogurt is a fermented, slightly acidic food product made from milk. Yogurt is usually made from a concentrated milk and is soured by a specific bacillus, *Lactobacillus bulgaricus*. As a food, yogurt is a rich source of protein, and contains all of the vitamins and minerals found in milk. Live yogurt, which contains active bacteria including *Lactobacillus acidophilus*, is most often used therapeutically, and should be eaten to increase the healthy bacteria in the body, to help it fight infection.

DATA FILE

Properties
• Antifungal • Aids digestion • May help to reduce cholesterol
• Encourages the growth of healthy bacteria in the bowels
• Helps to produce vitamin B

Uses
• For two to three weeks following a course of antibiotics, live yogurt should be eaten daily to increase beneficial bacteria.
• Apply live yogurt to areas affected by thrush; it can also be used internally as a douche.
• Daily intake of yogurt may prevent heart disease.
• Cleanse the skin with yogurt, which is a natural moisturizer. Apply to the skin with cotton wool.
• Eat live yogurt for chronic constipation and dyspepsia.
• Can eliminate bad breath that has been caused by intestinal putrefaction.
• Eat daily as a cancer preventive.

Notes and Dosages
Buy unsweetened live yogurt, sometimes known as "bio yogurt." Make your own yogurt by adding 3 teaspoons of live yogurt to 1pt. (600ml.) of milk. Leave to set. If taking *acidophilus* in tablet form, keep the tablets in the refrigerator. It is not toxic and can be taken daily, with food, in unlimited amounts.

> **CAUTION**
> Live yogurt is not effective when mixed with sweeteners. For best effect, make your own yogurt and flavor with a little unpasteurized honey and a banana.

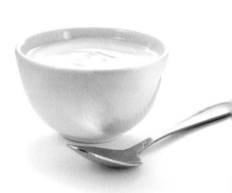

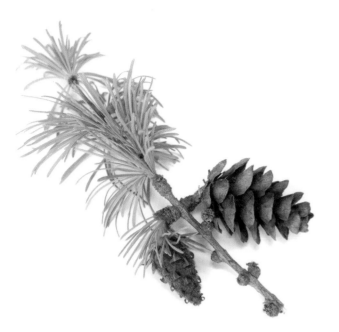

Larix decidua
LARCH

Larch is a tall conifer with needle-like leaves that are shed in the fall. Male and female flowers appear on the same tree in spring. It can grow to 100ft. (30m.) high, and the cones are small and erect. The flower remedy can help bring confidence and self-esteem, especially in teenage years.

DATA FILE

Properties
• Gives confidence • Strengthens willpower

Uses
• Larch is for those who lack confidence in themselves and fear failure, those who feel they are inferior. At times, lack of confidence may prevent them from even trying. They do not think they are worthy of success. Feelings of uselessness can lead to unhappiness and isolation.
• Larch increases confidence and strengthens personal will, helping us to appreciate our real worth.
• The remedy may be suitable for children starting a new school, who feel they will not be as clever as the other children and fear failure.

Notes and Dosages
The larch is the only cone-bearing tree to lose its leaves during the fall. Its timber has great strength. Prepare the flowers using the boiling method (see page 57). Feelings of worthlessness may hide deeper problems or a pattern of abuse, in which case other remedies and professional advice will also be useful.

Lavendula augustifolia
LAVENDER

Of the several varieties of lavender used medicinally, *Lavendula augustifolia* is the most important. Lavender is the most versatile, best loved, and most widely therapeutic of all essential oils. Lavender is a reviving yet soothing oil, an ideal ingredient for the bath or in a blend for massage.

DATA FILE

Properties
• Soothing • Antidepressant • Antiseptic • Antibacterial
• Analgesic • Decongestant • Antispasmodic • Tonic

Uses
• Apply the oil to cuts, wounds, burns, bruises, spots, and insect bites.
• Effective against colds, flu, throat infections, and catarrhal conditions.
• Eases digestive spasms, nausea, and indigestion.
• Helps treatment for rheumatism.
• Alleviates depression, insomnia, headaches, stress, and hypertension.

Notes and Dosages
Lavender is an evergreen woody shrub up to 3ft. (1m.) tall. Both the flowers and the leaves are highly aromatic, but only the flowers are used to make essential oil. The oil blends well with florals such as rose, geranium, ylang ylang, chamomile, and jasmine; citrus oils such as orange, lemon, bergamot, and grapefruit; and rosemary, marjoram, patchouli, clary sage, cedarwood, clove, and tea tree.

RECIPE

Bath or Massage Blend for Irritability
Add 3 drops lavender, 3 drops chamomile, and 2 drops neroli to a warm bath and disperse with your hand. Alternatively, add to 3 teaspoons (15ml.) grapeseed or sweet almond oil for a soothing massage.

> **CAUTION**
> Lavender is usually safe for all age groups, but some hay fever or asthma sufferers may be allergic. Dilute well if taking homeopathic remedies.

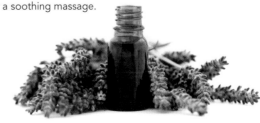

Ledebouriella seseloides

FANG FENG

Fang Feng belongs to a group of warm, acrid herbs that is used in traditional Chinese medicine to release exterior conditions: superficial illnesses caused by viruses, with symptoms in the skin or muscle layers. These herbs mainly cause sweating, or stop sweating where necessary.

DATA FILE

Properties
• Acrid • Sweet • Slightly warm • Analgesic

Uses
• Releases the exterior and expels wind: use for headaches, chills, and body aches from externally contracted wind cold.
• Alleviates pain: use for exterior wind damp painful obstruction, such as arthritis and rheumatic ailments.
• Fang Feng alleviates trembling and numbness of the hands and feet, particularly in Parkinson's disease.

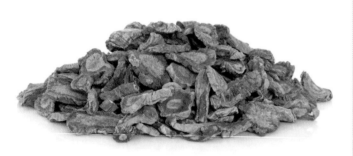

Notes and Dosages
In English, Fang Feng means "guard against wind," so it is used particularly in ailments where wind is predominant, according to traditional Chinese medicine. This means it causes sweating (acrid quality) in colds and flu. It is also useful in arthritis, where the pain moves about from joint to joint (wind-type arthritis).

> **CAUTION**
> Contraindicated in cases of deficient blood with spasms – it does not tonify the blood and produces sweating, so one would have to add tonifying blood herbs to stop it depleting the blood further. Contraindicated for cases of deficient yin with heat signs. Deficient yin can produce a "false heat" such as in menopausal sweats. As Fang Feng produces more sweat, it would deplete the yin fluid even further – it needs to be carefully combined.

Leonurus cardiaca

MOTHERWORT

A European wild plant with a tall spike of small pink flowers, motherwort self-seeds readily in the garden. Motherwort is especially good for female disorders – hence its name. Culpeper wrote, "... there is no better herb to drive melancholy vapours from the heart ... and make the mind cheerful, blithe and merry."

DATA FILE

Properties
• Calms the heart • Relaxes the womb • Antispasmodic
• Emmenagogue

Uses
• Take for anxiety with palpitations and irregular heartbeat.
• Use for tachycardia from an overactive thyroid.
• For tranquilizer withdrawal, take with skullcap or valerian.
• For anxiety from stress and overwork, take with vervain.
• For menopausal hot flushes, take with sage.
• For menstrual cramps, taken on a regular basis.
• Take daily during the last two weeks of pregnancy to help with the birth.

Notes and Dosages
Take standard herbalism doses of decoction or tincture (see page 39). It may take a few weeks to work.

RECIPE

Motherwort and Lemon Balm Tea
Motherwort and lemon balm tea combines motherwort's sedative effect and lemon balm's antidepressant qualities. Take as a regular tea for depression.
Mix together equal amounts of dried motherwort and lemon balm herbs. Store in a clean jar and label. Make an infusion, or tea, by pouring a cup of boiling water onto 1–2 teaspoonfuls of the dried herbs. Leave to infuse for 10–15 minutes. The tea should be drunk 3 times a day.

> **CAUTION**
> Avoid in pregnancy, except during the last two weeks.

Ligusticum chuanxiong

CHUAN XIONG

Also known as Szechuan lovage root, this herb invigorates (or "regulates") the blood, treating disorders associated with blood stasis. In traditional Chinese medicine, these problems include pain and internal masses or growths.

DATA FILE

Properties
• Acrid • Warm

Uses
• Invigorates the blood and promotes the circulation of qi: use for any blood stasis patterns, especially in gynecology, including dysmenorrhea (menstrual cramps), amenorrhea (lack of menstruation), difficult labor, or retained placenta.
• Used for chest, flank, and epigastric (above the navel) pain caused by stagnant qi and blood.
• A leading herb for externally caught wind disorders (viruses) with symptoms such as headaches, migraines, and dizziness.
• Helpful for arthritis and a variety of skin problems caused by wind, including itching.

Notes and Dosages
As Chuan Xiong moves the qi upward it is an essential herb used in combinations for treating all types of headaches. This herb enters the liver, gall bladder and pericardium.

> **CAUTION**
> Contraindicated in yin deficiency with heat signs (it is warming), headaches due to rising liver yang (unless combined carefully), qi deficiency (it does not tonify), or excessive menstrual bleeding (it moves blood further).

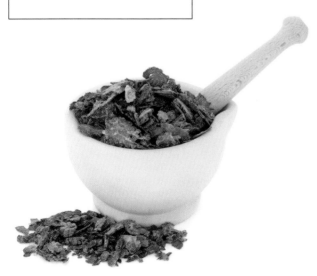

Linum usitatissimum

FLAXSEED

Flax is a group of annual and perennial plants from the Linaceae family. Several varieties of one species, *Linum usitatissimum*, are grown primarily for their fiber, used in making linen, or for their seeds, the source of linseed oil. The seeds contain a remarkable healing oil which can be used both internally and externally. Flaxseed is also known as linseed, but should not be confused with the "boiled" linseed oil available from building merchants. As far back as Hippocrates, flaxseed tea has been used to treat sore throats, hoarseness, and bronchial spasms.

DATA FILE

Properties
• Mildly laxative • Tonic for the kidneys • Encourages healing
• Analgesic • Antispasmodic

Uses
• Apply the oil to sprains to reduce inflammation and ease the pain.
• Mix flaxseed with lime water to reduce the pain of burns.
• Flaxseed tea can be used for mild constipation, and to encourage kidney function. The tea also works to ease kidney pains and cramping.
• The tea can be drunk during bouts of bronchitis to reduce inflammation of the lungs and prevent spasm.

Notes and Dosages
Add lemon and honey to flaxseed tea to encourage its action and improve taste.

> **CAUTION**
> Commercially produced linseed oil is used in protective coatings such as paints and varnishes because it has a drying action. It is not suitable for human consumption!

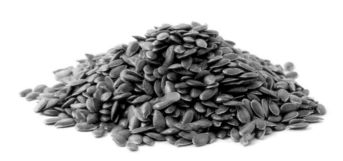

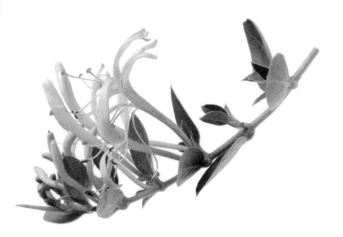

Lonicera caprifolium
HONEYSUCKLE

The honeysuckle flower remedy is prepared from the flowers of the Italian honeysuckle, *Lonicera caprifolium*. It is useful for the elderly, the bereaved, or for those suffering homesickness.

DATA FILE

Properties
• Integrates past experiences • Gives strength to face new challenges

Uses
• The honeysuckle flower remedy is for those who dwell too much on memories of the past, on the "good old days" and who do not expect to experience such happiness and companionship again. The past seems rosy and familiar; the future seems dark, bleak, forbidding, and unknown. Nostalgia may be a temporary sensation, a fleeting regret, or it may be a pattern that prevents further joy and expression.
• The flower remedy is also useful for grief and bereavement where these cause the person to dwell on the past.

Notes and Dosages
Prepare the honeysuckle flower remedy using the boiling method (see page 57). Honeysuckle flowers, with their almost sickly sweet scent, are seen in woodland and shaded hedges throughout the summer.

Lonicera japonica
JIN YIN HUA

Also known as honeysuckle flower, Jin Yin Hua is one of a group of herbs that is used in traditional Chinese medicine to clear heat: this includes febrile conditions and any illnesses with heat signs, such as fever, inflammation, red eyes, aversion to heat, and hot skin eruptions.

DATA FILE

Properties
• Sweet • Cold • Antibacterial

Uses
• Especially useful against salmonella (food poisoning), and is effective against many *streptococcus* or *staphylococcus* infections.
• Clears heat and relieves toxicity: use Jin Yin Hua for hot, painful sores, particularly of the breast (mastitis), throat (viral or bacterial tonsillitis), or eyes (conjunctivitis).
• Expels external wind heat: use for the early stages of febrile illnesses.
• Clears damp heat from the lower burner: use for dysentery or cystitis.

Notes and Dosages
This herb works through the large intestine, lung, and stomach channels.

> **CAUTION**
> Contraindicated in cases of diarrhea due to spleen and stomach deficiency: it is for strong infections and does not tonify weakness. Contraindicated in sores that do not have infected pus, but clear liquid inside.

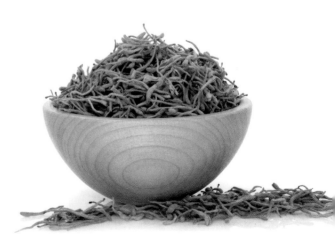

Lycium barbarum, Lycium chinense

GOU QI ZI

Also known as Chinese wolfberry fruit, in traditional Chinese medicine this herb treats patterns of blood deficiency. In TCM the two organs most affected by this disorder are the heart and liver, which direct and store the blood, respectively. In Western herbalism, this bright red fruit is used as a tonic for old age.

DATA FILE

Properties
• Sweet • Neutral • Tonic for old age and associated weakness

Uses
• In TCM, Gou Qi Zi is used for impotence, leaking of sperm, and diabetes, particularly in the elderly, when the yin is in decline.
• Good for failing or blurred vision, dizziness, and dry or sore eyes.
• Moistens the lungs.
• Use for aches and pains, especially backache, particularly in old age.
• Take for general weakness with vertigo, tinnitus, and recurrent headaches.
• Take during convalescence, with equal parts of schisandra: it improves skin color and restores strength.

Notes and Dosages
The wolfberry, also called the Duke of Argyle's tea plant, is the fruit of a deciduous Chinese shrub, grown in Europe as a hedging plant, reaching 8ft. (2.5m.) tall and spreading to about 15ft. (5m.). Lycium bears pinkish flowers and grows well even in poor soil. For a tincture, take ½fl.oz. (l5ml.) with a little water daily. When using the dried fruit, use ½oz. (10g.) daily chewed or in decoction. Traditionally the berries are added to soup to help strengthen eyesight.

RECIPE

Eye-Strengthening Soup
Take 1oz. (25g.) wolfberry fruit, 3 chopped carrots, and a sliced onion. Add to 1pt. (500ml.) soup stock made with chicken or vegetable stock cubes. Simmer until the vegetables are cooked. Strain and blend. Take regularly to nourish the vital essence and benefit vision.

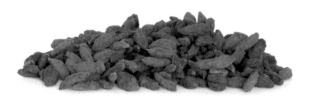

Lycopodium clavatum

LYCOPODIUM

Also known as club moss, wolf's claw, stagshorn moss, or running pine, this plant has long been used to treat stomach complaints and urinary disorders, and is grown in the mountains and forests of the northern hemisphere. Historically, Arab physicians used it to disperse kidney stones. For homeopathic use, the pollen dust is shaken out of the spikes of the fresh plant.

DATA FILE

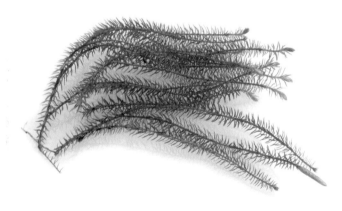

Properties
• Digestive • Calming

Uses
• This remedy is commonly used to treat digestive complaints, such as vomiting, indigestion, distended abdomen with flatulence, constipation, bleeding piles, and hunger which turns to discomfort after eating.
• Other problems that can be alleviated include swelling in the ankles, feet, or hands (edema); burst blood vessels in the eye; chronic catarrh; psoriasis on the hands; and pneumonia.
• In men, the remedy is helpful for an enlarged prostate; urine that has a reddish tinge and contains a sandy sediment due to kidney stones; and increased libido, but without the ability to achieve or sustain an erection.

Notes and Dosages
According to homeopaths, problems that can be eased by Lycopodium tend to occur on the right side of the body, and are accompanied by cravings for sweet food. Symptoms improve when in cool, fresh air, when wearing loose clothing, after hot food and drink, and at night. The remedy may also help emotional problems and anxiety caused by insecurity.

Malus pumila

APPLE

The apple has many uses in traditional medicine, and the old adage "To eat an apple going to bed will make the physician beg his bread" has been justified by its many health-giving properties. Research shows that apples are excellent detoxifiers, and apple juice – even store bought – may help to overcome viruses.

DATA FILE

Properties
• Cleans teeth and strengthens gums • Lowers cholesterol levels • Antiviral • Detoxifies • Neutralizes indigestion • Prevents constipation • Soothing • Antiseptic

Uses
• Eat raw apples regularly, as a detoxificant, for gout and rheumatism.
• To prevent viruses from settling in, and to reduce their duration, eat an apple (or drink a glass of apple juice) three times a day.
• Raw, peeled, and grated apples can be used as a poultice for sprains.
• For indigestion, heartburn, and other digestive disorders, eat an apple with meals.
• Use an apple poultice for treating rheumatic and weak eyes.
• Eating two apples a day may reduce cholesterol levels.
• As a treatment for intestinal infections, hoarseness, rheumatism, and fatigue, increase your daily intake to as much as 2lb. (1kg.).
• For curative purposes, as an alternative to eating the whole fruit, drink 1pt. (500ml.) of naturally sweet apple juice a day.
• Grated apple, mixed with live yogurt, may be helpful in cases of diarrhea.

Notes and Dosages
The highest benefits can be derived from fresh apples and freshly pressed apple juice, but ready-made juice is also good for the body.

> **CAUTION**
> Apple seeds can be toxic when taken in large amounts.

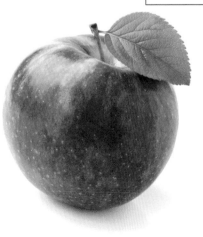

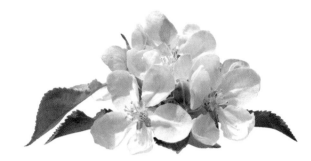

Malus sylvestris

CRAB APPLE

The fruits yielded by this plant are small, yellow, and very acid, although they are able to make a piquant preserve. The tree grows in hedges and on waste ground, providing a good show of color in the fall. The blossoms can be used to make a flower remedy.

DATA FILE

Properties
• Cleansing • Encourages self-acceptance

Uses
• This flower remedy is useful for those who feel self-condemnation and disgust, and are in need of detoxification. This may be a temporary feeling brought on by shame or remorse, or thoughts that are felt to be unclean. Those in need of crab apple may hurt, punish, cut, or otherwise abuse themselves. Crab apple cleanses both the mind and body.
• The remedy is also useful to encourage acceptance of spots or physical blemishes, and for a deep phobia or cleanliness fetish.

Notes and Dosages
Prepare the blossoms using the boiling method (see page 57). The remedy may be added to baths or to skin creams.

Matricaria chamomilla, Chamaemelum nobile

CHAMOMILE

Wild plants with small, daisy-like flowers, both German and Roman chamomile are used in Western herbalism, aromatherapy, and homeopathy. It is the flowers that are most often used for therapeutic purposes. In aromatherapy, it is usually Roman chamomile that is used to make the essential oil. It is one of the gentlest essential oils available, and particularly suitable for treating children. Homeopathically, the juice is extracted from the whole fresh plant when it is in flower in the late spring, and the remedy is given to those who are sensitive and have a low pain threshold, and is particularly good for children.

DATA FILE

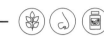

Properties
• Calming • Induces sleep • Anti-inflammatory • Antiseptic
• Antispasmodic • Digestive • Antidepressant • Stress relieving

Uses
• Take for anxiety, tension, headaches, and insomnia.
• Use to relieve the pain of toothache, menstrual cramps, arthritis, and neuralgia.
• Useful for any kind of digestive upset, such as acidity, heartburn, wind, and colic.
• Apply as a lotion, cream, compress, or in a bath, for itchy skin conditions, rashes, inflammation, cuts, boils, allergies, insect bites, and chilblains.
• Chamomile has a balancing effect on the menstrual cycle and reduces fluid retention.
• Useful for restless and overexcitable children, and for most children's complaints, including fevers and teething troubles.
• Massage with chamomile essential oil can soothe fretful or colicky babies, and the diluted oil can be rubbed into the cheek to relieve teething pain.

Notes and Dosages
Chamomile is a small perennial herb with daisy-like white flowers and feathery pennate leaves. In herbalism, chamomile may be taken freely, except during early pregnancy. As a sedative, make a double-strength tea, using 2 teaspoons of flowers or 1 tea bag. Use a covered vessel, so the steam does not escape. Linden flowers, chamomile, and four cloves make an effective drink before bed, relaxing the body and the mind, and bringing satisfying sleep. For infants, make an ordinary-strength tea and give them 2 or 3 teaspoons to drink, either directly or in some pure fruit juice. For times of severe stress, make a mixture of three parts chamomile to two parts sage and one part basil (a pinch of ginger powder is optional). Take twice a day to reduce tension and husband resources.

The essential oil blends well with lavender, geranium, bergamot, jasmine, rose, neroli, clary sage, sandalwood, and mandarin.

RECIPE

Chamomile Compress for Sore and Inflamed Eyes or Skin
Put a handful of dried chamomile flowers into a bowl. Slowly pour on boiled water, stirring all the time until they make a mush. Allow to cool. Wrap in a length of cotton and apply. Leave on for at least 15 minutes.

CAUTION
Do not use in the first three months of pregnancy. Do not allow chamomile essential oil to get into the eyes. Chamomile can cause an allergic rash, but this disappears on stopping use of the herb. German chamomile may be used instead of Roman chamomile, but not chamomile *Maroc ormenis multicaulis*, which is not true chamomile.

Medicago sativa

ALFALFA

Alfalfa is grown the world over, primarily as food for livestock. The ancient Chinese, noticing their cattle preferred grazing in alfalfa, started to sprout alfalfa shoots to use as a vegetable. Ancient Arabs fed it to their horses to increase speed and endurance. They called it *al-fac-facah*, "father of every food," and introduced it to the Spanish, who changed the name to alfalfa. Ayurvedics have used alfalfa to cleanse the liver, to detoxify the blood, and to treat ulcers, arthritis, and fluid retention.

DATA FILE

Properties

• Bitter • Astringent • Cooling properties • Detoxifying
• Antifungal • Promotes pituitary gland function

Uses

• Alfalfa leaves, brewed into a tea, help to reduce blood cholesterol levels and clean plaque deposits from arterial walls.
• It is a great detoxifier and can be used on a regular basis to cleanse the system and provide refreshing chlorophyll.
• Good for anemia, ulcers, colitis, diabetes, and hemorrhaging.
• Useful for arthritis, sciatica, rheumatism, and fluid retention.
• Sprouts help neutralize carcinogens in the colon, binding them and speeding their elimination from the body.
• Sip the infusion for a natural breath freshener.
• Alfalfa reduces both kapha and vátha, and has a neutral effect on pitta.

Notes and Dosages

Alfalfa has deep roots and so is resistant to drought. It has mauve flowers in summer. The leaves, petals, flowers, and sprouts may all be used. Take as a tea, a supplement, or in sprouts. To make tea, use 2 teaspoons of the herb to 1 cup of boiling water. Let it steep for 15 minutes. Drink up to 3 cups of the tea a day. Alfalfa combines well with fenugreek, garlic, ginger, saffron, and turmeric.

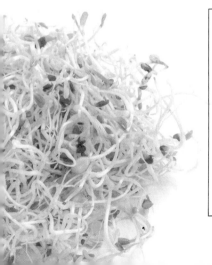

> **CAUTION**
> Pregnant and nursing women should consult a physician before use. Never eat alfalfa seeds because they contain high levels of the toxic amino acid canavanine. Over time, eating the seeds could result in impaired functioning of the platelets and white blood cells. The alfalfa plant contains saponins, chemicals that may affect red blood cells. In recommended doses, alfalfa is considered safe.

Melaleuca alternifolia

TEA TREE

This small tree or shrub is a traditional remedy among the Aboriginal people of Australia. Originally, the leaves were made into a tea, and hence its name. More recently, scientific research has shown that tea tree oil can combat many types of infection.

DATA FILE

Properties

• Antifungal • Antibacterial • Antiviral • Insecticide • Expectorant
• Anti-inflammatory • Immune stimulant • Reduces fever

Uses

• Use for skin problems such as spots, acne, warts, verrucae, athlete's foot, rashes, insect bites, burns, and blisters.
• Can be used to clean cuts and infected wounds, and it helps skin to heal by encouraging the formation of scar tissue.
• Effective against dandruff, cold sores, and urinary or genital infections such as cystitis and thrush.
• An excellent choice when fighting colds, flu, respiratory infections, catarrhal problems, and infectious illnesses.
• Effective against fleas and lice.
• Use as a deodorant.

Notes and Dosages

Tea tree is a small tree or shrub, with needle-like leaves similar to those of cypress, and stalkless yellow or purple flowers. Tea tree oil blends well with lavender, geranium, chamomile, myrrh, lemon, rosemary, marjoram, clary sage, pine, and spice oils such as clove and cinnamon.

RECIPE

Treatment Oil for Acne

Add 4 drops tea tree, 3 drops bergamot, and 3 drops lavender to 2 teaspoons (10ml.) jojoba oil. This mixture is excellent for inflamed or acne-prone skin. Dab onto the affected areas.

> **CAUTION**
> People with sensitive skin should introduce the oil with caution. Do not swallow mouthwashes or gargles.

Melaleuca cajeputi

CAJEPUT

In Malaysia, the Philippines, Indonesia, and Australia, wild cajeput is used extensively for all manner of ills, from colds to toothache. Closely related to tea tree, this oil is distilled from the leaves and buds of cajeput, and has a distinctly medicinal camphorous odor.

DATA FILE

Properties
• Antiseptic • Antimicrobial • Clears mucus • Analgesic • Energizing

Uses
• Cajeput is good to use in steam inhalations for colds, flu, sinusitis, asthma, bronchitis, and other respiratory infections.
• Eases the pain of headaches and sore throats, and can be used to good effect on muscular and arthritic pain.
• Used with care, it is effective against cystitis and other urinary infections.
• Cajeput can be used to soothe the stomach, counteract digestive spasms, and kill infections in the gastrointestinal system.
• Use on the skin for minor conditions such as insect bites and spots.
• Inhalation, which is one of the best ways to use this oil, helps to dispel mental fatigue and apathy.

Notes and Dosages
Cajeput is a tall evergreen tree, up to 100ft. (30m.) high, with thick pointed leaves and white flowers. The oil blends well with sandalwood, juniper, hyssop, lavender, rosemary, pine, lemon, eucalyptus, and marjoram.

RECIPE

Inhalation for Colds and Flu
Add 4 drops cajeput, 3 drops rosemary, and 2 drops eucalyptus to a bowl of steaming water. Cover your head with a towel, bend over the bowl, and inhale for 5–10 minutes.

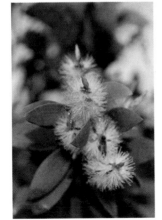

> **CAUTION**
> Dilute well, as cajeput is a skin irritant. Do not use as a gargle or as a vaginal wash as the oil can irritate the mucous membranes. Cajeput is a stimulant, and so is best avoided in the late evening.

Melaleuca viridiflora

NIAOULI

Closely related to cajeput and tea tree, niaouli is distilled from the leaves of a large tree grown in Australia and New Caledonia. It is a much more gentle oil than cajeput, and less likely to irritate the skin or mucous membranes. Niaouli, which has a strong medicinal odor, is sometimes labeled as "gomenol."

DATA FILE

Properties
• Antiseptic • Bactericidal • Encourages healing • Stimulates immune system • Antispasmodic • Balancing

Uses
• Good for cystitis and other urinary infections.
• A few drops added to cooled boiled water makes a healing antiseptic wash for cleaning minor wounds, cuts, or burns.
• Stimulates the healing of burns and promotes the growth of new tissue.
• Treats oily skin, spots, acne, and insect bites.
• Inhalations of niaouli are helpful in colds, flu, respiratory, and catarrhal conditions.
• Added to a chest rub, helps to alleviate infections and stimulate the immune system.
• Can benefit digestive problems.

Notes and Dosages
The niaouli tree has pointed linear leaves, and spikes of stalkless yellow, and occasionally red, flowers. Niaouli oil blends well with frankincense, basil, clary sage, geranium, lavender, neroli, ylang ylang, and other floral and citrus oils.

RECIPE

Chest Rub for Coughs
Add 3 drops niaouli, 2 drops hyssop, and 1 drop myrrh to 3 teaspoons (15ml.) of vegetable oil and rub into the chest.

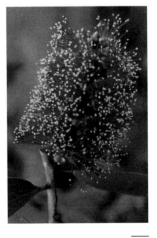

> **CAUTION**
> Dilute niaouli oil well, as it may irritate the skin of some people.

Melissa officinalis

LEMON BALM

Lemon balm, or "heart's delight," has been used medicinally since the 17th century. The fresh lemony essential oil, usually called melissa oil, is distilled from the leaves and flowering tops. Unfortunately, the plant yields very little essential oil, which is why true melissa oil is so expensive, and why most commercial oil is adulterated with other lemon oils.

DATA FILE

Properties
• Antispasmodic • Calming • Uplifting • Tonic • Antihistamine

Uses
• Helps to reduce high blood pressure and to calm palpitations and rapid breathing, making it a good remedy for mild shock.
• Use for menstrual problems: calms and regulates the menstrual cycle, helps to ease menstrual cramps, and alleviates scanty menstruation and amenorrhea.
• Reduces digestive spasms in colic, nausea, and indigestion.
• Relieves migraine and combats fever.
• Low dilutions can be beneficial for eczema and other skin problems.
• May help allergies affecting the skin and the respiratory system.
• Calms the nervous system, relieves anxiety, and has an uplifting effect on the emotions, dispelling sadness and loss, and counteracting hysteria.

Notes and Dosages
The lemon balm herb has bright green, serrated leaves and tiny white or pink flowers. Melissa oil blends well with lavender, geranium, patchouli, tea tree, bergamot, rosemary, hyssop, pine, and petitgrain.

RECIPE

Melissa Mind and Body Soother
For frazzled nerves, irritability, and exhaustion, dilute 3 drops melissa, 2 drops chamomile, and 2 drops bergamot in 1 teaspoon (5ml.) of sweet almond oil and add to your bath water.

CAUTION
Melissa, or lemon balm, oil is sometimes adulterated with other lemon oils.

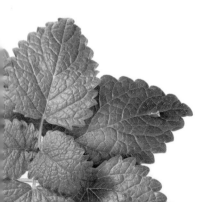

Mentha piperita

PEPPERMINT

Peppermint is best known as a remedy for digestive problems, particularly in the form of a tea. Apart from its many therapeutic applications, it is also used as a humane form of pest control.

DATA FILE

Properties
• Digestive • Mildly stimulating • Tonic • Expectorant • Analgesic • Antiseptic • Carminative • Antispasmodic • Emmenagogue

Uses
• Relieves indigestion, flatulence, spasms, diarrhea, nausea, stomach cramps, and travel sickness.
• Helps to tone the liver, intestines, and the nervous system.
• It is a valuable expectorant in the treatment of bronchitis and flu, and can reduce fevers by inducing sweating and cooling the body.
• Drink with elderflower and yarrow for colds, sinus problems, and blocked nose. Inhale the steam as you drink.
• Use as a painkiller, beneficial for toothache, menstrual cramps, headaches, and some migraines.
• For hot, itchy skin problems, a strong tea may be used as a lotion, which is also a useful antiseptic for acne and congested skin.
• Muscle and mental fatigue are both relieved by peppermint.

Notes and Dosages
The peppermint plant is easily grown in gardens, but is rather invasive. Try growing it in a bucket buried in the ground, with the bottom knocked out. The leaves are collected just before the flowers open. The herbal tea may be drunk freely. Adding a couple of drops of the essential oil to hot water, and drinking it, or sucking a peppermint sweet, is also effective in many cases. Peppermint oil blends well with lavender, chamomile, rosemary, lemon, eucalyptus, benzoin, sandalwood, and marjoram.

RECIPE

Peppermint Travel Oil
Add 5 drops peppermint, 5 drops lemon balm, 5 drops angelica, and 5 drops ginger to a dropper bottle containing 1fl.oz. (30ml.) of sweet almond oil. Inhale or massage a few drops into the temples or back of the neck to relieve jet lag or headaches. Massage clockwise round the abdomen for stomach ache.

CAUTION
Do not use during pregnancy. The amounts taken in food are harmless. Not suited to infants. The oil may irritate the skin of sensitive people. Do not use while taking homeopathic remedies. Do not use for long periods at a time.

Mimulus guttatus
MIMULUS

A pretty, water-loving plant common in damp places, mimulus has rich yellow flowers in midsummer that resemble the snapdragon. It grows to 2ft. (60cm.). The flowers are used to make a remedy for combating anxiety and fears.

DATA FILE

Properties
• Strengthening • Liberating

Uses
• Mimulus is for fear that can be identified, of known or worldly things: pain, accidents, poverty, being alone, and misfortune. These understandable fears dominate responses, either prodding people into hasty action or freezing them into inaction. Underneath, sufferers are fed by insecurity and a negative attitude toward past experience. Fear can lead to stammering, palpitations, indigestion, sleeplessness, and troubled dreams.
• This remedy is for shy, timid people who tend to avoid social occasions and large crowds of people.
• It liberates us from fear and helps us to understand the rhythms and balances of everyday life, to grow beyond the limits set by fear, and to have the courage and freedom to respond in appropriate ways.

Notes and Dosages
The mimulus or monkey plant is a bog plant, in need of shade and cool, damp conditions. Use the sun method to prepare (see page 56).

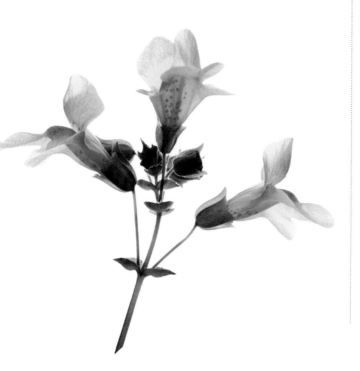

Myristica fragrans
NUTMEG

Known as "jaiphala" to the Ayurvedics, nutmeg is a tropical evergreen tree native to Indonesia. The brown, wrinkled fruit contains a kernel which is covered by a bright red membrane. The membrane produces the spice mace. The 2–4in. (5–10cm.) kernel provides us with nutmeg. Many healing remedies use mace and nutmeg together.

DATA FILE

Properties
• Warming • Rejuvenating • Calming • Sleep-inducing • Carminative

Uses
• Nutmeg is calming and sleep-inducing, making nutmeg tea before bed an excellent remedy for insomnia and other sleep disorders.
• Improves appetite and digestion while dispelling nausea, flatulence, or acid stomach.
• Eases menstruation.
• May ease kidney trouble.
• Increases kapha and vátha, and has a neutral effect on pitta.

Notes and Dosages
The kernel of the seed is used. Nutmeg is highly toxic and hallucinogenic when ingested in large doses, and is only recommended for use in small doses of 1 teaspoonful or less. May be taken whole or as a powder, as a tea, a spice, a massage oil, or an inhalation. The herb blends with balsam, bay, cinnamon, cumin, and lavender.

RECIPE

Nutmeg Stomach Tonic
This tonic will relieve gas, nausea, and indigestion. Take 1½ teaspoons of powdered slippery elm bark, ½ teaspoon of nutmeg, and 1½ teaspoons of mace. Mix thoroughly and add a little cold water to make a smooth paste with no lumps. Bring 1pt. (500ml.) of light cream or ½pt. (250ml.) each of cream and water to boiling point, remove from the heat, and quickly add the paste. Stir with a wooden spoon for 1 minute or until the powder is completely dissolved. Let cool until lukewarm. Drink ½ cup. You may take ½ cup up to three times daily, always warm.

> **CAUTION**
> Nutmeg can be very toxic and has hallucinogenic properties. Eating as few as two nutmeg kernels can cause death. Use only in the medicinal amount. Consult a physician before using nutmeg medicinally. Pregnant women and people in high pitta should avoid nutmeg.

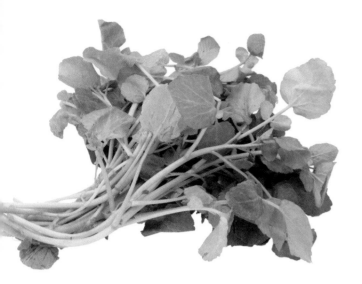

Nasturtium officinalis
WATERCRESS

Watercress is a floating or creeping water plant of the mustard family, Cruciferae. A perennial, it grows best in fresh water, particularly in cool streams and ponds, and in wet soil. It is a rich source of vitamin C.

DATA FILE

Properties
• Digestive • Anti-inflammatory • Diuretic • Expectorant
• Antiseptic • Antibiotic • Stimulates the immune system

Uses
• Stimulates digestion: eat with a meal if you have a tendency toward heartburn or dyspepsia.
• Eat the bruised leaves to help skin pimples and to fade freckling.
• Eat fresh watercress daily to help prevent migraine.
• Used to treat respiratory ailments such as coughs, catarrh, and bronchitis – eat fresh until symptoms improve. It can also be useful as a preventive measure for chronic respiratory conditions.
• Contains benzyl mustard oil, which is powerfully antibiotic, but does not harm our healthy bacteria.
• May help in the treatment of edema.
• Provides good supplies of the vitamins C, A, and B (thiamine and riboflavin), iron, potassium, and calcium.
• High levels of potassium may help to prevent insomnia – eat some fresh leaves an hour before bedtime, and often throughout the day.
• May strengthen the whole body system in cases of debility caused by chronic illness.

Notes and Dosages
Watercress's round, edible leaves are pungent to the taste, and commonly used as salad greens or as a garnish.

Natrum muriaticum
NAT. MUR.

Also known as rock salt, halite, or sodium chloride, salt has long been a valuable commodity. Many people add salt to food for flavor, but in fact we get more than enough salt naturally from what we eat. In conventional medicine, salt is used in the form of saline solution, for instance, during surgery to replace fluids. Homeopathically, the Nat. mur. remedy is made from rock salt which is formed through the evaporation of salty water, leaving a crusty crystalline solid. The remedy is used to treat a number of conditions resulting from emotional problems and ailments characterized by a discharge. It is also one of the 12 tissue salts identified by Dr. Wilhelm Schussler.

DATA FILE

Properties
• Relieves anxiety • Aids ailments accompanied by secretions

Uses
• May relieve emotional problems, such as distress, restlessness, and depression, which tend to occur because of the suppression of other emotions, such as fear and grief.
• May help conditions characterized by secretions or discharge, such as colds, catarrh, vaginismus, mouth ulcers, nasal boils, acne, cold sores, and other skin complaints such as hangnails, warts, and a cracked lower lip.
• In women, it may help with erratic menstruation; menstruation which has stopped due to stress, shock, or grief; malaise or swollen ankles before and after menstruation; and a dry or sore vagina.
• Headaches may also respond well.

Notes and Dosages
Sea salt and rock salt are the usual sources of Nat. mur.

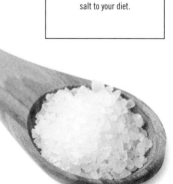

> **CAUTION**
> Contact your physician before adding additional salt to your diet.

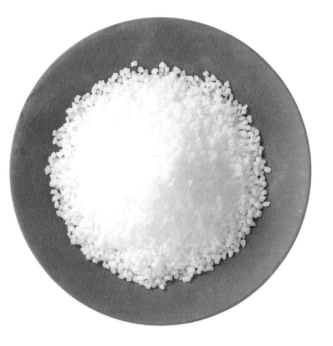

Natrum sulfuricum
NAT. SULF.

Sodium sulfate, a white crystalline compound, is found naturally in spa waters, saltwater lakes, and mineral water. It is also known as Glauber's salt. Sodium sulfate is used in the manufacture of paper, detergents, and glass. It is naturally present in the body and helps to maintain water balance. Homeopathically, it is one of the 12 tissue salts identified by Dr. Wilhelm Schussler.

DATA FILE

Properties
• Expectorant • Eases emotional problems

Uses
• Used to treat chest problems such as asthma, bronchitis, colds, and flu, where there is a build-up of thick yellowish catarrh, which comes from the nose.
• May help emotional trauma after an accident in which the head is injured, leading to depression and suicidal thoughts or other emotional changes; and headaches that have a vice-like grip at the back of the head and behind the forehead.
• Other conditions for which this remedy is prescribed homeopathically include dry mouth, with the tongue having a dirty coating; biliousness; and thirst and frequent urination, leading to an inability to deal with damp conditions and sharp liver pains.

Notes and Dosages
Glauber's salt, or sodium sulfate, is the source of this remedy. It occurs naturally as the mineral threnardite.

Nitroglycerin
GLON.

Nitroglycerin, known as Glonoinum to homeopaths, is a thick, clear, toxic liquid, discovered by the Italian chemist A. Sobrero in the mid-19th century. Two decades later, Swedish scientist Alfred Nobel used it as the explosive component in dynamite. In Victorian times, typesetters and printers who worked under the powerful heat of incandescent gas lamps used it to treat the severe headaches they suffered. In conventional medicine, nitroglycerin is used to treat heart disease.

DATA FILE

Properties
• Balances blood and circulation problems

Uses
• May be useful for heat exhaustion that causes flushes of heat and a painful bursting sensation in the head.
• Prescribed for headaches and migraine when the head feels very hot and blood vessels seem to be expanding, the patient feels like vomiting, and pressure on the head is unbearable; dizziness; and for headaches that are aggravated by heat or cold.
• Prescribed for the cessation of menstruation and the hot flushes often associated with the menopause.

Notes and Dosages
This remedy is a highly diluted form of nitroglycerin made from glycerin, nitric acid, and sulfuric acid.

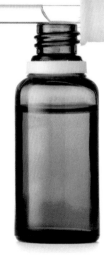

> **CAUTION**
> Although Glonoinum is highly diluted, nitroglycerin is both toxic and explosive. Consult with your physician before taking. Keep in a secure place and beyond the reach of children.

Ocimum basilicum

BASIL

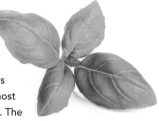

There are many different varieties of basil, but French basil is the most commonly used in aromatherapy. The uplifting and refreshing oil has a strong spicy-sweet smell that is often most appealing in a blend with other oils. Ayurvedics have used basil, known as "tulsi," to treat stomach, kidney, and blood ailments.

DATA FILE

Properties
• Expectorant • Antiseptic • Antibacterial • Antifungal • Stimulating
• Antidepressant • Antispasmodic • Carminative • Tonic
• Diaphoretic • Fever reducing • Stimulates the immune system

Uses
• Basil oil relieves mental fatigue, clears the mind, and improves concentration. It has a strong effect on the emotions, and can ease fear or sadness.
• The oil is good for chest infections, congested sinuses, chronic colds, and head colds.
• Basil relieves abdominal pains, indigestion, and vomiting.
• Massage with basil oil works well on tired muscles; it also eases arthritis, rheumatism, and gout.
• Basil oil kills intestinal parasites. A basil poultice can be used to treat ringworm.
• Wipe with basil tea to treat acne.
• In Ayurveda, basil reduces kapha and vátha, and increases pitta.

Notes and Dosages
Basil can be grown on a window-ledge if kept in a sunny position. Basil can be drunk as a tea or juice, cooked into medicated ghee, used as an inhalation, massaged as a therapeutic oil, or made into a compress or poultice. To make a tea, steep 3 teaspoons of dried leaves in 1 cup of boiling water for 20 minutes. Apply with a cotton ball to freshly washed skin to help acne, or drink up to 3 cups of the tea per day as an internal antibacterial treatment.

Basil oil blends well with lavender, bergamot, cedarwood, lemon, juniper, rosemary, tea tree, eucalyptus, geranium, clary sage, lime, and citronella.

RECIPE

Vaporizer Blend for Migraine
Add 3 drops basil, 4 drops lavender, and 3 drops peppermint to a vaporizer. Relax in a darkened room and inhale deeply.

CAUTION
Do not use during pregnancy, as basil has been used as a menstruation promoter and labor inducer. Basil oil may irritate people with sensitive skin. Do not use the oil from exotic basil, which is slightly toxic.

Olea europea

OLIVE

The olive is a long-lived, evergreen, subtropical tree, and has been cultivated for at least 4,000 years for its edible fruit and its valuable oil. It is native to the eastern Mediterranean region. Its leaves and the oil of its fruit are used in cooking and medicinally, and studies show that it has powerful anticholesterol action in the body, making it a useful addition to any home medicine cabinet. Only cold-pressed olive oil is suitable for therapeutic use. Olive is also used as a flower remedy.

DATA FILE

Properties
• Antioxidant • Emollient • Soothing • Lowers cholesterol levels
• Renewing

Uses
• Olive oil or fresh olives can be used to treat constipation.
• Olive oil soothes the itching of eczema, and moisturizes dry skin, hair, and scalp.
• Olive oil is rich in vitamin E, and may help to lower cholesterol levels. Taken daily, it can reduce the risk of heart disease and help to slow down the degenerative effects of aging.
• Drink a little extra virgin olive oil to cure a hangover.
• Olives are said to counteract poisoning from mushrooms or fish: drink a little extra virgin, cold-pressed oil when symptoms present themselves.
• The flower remedy is for all physical and mental tiredness after some effort or struggle. Olive helps restore vitality by helping people to relax and take a more balanced attitude toward life, making sure they allow themselves "quality" time for unwinding, rest, and spiritual renewal.

Notes and Dosages
Olive is a small evergreen common in southern Europe. The fruits yield olive oil. The flower remedy is prepared using the sun method (see page 56).

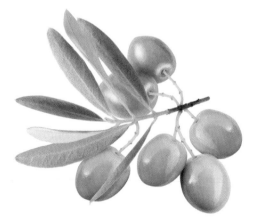

Ophiopogon japonicus
MAI MEN DONG

In traditional Chinese medicine, this herb tonifies the yin, and it therefore moistens and nourishes fluids. Any of the major organs may suffer from a yin deficiency, and Mai Men Dong is an important herb for their revitalization.

DATA FILE

Properties
• Sweet • Bitter • Slightly cold • Moistening • Tonic

Uses
• Moistens the lungs and eases coughing.
• Tonifies the stomach yin and generates fluid, making it useful for stomach aches, "dry" vomiting, and a shiny tongue with little coating.
• Use after febrile illness when the mouth is parched, and there is severe thirst or recurring fever.
• Use for an irregular pulse and palpitations from injury to the fluids or blood.
• May be prescribed for diabetes, as well as to brighten the vision and strengthen the lower back.

Notes and Dosages
This remedy is the tuber of the dwarf lilyturf plant. Like Tu Su Zi, it is added to prescriptions to moisten, but only in yin-deficient patterns. It works through the lung, stomach, and heart channels.

> **CAUTION**
> Contraindicated in cases of deficiency without heat signs. Like all tonifying yin herbs, it aids dampness and should therefore not be used for cold phlegmy coughing or deficient spleen with loose stools or a thick, greasy tongue coating.

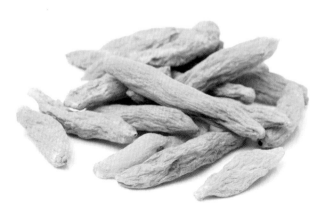

Origanum majorana
SWEET MARJORAM

In ancient times, marjoram was reputed to promote longevity, a belief that encouraged the ancient Greeks to include it in perfumes, cosmetics, and medicine. In folk tradition, marjoram was believed to bring joy to newlyweds and peace to the dead. The essential oil, with its warm spicy scent, is still used to relieve agitation, dispel grief, and restore calm.

DATA FILE

Properties
• Warming • Analgesic • Antispasmodic • Sedative • Tonic
• Antiviral • Antibacterial • Expectorant • Vasodilator • Digestive

Uses
• Use for muscle spasms and strains.
• Relieves nervous tension and promotes restful sleep.
• Inhaling marjoram can help to relieve headaches and migraine.
• Helps to fend off colds and infections, and works as an expectorant in a steam inhalation for chest infections.
• Massaged into the chest or throat, can relieve painful coughs.
• Beneficial in treating high blood pressure and improving circulation.
• Calms digestion, strengthens intestinal peristalsis, and eases menstrual cramps.
• Marjoram is a comforting oil that reduces sexual desire.

Notes and Dosages
Sweet marjoram is a strongly scented, tender perennial herb, grown as an annual in colder climates. The oil blends well with bergamot, chamomile, frankincense, rose, sandalwood, lavender, rosemary, cedarwood, juniper, eucalyptus, and tea tree.

RECIPE

Marjoram Cold Cure
Add 4 drops marjoram and 2 drops eucalyptus to a hot bath to relieve cold symptoms, or add 2 drops to 1 teaspoon (5ml.) of vegetable oil and use as a chest rub.

> **CAUTION**
> Do not use in pregnancy.

Ornithogalum umbellatum

STAR OF BETHLEHEM

The delicate flowers of this wild lily are like six-pointed stars and bloom in late spring. Star of Bethlehem is one of the five ingredients in Rescue Remedy, which can be carried with you for all emergencies.

DATA FILE

Properties
• Calming • Comforting

Uses
• Star of Bethlehem neutralizes the effects of shock, so that the body and mind can again find equilibrium and comfort. This may be the shock of bad news, of loss, of an accident, even of being born. People "jump" with shock: waves ripple outward through the body, affecting every cell and tissue. Time is needed for everything to settle, to be comfortable in the body, but sometimes the trauma may be so extreme, or the shock unrealized or repressed, that the effects continue to resonate years later. Long-repressed shock or trauma may lead to psychosomatic symptoms. Star of Bethlehem neutralizes the effects so that the body is able to harmonize.

Notes and Dosages
Star of Bethlehem grows wild in Asia and North Africa, and as far north as the U.K. Prepare the flowers using the boiling method (see page 57).

RECIPE

Homemade Rescue Remedy
Rescue Remedy can be bought as a liquid or as a cream. It is made from equal amounts of these five essences: cherry plum, for feelings of desperation; rock rose, to ease terror, fear, or panic; impatiens, to soothe irritability and agitation; clematis, to counteract the tendency to drift away from the present; and star of Bethlehem, to address the mental and physical symptoms of shock. Together, these flower essences make a safe mental sanctuary in which to recover. Carry Rescue Remedy with you for all emergencies, such as a shock, an accident, or an argument; or to take before a trying event, such as an examination, court appearance, or operation.

Make a treatment bottle of Rescue Remedy by adding 2 drops of each constituent flower remedy to a 1fl.oz. (30ml.) bottle of brandy. A cream can be made at home by adding 4 drops of stock Rescue Remedy to a favorite skin cream or neutral base, then adding 2 drops of crab apple.

Rescue Remedy is the only Bach Flower Remedy that is usually taken neat, straight from the bottle. Put 4 drops directly onto or under the tongue. Repeat dosage as often as needed. Put 4 drops into a glass of water and sip throughout the day until you feel more settled. A startled infant or baby can be reassured by putting 4 drops into the evening bath.

Oryza sativa

RICE

Rice is the cereal that is a staple food to more than half of the world's peoples. It also has important medicinal uses, for which the rhizomes, seeds (the grains), and germinated seeds are used. White rice is the grain that is left after the bran and germ have been removed; brown rice retains the bran and germ. Rice is available as a breakfast cereal (the grains are "puffed" during manufacture), and is fermented to produce rice wine, called saki by the Japanese.

DATA FILE

Properties
• Tonic • Diuretic • Digestive • Lowers blood pressure
• Anti-inflammatory

Uses
• Eat rice daily if you suffer from chronic dyspepsia: it is excellent for heartburn, particularly that associated with pregnancy.
• Use rice bran for the treatment of hypercalciuria.
• Use rice flour to make a poultice for relieving inflammation of the skin, including acne, measles, burns, and hemorrhoids.
• Increase your intake prior to menstruation if you suffer from bloating and symptoms of premenstrual syndrome. Eaten regularly, rice can prevent edema.
• Rice water helps to overcome stomach upsets.
• Germinated rice seeds may help in the treatment of abdominal bloating, lack of appetite, and indigestion.
• Nutritionally, rice contains high levels of carbohydrates, B vitamins (folic acid and pyridoxine), iron, and potassium. Brown rice also contains the B vitamin thiamine, which is present in the bran.

Notes and Dosages
Brown, unpolished rice contains more vitamins and fiber.

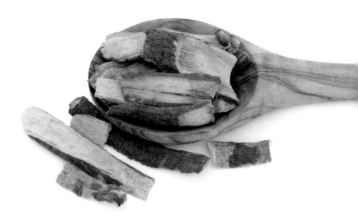

Paeonia lactiflora

BAI SHAO

Known in the West as white peony root, Bai Shao is a cooling herb with a sinking action, which means it takes qi down strongly. It is useful when the liver is not fulfilling its function of making the blood and qi flow smoothly.

DATA FILE

Properties
• Bitter • Sour • Cool • Antispasmodic • Balances the menstrual cycle

Uses
• Treats headaches and dizziness due to rising liver yang, and flank, chest, and abdominal pain from constrained (stuck) liver qi, or disharmony between the liver and spleen, which normally have a close relationship in the upper abdomen.
• "Softens" the liver, treating spasms in the abdomen, or cramps in the hands or feet.
• Good for menstrual irregularity or pain, or uterine bleeding, and, as it preserves the yin fluids, treats vaginal discharge and leaking of sperm.
• Treats excessive sweating in an external illness, or night sweating in yin deficiency.
• Adjusts the ying and wei, balancing the inner and outer qi levels, which control the opening and closing of the pores.

Notes and Dosages
Bai Shao has many uses and is an important herb, working through the liver and spleen channels.

> **CAUTION**
> Exercise caution with diarrhea due to cold from deficiency, as it is a cold herb.

Panax ginseng
GINSENG

Named Ren Shen in traditional Chinese medicine, ginseng is a famous tonic of the Far East, where it is very widely used for stress. The root is also used in Western herbalism, to treat weakness and strengthen the immune system.

DATA FILE

Properties
• Sweet • Slightly bitter • Energizing • Strengthens the immune system • Adaptogenic • Increases concentration • Reduces stress

Uses
• Take for convalescence, exhaustion, jet lag, lack of concentration, and weakness in old age.
• Take with other strengthening herbs for getting rid of infections.
• May help loss of sex drive in men.
• May help the body cope with the side-effects of chemotherapy.
• Ren Shen is good for lung problems such as labored breathing and wheezing, and spleen qi deficient problems such as lethargy, lack of appetite, bloating, and diarrhea.
• Ren Shen calms the heart when there are palpitations, and in cases of anxiety, insomnia, or forgetfulness.

Notes and Dosages
Note that Siberian ginseng, *Eleutherococcus senticosus*, is sometimes sold as ginseng. It may have some of the same medicinal properties. In TCM, Ren Shen is an expensive herb as it takes six or seven years to cultivate. It is usually substituted by Dang Shen in prescriptions. The recommended dosage in Western herbalism is 100mg. of powdered root, 300mg. of cut root in decoction, or 20–30 drops of the tincture twice daily. Many preparations are available in stores: follow the dose on the packet.

> **CAUTION**
> Do not take in pregnancy. May aggravate anxiety and irritability. Avoid with high blood pressure. Do not take large doses in conjunction with stimulants. Do not take consistently without professional advice. Not for children. Ren Shen is contraindicated for yin deficiency with heat signs (it is slightly warming), heat excess or no significant qi deficiency.

Panax notoginseng
SAN QI

Also known as notoginseng or pseudoginseng root, this herb is used for bleeding or hemorrhage. Generally this herb is not used alone, but with other herbs that treat the cause of the bleeding, such as hot blood, yin deficiency, spleen deficiency, or stasis of the blood.

DATA FILE

Properties
• Sweet • Slightly bitter • Warm

Uses
• Stops bleeding without causing blood stasis: use for nosebleeds, uterine bleeding, or trauma-induced bleeding.
• Reduces swelling and alleviates pain, particularly after injuries, falls, fractures, bruises, and sprains.
• Good for chest and abdominal pain, as well as joint pain caused by congealed blood.

Notes and Dosages
San Qi has long been used in battle: soldiers carried this black powder with them to stem wounds. It may be taken on its own or in a prescription.

> **CAUTION**
> Contraindicated during pregnancy. All unexplained bleeding, unstoppable bleeding, or chest pain should be investigated by a physician. Use with caution in patients with blood or yin deficiency.

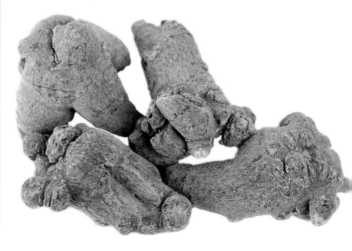

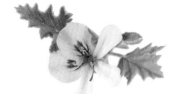

Pelargonium graveolens
GERANIUM

Potted geraniums have a long history of medicinal use. Over 700 varieties exist, and their essential oils differ depending on where the plant is grown. Fresh and floral in fragrance, geranium was traditionally regarded as a feminine oil, a powerful healer, and a valuable insect repellent.

DATA FILE

Properties
- Uplifting • Refreshing • Balancing • Anti-inflammatory
- Soothing • Astringent • Antiseptic • Diuretic • Insect repellent

Uses
- Alleviates apathy, anxiety, stress, hyperactivity, and depression.
- Use topically for arthritis, acne, diaper rash, burns, blisters, eczema, cuts, and congested pores.
- Geranium's antiseptic properties make it useful for cuts and infections, sore throats, and mouth ulcers.
- Relieves swollen breasts and fluid retention, and stimulates sluggish lymph and blood circulation.
- Massage with geranium oil to relieve premenstrual pain and tension, and to treat menopausal problems, as it has a balancing effect on mind and body.

Notes and Dosages
Geranium oil is extracted from the leaves, stalk, and flowers of the plant. It blends well with lavender, bergamot, rose, rosewood, sandalwood, patchouli, frankincense, lemon, jasmine, juniper, tea tree, benzoin, basil, and black pepper.

RECIPE

Massage Blend for Premenstrual Syndrome
Add 10 drops geranium, 10 drops clary sage, and 10 drops bergamot to a bottle containing 1fl.oz. (30ml.) or 6 teaspoons of vegetable oil and shake well. Put 6–8 drops in your bath or use a little as a body oil to massage around your abdomen, hips, and lower back.

> **CAUTION**
> Do not use during the first three months of pregnancy and not at all if there is a history of miscarriage.

Persica americana
AVOCADO

Avocados are the fruit of a small, subtropical tree. They are rich in vitamins A, some B-complex, C, and E vitamins, and potassium, and because they contain some protein and starch, as well as being a good source of monounsaturated fats, they are considered to be a perfect – or complete – food. Traditionally avocados have been used for skin problems. The pulp has both antibacterial and antifungal properties.

DATA FILE

Properties
- Antioxidant • Benefits circulation • Digestive • Antibacterial
- Antifungal • Soothing

Uses
- Eat an avocado each day as a restorative, particularly during convalescence.
- The pulp, applied to grazes and shallow cuts, and covered with sterile gauze, can prevent infection entering the body and encourage healing.
- An avocado paste can be applied to rashes, eczema, and rough skin to soothe and smooth.
- To make a face mask, mash a ripe avocado with a little olive oil and apply to the skin. Leave on for 15 minutes.
- Eat regularly for digestive and circulatory problems.
- The flesh of a ripe avocado soothes sunburned skin. Cut an avocado in half and rub gently over the affected area.
- May help sexual problems.
- Avocado oil can be used as a base oil for massage.

Notes and Dosages
Avocados are full of vitamins and minerals, but they also have a high fat content.

> **CAUTION**
> Do not eat avocados or take any product containing avocado if you have been prescribed MAOI antidepressants.

Petroselimum sativum

PARSLEY

Common garden parsley is not only rich in vitamins, but also has significant therapeutic properties. The root is used in herbalism for digestive disorders, while the herb and seeds are used mainly for kidney and bladder problems. The essential oil, distilled mainly from the seeds, has a warm, spicy, herbaceous scent.

DATA FILE

Properties
- Diuretic • Antiseptic • Tonic for the reproductive system
- Stimulates appetite • Digestive • Mildly laxative • Antirheumatic

Uses
- As a diuretic, parsley helps fluid retention, premenstrual syndrome, and cellulite.
- Its antiseptic effect makes it helpful for cystitis.
- Sometimes used for massage during labor and to regulate the menstrual cycle.
- May shrink small blood vessels and is helpful in treating piles, broken or thread veins, and bruising.
- Use to stimulate appetite, as a mild laxative for sluggish digestion, and to relieve flatulence, stomach cramps, and indigestion.

Notes and Dosages
Parsley has crinkly green foliage and small greenish-yellow flowers that produce small brown seeds. Parsley oil blends well with geranium, rose, rosemary, lavender, bergamot, lemon, neroli, clary sage, tea tree, and spice oils.

RECIPE

Parsley Bath for Water Retention
Add 2 drops parsley oil, 3 drops geranium oil, and 3 drops fennel oil to a warm bath and swirl through the water with your hand.

CAUTION
Use parsley oil in moderation, as it can be toxic and irritant. Do not use during pregnancy. The quantities of parsley used in cookery are not harmful.

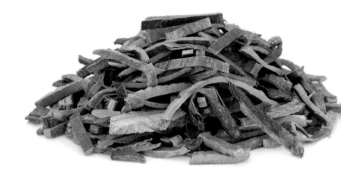

Phellodendron amurense

HUANG BAI

This herb is one used by traditional Chinese practitioners to clear heat: this includes febrile conditions and any illnesses with heat signs. It is one of the "Three Yellows," which are often used together for severe infections. Western names for the herb include Amur cork tree bark.

DATA FILE

Properties
- Bitter • Cold • Antimicrobial • Detoxifying

Uses
- Drains damp heat, particularly in the lower burner: use for damp heat leukorrhea (vaginal discharge) and foul-smelling diarrhea.
- Drains kidney fire: use for ascending kidney fire with deficient yin signs, such as menopausal hot sweats, night sweating, and sweats from withdrawing from illicit drugs.
- Detoxifies fire-poison, for example sores with pus in them.
- Use for red, swollen, and painful legs, as well as leg ulcers that require antibiotics.

Notes and Dosages
Phellodendron amurense has dark, cork-like bark when the tree is old. Huang Bai is a weaker (and cheaper) version of Huang Lian in its antimicrobial effects. It works through the kidney and bladder channels.

CAUTION
Contraindicated in cases of spleen deficiency, with or without diarrhea (spleen deficiency must be diagnosed by a TCM practitioner).

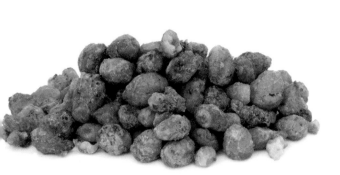

Pinellia ternata

BAN XIA

Ban Xia, also known as pinellia rhizome, is a herb that transforms phlegm, which in traditional Chinese medicine is the accumulation of thick fluid mainly in the respiratory and digestive tracts, but which may occur in the muscles and other body tissues.

DATA FILE

Properties
• Acrid • Warm • Drying • Anti-emetic

Uses
• Transforms phlegm and helps rebellious qi to descend, so is one of the main herbs for coughs with sputum.
• Harmonizes the stomach and stops vomiting, also helping abdominal and epigastric (upper abdominal) bloating.
• Use for nodules caused by phlegm lingering, such as goiter.

Notes and Dosages
Ban Xia is one of the main herbs for drying damp, and can be added to prescriptions to avoid nausea from other herbs.

> **CAUTION**
> Contraindicated in bleeding, coughs due to yin deficiency (dry coughs) or depleted fluids. Use with caution in heat cases. In very large amounts, it is somewhat toxic (causing nausea), but can be cured by ginger.

Pinus sylvestris

SCOTCH PINE

Perhaps one of the best-known natural fragrances is the fresh, invigorating aroma of pine. The Arabs, Greeks, and Romans all made use of its medicinal properties, while Native Americans are believed to have used pine to prevent scurvy and infestation with lice and fleas.

DATA FILE

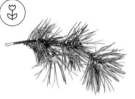

Properties
• Expectorant • Antiseptic • Antiviral
• Insecticidal • Deodorant • Invigorating

Uses
• Inhalations of pine are wonderful for colds, catarrhal conditions, including hay fever, sore throats, chest infections, and blocked sinuses.
• Stimulates the circulation and helps to relieve rheumatic and muscular aches, pains, and stiffness.
• Pine is also deodorizing, making it good for excessive perspiration.
• Use for clearing lice and scabies.
• The refreshing aroma dispels apathy, and relieves mental fatigue, nervous exhaustion, and stress-related problems.
• The pine flower remedy is a very specific remedy for those who blame themselves and are suffering from self-reproach. Even when successful, they are never content, and always feel that they could have done better. They blame themselves even when the fault is someone else's. Pine helps us understand that if we respond honestly and freely there is no need for blame and we can move on.

Notes and Dosages
Scotch pine has long, stiff needles that grow in pairs, and pointed, brown cones. The essential oil blends well with lavender, rosemary, cedarwood, eucalyptus, tea tree, juniper, and sandalwood. The flower remedy is prepared using the boiling method (see page 57).

RECIPE

Inhalation for Sinusitis and Stuffy Colds
Add 2 drops pine, 2 drops eucalyptus, and 2 drops peppermint essential oils to a bowl of steaming water. Cover your head with a towel and inhale for 5–10 minutes. Do this 5 or 6 times a day.

> **CAUTION**
> Use only small amounts of pine oil in the bath or massage. Do not use if you have sensitive skin. Always check the source of your oil, as oils are distilled from several species, some of which are unsuitable for aromatherapy.

Piper longum

LONG PEPPER

Native to India and Java, these peppers are gathered and stored to ripen for use, in order to preserve the greatest heat potency. Long pepper, or pippali, is the primary ingredient in Ayurvedic medicine to treat kapha disorders. Together with ginger and black pepper, long pepper is used as a component in the Ayurvedic blend Trikatu.

DATA FILE

Properties
- Pungent • Heating • Digestive • Carminative • Emetic
- Decongestant • Expectorant • Analgesic • Stimulates circulation

Uses
- Internally, long pepper is taken for asthma, bronchitis, colds, throat problems, and as a treatment for fever and toothache.
- Externally, long pepper can be used for arthritis and muscle soreness.
- Taken internally, long pepper is useful as a digestive aid, helping both diarrhea and constipation.
- Long pepper restores kapha and vátha to balance, and its warming action increases pitta.

Notes and Dosages
The fruit may be taken as a powder, a tea or infusion, a food, or an oil. The herb combines well with black pepper, fenugreek, ginger, and turmeric.

RECIPE

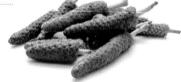

Long Pepper Tea
Use this long pepper and rock salt tea to clear sore throats, sinus congestion, coughs, and hiccups. To a large mug, add 1½ cups of boiling water, ½ teaspoon of long pepper powder, and ½ teaspoon of rock salt. Cover and let steep for 15 minutes. Pour the tea into another cup, leaving the sediment behind. Drink while warm.

CAUTION

Long pepper should not be given to children under two years old. Use rubber gloves when chopping peppers, as it may burn the fingertips. If burning should occur, wash with vinegar several times, rinsing carefully. Pepper oil can linger for several hours, and will cause severe pain if it comes in contact with sensitive tissues, such as eyes or genitals.

Piper nigrum

BLACK PEPPER

Black pepper, a traditional seasoning for food, is a warm, aromatic, and comforting spice with therapeutic uses. The fruit, or corns, of the vine and the essential oil extracted from them are used. Black pepper is the whole, sun-dried, unripened fruit of the vine; white pepper is the ripe fruit, from which the skins have been removed. In Ayurvedic traditions, black pepper or marich is named after the Sanskrit word for the sun.

DATA FILE

Properties
- Heating • Drying • Pungent • Bitter
- Stimulant • Digestive • Decongestant
- Expectorant • Stimulates circulation • Analgesic

Uses
- Use in cooking as a stimulant: black pepper's qualities are enhanced by heating.
- Add black pepper to food daily to treat indigestion and flatulence.
- The essential oil eases muscular aches and pains. Black pepper contains piperine, which helps to relieve pain.
- Pepper is an effective expectorant, and can be taken internally, or rubbed onto the chest (a tiny amount of oil in a carrier oil).
- Pepper has a laxative effect, tones the muscles of the colon, soothes the stomach, and stimulates the appetite.
- In Ayurvedic medicine, black pepper mixed with ghee is used to treat nasal congestion, sinusitis, and inflammation of the skin.
- Can stimulate the circulation to help warm cold hands and feet.
- In Ayurveda, black pepper reduces kapha, and increases pitta and vátha.

Notes and Dosages
The pepper kernel can be take as a spice, as an oil, a tea, or in a compress. In Ayurvedic tradition, black pepper combines well with orange, ginger, cypress, anise, sandalwood, lemon, and basil. The essential oil blends well with frankincense, lavender, rosemary, marjoram, lemon, benzoin, cedarwood, parsley, fennel, and florals.

RECIPE

Compress for Painful Joints
Add 3 drops black pepper essential oil, 2 drops chamomile oil, 2 drops marjoram oil to a bowl of hot or cold water and apply to the affected area as directed. Use hot or cold as preferred.

CAUTION

The essential oil may irritate those with sensitive skin: dilute well. Large amounts of black pepper used regularly may result in overstimulation of the kidneys. When using black pepper for medicinal purposes, follow the recommended dosage. Do not use the oil while taking homeopathic remedies. Overuse of stimulant herbs can impair your body's natural balance.

Plantago major, Plantago lanceolata

PLANTAIN LEAF

The broadleaf and narrowleaf plantains, not related to the cooking banana, are common weeds of pathways and lawns. The broadleaf plantain was said to spring up wherever the English established a colony, giving rise to its common name of "white man's foot."

DATA FILE

Properties
- Soothing • Healing • Astringent

Uses
- Plantain tea eases a running nose from allergies, irritation, and colds.
- Take internally for irritable bowel and irritable bladder.
- Use as a compress or lotion for insect bites, allergic rashes, and infected eczema, and for cleaning wounds, drawing stings, and splinters.
- Soothes neuralgic pains and shingles rash.
- Use as a cream or ointment for bleeding piles.
- The tea is a cooling drink for persistent fevers and is a useful addition to any medicine given to "hot" people.
- Add to a mouthwash for sore and bleeding gums.

Notes and Dosages
Make a double-strength tea (2 teaspoons per cup) for most purposes. Take it freely.

RECIPE

Plantain Lotion
Finely chop sufficient fresh plantain leaves to fill a small jar. Add sufficient glycerin to cover the leaves. Stand for 2 weeks, stirring from time to time. Strain and store in a dark bottle.

Use as a soothing and healing lotion for weeping and itchy rashes, and insect bites.

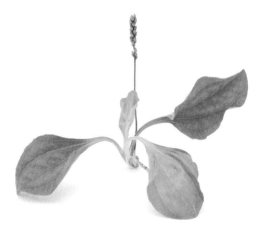

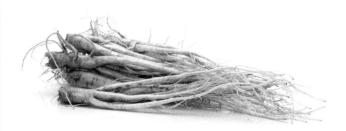

Platycodon grandiflorus

JIE GENG

The balloon flower root relieves coughing and wheezing. Like other Chinese cough remedies, it treats the manifestation (presenting symptoms) of the problem, and therefore needs to be combined with other herbs that treat the root cause.

DATA FILE

Properties
- Bitter • Acrid • Neutral • Expectorant • Expels pus

Uses
- Circulates the lung qi, expels phlegm and stops coughing: Jie Geng can be used to treat a wide variety of coughs, depending on the other herbs with which it is combined.
- Use for sore throat and loss of voice, especially those caused by external heat.
- Use for expelling pus associated with lung or throat abscess.

Notes and Dosages
Jie Geng works on the Lung meridian, treating chest complaints. Like Xing Ren, Jie Geng can be used for a wide variety of coughs, especially for coughs caused by external pathogens, either wind cold or wind heat. The herb is also often put into other prescriptions to direct herbs to the chest and head areas.

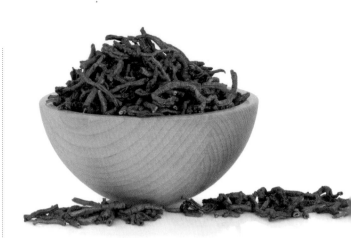

Pogostemon cablin
PATCHOULI

The distinctive exotic and earthy aroma of patchouli is one that you either love or hate. Smell is important to the success of aromatherapy, so only use this oil if you like its scent. Patchouli has many uses, and is especially pleasant when used as part of a blend. It is an intense odor, which improves with age.

DATA FILE

Properties
- Antidepressant • Nervous tonic • Aphrodisiac • Astringent
- Antiviral • Antiseptic • Anti-inflammatory • Diuretic

Uses
- Use to treat mild depression, anxiety, nervous exhaustion, lack of interest in sex, and stress-related problems.
- Good for chapped or cracked skin and open pores, and is also effective for acne, eczema, dermatitis, dandruff, and fungal infections of the skin.
- It is a cell regenerator, good for aging skins, and promotes wound-healing.
- Try for cellulite and as a general tonic.

Notes and Dosages
Patchouli is a perennial herb with large, fragrant, furry leaves. The oil is extracted from dried patchouli leaves. Patchouli oil blends well with rose, geranium, bergamot, neroli, ylang ylang, lemon, sandalwood, clary sage, clove, cedarwood, and lavender.

RECIPE

Antiwrinkle Night Oil
Add 2 drops patchouli, 3 drops lemon, and 5 drops rose to 2 drops evening primrose oil and 1 teaspoon (10ml.) sweet almond or hazelnut oil. Blend well and apply to the face and neck at night.

> **CAUTION**
> Keep all essential oils out of the reach of children.

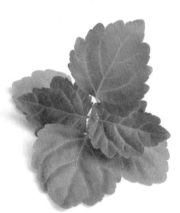

Polygala tenuifolia
YUAN ZHI

Chinese senega root, also called polygala, is used in traditional Chinese medicine to nourish the heart and calm the spirit, or shen, which is said to reside in the heart. When the shen is calm, personality is at its most potent.

DATA FILE

Properties
- Bitter • Acrid • Slightly warm • Releases emotions • Expectorant
- Anti-inflammatory

Uses
- Use for the release of pent-up emotions: take for insomnia, anxiety, palpitations, forgetfulness, and for many emotional problems.
- Use for coughs with copious sputum, especially when difficult to expectorate.
- To reduce abscesses, dissipate swellings, and relieve swollen breasts, use in powdered form, applied topically or mixed into a glass of wine.

Notes and Dosages
This herb works through the heart, lung, and kidney channels.

> **CAUTION**
> Contraindicated for yin deficiency with heat signs. Caution should be exercised with ulcers or gastritis.

Polygonum multiflorum

HE SHOU WU

In traditional Chinese medicine, the fleeceflower root treats patterns of blood deficiency, and the two organs most affected by this disorder are the heart and liver, which direct and store the blood, respectively.

DATA FILE

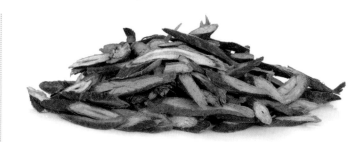

Properties
• Bitter • Sweet • Astringent • Slightly warm • Laxative • Firms the jing • Detoxifying • Tonic • Rejuvenating

Uses
• Helps to prevent signs of aging: particularly used for premature graying or when the hair falls out (the name means "black hair"), as well as for dizziness, blurred vision, spots in front of the eyes, and a weak lower back and knees.
• Stops premature ejaculation, leaking of sperm, and vaginal discharge.
• Used raw, it is good for goiter, neck lumps, carbuncles, and sores.
• Take for constipation.
• Expels wind from the skin by nourishing the blood: use for rashes that appear suddenly.
• May treat chronic malaria and prevent hardening of the arteries.

Notes and Dosages
He Shou Wu is very commonly used, as it both tonifies and preserves the kidney jing-essence without being cloying.

CAUTION
Contraindicated for spleen deficiency, phlegm, or diarrhea. Consult with your physician before taking fleeceflower.

Polygonum multiflorum

YE JIAO TENG

Made from the dry vine stem of the fleeceflower, this herb nourishes the heart and calms the spirit. It is useful in tackling disturbed emotions.

DATA FILE

Properties
• Sweet • Slightly bitter • Neutral • Soothing
• Stimulates circulation

Uses
• Use for yin- or blood-deficiency patterns with insomnia, irritability, emotional weakness, and dream-disturbed sleep.
• Make into a decoction and use as an external wash to alleviate itching and rashes.
• Nourishes the blood in the limbs when the circulation is blocked or weak due to deficiency, and is used for such symptoms as generalized weakness, soreness, and aching or numb limbs.

Notes and Dosages
This herb works through the heart and liver.

CAUTION
Contraindicated with diarrhea. Consult with your physician before taking.

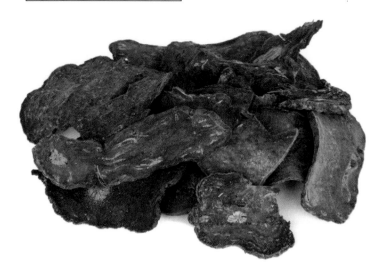

Populus tremula

ASPEN

Aspen is a slender, silver-barked, deciduous tree. It grows to 30ft. (10m.), its almost circular leaves trembling in the slightest breeze.

DATA FILE

Properties
• Calming • Gives courage

Uses
• Aspen is suitable for vague or unexplained fears. The fear can be so deep that it is too frightening to express, and the sufferer feels burdened by doom, and inexplicable terror. Fear may be extreme enough to affect appetite, produce palpitations, and interrupt sleep patterns, bringing nightmares.
• Suitable for easing the fears and nightmares of children where they cannot describe what they are frightened of.
• This remedy brings reassurance that there is nothing to fear. It helps us to face the unknown with courage and trust.

Notes and Dosages
Aspen is a type of poplar with gray-green leaves that flutter in the breeze. It also has cottony catkins. Prepare this flower essence using the boiling method (see page 57).

Poria cocos

FU LING

This fungus, also known as tuckahoe, hoelen, and bread root, is a widely used herb in traditional Chinese medicine. It transforms dampness that creates stagnation in the middle burner, with various digestive or fluid-retaining effects.

DATA FILE

Properties
• Sweet • Bland • Neutral • Diuretic • Calming

Uses
• Good for difficulty with urination, diarrhea or edema (water retention), all symptoms of dampness in the system.
• Helps with loss of appetite or bloating.
• Calms the spirit, making it good for palpitations, insomnia, or forgetfulness.
• Strengthens the spleen and transforms phlegm – congested fluids which can cause heart palpitations, headaches, or dizziness.

Notes and Dosages
Fu Ling is a neutral herb that is added to many prescription mixes. It is a main ingredient in the qi-strengthening prescription Si Jun Zi Wan ("Four Gentlemen") and is also essential in the main yin-tonifying prescription, where it stops a person becoming too moist from the yin (fluid) tonifying herbs.

> **CAUTION**
> Contraindicated for copious urine from deficient cold.

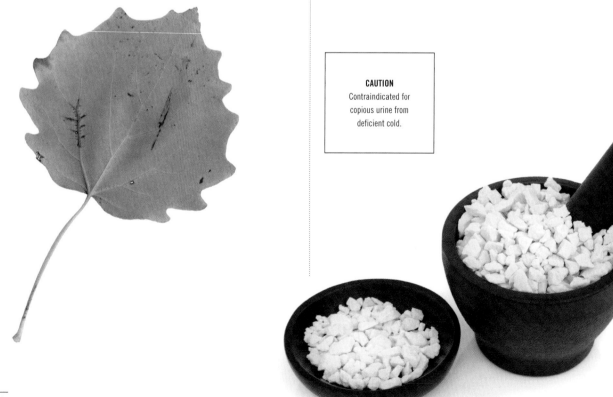

Prunus amygdalus dulcis,
Prunus amygdalus amara

ALMOND

The almond tree produces the oldest and most widely grown of all of the world's nut crops, and is indigenous to western Asia and North Africa. Of the two major types of almonds grown, the sweet almond (*P. dulcis*) is cultivated for its edible nut. The bitter almond (*P. amara*) is inedible but contains an oil – also present in the sweet almond, and in the ripe kernels of the apricot and peach – which, when combined with water, yields hydrocyanic (prussic) acid and benzaldehyde. The oil is used in making flavoring extracts and in some sedative medicines.

DATA FILE

Properties
• Anti-inflammatory • Aids respiration • Digestive • Lowers fever

Uses
• Almonds are rich in protein, fat, zinc, potassium, iron, B vitamins, and magnesium.
• Add ground almonds to water to prevent fevers.
• Almond milk is an excellent tonic during convalescence.
• Drink almond milk daily to reduce frequency of digestive disorders, and to relieve respiratory problems.
• Combine almond milk with barley water for urinary problems.
• Take for bronchitis.

Notes and Dosages
Almonds are the kernel of the stone in the fruit of the almond tree. Eat almonds with foods rich in vitamin C to encourage maximum absorption.

RECIPE

Almond Milk
Almond milk helps digestive, respiratory, and urinary problems. Drink it every day for the best results. Blend 6 tablespoons of almonds in a food processor with 1pt. (500ml.) water. Grind until smooth. Add 1 teaspoon of honey for flavor. Strain the mixture through a sieve or fine cloth to drink. Store in a refrigerator.

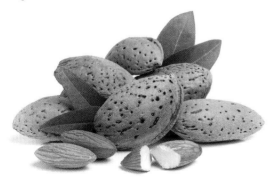

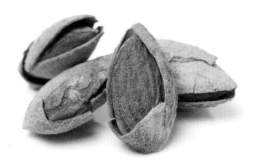

Prunus armeniaca

XING REN

This herb, obtained from apricot kernels, is primarily used to treat coughing and wheezing. As it treats the manifestation (presenting symptoms) of the problem, it needs to be combined with other herbs that treat the root cause.

DATA FILE

Properties
• Bitter • Slightly warm • Slightly toxic • Relieves breathing
• Laxative

Uses
• Stops coughing and calms wheezing: used for many kinds of coughs, whether from heat or cold, exterior or interior, depending on the combination with other herbs.
• Moistens intestines and unblocks the bowels

Notes and Dosages
Xing Ren is a valuable constituent of various herbal cough remedies. It may be combined with Huo Ma Ren or Dang Gui for constipation due to deficient qi and dry intestines. It works in the lung, and large intestine channels.

> **CAUTION**
> Use with caution for children and in cases of diarrhea.

Prunus cerasus
CHERRY PLUM

A small tree with red or yellow fruit, cherry plum is often grown as hedging and windbreaks. It flowers from early spring, with delicate pale pink flowers.

DATA FILE

Properties
• Encourages to let go of fear • Helps to regain control of the emotions

Uses
• Cherry plum is for the fear of letting go or of losing control. The fearful thoughts may be of a suicidal, compulsive, or destructive nature. This mental pain and turmoil may happen during a period of great emotional or physical change, when the person is worn and stressed.
• This remedy is also useful for uncontrolled tantrums in children, when they are frightened by their own loss of temper.
• Cherry plum restores control and trust of the mind and emotions.

Notes and Dosages
The wild cherry plum is in flower almost before the arrival of spring. Flowering twigs are used for the remedy. Prepare them using the boiling method (see page 57).

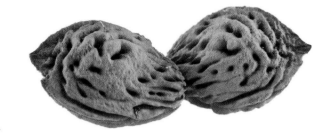

Prunus persica
TAO REN

Made from peach kernels, this traditional Chinese remedy invigorates (or "regulates") the blood, treating problems associated with blood stasis. In TCM these disorders include pain and internal masses or growths.

DATA FILE

Properties
• Bitter • Sweet • Neutral • Laxative • Stimulates circulation of blood

Uses
• Like many seeds, Tao Ren is useful for constipation caused by dry intestines.
• Treats disorders of the blood and congealed blood amenorrhea and abdominal pain, or pain from injuries.
• Use for abscesses.

Notes and Dosages
Tao Ren is a very strong herb, working through the heart, liver, lung, and large intestine channels.

> **CAUTION**
> Do not use during pregnancy.

Ptilotus atriplicifolius

MULLA MULLA

A small plant from desert regions, mulla mulla responds to the weather, and sends out clusters of pink, long-lasting flowers when conditions are favorable. All but one of the many species of *Ptilotus* are exclusive to Australia.

DATA FILE

Properties
• Rejuvenating • Protects from the damaging effects of heat

Uses
• For those suffering the effects of fire, heat, or radiation, in reality and symbolically. People who need mulla mulla may have burns, sunburn, or hot rashes; they may be suffering exhaustion from heat, or from working in over-hot conditions, or a hot climate; or they may be having laser treatment.
• Mulla mulla helps the body recover from damage and protects it from harmful rays.

Notes and Dosages
Like many desert plants, mulla mulla has stunning flowers which seem to symbolize hope and life. Prepare them using the sun method (see page 56).

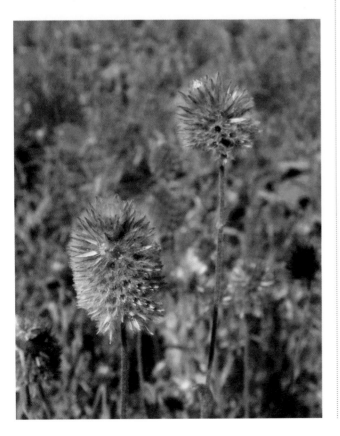

Quercus robur

OAK

Quercus robur is the common oak. Most people recognize the acorns, but the flowers are less familiar. Male and female flowers are borne on the same tree and appear from April onward.

DATA FILE

Properties
• Encourages adaptability and flexibility

Uses
• Oak people are strong and brave fighters. They struggle through events and physical illnesses even when there is no hope, never thinking of surrender. Their strength may sometimes be inappropriate, and they can exhaust themselves by pushing blindly on in one narrow direction. Strength is a virtue, but it is pointless pushing against an immovable object. Oak helps us surrender, step back, look around, and to consider some different answers.
• Oak restores the true inner strength, which is flexible and adaptable.

Notes and Dosages
Pick the small, female catkins only. Prepare them using the sun method (see page 56).

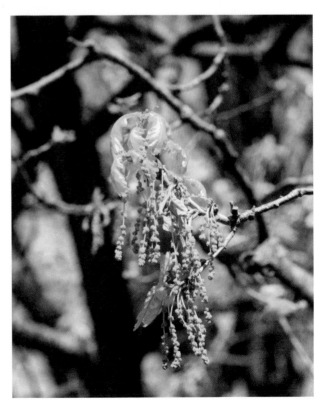

Rehmannia glutinosa
SHENG DI HUANG

Sheng Di Huang is one of a group of herbs that is used in traditional Chinese medicine to clear heat: this includes febrile conditions and any illnesses with heat signs. It can be used to treat diabetes by addressing the heat cause. The remedy is obtained from the root of the Chinese foxglove.

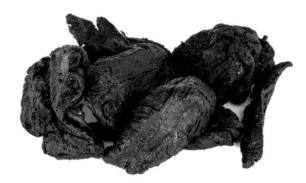

DATA FILE

Properties
- Sweet • Bitter • Cooling • Generates fluid • Soporific
- Mildly laxative

Uses
- Use in febrile illnesses where the heat has dried up the fluids in the body, causing thirst, irritability, and a scarlet tongue.
- Nourishes the yin and generates fluids: treats constipation.
- Cools heart fire blazing: use for mouth and tongue ulcers, and insomnia.
- May be prescribed for diabetes.

Notes and Dosages
This herb works through the heart, liver, and kidney channels.

> **CAUTION**
> Contraindicated in cases of spleen deficiency with dampness, as Sheng Di Huang is too moistening. Also contraindicated in the presence of phlegm.

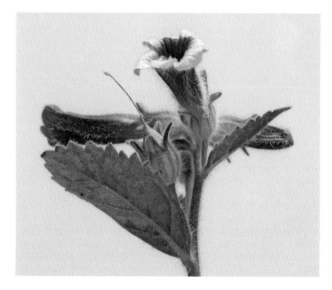

Rehmannia glutinosa
SHU DI HUANG

Like Sheng Di Huang, this remedy is obtained from the Chinese foxglove root, but in Shu Di Huang the root is cooked in wine. This herb treats patterns of blood deficiency, and in TCM the two organs most affected by this disorder are the heart and liver.

DATA FILE

Properties
- Sweet • Slightly warm

Uses
- Treats blood-deficient symptoms, such as a pale complexion, dizziness, palpitations, and insomnia.
- Helps menstrual problems such as irregular bleeding, uterine bleeding, and amenorrhea (no menstruation).
- Prescribed for kidney yin-deficient patterns, including night sweats, heat in the bones, nocturnal emissions (wet dreams), diabetes, and tinnitus (ringing in the ears).
- Also prescribed for jing deficiency, including such kidney symptoms as low back pain, weakness of the knees and legs, lightheadedness, deafness, and premature graying of the hair.

Notes and Dosages
Shu Di Huang is a very important herb, as it is both a blood and a yin tonic. It works through the heart, kidney, and liver channels.

> **CAUTION**
> Use with caution in cases of spleen and stomach deficiency, or stagnant qi or phlegm. As with many tonifying herbs, it nourishes the moist substances in the body, so overuse can lead to bloating and loose stools: it must be carefully combined.

Rheum palmatum, Rheum officinale

CHINESE RHUBARB

Chinese rhubarb, also called turkey rhubarb, closely related to edible garden rhubarb, is used in both traditional Chinese medicine and Western herbalism. In Chinese medicine, the root and rhizome are used to make Da Huang, which comes into the category of descending downward: it facilitates the expulsion of stools in cases of constipation. This downward action clears heat.

DATA FILE

Properties
• Bitter • Cooling • Laxative • Astringent • Tonic

Uses
• Take for constipation, feelings of congestion and fullness in the stomach, and stomach acidity.
• Use either topically or internally for boils, sores, burns, or hot skin lesions (red lesions, giving off heat).
• Take for gastroenteritis and diarrhea from food poisoning.
• May be prescribed for cystitis, gout, and acute liver and gall bladder diseases.
• Take for bleeding hemorrhoids (piles) and nosebleeds.
• Good for stagnant blood complaints such as endometriosis and amenorrhea (lack of menstruation).

Notes and Dosages
Rheum palmatum is a perennial growing to a height of 6ft. (2m.), with 2ft. (60cm.) leaves. Note that consuming rhubarb root may cause the urine to take on a reddish tinge. In TCM, Da Huang is a cold herb, used to treat heat conditions by purging the body. It works through the heart, large intestine, liver, and stomach channels.

In Western herbalism, half the standard dose is used: ½ teaspoon to 1 cup of water for decoction, or 30–40 drops of the tincture, 3 times daily.

RECIPE

Laxative Wine
Warm a glass of white wine (don't boil). Pour the wine onto 1 teaspoon of chopped rhubarb root. Add a good pinch of cinnamon powder and stand overnight. Strain and drink.

CAUTION
Do not take during pregnancy. Exercise care if taking during menstruation, and postpartum (after birth). Do not use in the first stage of infectious diseases, in bowel spasm, or when colicky pains are present. Avoid taking laxatives for long periods. Do not eat rhubarb leaves. Also contraindicated for qi or blood deficiency – it doesn't tonify weakness but may be added to a tonifying prescription to clear heat. Contraindicated for cold.

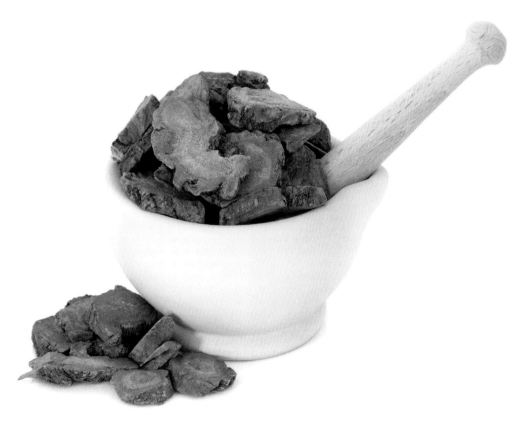

Ricinocarpos pinifolius
WEDDING BUSH

Ricinocarpus pinifolius is a small bush with abundant, six-petaled white flowers. Male and female flowers grow on the same bush. The flowers were traditionally used for wedding decorations, giving the bush its name.

DATA FILE

Properties
• Encourages commitment and dedication • Takes away passivity

Uses
• Wedding bush is for those who doubt their ability to commit or accept the responsibility of deep caring; for those with a pattern of starting but not finishing, and running away from the self in all aspects of life; for those who are an "emotional rolling stone." They may be in love with love (or the newness of love) and move from one affair to another, or they may have one job after another.
• Wedding bush encourages the confidence to commit, to feel the comfort rather than the burden of responsibility, and to make a long-term dedication to life and its purpose. It reminds us that commitment is an attitude of mind involving self-worth.

Notes and Dosages
Despite its delicate and fragrant flowers, the wild rose is vigorous and thorny. Pick both male and female flowers. Prepare the flower remedy using the sun method (see page 56).

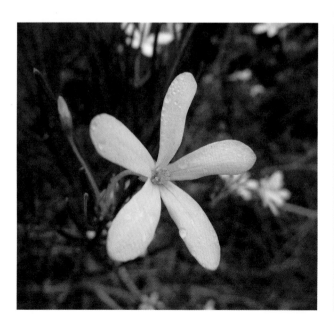

Rosa species
ROSE

The common wild rose, *Rosa canina*, is used to make the wild rose flower remedy. The plant can be seen rambling over country hedges, with the flowers appearing in early summer and varying in color from almost white to deep pink. The fruit, or rosehip, is a striking scarlet. Most of the rose oil used in aromatherapy is produced from two types of rose: *Rosa centifolia* and *Rosa damascena*. They vary slightly in color and fragrance, but have similar properties and uses.

DATA FILE

Properties
• Aphrodisiac • Sedative • Tonic • Antidepressant
• Antiseptic • Detoxifying • Digestive

Uses
• Rose essential oil has an affinity with the female reproductive system, helping to regulate the menstrual cycle and alleviate premenstrual syndrome or postnatal depression.
• The oil benefits stress-related conditions such as insomnia and nervous tension.
• Use the oil to protect against viruses and bacteria.
• Rose oil acts as a tonic for the heart, circulation, liver, stomach, and uterus, and helps to detoxify the blood and organs.
• Rose oil regulates the appetite, and prevents and relieves digestive spasms, constipation, and nausea.
• Used topically, the oil soothes cracked, chapped, sensitive, dry, inflamed, or allergy-prone skin, stops bleeding, and encourages wound-healing. Broken veins and aging skin also benefit.
• Wild rose flower remedy is for the fatalist. This person glides through life passively, taking it as it is, without motivation or expectation. Wild rose stimulates interest and an appreciation of life's color and joy. The remedy encourages action, and a purposeful pleasure in being and doing.

Notes and Dosages
Rose essential oil blends well with clary sage, lavender, sandalwood, geranium, bergamot, and ylang ylang. Prepare the flower remedy using the boiling method (see page 57).

RECIPE

Comforting Massage Blend for Grief
Add 4 drops rose essential oil, 2 drops frankincense, 4 drops chamomile to 3 teaspoons (15ml.) of sweet almond or grapeseed oil.

> **CAUTION**
> Do not use rose essential oil during the first three months of pregnancy and not at all if there is a history of miscarriage.

Rosmarinus officinalis

ROSEMARY

Rosemary was one of the first herbs to be used medicinally. Traditionally it was used to ward off evil, to offer protection from the plague, and to preserve and flavor meat. This strong distinctively scented oil is one of the most valuable of all essential oils.

DATA FILE

Properties

- Gentle bitter tonic • Stimulates circulation • Antiseptic
- Antibacterial • Antifungal • Diuretic • Relieves stress
- Lifts the spirits • Tones skin • Digestive • Antispasmodic

Uses

- Rosemary vinegar is a powerful disinfectant.
- Regular rosemary infusions may help to lift mild depression.
- Take rosemary with chamomile for stress-related headaches.
- Use as a gargle for sore throats, making a useful substitute for sage during pregnancy.
- Two cups of rosemary tea a day will prevent hair loss through poor circulation and restimulate growth after chemotherapy.
- Drink with horsetail for hair loss due to stress and worry.
- Drink rosemary tea for poor digestion, gall bladder inflammation, gallstones, and general feeling of liverishness.
- Rosemary tea can be used as a conditioning hair rinse.
- Rinse hair and scalp with rosemary vinegar for dandruff and for gloriously glossy hair (especially for dark hair).
- Refreshing rosemary oil, as well as rosemary tea, are circulation stimulants, excellent for low blood pressure, muscle fatigue, poor circulation, aches, pains, and strains.
- When used in massage, the oil relieves stress-related disorders, mental exhaustion, and promotes mental clarity.
- Applied topically, rosemary oil tones the skin and helps acne, eczema, dandruff, lice, and hair loss.
- Helps fluid retention, relieves painful menstruation, and clears vaginal discharge.
- Rosemary oil prevents and reduces digestive spasms, relieves wind, and regulates digestion.
- Inhalations of rosemary oil may help to clear catarrh, coughs, colds, and headaches.

Notes and Dosages

Rosemary is an aromatic, evergreen bush, with silvery green leaves and pale blue flowers. For herbal remedies, take standard doses, used freely.

The oil is usually extracted from fresh flowering tops. Rosemary oil blends well with frankincense, petitgrain, basil, thyme, bergamot, lavender, peppermint, pine, cedarwood, cypress, spice oils such as cinnamon, clove, ginger, and black pepper. Add 15 drops of essential oil to a bath to ease muscular tension, improve circulation, and boost spirits.

RECIPES

After-Sport Shower Formula

Add 2 drops rosemary essential oil, 2 drops pine, and 4 drops of lemon to a large dollop of a gentle, unscented shower gel. Step into a hot shower and work into a lather using a sponge or flannel.

Rosemary Vinegar

Take 1oz. (25g.) rosemary and 2pt. (1l.) cider vinegar.
Leave the rosemary to steep in the vinegar for two weeks.
Shake occasionally. After two weeks, strain, bottle, label, and date.
Use 1–2 dessertspoons in the final rinsing water when washing hair.
For dandruff, massage rosemary vinegar thoroughly into the scalp 20 minutes before washing.

CAUTION

Do not use during pregnancy. Rosemary is not suitable for people with epilepsy or high blood pressure. Do not use for treating headaches and migraines that feel "hot." The amounts taken in food are harmless.

Rubus idaeus
RASPBERRY

The leaves from the raspberry bush are used to make a herbal tea often taken by women in the last weeks of pregnancy, to promote an easy birth. Raspberries grow best in rich, moist, well-drained soil, and prefer a sunny position.

DATA FILE

Properties
• Astringent • Antispasmodic • Especially applicable to the womb

Uses
• Drink raspberry leaf tea in the last 2 months of pregnancy to promote an easy birth by tonifying the uterus. Continue for 3 or 4 weeks afterward to re-tone the womb quickly.
• Use raspberry leaf tea as a mouthwash for sore mouths, sore throats, weak gums, and mouth ulcers.
• Raspberry vinegar can be taken as a gargle for sore throats.
• Take the leaves with marshmallow and peppermint for diverticulitis.
• For children's diarrhea and oral thrush, put raspberry leaf tea in a sterilized spray bottle and spray into the mouth 3 or 4 times daily.

Notes and Dosages
When picking your own leaves or fruit, make sure that the bush has not been sprayed with pesticide. To prepare your own remedies from the leaves, use standard doses. For tablets, follow the dose on the packet.

RECIPE

Raspberry Vinegar
Fill a large jar with fresh raspberries, just the fruit. Cover with cider vinegar and stand in a cool place for two weeks. Strain and store in clean bottles. As a gargle for throats, dilute the vinegar with two parts of water.

> **CAUTION**
> Avoid raspberry leaves in early pregnancy except with professional advice: the remedy is best taken during the last three months.

Rumex crispus
YELLOW DOCK

The dried root of this common wild plant is often used for blood and skin diseases. It contains anthraquinones, which act on the bowel and relieve constipation.

DATA FILE

Properties
• Astringent • Laxative • Bitter tonic • Alterative

Uses
• Use the decoction, tincture, or syrup to treat constipation.
• Take for liver congestion with poor fat digestion, and for feelings of heaviness which come on after eating.
• Use for stomach acidity, and for irritable bowel syndrome with constipation.
• Take for food poisoning and intestinal infections.
• Drink with burdock for the relief of chronic, hot, and itchy skin diseases.

Notes and Dosages
The dried root of the plant, which is dug up in the fall, is used for all remedies. Yellow dock is also known as curled dock, because of its twisting leaves. Make the decoction using ½oz. (12g.) yellow dock root to 1pt. (500ml.) water. For constipation, take 1 cup of decoction or 2 teaspoons of tincture daily, but more might be needed for short periods. Use half this dose for chronic conditions, for children, and for constipation in pregnancy.

RECIPE

Laxative Syrup
Take ½oz. (12g.) dried root, ½pt. (250ml.) of water and one stick of cinnamon. Simmer together for 20 minutes, then strain out the solids. Reduce the liquid over low heat to 2fl.oz. (50ml.). Add 4oz. (100g.) sugar. Stir over low heat until dissolved. Take 6 dessertspoons for adults, and 3 for children and pregnant women.

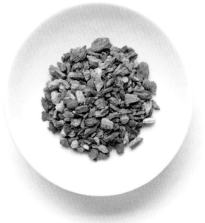

Salix alba

WHITE WILLOW

The bark from the white willow tree is used to treat arthritis and back pain, and to lessen sexual desire. The tree's twigs and leaves are also used to make a flower remedy to encourage maturity.

DATA FILE

Properties
• Anti-inflammatory • Mild painkiller • Anaphrodisiac • Tonic

Uses
• A decoction or tincture treats all types of arthritis and gout. Mix with celery seed for multiple painful joints.
• Take a decoction with cramp bark for inflammatory back pain and lumbago.
• Sip a decoction for chronic diarrhea.
• Take together with rosemary for headaches.
• May help sexual overstimulation, wet dreams, and premature ejaculation.
• Take decoction or tincture for convalescence.
• People who need the willow flower remedy may be sulky and selfish, embittered with self-pity, and ungrateful for help. Willow encourages a more positive and mature attitude.

Notes and Dosages
Salix alba is a 50ft. (15m.) silver-gray deciduous tree. Use willow bark to prepare herbal remedies, using standard doses (see page 39) – and persist. Willow bark contains aspirin-like compounds, but it does not upset the stomach. Prepare the flower remedy using the boiling method (see page 57).

RECIPE

Willow Bark and Ginger Decoction
Add 2 heaped teaspoons of dried willow bark and 1 heaped teaspoon ginger powder to 2 cups of water. Simmer together for 10 minutes. Strain. Add honey to taste, then drink. Take freely for chills, diarrhea, and in convalescence.

> **CAUTION**
> Do not take willow bark when pregnant or breastfeeding. Avoid if allergic to salicylates (aspirin). Not suitable for children.

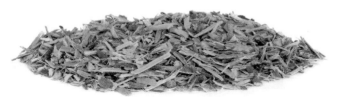

Salvia officinalis

SAGE

The leaves of the common garden and cooking herb are also used in Western herbalism. The purple or red variety is stronger, but any variety will suffice. Sow seeds in late spring, in well-drained soil. Choose a sunny position. The plant grows to about 2ft. (60cm.).

DATA FILE

Properties
• Astringent • Stimulant • Antiseptic • Carminative
• Antispasmodic • Nervine • Strengthening • Tonic for women

Uses
• Take for depression and nervous exhaustion, post-viral fatigue, and general debility.
• Use for anxiety and confusion in elderly people, or accompanying exhaustion and weakened states.
• Drink sage tea for indigestion, wind, loss of appetite, and mucus on the stomach.
• Take cold tincture for excessive sweating and night sweats, or weak lungs with persistent and recurrent coughs and allergies.
• Use as a tea or compress for menopausal hot flushes, menstrual cramps, and premenstrual painful breasts.
• Cold sage tea taken every few hours will usually dry up breast milk.
• Use as a gargle and mouthwash for sore throats, laryngitis, tonsillitis, mouth ulcers, and inflamed and tender gums.
• Use as an antiseptic wash for dirty wounds that are slow to heal.

Notes and Dosages
Use the leaves in standard doses (see page 39). Traditionally, 1 cup a day maintains health in old age. For an extra-strength gargle, add 5 drops of tincture of myrrh (from pharmacies or herb stores) to 1 cup of sage tea. Sage tincture can be taken, instead of the cold tea, for stopping night sweats: 4 teaspoons daily, in a little water. Sage leaves may be added to meat, fish, egg, and vegetable dishes.

RECIPE

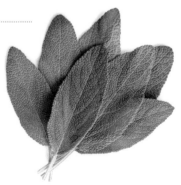

Sage and Vinegar Poultice
Bruise a handful of fresh sage leaves by flattening them with a rolling pin. Place in a pan and cover with cider vinegar. Simmer very gently until the leaves are soft. Wrap the leaves in a cloth and apply warm for bruises, swellings, and stings.

Salvia sclarea
CLARY SAGE

Affectionately known as "clear eye," clary sage was used in medieval times for clearing foreign bodies from the eyes. It remains popular in aromatherapy because of its gentle actions and pleasant nutty fragrance. The oil is extracted from the flowering tops and leaves.

DATA FILE

Properties
• Antidepressant • Muscle relaxant • Digestive • Astringent
• Antibacterial • Encourages menstruation • Aphrodisiac

Uses
• Helps to regulate the nervous system and is most beneficial in treating anxiety, depression, and stress-related problems.
• Acts as a powerful muscle relaxant, helping to ease muscular aches and pains.
• Benefits digestion, relieving indigestion and flatulence.
• Useful for oily skin and scalp conditions.
• Inhalations may help with throat and respiratory infections.
• May be recommended for scant or absent menstruation and for premenstrual syndrome.
• Massage may act as an aphrodisiac.

Notes and Dosages
Clary sage is a biennial or perennial herb with large, hairy leaves. The essential oil blends well with lavender, frankincense, sandalwood, cedarwood, citrus oils, geranium, ylang ylang, juniper, and coriander.

RECIPE

Premenstrual Bath Blend
Add 3 drops clary sage, 2 drops chamomile, 2 drops geranium to a warm bath. Disperse with your hand, and relax for at least 10 minutes.

CAUTION
Do not use during pregnancy. Do not use when drinking alcohol as it can make you drunk, drowsy, and can cause nightmares.

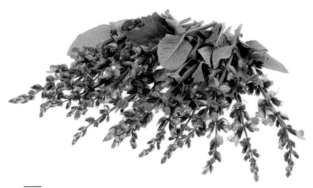

Sambucus nigra
ELDERFLOWER

The creamy white flowers from this small tree, common in hedgerows, are used in Western herbalism. The tree is in flower for only three weeks in summer. Elderflower ointment has long been a remedy for chilblains and chapped hands.

DATA FILE

Properties
• Restorative for mucous membrane and sinuses • Diaphoretic
• Diuretic • Anti-inflammatory

Uses
• Take the tea or tincture for sinusitis, colds, hay fever, and flu.
• Take to break a fever with hot, dry skin: it will induce sweating, bring down the temperature, and protect the kidneys.
• Suitable for use in children's fevers as a tea and as a lotion to soothe the rashes that often come with them.
• Apply as a lotion or compress for sore and runny eyes, eyestrain, and sunburn.
• Use in a cream for chapped and discolored skin.
• Eating fresh elderflowers will relieve the symptoms of hay fever, as will drinking a tea made with equal parts of elderflowers and eyebright (*Euphrasia officinalis*).
• For colds and runny noses in infants, add 3 or 4 cups of elderflower tea to their daily bath.

Notes and Dosages
The hot tea is taken freely, up to 1 cup every 2 hours, for colds and fevers; 3 cups a day for chronic colds and sinusitis. For children over five, use half doses. To prevent hay fever, take 3 cups a day, starting two months before your regular season.

RECIPE

Hayfever Nose Wash
Elderflower nose wash is useful for sinusitis and hay fever. Make a cupful of a strong infusion, allow it to cool to blood heat, and add a pinch of salt. Sniff the mixture up each nostril in turn, then allow it to run out or use a special nasal bath. Use daily during the hay fever season.

Santalum album

SANDALWOOD

Sandalwood is a small tree which grows primarily in southern Asia. While the aromatic wood is used to make scented carvings, the medicinal properties are in the oil, which can be pressed from the wood, or extracted with alcohol or water.

DATA FILE

Properties
- Bitter • Sweet • Astringent • Cooling • Moisturizing
- Alterative • Hemostatic • Antipyretic • Antiseptic
- Antibacterial • Carminative • Sedative • Antispasmodic
- Aphrodisiac • Nervine • Expectorant • Diuretic • Disinfectant
- Helps to regenerate tissues

Uses
- Sandalwood is effective for treating urinary disorders, and particularly cystitis.
- Sandalwood can cure skin problems that are bacterial in origin, as well as acute dermatitis, dry skin, shaving rash, psoriasis, eczema, and acne.
- Encourages wound healing.
- May ease depression, insomnia, nervousness, anxiety, and impotence.
- Clears catarrh and is effective for bronchitis, laryngitis, coughs, and sore throats.
- May be used as an insect repellent.
- Soothes the stomach, reduces digestive spasms, relieves fluid retention, and reduces inflammation.
- Reduces pitta and vátha, and has a neutral effect on kapha.

Notes and Dosages
Sandalwood oil is pressed or extracted from the wood. The oil can be used in perfumes, massage oils, inhalations, and baths, while the decoction can be used as a gargle, lotion, compress, or douche. In Ayurvedic practice, sandalwood works well with clove, geranium, musk, myrrh, tuberose, and vetiver.

RECIPES

Sandalwood Decoction
A sandalwood decoction will reduce fever if taken internally or externally and it can be used to treat acne and other skin problems. Boil 1 heaped teaspoon of sandalwood in 1 cup of water. Cover and boil for several minutes. Strain and cool. Drink 1 or 2 cups a day, a tablespoon at a time. For external use, apply to freshly washed skin, and let dry. Repeat three times a day or as needed.

Aftershave Soother
Add 4 drops of sandalwood oil, 6 drops benzoin, and 4 drops chamomile to a bottle containing 4 teaspoons (20ml.) hazelnut oil. Warm a tiny amount in your hands and smooth into the face after shaving.

> **CAUTION**
> Do not use undiluted sandalwood oil on the skin.

Schisandra chinensis

SCHISANDRA BERRIES

Known in traditional Chinese medicine as Wu Wei Zi, this herb is used to stabilize and bind. The red berries are the fruit of an ornamental vine grown in China.

DATA FILE

Properties
• Sour • Warm • Astringent • Nourishing • Soothing expectorant

Uses
• Absorbs the leakage of lung qi and eases dry and chronic coughs, and asthma.
• Firms the kidneys, binds up jing-essence and stops bouts of diarrhea, leaking of sperm, urinary frequency or incontinence, and vaginal discharges, especially watery and white (cold).
• Absorbs sweating and generates fluids.
• Quietens the spirit and calms the heart, treating symptoms such as panic attacks, palpitations, irritability, dream-disturbed sleep, insomnia, forgetfulness, fear of ghosts, and of going outside.
• Take for weakness with nervous exhaustion, or exhaustion from prolonged hard work.
• Use for loss of sex drive in women and men.
• Restores softness to the skin.

Notes and Dosages
In common with other Chinese herbs in this category, Wu Wei Zi is not for sweat caused by outside infections. In Western herbalism, take 1 teaspoon three times daily of the tincture; or take ½oz. (10g.) daily of the dried berries by decoction.

RECIPE

Schisandra Wine
Add 4oz. (100g.) dried schisandra berries to a bottle of rice wine. Store in a cool place for four weeks. Drink a small wine glass twice daily. Take for weak lungs with recurrent coughs, and to keep skin soft in old age.

> **CAUTION**
> Contraindicated for external conditions, and the early stages of coughs and rashes: it will keep the "exterior pathogenic factor" inside.

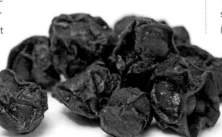

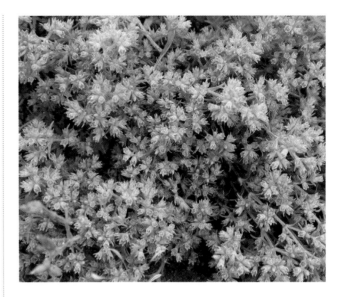

Scleranthus annuus

SCLERANTHUS

Scleranthus is a small, bushy, spreading plant that grows to 4in. (10cm.) on sandy soils and in cornfields. The plant's green flowers have no petals and grow at the forks and ends of the stems.

DATA FILE

Properties
• Encourages stability and balance • Enables decision-making

Uses
• For those who are unable to decide and who suffer much from hesitation, confusion, and uncertainty. People who need Scleranthus need to learn to decide for themselves; it is important that they do so, but they cannot. They are uncertain, indecisive, vacillate, and subject to erratic mood swings.
• Scleranthus gives the stability to listen to the inner self, and integrate the emotional and intellectual extremes (which sometimes seem contradictory) into balanced and sustained action.

Notes and Dosages
This branching annual plant has tiny green flowers from early spring to late summer. Prepare them using the sun method (see page 56).

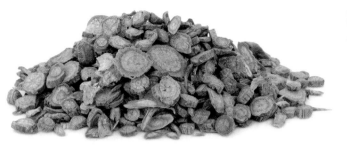

Scutellaria baicalensis
HUANG QIN

Huang Qin is made from the roots of skullcap, a summer-flowering perennial. This herb is one that clears heat: this includes febrile conditions and any illnesses with heat signs. It is one of the "Three Yellows," which are often used together for severe infections.

DATA FILE

Properties
• Bitter • Cold

Uses
• Huang Qin mainly clears heat in the chest and abdominal areas, so it is used for virulent diseases with high fever, irritability, thirst, cough, and expectoration (coughing up) of thick, yellow sputum.
• Can also be used topically on a dressing to clear red, hot swellings.
• Clears damp heat, especially in the stomach or intestines: take for smelly diarrhea.
• Use for damp heat in the lower burner, with symptoms such as cystitis.

Notes and Dosages
This herb works through the heart, lung, gall bladder, and large intestine channels.

Scutellaria laterifolia, Scutellaria galericulata
SKULLCAP

Blue skullcap, which is easily grown in gardens, and common skullcap, which grows wild on riverbanks, are used in Western herbalism to calm nerves and ease tension.

DATA FILE

Properties
• Strengthens and calms the nervous system • Antispasmodic

Uses
• Take for anxiety, tension headaches, and premenstrual syndrome; for examination nerves, and to help fight off post-examination depression.
• Take with valerian or chamomile and linden flowers for insomnia and disturbed sleep, and for tranquilizer withdrawal.
• Take with vervain for workaholics, the mixture being relaxing without sedative effects.

Notes and Dosages
Skullcap prefers a sunny, open position in ordinary soil. The plant lives for about three years. Take standard herbalism doses (see page 39). There are many relaxing tablets containing skullcap and other herbs, available at various stores. Follow the dosage on the box.

RECIPE

Examination Tea
Mix together equal parts of dried skullcap, linden flowers, and sage leaf. Store in a jar in a dark place. Make a tea in the normal way, using 1 teaspoon of the mixture to 1 cup of boiling water. Drink 1 cup before examinations or 3 cups a day while studying.

> **CAUTION**
> Some years ago, commercial preparations were found to contain germander, which is poisonous. Always buy your herbs and herbal preparations from a reputable firm.

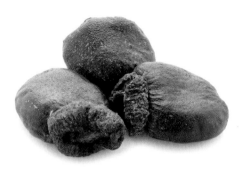

Semecarpus anacardium
ANACARD. OR.

Grown in the East Indies, the acrid black juice of the marking nut tree was used by the Ayurvedics to burn away moles, warts, and other skin complaints. The Arabs used the juice for a number of conditions, such as mental illness, memory loss, and paralysis. Homeopathically, cardol, the juice extracted from the pith between the shell and kernel, is used to make the remedy that is given for "tight" feelings of pain.

DATA FILE

Properties
• Analgesic

Uses
• This remedy is useful when there is a feeling of tightness or constricted pain.
• Other conditions that may be relieved are itchy skin, piles, constipation, indigestion, rheumatism, and duodenal ulcers.
• May be prescribed for those who suffer an inferiority complex and who want to prove themselves.

Notes and Dosages
According to homeopaths, symptoms that may be eased by Anacard. or. improve immediately after eating, when lying on the affected part, after rubbing, and worsen around midnight, after washing in hot water and using a compress.

Sepia officinalis
SEPIA

Historically, cuttlefish ink has been used medicinally to treat conditions such as kidney stones, hair loss, and gonorrhea. It is also used as a pigment in paint. Today, the homeopathic remedy Sepia is most commonly taken by women, and is used to treat complaints such as menstrual problems and hormonal imbalances.

DATA FILE

Properties
• Relieves menstrual problems • Balances hormones
• Strengthening

Uses
• Useful for women who feel "dragged down," both physically and emotionally.
• Useful for complaints relating to the vagina, ovaries, and uterus, such as heavy or painful menstruation, premenstrual syndrome, menopausal hot flushes, thrush, and the feeling of a sagging abdomen, where the woman feels the need to cross her legs.
• Pain during sex, aversion to sex, or exhaustion afterward can also be treated.
• Useful for headaches with nausea, hair loss, dizziness, offensive sweating, indigestion, skin discoloration, and circulatory problems.

Notes and Dosages
The cuttlefish is the source of sepia used to color ink, and to make the Sepia remedy. Although Sepia is mainly a women's remedy it is sometimes used for hair loss in either sex.

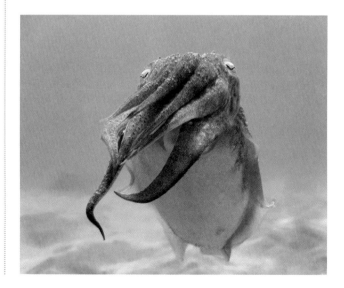

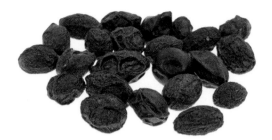

Serenoa repens
SAW PALMETTO

The dried fruit of a small palm-like plant grown in the West Indies and U.S. are used in Western herbalism. The berries are gathered from early fall to the middle of winter, and dried for storage.

DATA FILE

Properties
• Strengthening tonic • Urinary antiseptic • Diuretic • Alterative
• Stimulates sex hormones

Uses
• Take for prostate enlargement and cystitis.
• Take with damiana for weakness and impotence in men.
• Helps restore weight after severe illness.
• May help failure to thrive in children, with marshmallow: take 10–15 drops of the combined tincture 3 times daily in juice.

Notes and Dosages
For a decoction, use ½ teaspoon of the crushed berries to 1 cup water. Adults can take 1 or 2 cups daily. When using the tincture (available from specialist herb stores), take 20–40 drops, in water, 3 times daily.

RECIPE

Saw Palmetto and Nettle Root Tincture
Dig up, wash, and finely chop two or three handfuls of fresh nettle roots. Place in a jar and cover with saw palmetto tincture. Leave for two weeks, shaking from time to time. Strain and bottle. For prostate problems, take 30 drops, 3 times daily.

> **CAUTION**
> Do not use in early pregnancy. Always have suspected prostate problems medically checked.

Silybum marianum
MILK THISTLE

This tall, beautiful thistle can be grown easily. The seeds, which are used in Western herbalism, resemble sunflower seeds. The seedheads are stored in a warm place to release the seeds.

DATA FILE

Properties
• Strengthens and clears the liver and gall bladder
• Antidepressant • Anti-inflammatory • Lactagogue

Uses
• Promotes milk production in nursing mothers.
• Take for "liverishness" and liver disease, poor fat tolerance, pale stools, and to protect the liver when taking strong drugs and medicines.
• Use for mild depression that comes on following hepatitis.
• Helps in the treatment of gallstones and for inflammation.
• Useful for *Candida* and food allergies.
• May ease high blood pressure with liverish symptoms.

Notes and Dosages
The seeds of the thistle are used. For a standard decoction, take ½ cup 3 times daily for at least six months. Tablets are also available: follow the instructions on the box.

> **CAUTION**
> Liver disease should be treated by a physician.

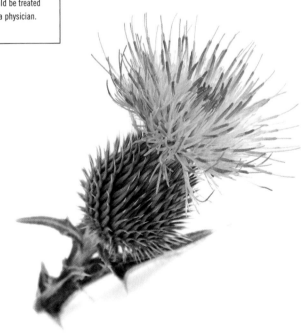

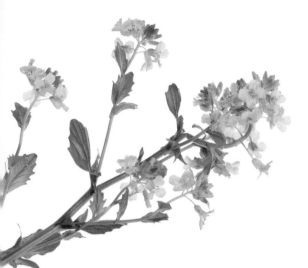

Sinapis arvensis
WILD MUSTARD

The common wild mustard, also called charlock mustard, found growing in hedges and on waste ground has large yellow flowers that appear in early summer. This annual plant grows to about 2ft. (60cm.) and self-seeds readily.

DATA FILE

Properties
• Encourages hopefulness

Uses
• The mustard flower remedy is used for dark clouds of gloom or deep, black depression that seems to come from nowhere. It is for the feeling of being under a cloud that blocks out the warming rays and optimism of the sun. It may lift just as suddenly as it arrived.
• This remedy restores hope and a sense of pleasure in living. It lightens our mood, giving us the faith and hope to carry on.

Notes and Dosages
Prepare the flowers using the boiling method (see page 57).

(see page 57)

CAUTION
If depression is continual or severe episodes of depression occur frequently, seek professional assistance. It is important to seek the physiological or psychological root.

Solanum tuberosum
POTATO

The potato plant is native to the Americas. Potatoes have been used for medicinal purposes for hundreds of years, and are extremely nutritious, supplying fiber, B vitamins, minerals, and vitamin C. The peels are high in potassium, and potato-peel tea has been traditionally used for high blood pressure.

DATA FILE

Properties
• Alkaline, which helps to detoxify the body • Antiulcer
• Anti-inflammatory • Analgesic • Stimulates circulation

Uses
• The juice of the raw potato can be used for stomach ulcers and to relieve the inflammation of arthritis.
• Make a potato poultice for healing a bruise or sprain of any kind.
• Raw, grated potatoes can relieve the pain of a burn.
• Apply hot baked potato pulp for tennis elbow and other joint pain.
• Boiled potato peel is said to be useful for inflammation of the prostate. Apply as a poultice to the affected area.
• Eaten daily, potatoes can help to prevent premature aging and heart disease.
• Regular consumption can prevent constipation and help to ease inflammation associated with irritable bowel syndrome.

Notes and Dosages
The juice of raw potatoes is most useful, and can be added to soups, fruit juices, or stews to disguise the taste.

CAUTION
Poisonous alkaloids are present in most nightshade plants, including the common potato, but it is safe to eat if cooked, and in small amounts when raw. Sprouting potatoes are poisonous and should not be eaten.

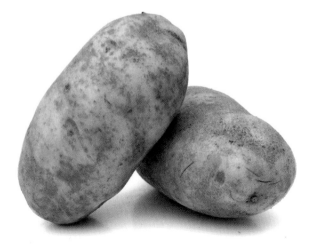

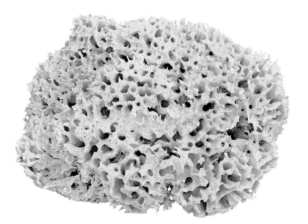

Spongia species
SPONGIA

Sea sponge was first treasured for its medicinal properties more than 600 years ago, when it was used as a treatment for goiter, the swelling of the thyroid gland, which is brought on by a deficiency of iodine. Although it was not known then, sponge contains useful amounts of iodine and bromine. Homeopathically, the Spongia tosta remedy is made by toasting and powdering the sponge, which is harvested from the waters of the Mediterranean.

DATA FILE

Properties
• Helps dry coughs • Soothes sore throats

Uses
• This remedy works particularly well for sneezing and a hoarse, dry barking cough, with the patient waking in alarm with the feeling of suffocation, later followed by thick mucus which is difficult to bring up.
• Also helps associated symptoms of coughs, such as hoarseness, dryness of the larynx from a cold, headaches which are worse when lying down, but improve when sitting up, dry mucous membranes, and feelings of heaviness and tiredness.

Notes and Dosages
Those who may benefit from Spongia usually find that their symptoms are soothed by warm drinks.

Stephania tetrandra
HAN FANG JI

Like Wu Jia Pi, this Chinese herb, obtained from stephania root, dispels wind dampness from the muscles, joints, and bones. Whereas Wu Jia Pi is a warm herb, however, Han Fang Ji is cold. Wind damp causes rheumatic and arthritic ailments.

DATA FILE

Properties
• Bitter • Acrid • Cold • Antirheumatic • Anti-inflammatory
• Analgesic • Eases edema • Diuretic

Uses
• As a cold herb, Han Fang Ji treats hot, painful swollen joints, such as in an acute attack of rheumatoid arthritis.
• Promotes urination, so very effective at reducing edema, especially of the lower body and legs.
• Relieves the pain of rheumatism.

Notes and Dosages
This herb works through the bladder, spleen, and kidney channels.

> **CAUTION**
> Use with caution in cases of yin deficiency, as it is very drying.

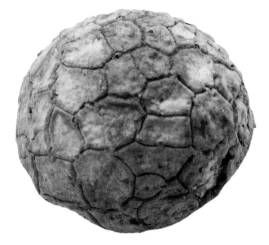

Styrax benzoin
BENZOIN

Benzoin has been used in the East since antiquity as a medicine and as incense. It came into use in the West in the Middle Ages as a remedy for respiratory complaints. The oil, which has a sweet vanilla-like scent, is extracted from the resin of the tropical benzoin tree. It is not strictly an essential oil, but a resinoid dissolved in alcohol.

DATA FILE

Properties
• Warming • Decongestant • Soothing • Anti-inflammatory
• Diuretic • Antiseptic • Stimulates the circulation

Uses
• Inhaled, benzoin is helpful for colds and flu, and for clearing mucus from the system, can soothe sore throats and help to restore a lost voice.
• Benzoin blended with cream or oil and rubbed into the skin soothes chapped or irritated skin on the hands, as well as cuts and skin inflammation.
• Good for urinary tract infections.
• Helps to alleviate arthritis and rheumatism.
• Emotionally calming in a crisis, warming and comforting in times of loneliness, and helps to dispel depression, anxiety, and nervous tension.

Notes and Dosages
Crude benzoin is collected from the tree directly and made into benzoin resinoid using solvents, which are then removed. Benzoin blends well with sandalwood, lemon, rose, juniper, myrrh, frankincense, jasmine, cypress, and spice oils.

RECIPE

Warming Winter Bath
Add 2 drops benzoin, 3 drops marjoram, and 2 drops clary sage to a warm bath. Disperse with your hand, close the bathroom door to keep in the steam, and soak for at least 10 minutes.

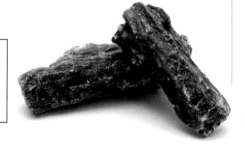

> **CAUTION**
> Can cause irritation in some sensitive individuals.

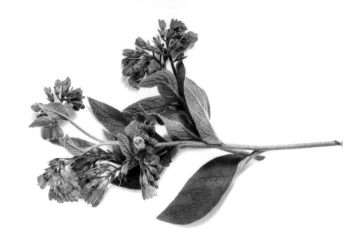

Symphytum officinale
COMFREY

Comfrey is a common wild plant with large, bristly leaves and clusters of purple flowers. The root and leaves are used for herbal treatments, although preparations of the root should not be taken internally. One common name for comfrey is "knitbone," testifying to its healing powers.

DATA FILE

Properties
• Healing • Mucilaginous

Uses
• Comfrey promotes rapid healing of cuts, wounds, sprains, and broken bones when taken as a tea or tincture, or used in poultices, creams, ointments, and liniments. Clean wounds well before applying comfrey.
• Use as a cream for cracked, dry skin.
• Add a few drops of a warming essential oil such as black pepper to the infused oil to make a good liniment for arthritis, bunions, and aches and pains arising from old injuries.
• Take with chamomile and meadowsweet for hiatus hernia and stomach ulcers.

Notes and Dosages
Comfrey grows to about 3ft. (1m.) high and bears purplish or cream flowers. Use standard doses (see pages 39 and 41).

> **CAUTION**
> There has been suspicion of liver damage from using comfrey root and from eating large amounts of the herb. The herb tea and tincture are believed safe to use, but it is sensible to avoid them in pregnancy, during breastfeeding, and for infants. Preparations of the root are not taken internally.

Tabebuia avellanedae
PAU D'ARCO

A tree from the South American rainforest, pau d'arco is also called lapacho and taheebo tree. Its bark may be useful in the treatment of immunodeficiency diseases.

DATA FILE

Properties
- Immune tonic • Antibiotic • Antifungal

Uses
- Use for immune deficiency with susceptibility to infections.
- Good for diarrhea and intestinal infections.
- For oral thrush, take as a mouthwash; and to treat candidiasis, take as a decoction.

Notes and Dosages
Make half-strength decoctions, ½oz. (12g.) pau d'arco to 1pt. (500ml.) water. Drink 3 cups daily. Tablets and capsules are available: follow the doses on the packet. Some believe that this herb may be helpful for breast, liver, and prostate cancers, but research has not proved this conclusively. The dose required to be effective could have toxic side-effects.

RECIPE

Tonic Soup
Make a decoction with ½oz. (12g.) pau d'arco and 2pt. (1l.) water. Strain. Chop a small onion, two cloves of garlic, and a dozen oyster fungi. Simmer in the decoction until soft. Chop a small bunch of watercress and add to the soup just before serving. Eat daily for a weak immune system.

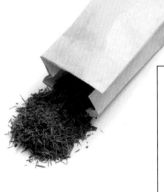

> **CAUTION**
> Do not give to children. Do not take during pregnancy and breastfeeding. Consult with your physician before taking large doses of this herb, as it can cause internal bleeding and vomiting. People with blood-clotting disorders should seek professional advice. Pau d'arco may interfere with prescription medications.

Tanacetum parthenium
FEVERFEW

This small-flowered daisy is easily grown in gardens. Use the leaves, which should be picked just before the plant flowers. Feverfew is good for period pains, vertigo, and arthritis. The name is a corruption of the word "febrifuge."

DATA FILE

Properties
- Anti-inflammatory • Antispasmodic • Emmenagogue • Analgesic

Uses
- Take the tincture for migraine and arthritis.
- Combine with valerian for migraine linked with anxiety and tension.
- Combined with skullcap, feverfew relieves persistent headaches.

Notes and Dosages
The best preparation is the tincture made from the fresh plant. Take 1 teaspoon in a little water at the first signs of a migraine; repeat after 2 hours if necessary. For repeated attacks and as a treatment for arthritis, take 1 teaspoon every morning. If you have a plant, 2 or 3 medium-sized leaves equal 1 teaspoon of tincture.

RECIPE

Feverfew Migraine Sandwiches
If it is not possible to keep a feverfew plant, make fresh feverfew sandwiches and keep them in the freezer. Butter the bread. Cover one slice with a double layer of fresh feverfew leaves. Put on the top slice and press. Cut the sandwiches into small cubes. Each cube should have two or three medium-sized feverfew leaves. Wrap each cube in plastic wrap. Label, date, and freeze. Take one cube at the first sign of headache, then every two hours until the headache is over.

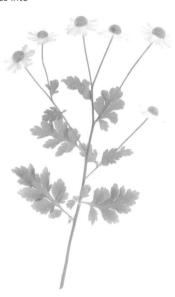

> **CAUTION**
> Not to be taken in pregnancy or during breastfeeding. Do not give to children. Do not take if using blood-thinning drugs such as warfarin. Chewing the leaf can cause mouth ulcers in some people; if this is the case, use the tincture or capsules.

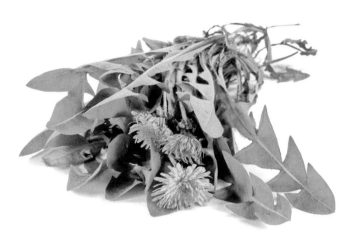

Taraxacum officinalis
DANDELION LEAVES

The leaves of the familiar weed can be picked at any time. They can be cooked and eaten like spinach, and are good for a springtime cleansing tonic. Dandelion leaf tea relieves edema and water retention.

DATA FILE

Properties
• Powerful diuretic • Nourishing • Digestive

Uses
• Take tea for all types of water retention and edema, especially for swollen ankles that are associated with circulatory problems.
• Take with uva ursi or thyme for cystitis.
• Contains vitamins A and C and many trace minerals, and is especially high in potassium.

Notes and Dosages
Use 2 or 3 teaspoons of the dried herb to 1 cup of boiling water. Drink freely. Take sufficient to produce a good flow of urine. The fresh leaves are a tasty salad ingredient.

RECIPE

Blanched Dandelion Leaf
This stimulates digestion and is excellent to include in a daily salad for cases of poor appetite, weak digestion and liver, and for general convalescence. Put a large pot upside down over a growing plant to keep out the light. Leave for two weeks or until the leaves are white. Eat two leaves daily.

Taraxacum officinalis
DANDELION ROOT

The bitter dandelion root is a favorite in folk medicine, and particularly useful for stimulating a sluggish liver. The root of the dandelion is more effective than the leaves and stem in the treatment of liver problems. Coffee made from dandelion root is available, and it is thought to have a tonic effect on the pancreas, spleen, and female organs.

DATA FILE

Properties
• Liver tonic • Digestive • Alterative • Diuretic

Uses
• Take for all types of liver and gall bladder problems.
• Use for indigestion, loss of appetite, and constipation in pregnancy.
• For arthritis and stubborn skin disease, take in combination with burdock.
• The liver plays a crucial role in detoxification and nutrition, so dandelion root is helpful in most chronic and wasting diseases, and helps the body to cope with strong chemical drugs.

Notes and Dosages
The decoction is best for liver problems. To feel an effect, take at least 3 cups of decoction a day for 6 months. Using a tincture, take 4–6 teaspoons daily.

RECIPE

Dandelion Coffee
Although dandelion is a wonderful plant, it does not always grow where it is wanted. When weeding, keep the long taproots. Scrub all the dirt off the roots, chop into pieces, and roast in a medium oven until dry and slightly burnt. Make a decoction and take 1 or 2 cups a day as a liver strengthener and tonic.

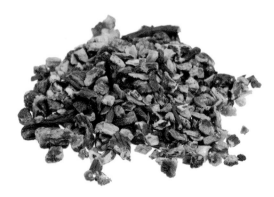

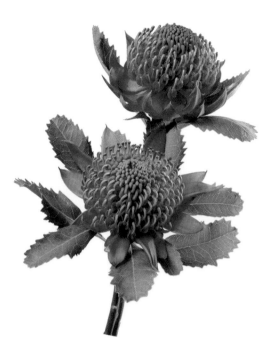

Telopea speciosissima

WARATAH

Waratah is the Australian Aboriginal word for beautiful. It is a shrub with magnificent red flowers packed together into a globe measuring 5in. (12cm.) across. It is a very striking plant, used for a powerful flower remedy.

DATA FILE

Properties
• Gives the courage to be courageous

Uses
• Waratah is a very powerful and fast-acting flower remedy. It should be taken for despair, deep distress, and any emotional or physical crisis. Physical signs may be exhaustion, interrupted or prolonged sleep, and loss of the ability or interest to care for oneself.
• The globe of the flowers reflects how the remedy brings everything in the personality together: strength, old and forgotten skills and lessons, trust, and love. This remedy gives us the faith and confidence to hold our head up in all weathers, to stand erect and just be ourselves – blooming, obvious, and beautiful.

Notes and Dosages
Prepare the flowers using the sun method (see page 56).

Tetratheca ericifolia

BLACK-EYED SUSAN

This small scrubby plant of the Australian woodland is called "black-eyed" as the drooping, bell-like flowers have a core of black pollen-covered stamens surrounded by four mauve petals. It is used to make a flower remedy to encourage inner peace.

DATA FILE

Properties
• Releases stress • Helps us slow down

Uses
• Black-eyed Susan is for people who are always rushing and striving, for the workaholic who does not have time for himself or herself or the people around, and is expending all his or her energy at a fast rate. Accompanying physical symptoms are irritability, poor digestion, restless sleep, and general tension and stress. They may also have nervous rashes.
• Just as this plant's petals draw attention to the dark centers of the flowers, so the remedy can help people to focus on their inner core. The flowers' petals protect the black center, so the remedy helps us turn inward, slow down, and pay attention to our inner rhythm.

Notes and Dosages
Prepare the flowers using the sun method (see page 56).

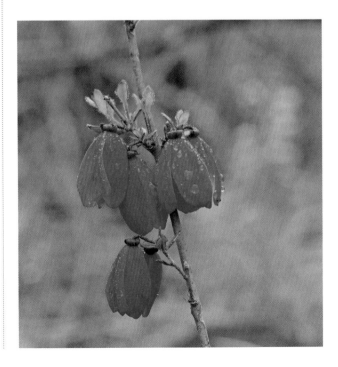

Thymus vulgaris

THYME

Thyme is an attractive small perennial herb. It is easy to grow and thrives in the rock garden or a sunny, well-drained border. There are many different garden varieties. The herb is used in both Western herbalism and aromatherapy. The oil, distilled from the leaves and tiny purple flowering tops, has a fresh green scent.

DATA FILE

Properties

• Antiseptic • Antibacterial • Antifungal • Expectorant • Digestive tonic • Antirheumatic • Soothing • Rubefacient • Diuretic

Uses

• Take decoction or tincture for any cough with infected or tough phlegm.
• May be helpful, if taken regularly, in asthma, but consult with your physician before use. Try ground thyme, with sage and chamomile, inhaled on a charcoal block.
• A thyme decoction or syrup eases indigestion, wind, and intestinal infections.
• For cystitis, take in a decoction along with marshmallow.
• A strong tea fights distressing intestinal worms in children.
• Drink weak tea for nightmares.
• Thyme vinegar is an antifungal treatment for athlete's foot.
• Use thyme vinegar, diluted with an equal amount of water, for washes and douches for thrush.
• Thyme oil has an uplifting fragrance, which can relieve depression, headaches, and stress.
• The diluted oil is good for cleaning wounds, burns, bruises, and clearing lice. Used as a mouthwash it helps to soothe and heal abscesses and gum infections.
• Used in massage, the oil's antirheumatic and antitoxic properties are beneficial in treating arthritis, gout, and cellulite. Rubefacient and stimulant actions also help with muscle and joint pain, and poor circulation.
• Used in inhalations, thyme oil stimulates the immune system to effectively fight off colds, flu, and catarrh, and ease coughing.

Notes and Dosages

Take freely, bearing in mind the cautions below. Large doses might be needed for coughs. For infants' coughs, give 2 or 3 teaspoons of syrup up to 4 times daily. Make a chest rub from the infused oil. For children's worms, give ¼–½ cup of strong tea before breakfast, for 1 week.

Thyme essential oil blends well with lemon, bergamot, rosemary, lemon balm, lavender, pine, black pepper, tea tree, lime, cedarwood, and grapefruit.

RECIPES

Thyme Cough Syrup

Thyme makes an ideal antiseptic expectorant cough syrup. It tastes pleasant and appeals to children. This recipe is for a tight chest and restless unproductive cough. Take ½oz. (12g.) thyme, 1oz. (25g.) chamomile, 1 teaspoon cinnamon, and a pinch of cayenne or ginger (optional). Make a decoction, reduce, and add sugar or honey. Take as directed.

Antiseptic Mouthwash

Add 10 drops thyme oil, 15 drops peppermint, 5 drops fennel, and 5 drops myrrh to a bottle containing 4fl.oz. (125ml.) of inexpensive brandy. Shake well and add 2 teaspoons (10ml.) of the mix to a glass of warm water. Rinse the mouth thoroughly, but do not swallow.

CAUTION

Do not take internally or use externally during pregnancy. The amounts taken in food are harmless. Asthma is a serious condition and should always be treated by a physician. Dilute thyme oil well, as it may cause irritation and sensitization in some people. Do not use if you have high blood pressure. Do not use if you are taking homeopathic remedies.

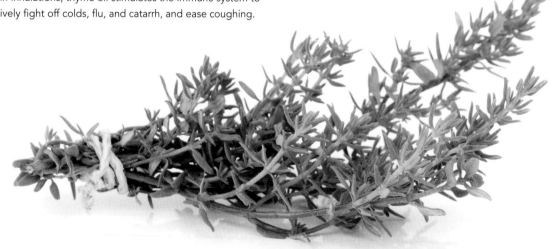

Tilia europea

LINDEN

A tree often grown in parks and along streets, the linden, also called lime, has wood that is good for carving, as it will take fine detail. Use the flowers, which are also called limeflowers, for soothing herbal remedies. *Tilia europea* grows to 120ft. (35m.).

DATA FILE

Properties
• Calming • Soothing • Strengthens nerves • Antispasmodic
• Diaphoretic

Uses
• Drink tea for anxiety, irritability, and insomnia. Long-term use improves tolerance of stress.
• Improves digestion, particularly nervous indigestion.
• Tea, used at standard tea strength and taken freely, induces sweating and reduces temperature in fevers.
• Take linden with hawthorn tops as a tea for mild high blood pressure.
• Linden flowers combined with elderflowers treat colds.
• Take with hops to treat nervous tension.

Notes and Dosages
Use standard doses (see page 39). May be taken freely. Linden is a popular everyday tea in France and mixes well with other herb teas.

RECIPE

Linden Flower Bath for Infants
This recipe is specially good for dry skin and eczema with irritability. Add ½oz. (12g.) of dried linden flowers to 1pt. (500ml.) of water. Bring to the boil, cover, and allow to stand for 15 minutes. Add to the baby's bath.

> **CAUTION**
> Old or improperly dried flowers are said to be somewhat narcotic. Reject stale-smelling and discolored flowers. Store carefully.

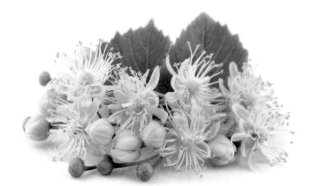

Trigonella foenum-graecum

FENUGREEK

Known as *"methica"* in Ayurvedic practice, fenugreek is a healing herb whose qualities were brought to the attention of humans by animals. Farmers noticed that sick cattle would eat fenugreek plants even when they would not eat anything else. Fenugreek began to be used as a digestive aid and laxative. Fenugreek seeds contain a lot of bulk and mucilage, and, when mixed with water or saliva, become gelatinous and ease sluggish bowels.

DATA FILE

Properties
• Digestive • Laxative • Antiseptic • Warming • Expectorant
• Anti-inflammatory • Antiseptic • Soothing • Lactagogue

Uses
• Take for indigestion, constipation, and other digestive disorders.
• Helps bronchitis, inflamed lungs, and fevers.
• Gargling a fenugreek decoction will soothe sore throats.
• Helps asthma and sinus problems by reducing mucus.
• Apply as a poultice to wounds, boils, and rashes.
• Stimulates the uterus, bringing on menstruation, reduces blood sugar levels, and lowers cholesterol.
• Decoctions can treat arthritis and aching joints.
• The seeds can be eaten by nursing mothers to increase milk production.
• Reduces kapha and vátha, and increases pitta.

Notes and Dosages
Fenugreek seeds should be gathered in the fall. The seeds may be used as a spice, a tea, a massage oil, an inhalant, a poultice, or plaster. Fenugreek can be taken with peppermint, lemon, and anise.

RECIPE

Sore Throat Decoction
Bruise 2 tablespoons of fenugreek seeds. Add 4 cups of water. Bring to a boil, then cover and simmer for 10 minutes. Drink up to 3 cups a day. Add honey, lemon, or licorice to sweeten.

> **CAUTION**
> Because of its use as a uterine stimulant, fenugreek should not be taken by pregnant women. Fenugreek seeds may cause water retention and weight gain. Do not give fenugreek to children under two years.

Turnera diffusa

DAMIANA

The leaves of this small, strongly aromatic shrub, grown in South America, are used for therapeutic purposes. They treat depression, anxiety, poor digestion, cystitis, and are a tonic for the reproductive system.

DATA FILE

Properties
• Stimulant tonic for the nerves and reproductive system in both sexes • Aphrodisiac

Uses
• Take for impotence and sterility associated with anxiety, especially in men.
• Use for physical weakness, depression, mental stupor, and nervous exhaustion in both sexes.
• Take for prostatitis and relief of chronic cystitis.

Notes and Dosages
Damiana leaves and stems are gathered when the plant is in flower, then dried. Take ½ cup of the tea or 1 teaspoon of the tincture twice daily. Alternatively, combine damiana with other herbs, such as wild oats or saw palmetto, and use 1 cup of the combination tea, or 1 teaspoon of tincture, twice daily.

RECIPE

Damiana Combination for Herpes
Combine equal parts of tinctures of damiana and echinacea. Take 1 teaspoon every four hours. This will often avert an attack, if taken at the first signs. Alternatively, make a decoction with equal parts of the herbs and take ½ cup every four hours.

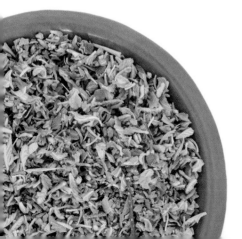

> **CAUTION**
> Do not exceed the recommended dose, as damiana is quite stimulating.

Ulex europaeus

GORSE

Gorse is a bushy shrub with pea-like yellow flowers. It is abundant on poor, stony soils and heaths. It is almost leafless, but its green, spiny stems give it an evergreen appearance. The flowers are used to make a flower remedy to ease despair.

DATA FILE

Properties
• Encourages hope • Restores the feeling that anything is possible

Uses
• Gorse is taken for strong feelings of hopelessness and despair. People who need gorse may seek help in order to please others, but underneath feel that nothing more can be done for them. They have lost the will to strive, perhaps in response to a life event, an accident, a medical diagnosis, or a long-standing illness or fear. They are caught up in negativity, unwilling to try new avenues, and unwilling to hope.
• Gorse gives the courage to try, building renewed hope, and giving the will to continue the fight toward recovery.

Notes and Dosages
The prickly gorse or furze has headily scented yellow flowers almost the whole year round. Use the sun method to prepare them (see page 56).

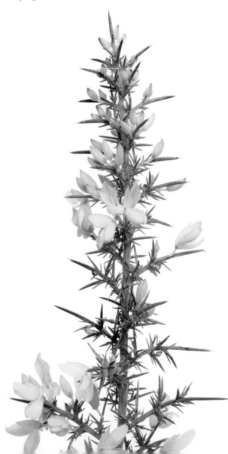

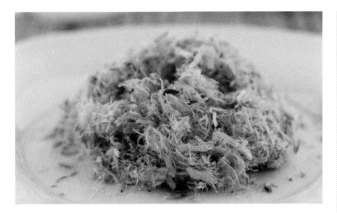

Ulmus fulva
SLIPPERY ELM

The inner bark of this small U.S. tree is usually sold powdered. It smells rather like fenugreek, but tastes bland. The bark is very nutritious, as well as having healing properties.

DATA FILE

Properties
• Soothing • Mucilaginous • Digestive

Uses
• Take for any sort of inflammation or irritation in the digestive tract: nausea, indigestion, wind, food allergies, stomach ulcers, acidity, heartburn, hiatus hernia, colitis, diverticulitis, and diarrhea.
• Mix with sufficient water to make a paste for drawing splinters.
• Use with chamomile in a poultice to ease swelling.
• Often prescribed during convalescence.

Notes and Dosages
Tablets flavored with carminative herbs are especially useful. Take 1 or 2 with a glass of water or milk before meals. For travel sickness and nausea in pregnancy, suck one tablet slowly. Stir 1 level teaspoon of powder into a drink, and take 3 times daily before meals. Slippery elm is often used to back up other remedies.

RECIPE

Slippery Elm and Chamomile Poultice
To make a soothing and healing poultice for any kind of painful swelling, mix together 2 dessertspoons each of slippery elm powder and dried chamomile flowers. Add hot water, slowly, stirring all the time to make a paste. Wrap the warm paste in light cotton and apply. Leave in place for a half-hour.

Ulmus procera
ELM

The magnificent English elm, once common in hedgerows and fields, is now sadly rare due to Dutch elm disease. It grows to a towering 120ft. (35m.) and spreads to 50ft. (15m.).

DATA FILE

Properties
• Restores confidence

Uses
• The elm flower remedy is for temporary feelings of inadequacy. People who benefit from elm do good work and are proud of themselves and their calling. They seek and aim for perfection. When this goal seems unattainable, they can become overwhelmed. Elm is for brief faltering moments of despair and lack of confidence, when the task seems too much.
• Elm restores faith in ability, so that we do not strive for unattainable perfection, but instead appreciate the worth of our own actions. Elm gives the strength to balance responsibilities with the practical needs of everyday reality and carry on.

Notes and Dosages
The English elm has clusters of small green flowers with long purple-pink stamens that appear before the leaves open. Prepare them using the boiling method (see page 57).

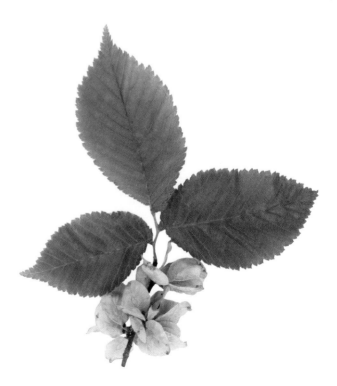

Urtica dioica

NETTLE

The common stinging nettle grows all over the world. Plants have either male or female flowers, which is suggested by the species name *dioica*, meaning "two houses." Nettles are used in both herbal and homeopathic remedies. The Urtica Urens homeopathic remedy is used both internally and externally.

DATA FILE

Properties
• Iron tonic • Mild diuretic • Antihistamine • Strengthening
• Styptic • Soothes the skin

Uses
• Drink nettle tea for iron deficiency anemia, lethargy, weakness, and during convalescence.
• Apply topically as a juice, tea, or lotion for nettle rash, allergies to strawberries, insect bites, and nervous eczema.
• Treats urinary gravel and water retention.
• May ease arthritis.
• Take a decoction with cleavers as a spring tonic.
• Urtica Urens cream is useful for skin conditions, particularly if the skin is stinging: rashes where the skin is blotchy, such as urticaria (hives), for bee stings, and allergic reactions.
• Urtica Urens may also be prescribed for rheumatism, neuralgia, gout, and blocked milk ducts.

Notes and Dosages
The small plant is covered in soft, spiny hairs which secrete a sap that causes itching and inflammation if touched. Take standard herbalism doses (see pages 39 and 41). Leave the tops or leaves to infuse for 15 minutes for best effect. The tops can be cooked as spinach or made into soup.

RECIPE

Nourishing Nettle Soup
Pick 1pt. (500ml.) of the tops of young nettles, avoiding too much stem. Chop two medium potatoes, a carrot, and a small onion. Add the ingredients to twice as much water and boil until the potatoes are soft. Blend in a food processor. Serve seasoned to taste.

> **CAUTION**
> Nettles teas may be too drying for some people, in which case take with marshmallow.

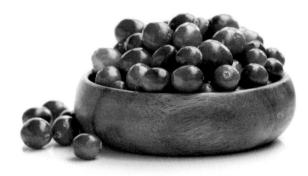

Vaccinium oxycoccos, Vaccinium macrocarpon

CRANBERRY

Cranberries are small acidic berries which are rich in vitamins C and A, and contain an excellent infection-fighting ingredient. The berries are used in sauces and jellies served with savory and sweet foods and in a variety of fruit juices.

DATA FILE

Properties
• Urinary antiseptic • Stimulates circulation • Aids respiratory system

Uses
• A daily glass of cranberry juice will prevent and treat cystitis.
• Fresh cranberry juice can help with urinary problems caused by the prostate gland in later life.
• Crushed cranberries, boiled in distilled water and skinned, can be added to a cup of warm water to overcome an asthma attack.
• The juice extracted from cranberries contains oxalic acid, which discourages the formation of kidney stones.

Notes and Dosages
Cranberries are the fruits of an ericaceous shrub. They prevent harmful bacteria attaching to the bladder walls.

> **CAUTION**
> Cranberries contain large amounts of oxalic acid, and should not be eaten raw. Asthma is a serious condition that should always be treated by a physician.

Valeriana officinalis

VALERIAN

The root of the wild valerian plant is used in herbalism. In the Middle Ages, valerian root was used as a spice and a perfume, as well as a medicine.

DATA FILE

Properties
- Sedative • Nerve restorative • Calms the heart • Antispasmodic
- Carminative

Uses
- Drink valerian decoction for anxiety, confusion, migraines, insomnia, and depression with anxiety.
- Tincture or decoction is helpful for withdrawal from tranquilizers.
- Take for high blood pressure or palpitations caused by stress.
- Take with chamomile for colic and nervous indigestion.

Notes and Dosages
Valerian grows in damp ground, reaching 3ft. (4m.). The roots of the plant are used, and are dug up in the fall. The cold decoction is best: soak 1 teaspoon of valerian root in 1 cup of cold water overnight. Take ½–1 cup daily. Take 20–60 drops of the tincture 3 times daily. More may be needed to help with tranquilizer withdrawal. Relaxing tablets containing valerian are widely available.

RECIPE

Valerian Sleeping Mixture
Mix together equal amounts of tinctures of valerian root, dandelion root, and chamomile flowers (some specialist stores will make up the mixture for you). Store in a dark bottle and label. Adults should take 1–3 teaspoons in a little water before bed for sleeplessness with tension or from indigestion.

> **CAUTION**
> Valerian causes hyperactivity in some people. Very large doses can cause temporary giddiness. Do not take for long periods without examining why you are so tense. Tranquilizer withdrawal should only be undertaken with psychological support.

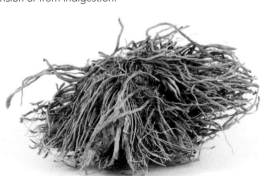

Verbascum thaspus

MULLEIN

Mullein is a beautiful wild flower with a tall, thick spike of yellow flowers. Use the leaves and flowers to prepare herbal remedies. Mullein was once known as "bullock's lungwort" because it cured cattle's lung diseases.

DATA FILE

Properties
- Soothing expectorant • Healing • Demulcent • Emollient
- Astringent

Uses
- Drink tea for deep and ticklish coughs, asthma, bronchitis, and diarrhea.
- Use mullein flower infused oil as a salve for itchy eyelids.
- Mullein flower and garlic infused oil can soothe the pain of acute earache.
- Two drops of mullein flower infused oil, in a little juice, three times daily, is helpful for bedwetting.

Notes and Dosages
The tea gives the best results for coughs. Allow the mullein to infuse for a long time and drink freely.

RECIPE

Mullein and Garlic Infused Oil
Use this oil for itchy ears, earache, and ear infections. Pick the spike from a mullein in full flower. Make an infused oil (see the instructions on page 41). Fill a small jar with chopped garlic and cover it with the mullein oil. Leave overnight. Strain and use as eardrops.

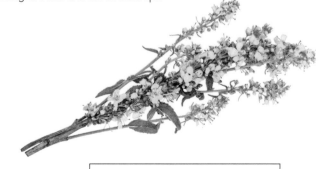

> **CAUTION**
> Do not use eardrops if the eardrum has burst. Asthma is a serious condition that should always be treated by a physician.

Verbena officinalis

VERVAIN

Vervain, sometimes called verbena, is a common wayside perennial found in meadows, on the roadside, and in dry, sunny places. It bears spikes of small, unscented pale pink or lilac flowers. Vervain has many uses in herbalism and is known as the "herb of grace." The flowers are also used to prepare a flower remedy for those who have very fixed ideas and principles.

DATA FILE

Properties
- Tonic • Reduces fever • Nerve restorative • Antispasmodic
- Carminative • Diuretic • Lactagogue • Emmenagogue

Uses
- Take vervain tea as a tonic for exhaustion, post-viral fatigue, post-operative tiredness, and tiredness from overwork.
- Use the tea for nervous depression, postnatal depression, and insomnia.
- Take for fevers and flu, especially accompanied by headaches and nervous symptoms.
- Take for indigestion and for digestive discomfort following treatment for intestinal parasites.
- Use for "liverishness" with nausea, heavy headaches, and depression.
- May relieve irritable bowel syndrome with mucus in the stools.

- Sip the tea throughout labor to encourage regular contractions. Continue taking it after the birth to encourage milk flow.
- May be helpful in relieving chest tension in asthma, alongside conventional treatment.
- Eases menstrual cramps and may restore menstruation stopped by stress.
- Use as a compress for inflamed eyes.
- The vervain flower remedy is for people who are strong-willed and rarely change their views; they think they are right and obstinately maintain a stance, or fight on when others would have conceded. They wish to convert all those around them. They strive with mental energy and willpower, but the effort of trying to persuade others is extremely stressful. They may experience stress-related illnesses, including anxiety, indigestion, and sleep disorders. Vervain brings calm and the ability to see the other point of view.

Notes and Dosages
Both the leaves and the flowers of the vervain plant are used to make herbal remedies. Take standard-strength teas every two hours in fevers, or 3 cups a day for chronic complaints. For worms and parasites, make double-strength tea and drink before breakfast for some weeks or until better. The flower remedy is prepared using the sun method (see page 56).

RECIPE

Combined Vervain Remedy for Overwork
Prepare the vervain flower remedy using the boiling method, or buy a bottle of the prepared flower remedy stock. Add 4 drops of this remedy to 1 cup of vervain tea, standard strength. Drink 2 or 3 cups daily to relieve tiredness and tension resulting from overwork.

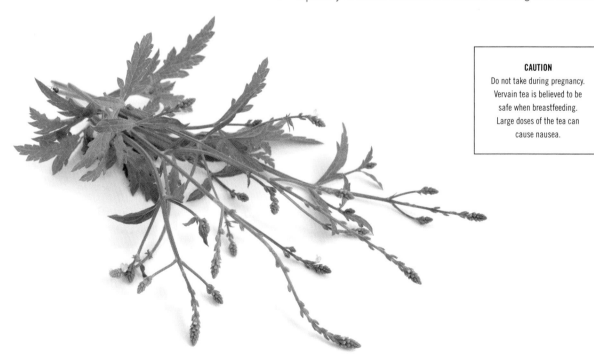

> **CAUTION**
> Do not take during pregnancy.
> Vervain tea is believed to be
> safe when breastfeeding.
> Large doses of the tea can
> cause nausea.

Vetiveria zizanioides

VETIVER

Vetiver is a grassy plant known for its grounding, centering properties. In Ayurveda, the herb is used externally during emotionally stressful times and as a tonic for women suffering from premenstrual syndrome. The deep, smoky, earthy aroma of vetiver essential oil is wonderfully grounding and relaxing.

DATA FILE

Properties
• Warming • Sweet • Bitter • Sedative • Antiseptic • Tonic
• Grounding • Regenerating • Aphrodisiac • Moth repellent

Uses
• Vetiver is used in massage and in baths to relieve stress, anxiety, nervous tension, and insomnia.
• Massage with vetiver can provide relief from arthritis or rheumatism, and general muscular aches and pains.
• Helps to clear acne, assists with wound-healing, and benefits aging skin.
• Vetiver reduces vátha, and increases both kapha and pitta.

Notes and Dosages
Vetiver is a tall, tufted, perennial, scented grass with straight stems and long, narrow leaves. The leaves and roots of the plant can be used externally as a lotion, in the bath, as a massage oil, and in patches and perfumes. In aromatherapy, the essential oil is distilled from the dried roots. It has a very strong smell. Do not allow it to overpower any blend you are making.

RECIPE

Vetiver Travel Oil
Vetiver oil is particularly useful for jet lag, and for grounding and clarity while traveling.Use 2fl.oz. (60ml.) apricot kernel oil as a base. Add 5 drops vetiver oil, 5 drops geranium oil, and 2 drops juniper or grapefruit oil. Apply this mixture liberally all over your skin before travel. Once traveling, carry a damp washcloth to which the oils have been added.

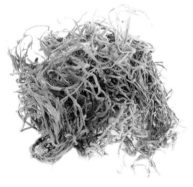

> **CAUTION**
> Do not take internally.
> Keep out of the eyes.
> Keep away from children.

Viburnum opulus

CRAMP BARK

This bark is taken from the wild form of the guelder rose. It is used in Western herbalism to treat nervous complaints, cramp, spasms, heart disease, and rheumatism.

DATA FILE

Properties
• Relaxant • Antispasmodic • Mildly sedative

Uses
• Use for any sort of cramping pains, colic, menstrual cramps, muscle spasm, and shoulder and neck tension.
• Take when back pain involves some muscle spasm.
• May be helpful for children when bedwetting is associated with tension and anxiety.

Notes and Dosages
The bark has a strong smell and is sold in flakes or thin strips. It is produced mainly in northern Europe. It is best taken freely, 1 cup of the decoction or 1–2 teaspoons of the tincture 4 or 5 times daily. May be improved by the addition of a little ginger. For children, give 30 drops of tincture, in fruit juice, 3 times daily.

RECIPE

Cramp Bark Capsules for Menstrual Cramps
Grind 1oz. (30g.) cramp bark and 1 teaspoon ginger powder together in a coffee grinder until you have a fine powder. Fill standard-sized gelatin capsules, available from herb suppliers. Take 2 or 3 capsules as required for quick relief from pain.

> **CAUTION**
> Some people find that large doses will lower their blood pressure, making them feel a little faint.

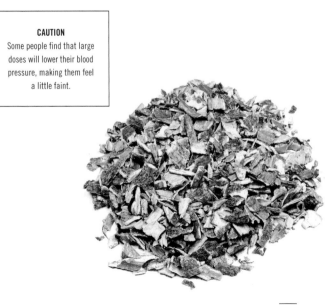

Vitex agnus-castus

AGNUS CASTUS

The dried berries of this pretty, half-hardy Mediterranean shrub, also known as chaste tree, are used in herbalism both to increase sex drive and to damp it down, as indicated by its name! Agnus castus is still used in monasteries to help the monks keep their vow of chastity, by balancing excess male hormones.

DATA FILE

Properties
• Balances hormones

Uses
• Take for premenstrual syndrome with irritability, breast pain, and water retention.
• Use for menopausal symptoms, especially with mood swings and depression. Take with sage for hot flushes.
• Helps restore a regular menstrual cycle when coming off the contraceptive pill or when the cycle has been disrupted.

Notes and Dosages
Berries should be picked in the fall then dried. The best time to take the berries is first thing in the morning, before breakfast. One cup of the decoction or 20–30 drops of the tincture in a little water, taken daily, will usually suffice.

RECIPE

Agnus Castus Pepper
The dried berries have a pleasant, peppery taste, and may be powdered in a coffee grinder and sprinkled onto meals. Take 2 good pinches or ¼ flat teaspoon.

CAUTION

Do not take during pregnancy. May cause changes in the menstrual cycle. This is a natural part of the way the herb works. Agnus castus may be taken in conjunction with hormone drugs, but it is best to seek the advice of a professional herbalist before doing so. Not to be taken with progesterone.

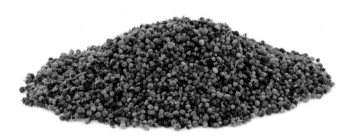

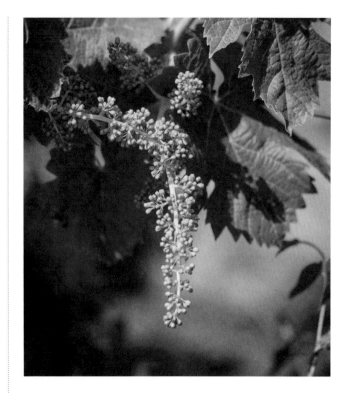

Vitis vinifera

GRAPEVINE

The grapevine is a thick-trunked shrub that climbs by means of tendrils. The flower clusters are small and green, and give way to the well-known fruit – green or purple berries. The flowers produce a remedy for those who are bossy or over dominant.

DATA FILE

Properties
• Encourages respect for others

Uses
• Vine flower remedy is for capable, confident, and successful people; for those who would be "king" (or "queen"). They believe they know best and that others would be happier if they followed. They can bully and dominate, disempowering others, and gaining authority at the expense of their confidence. Even in illness, from the sickbed, they can be ruthless and dominating.
• Vine encourages recognition of equality, and the respect due to everyone. It enables us to lead through consent rather than fear. Vine allows us to stand back and let others express themselves, to respect the absolute authority of each person over their own inner life, and to acknowledge their personal choices.

Notes and Dosages
Prepare the flower remedy using the sun method (see page 56).

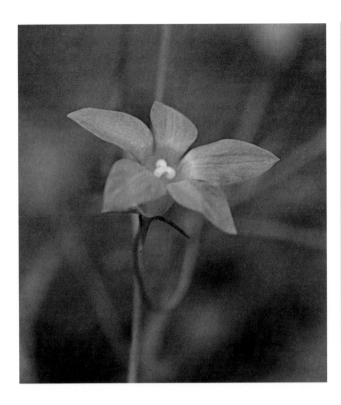

Wahlenbergia gloriosa,
Wahlenbergia stricta

BLUEBELL

These small perennial bluebells are native to Australia. The small, blue flowers appear in spring. *Wahlenbergia* species thrive best in partial shade, and prefer a well-drained soil.

DATA FILE

Properties
• Encourages sharing • Enables wholehearted love

Uses
• Bluebell is a remedy for the heart: it opens the heart to the flow of the universe. People who need bluebell are emotionally closed and fearful. The heart may be closed through hurt, fear, or loneliness. They fear that love will run out and they will be left with nothing. They may be possessive and greedy, with objects representing love. They may also have congestive and containing symptoms such as indigestion, cramps, constipation, or hemorrhoids.
• This remedy helps to conquer greed and possessiveness, and brings a will to love and share.

Notes and Dosages
Prepare the flowers using the sun method (see page 56).

Wisteria sinensis

WISTERIA

Chinese wisteria is a large, woody vine, originally from China. The flowers come before the leaves in spring, and hang in large drooping plumes of pale lilac and mauve. This climber can grow to 100ft. (30m.).

DATA FILE

Properties
• Encourages comfortableness with own sexuality • Aids intimacy and trust

Uses
• In Western culture, sex and gender issues are sometimes seen as a matter of power and control. Women who need wisteria may have a touch taboo or not enjoy sex. Men who need wisteria may be equally fearful and "role-bound," being macho or a "New Man," when they should let go and be themselves.
• Wisteria helps people to overcome the inhibitions, blocks, and emotional conflicts produced by this combative attitude. Wisteria helps to transcend traditional gender roles and to be comfortable with one's own sexuality. Wisteria can enable us to be open, express ourselves, and experience the intimate power and passivity of the orgasm.

Notes and Dosages
The soft lilac racemes of wisteria have a gentle perfume that is found to be very soothing. Prepare the flowers using the sun method (see page 56).

> **CAUTION**
> If there is a history of abuse or relationship problems, professional help should be sought.

Zea mays

CORN

The kernels of corn have a translucent, horny appearance when immature and are wrinkled when dry. The ears are eaten fresh or frozen, or are canned. Corn, or maize, is known primarily as a staple food, but it also has therapeutic properties. The corn silk (stigmas and styles of female flowers), fruit, seeds, and oil are used. Corn is particularly useful as a remedy for urinary problems.

DATA FILE

Properties
• Stimulating • Cooling • Benefits urinary system
• Cleanses the kidneys

Uses
• Corn provides carbohydrates, B vitamins (thiamine and riboflavin), vitamin C, vitamin A, potassium, and zinc.
• A tea made by infusing corn silk in hot water may help in the treatment of kidney stones. Drink three times a day.
• A little corn silk eaten raw, with or without the corn kernels, will benefit the urinary system and may help prevent cystitis.
• Corn and its products may be beneficial in the treatment of bedwetting in children, disorders of the prostate and cystitis, and inflammation of the urethra.
• Cornstarch, manufactured from the inner part of the corn kernel, makes a fine powder suitable for use as a face or bath powder.

Notes and Dosages
Corn silk refers to the hairs covering the corn: save these for making into herbal tea.

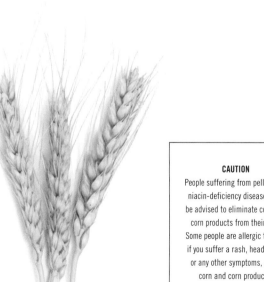

CAUTION
People suffering from pellagra (a niacin-deficiency disease) may be advised to eliminate corn and corn products from their diet. Some people are allergic to corn: if you suffer a rash, headaches, or any other symptoms, avoid corn and corn products.

Zingiber officinale

GINGER

Ginger is the spice made from the rhizome, or enlarged underground stem, of the herbaceous perennial plant *Zingiber officinale*, a member of the ginger family. Native to southern Asia, ginger is a warming, stimulating herb which is especially good for the circulation. It is used in Ayurvedic practice, Western herbalism, and aromatherapy. The essential oil distilled from the root smells similar to fresh root ginger.

DATA FILE

Properties
• Pungent • Sweet • Warming • Drying • Carminative
• Antispasmodic • Diaphoretic • Anti-emetic • Rubefacient
• Analgesic • Antiseptic • Antioxidant • Expectorant
• Promotes sweating • Antidepressant • Stimulant

Uses
• Chew crystallized ginger, take ginger capsules, or drink ginger tea, for nausea and the nausea of pregnancy and travel sickness. Alternatively, put a few drops of ginger oil on a small bandage and place behind the ear.
• Take internally for wind, colic, and irritable bowel.
• Good for chills, colds, flu, and sore throats.
• For fevers, add to elderflower or yarrow tea.
• For menstrual cramps, take with cramp bark and as a compress of grated root.
• Massage with diluted ginger oil for arthritis, rheumatism, muscle pain, and poor circulation.
• Massaged around the stomach and abdomen, diluted ginger oil calms the digestion, tones and soothes the stomach, and stimulates the appetite.
• When inhaled, ginger essence eases mental confusion, and helps to relieve fatigue and nervous exhaustion.
• In Ayurveda, ginger increases pitta in the body, reducing both kapha and vátha.

CAUTION
Avoid taking ginger in acute inflammatory conditions, in high fever, or if ulcers are present. Do not use locally on hot and inflamed areas. Use ginger oil sparingly, as high concentrations can cause irritation in sensitive people. Ginger in large doses can bring on menstruation. Pregnant women with a history of miscarriage should exercise caution and consult their physician before use.

Notes and Dosages

Ginger root is dug up when the leaves have dried. It is then thoroughly washed. The fresh root may be dried and powdered for convenience. Ginger can be taken as a food, a tea, a gargle, and a compress, or used as a massage oil. Taken internally, it is more easily tolerated than cayenne. It may be added to most remedies to improve absorption and activity. A mixture of ½ teaspoon of powder to 1 cup boiling water may be taken freely. If using the tincture, add 5–20 drops in any herb tea.

Ginger essential oil blends well with rose, cedarwood, rosewood, frankincense, vetiver, patchouli, petitgrain, neroli, lime, and other citrus oils.

RECIPES

Crystallized Ginger for Travel Sickness and Nausea

Peel a large piece of fresh ginger and chop it into small cubes. Make a syrup by dissolving 1 cup of sugar in 4 cups of water. Add the ginger and simmer gently until the root is soft. Leave in the syrup overnight, drain, and pack in sterilized jars.

Ginger Throat Gargle

Add 2 drops of ginger oil to 1 teaspoon (5ml.) of vodka and dilute with hot water. When it has cooled sufficiently, use it as a gargle for a sore throat.

Ziziphus spinosa
SUAN ZAO REN

The seeds of the sour jujube are used in traditional Chinese medicine to nourish the heart and calm the spirit. Research has shown that Suan Zao Ren has a sedative effect. It is used to treat emotional problems.

DATA FILE

Properties
• Sweet • Sour • Neutral • Reduces sweating • Calming • Sedative

Uses
• Treats symptoms such as irritability, insomnia, palpitations, and anxiety.
• Good for both spontaneous and night sweating, and may help with menopausal hot flushes.
• May be prescribed for fighting dependence on addictive drugs.

Notes and Dosages
Suan Zao Ren works through the liver, gall bladder, heart, and spleen channels.

CAUTION
Caution should be exercised in cases of severe diarrhea or heat excess. Always seek help from physicians and trained drug counselors when withdrawing from addictive drugs.

BAKING SODA

Also called bicarbonate of soda, baking soda is a white powder that is traditionally used as a raising agent for baking. It is used in many natural remedies, and on its own for its soothing and neutralizing properties.

DATA FILE

Properties
• Anti-inflammatory • Bleaches teeth • Alkaline (neutralizes acids)
• Soothing

Uses
• Apply a paste of baking soda and water to diaper rash to reduce skin inflammation and irritation.
• Drink a solution of baking soda and hot water (1 teaspoon to ½pt. [250ml.]) to reduce flatulence and ease indigestion.
• For bee stings, extract the sting by scraping with a credit card, then apply a paste of baking soda and water to neutralize.
• The juice of half a lemon mixed with 1 teaspoon of baking soda and warm water will help ease a headache. Drink every 15 minutes until the pain begins to recede.
• Brush your teeth with baking soda, a natural whitener which reduces agents causing bad breath.
• Take a teaspoonful in water to treat cystitis.

Notes and Dosages
When using baking soda medicinally, stick to the dosages above, and bear in mind the cautions detailed here.

> **CAUTION**
> Baking soda should be used only externally on children and babies. Consult a physician before taking baking soda if you have high blood pressure or heart trouble.

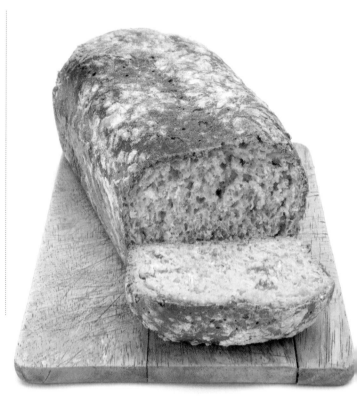

BREAD

Bread, particularly wholegrain bread, is an excellent source of carbohydrates and B-complex vitamins, which maintain the health of the nervous system and ensure the healthy functioning of body systems. Traditionally, bread was used as a poultice, and applied as a styptic to stop the bleeding of wounds.

DATA FILE

Properties
• Nutritious • Anti-inflammatory • Styptic

Uses
• Apply cold bread to closed eyes to reduce the inflammation of conjunctivitis and soothe itching.
• Apply a warm bread poultice to infected cuts to reduce itching and pain.
• Apply fresh bread to shallow wounds to help stop the bleeding.
• Ease the pain, and help to bring out a boil, by applying a hot bread poultice.
• Eat wholegrain bread while convalescing and when under stress: it is rich in B vitamins that feed the nervous system.

Notes and Dosages
Wholegrain bread contains three times as much fiber as white bread.

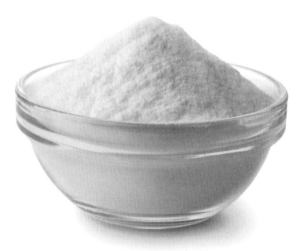

HONEY

Honey is the sweet liquid produced by bees from the nectar of flowers. For centuries, honey has been used as an antiseptic, for external and internal conditions, and as a tonic for overall good health. Each country has distinctive types of honey, dependent on the local flowers upon which the bees feed. All honeys are complex mixtures of the sugars fructose and glucose with water, organic acids, and mineral and vitamin traces, as well as some plant pigments. In homeopathy, the whole live honey bee is used, including the sting, and dissolved in alcohol, to make the Apis mellifica remedy.

DATA FILE

Properties
• Soothes raw tissues • Helps to retain calcium and balance acid accumulations • Sedative • Antifungal • Antibacterial • Possibly aphrodisiac • Nourishing • Moisturizing

Uses
• Honey water can be used as an eye lotion, which is particularly good for conjunctivitis and other infectious conditions.
• Gargle with honey water to soothe a sore throat and ease respiratory problems.
• Honey and lemon mixed together are a traditional remedy for coughs.
• Mix with apple cider vinegar as a tonic or "rebalancer." This may also help to relieve the symptoms of arthritis and reduce arthritic deposits.
• Honey ointment can soothe and encourage healing of sores in the mouth or vagina.
• Honey is an excellent moisturizer, and can be rubbed into the skin as a revitalizing mask.
• Honey warmed with a little milk can be used as a gentle sedative.
• Eating a little local honey may desensitize you to pollens in the area, acting as a remedy for hay fever and its symptoms.
• Apply a honey compress to cuts and bruises to soothe, encourage healing, and prevent infection.
• Smear set honey on ringworm or athlete's foot several times a day. Leave the foot uncovered.
• In homeopathy, Apis is prescribed for hot, stinging pain; violent headaches; fever; and smarting, watery swellings that are sensitive to touch.

Notes and Dosages
Ensure that you buy cold-pressed honey, because heated honey contains additives and loses its healing properties.

CAUTION
Honey should not be given to infants aged under one year. Unpasteurized honey should not be eaten by pregnant women, and only sparingly by children. Do not take the Apis homeopathic remedy during pregnancy.

VINEGAR

Vinegar (from the French vinaigre, "sour wine") is an acidic liquid obtained from the fermentation of alcohol, and used either as a condiment or a preservative. Vinegar usually has an acid content of 4–8 percent; in flavor it may be sharp, rich, or mellow. Vinegar is often used to preserve herbs, and used on its own for medicinal purposes.

DATA FILE

Properties
- Strengthens bones and nails • Antiseptic • Antifungal • Antibacterial
- Astringent • Antispasmodic • Balances metabolic activity • Tonic

Uses
- Helps to make more efficient use of calcium in the body, and can help to encourage strong bones, hair, and nails.
- Gargling with apple cider vinegar can help relieve a sore throat.
- Sip first thing in the morning, and just prior to meals to reduce appetite and encourage efficient digestion.
- Simmer cider vinegar in a pan, cover with a towel, and inhale to reduce the spasms of bronchitis and to help reduce any excess catarrh.
- Drink a glass of warm apple cider vinegar with honey a half-hour before bed to encourage restful sleep.
- Vinegar can be drunk (warm with a little honey) to treat digestive disorders and urinary infections.

- Apply vinegar to wasp stings to reduce swelling and ease discomfort.
- Coughs, colds, and infections will respond to a cup of warm water with 2 tablespoons of vinegar and some honey. Arthritis and asthma may also be treated with the same drink, adding slightly more vinegar.
- Apply cider vinegar to the skin to treat athlete's foot, ringworm, and eczema.
- Drink vinegar daily to treat thrush, and apply to the exterior of the vagina (mixed with a little warm water) to ease itching.
- Add vinegar to bath water to soothe skin problems, help to draw out toxins from the skin, and ease thrush.

Notes and Dosages
Malt, wine, and honey vinegars are among the many types of vinegars available. Apple cider vinegar is the most useful medicinally.

RECIPE

Cider Vinegar Inhalation
Inhaling the steam given off by hot cider vinegar will ease catarrh and soothe the bronchospasms common to bronchitis sufferers. Pour some apple cider vinegar into a pan and put it on the cooker to heat. Bring to the boil and simmer for a few minutes. Remove from the heat and pour into a medium-sized bowl. Drape a large towel over your head and the bowl, making a tent. Inhale deeply while the steam continues to be produced.

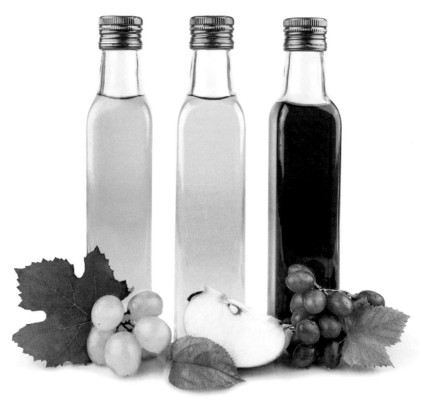

ROCK WATER

Water taken from a natural well or spring, preferably one with a traditional reputation for healing, is one of the flower remedies. The water should be open and free-flowing. There are many half-forgotten springs and wells. Choose one that is open to the air and sunshine, and is as natural as possible.

DATA FILE

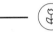

Properties
• Encourages harmony • Aids flexibility

Uses
• Rock water is for people who are very strict with themselves and unforgiving – like the rock. They practice self-discipline, have high ideals, and deny themselves anything that might distract them from their goal. However, true self-discipline does not involve denial. Denial is only necessary when the person is not acting from the heart and has a narrow view of his or her goal.
• This remedy gives the flexibility of water, a pure spring flowing toward the sea. It encourages harmony with the natural order of the world.

Notes and Dosages
Do not use water from a well dedicated to a saint, or within a church or shrine.

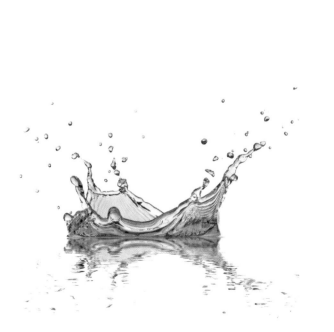

WATER

Water is the most common substance on the Earth's surface, covering more than 70 percent of the planet and present in the atmosphere as water vapor or steam. Human beings are comprised of about 75 percent water. Water is necessary for maintaining the correct osmotic pressure in cells, and is needed for many other body processes, such as transporting nutrients and waste products around the body in the blood (blood is about 80 percent water). Water that has been cooled or heated to form ice, hot water, or steam can be used to treat minor complaints.

DATA FILE

Properties
• Essential for life • Dilutes and expels toxins • Diuretic
• Aids kidney action • Prevents constipation • May contain some naturally occurring fluoride • Prevents dehydration

Uses
• Drink plenty of fresh water if you suffer from edema.
• Drink water to counter the effects of a hangover, and during illness to encourage the expulsion of toxins.
• When sufficient fluoride is present, tap water can help to prevent tooth decay.
• Water is a mild laxative: it adds water to stools and may stimulate muscle contraction in the digestive tract.
• Ice reduces swellings and helps sprains and backache.
• Salt water is a useful antiseptic for cuts and scrapes.
• For croup, place a cold compress around the throat, or remain in a steamy bathroom, which is best achieved by running the hot water faucet or the shower.
• Swallowing cracked ice may relieve morning and motion sickness.
• A hot compress can help to reduce skin inflammations caused by infection. Dip a face cloth or other thick cloth in hot water and wring out before applying.
• A warm bath can encourage relaxation and soothe muscular aches and pains.
• A cool bath can be soothing for sufferers of prickly heat.

Notes and Dosages
All adults, and particularly people who smoke or drink excessive amounts of alcohol or coffee, should drink at least eight glasses of water daily.

CAUTION
Water should be filtered if it contains impurities. Bottled mineral waters may be high in sodium.

VITAMINS, MINERALS, AND SUPPLEMENTS

U.S. RDA 3mg. E.U. RDA 800mcg.
VITAMIN A

Vitamin A is a fat-soluble vitamin that comes in two forms: retinol, which is found in animal products such as liver, eggs, butter, and cod liver oil; and beta-carotene, which our body converts into vitamin A when we need more. Beta-carotene is found in any brightly colored fruits and vegetables.

Vitamin A was for many years called a "miracle" vitamin because of its effect on the immune system and growth. It is necessary for healthy skin and eyes, and allows us to see in the dark. Beta-carotene is an antioxidant (see page 65), and it has anticarcinogenic properties.

DATA FILE

Properties
- Anticarcinogenic.
- Prevents and treats skin disorders and aging of skin.
- Improves vision and prevents night blindness.
- Improves the body's ability to heal.
- Promotes the growth of strong bones, hair, teeth, skin, and gums.
- May help in the treatment of hyperthyroidism.

Best Sources
Vitamin A: cod liver oil, liver, kidney, eggs, dairy produce.
Beta-carotene: carrots, tomatoes, watercress, broccoli, spinach, cantaloupe, apricots.

Dosages
The RDA is very much a minimum, and people with special needs (following illness, suffering from infections, with diabetes, for example) should have a higher level. Taken as vitamin A, up to 6,000mcg. is permissible if you are not pregnant. Taken as beta-carotene, 15mg. can be taken as a preventative measure against illness.

> **CAUTION**
> Vitamin A as retinol is toxic and should not be taken at all as a supplement by pregnant women, as it can cause birth defects in the unborn child.

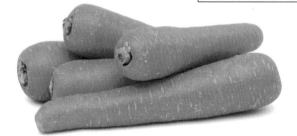

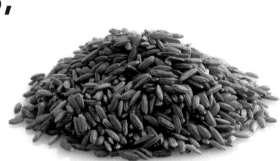

U.S. RDA 1.2–1.5mg. E.U. RDA 1.4mg.
B1 (THIAMINE)

Thiamine is involved in all key metabolic processes in the nervous system, the heart, the blood cells, and the muscles. It is useful in the treatment of nervous disorders, and can protect against imbalances caused by alcoholism.

There are more cases of vitamin B1 deficiency than of any other nutritional element – this has been said to be due to a growth in alcoholism. Thiamine is found in all plant and animal foods, but good sources are whole grains, brown rice, seafood, and pulses.

DATA FILE

Properties
- Protects against imbalances caused by alcohol consumption.
- B1 may be useful in treating heart disease.
- May be beneficial in the treatment of neurological disease (particularly when caused by B1 deficiency).
- May help to treat anemia.
- May improve people's mental agility.
- May help to control diabetes, which has been linked to deficiency.
- Useful in the treatment of herpes and infections.
- Helps to convert sugar to energy, in the muscles and the bones.

Best Sources
Pork, milk, eggs, whole grains, organ meats, brown rice, barley, seafood.

Dosages
Heavy drinkers, smokers, pregnant women, or those taking the pill should increase normal dosage to up to 100–300mg. per day. Increase intake in stressful conditions. Will be most effective as part of a good B-complex supplement.

> **CAUTION**
> Thiamine is nontoxic, but it is recommended that you do not take more than 400mg. daily.

U.S. RDA 1.7mg. E.U. RDA 1.6mg.

B2 (RIBOFLAVIN)

Riboflavin is a water-soluble member of the B-complex family of vitamins. It is crucial to the production of body energy and has antioxidant qualities. Riboflavin is not stored in any significant amount in the body, and deficiency is common.

Riboflavin is necessary for healthy skin, hair, and nails. Because it is destroyed by sunlight, it is recommended that you keep foods containing this vitamin in a dark, cool place. In particular, milk loses its riboflavin content after only two hours' exposure to sun.

DATA FILE

Properties
- Works with enzymes to metabolize fats, protein, and carbohydrates.
- Aids vision.
- Promotes healthy skin, hair, and nails.
- Promotes healthy growth and reproductive function.
- Boosts athletic performance.
- Protects against cancer.
- Protects against anemia.

Best Sources
Milk, eggs, cheese, fortified breads and cereals, green leafy vegetables, fish.

Dosages
Pregnancy, breastfeeding, taking the pill, and heavy drinking all call for an increased intake. Take as part of a B-complex supplement, and increase dosage in stressful situations. Taking 100–300mg. per day is commonly suggested.

> **CAUTION**
> Riboflavin is nontoxic in most doses, but it is recommended that you do not take in excess of 400mg. per day unless supervised by a registered practitioner.

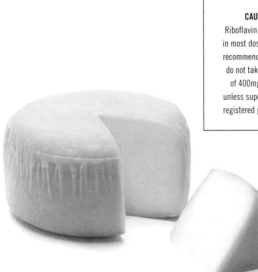

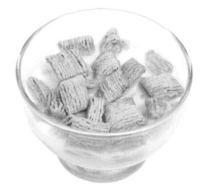

U.S. RDA 13–18mg. adults, 5–6mg. infants, 9–13mg. children under ten. E.U. RDA 15–18mg.

B3 (NIACIN)

Niacin is one of the water-soluble B-complex vitamins, and it is essential for the synthesis of sex hormones and a healthy nervous system. Niacin may also be valuable in helping to prevent and treat schizophrenia, and in acting as a detoxicant, ridding the body of toxins, pollutants, and drugs. Niacin takes the form of nicotinic acid and nicotinamide, and is a fairly recent addition to the family of B-complex vitamins, named as a vitamin only in 1937. Niacin has been shown to lower blood cholesterol and other body fats, and is useful in the prevention of heart disease. It may help to prevent diabetes.

DATA FILE

Properties
- Prevents and treats schizophrenia.
- Aids in cell respiration.
- Produces energy from sugar, fat, and protein.
- Maintains clear, healthy skin, nerves, tongue, and good digestion.
- May lower cholesterol and therefore protect against heart disease.
- Believed to be antioxidant.
- May help prevent migraine headaches.
- Reduces blood pressure.
- May alleviate arthritis.

Best Sources
Meat, fish, wholegrain cereals, eggs, milk, cheese.

Dosages
Large doses may be used therapeutically, but should be taken under the supervision of a physician or health practitioner. Doses of 20–100mg. of niacin, taken daily, may be beneficial. Best taken as part of a B-complex supplement.

> **CAUTION**
> In high doses, niacin may cause depression, liver malfunction, flushing, and headaches. Avoid doses larger than about 120mg. unless you are under the supervision of a registered practitioner.

U.S. RDA 10mg. E.U. RDA 6mg.

B5 (PANTOTHENIC ACID)

Pantothenic acid is a water-soluble member of the B-complex family of vitamins that helps maintain normal growth and the health of the nervous system. Pantothenic acid has become a popular supplement over the past decade for its ability to boost energy levels and improve immune response.

There is also evidence that pantothenic acid can lower cholesterol and protect against heart disease. Pantothenic acid is useful in reducing the effects of stress on the body, and is needed to convert choline into acetylcholine, which is necessary for brain functioning.

DATA FILE

Properties

- B5 encourages the healing of wounds.
- Helps the body in the production of energy.
- Reduces stress levels.
- Controls the metabolism of fat.
- Encourages functioning of the immune system.
- Prevents fatigue.
- Lowers cholesterol levels and so protects against heart disease.
- Prevents arthritis, and also treats it.
- May prevent hair loss and graying of hair.

Best Sources

Yeast, organ meats, eggs, brown rice, wholegrain cereals, molasses.

Dosages

Best taken in B-complex formulas, up to 300mg. per day for therapeutic use. The normal dosage, which should help to prevent disease, is about 100mg. per day.

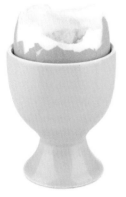

> **CAUTION**
> No known toxicity, although doses of over 300mg. per day should be supervised by a practitioner. Some people report stomach upsets at doses higher than 10mg.

U.S. RDA 2mg. E.U. RDA 1.6–2mg.

B6 (PYRIDOXINE)

Pyridoxine is a water-soluble B-complex vitamin which is necessary for the production of antibodies and white blood cells. B6 is necessary for the absorption of vitamin B12. It is also required for the functioning of more than 60 enzymes in the body and for protein synthesis.

Of all the B vitamins, B6 is the most important for a healthy immune system, and it is thought to protect the body against some cancers. B6 is widely used for relieving the symptoms of PMS and menopause, and may cure some forms of infertility. This vitamin is also used to prevent skin inflammation, and maintain healthy teeth and gums.

DATA FILE

Properties

- Boosts immunity.
- Helps to control diabetes.
- B6 assimilates proteins and fats.
- Helps prevent skin and nervous disorders.
- Alleviates nausea.
- Treats symptoms of PMS and menopause.
- Reduces muscle cramps and spasms.
- Acts as a natural diuretic.
- Protects against cancer.

Best Sources

Meat, fish, milk, eggs, wholegrain cereals, fresh vegetables.

Dosages

Should always be taken as part of a B-complex supplement, and in equal amounts with B1 and B2. Time-release formulas are best because it lasts for only eight hours in the body.

> **CAUTION**
> Vitamin B6 is toxic in high doses, causing serious nerve damage when taken at quantities of more than 2g. per day. Some people report side-effects with doses as low as 100mg.

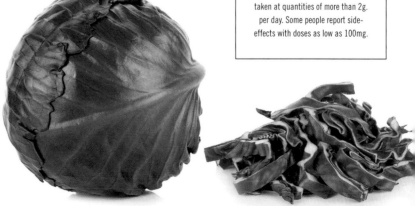

U.S. RDA 400mcg. E.U. RDA 200–360mcg.

B9 (FOLIC ACID)

Folic acid is a water-soluble vitamin that forms part of the B-complex family. It is also known as vitamin Bc or vitamin B9. Low levels of folic acid may lead to anemia. Folic acid is essential for the division of body cells, and it is also necessary for the utilization of sugar and amino acids.

Findings indicate that folic acid can prevent some types of cancer and birth defects, and it is helpful in the treatment of heart disease. Most folic acid deficiency is the result of a poor diet, because it is abundant in foods such as leafy green vegetables, yeast, and liver. Taken from just before conception, and particularly in the first trimester of pregnancy, folic acid can help to prevent spina bifida.

DATA FILE

Properties
• Improves lactation.
• May protect against cancer.
• Improves skin condition.
• Natural analgesic.
• Increases appetite in debilitated patients.
• Needed for metabolism of RNA and DNA.
• Helps form blood.
• Builds up babies' resistance to infection.
• Essential for transmission of genetic code.
• Prevents spina bifida.

Best Sources
Green leafy vegetables, wheat germ, nuts, eggs, bananas, oranges, and organ meats.

Dosages
There are many people at risk of deficiency, including heavy drinkers, pregnant women, the elderly, and those on low-fat diets. Supplementation at 400–800mcg. is recommended for those at risk. It is best taken with a good multivitamin and mineral supplement.

> **CAUTION**
> Folic acid is toxic in large doses and can cause severe neurological problems. High doses may cause insomnia and interfere with the absorption of zinc in the body.

U.S. RDA 3mcg. E.U. RDA 2mcg.

B12 (COBALAMIN)

Cobalamin is a water-soluble member of the B-complex vitamin family, and it is the only vitamin that contains essential minerals. B12 is essential for the healthy metabolism of nerve tissue, and deficiencies can cause brain damage and neurological disorders. Vitamin B12 was once considered to be a "wonder drug" and was given by injection to rejuvenate. B12 may also reduce the risk of cancer and the severity of allergies, as well as boosting energy levels. Low levels of this vitamin result in anemia.

DATA FILE

Properties
• Needed for maintenance of the nervous system.
• Improves memory and concentration.
• Required to utilize fats, carbohydrates, and proteins.
• Increases energy.
• Promotes healthy growth in children.
• May protect against cancer.
• Protects against allergens and toxic elements.

Best Sources
Liver, beef, pork, eggs, cheese, fish, milk.

Dosages
Dosages of 5–50mcg. should be adequate for most people; higher dosages should be supervised. Best taken as part of a B-complex supplement.

> **CAUTION**
> Although vitamin B12 is not considered to be toxic, it is recommended that you do not take more than 200mg. daily unless you are under the supervision of a registered practitioner.

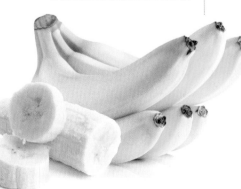

U.S. RDA 60mg. E.U. RDA 60mg.

VITAMIN C

Vitamin C is water soluble, which means that it is not stored by the body and we need to ensure that we get adequate amounts in our daily diet. More people take vitamin C than any other supplement, and yet studies show that a large percentage of the population have deficiencies.

Vitamin C is also known as ascorbic acid, and it is one of the most versatile of the vitamins we need to sustain life. It is one of the antioxidant vitamins (see page 65) and is believed to boost immunity, and to fight cancer and infection.

DATA FILE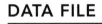

Properties
- Reduces cholesterol and helps prevent heart disease.
- Speeds up the healing of wounds.
- Maintains healthy bones, teeth, and sex organs.
- Acts as a natural antihistamine.
- May help to overcome male infertility.
- Fights cancer.
- Boosts immunity and reduces the duration of colds and other viruses.
- Helps maintenance of good vision.
- Antioxidant.

Best Sources
Rosehips, blackcurrants, broccoli, citrus fruits, all fresh fruits and vegetables.

Dosages
At least 60mg. per day is necessary for health, but more is required by smokers (25mg. is depleted with every cigarette), and people who are under stress, taking antibiotics, suffering from an infection, drink heavily, as well as after an accident or injury. Daily dosages of up to 1,500mg. per day appear to be safe, but take this in three doses, preferably with meals, and use a time-release formula.

> **CAUTION**
> Vitamin C may cause kidney stones and gout in some individuals. Some people suffer from diarrhea and cramps at high dosages, although the vitamin is considered to be nontoxic at even very high levels.

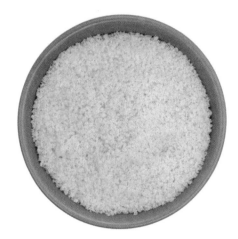

U.S. RDA 10mcg. E.U. RDA 5mcg.

VITAMIN D

Vitamin D is a fat-soluble vitamin that is found in foods of animal origin and is known as the "sunshine" vitamin. Vitamin D can be produced in the skin from the energy of the sun, and it is not found in rich supply in any food.

Vitamin D is important for calcium and phosphorus absorption, and helps to regulate calcium metabolism. Recent research suggests that it could have a role in protecting against some cancers and infectious diseases. Deficiency is caused by inadequate exposure to sunlight, and low consumption of foods containing vitamin D.

DATA FILE

Properties
- Protects against osteoporosis.
- May help in the treatment of psoriasis.
- Boosts immune system.
- May be useful in the treatment of cancer.
- Protects against cancer.
- Necessary for strong teeth and bones.

Best Sources
Animal produce, such as milk, eggs, oily fish, butter, cheese, cod liver oil.

Dosages
Supplementation of 5–10mcg. is suggested for those at risk of deficiency.

> **CAUTION**
> Vitamin D is the most toxic of all the vitamins, causing nausea, vomiting, headache, and depression, among other problems. Do not take in excess of 10mcg. daily.

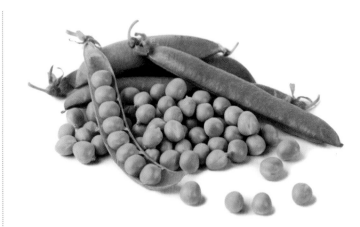

U.S. RDA 20mg. E.U. RDA 10mg.

VITAMIN E

Vitamin E is fat soluble and one of the key antioxidant vitamins (see page 65). Its key function is as an anticoagulant, but its role in boosting the immune system and protecting against cardiovascular disease is becoming increasingly clear.

Apart from its crucial antioxidant value, vitamin E is important for the production of energy and the maintenance of health at every level. Unlike most fat-soluble vitamins, vitamin E is stored in the body for only a short period of time, and up to 75 percent of a daily dose is excreted in the feces.

DATA FILE

Properties
- Antioxidant, so helps to slow the process of aging.
- Protects against neurological disorders.
- Boosts immunity.
- Protects against cardiovascular disease.
- Alleviates fatigue.
- Accelerates healing, particularly of burns.
- Reduces the various symptoms of PMS.
- Treats skin problems and baldness.
- Helps prevent miscarriage.
- Acts as a natural diuretic.
- Prevents formation of thickened scars.

Best Sources
Wheat germ (fresh), soybeans, vegetable oils, broccoli, leafy green vegetables, whole grains, peanuts, eggs.

Dosages
Vitamin E is available in many forms (the dry form is best for people with skin problems or oil intolerance). Daily dosage may be 250–280mg., but you may be advised to take higher doses in some cases.

> **CAUTION**
> Vitamin E is nontoxic, even in high doses, but it is suggested that you do not take in excess of 350mg. unless supervised by a registered practitioner.

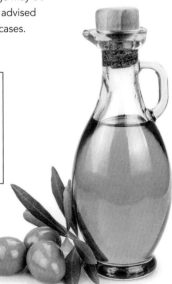

U.S. RDA none. E.U. RDA none.

VITAMIN K

The K vitamins are fat soluble, and are necessary for normal blood clotting. They are often used to treat the toxic effects of anticoagulant drops, such as warfarin, and in people who have a poor ability to absorb fats.

Vitamin K occurs naturally in foods such as wholegrain cereals as vitamin K1, and is produced by intestinal bacteria as vitamin K2. Synthetic vitamin K is known as K3. Vitamin K injections or oral drops are routinely given to babies soon after birth to prevent hemorrhage.

DATA FILE

Properties
- Controls blood clotting.

Best Sources
Cauliflower, spinach, peas, wholegrain cereals.

Dosages
We need an estimated 500–1,000mcg. of vitamin K from our diet per day.

> **CAUTION**
> There are no reports of toxicity, but because of the possibility that injected vitamin K may be related to childhood leukemia, oral drops are suggested for newborns.

U.S. RDA 300mcg. E.U. RDA 0.15mg.

BIOTIN (VITAMIN H)

Biotin is not a true vitamin, but it works with B-complex vitamins and is often called vitamin H, or co-enzyme R. Biotin is water soluble and is found in many common foods. It is essential for breaking down and metabolizing fats in the body.

Biotin is depleted in the body by alcohol, cooking or refining food, antibiotics, and when taken with raw egg whites, which contain avidin, a protein that prevents biotin absorption. Biotin works more effectively with vitamins B2, B6, B3, and A.

DATA FILE

Properties
- Prevents the hair from turning gray.
- Eases various muscular aches and pains.
- Treats eczema, dermatitis, and other skin conditions.
- Helps to prevent baldness.
- Essential for energy release from fats.

Best Sources
Nuts, fruits, beef liver, chicken liver, egg yolks, milk, kidneys, unpolished rice, brewer's yeast.

Dosages
Biotin is normally included in most readily available B-complex supplements.

U.S. RDA none. E.U. RDA none.

B BORON

Boron is a trace mineral found in most plants, and it is essential for human health. Recent research has reported that boron added to the diet of post-menopausal women prevents calcium loss and bone demineralization – a revolutionary discovery for sufferers of osteoporosis.

It is also claimed that boron will raise testosterone levels and build muscle in men, and boron is therefore often used by athletes and bodybuilders. Boron is found in most fruit and vegetables, and does not appear in meat and meat products. Boron supplements are usually taken in the form of sodium borate.

DATA FILE

Properties
- Assists in the external treatment of bacterial and fungal infections.
- Helps to lower the incidence of arthritis.
- Prevents osteoporosis.
- Used to build muscles.

Best Sources
Root vegetables (such as potatoes, parsnips, and carrots) grown in soil that is rich in boron.

Dosages
No RDA, but it is suggested that 3mg. should be taken daily to prevent osteoporosis.

> **CAUTION**
> Boron can be toxic, with symptoms including a red rash, vomiting, diarrhea, reduced circulation, shock, and then coma. A fatal dose is 15–20g., 3–6g. in children. Symptoms appear at about 100mg.

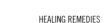

U.S. RDA 800–1,200mg. E.U. RDA 800mg.

CA CALCIUM

Calcium makes up bones and teeth, and is crucial in the maintenance of the immune system. There are many groups at risk of calcium deficiency – in particular the elderly – and because it is so important to body processes our bodies take what they need from our bones, which causes them to become brittle. The homeopathic remedies Calc. carb., obtained from the mother of pearl in oyster shells; Calc. phos., a mineral salt; and Hep. sulf., also known as calcium sulfide, contain very small quantities of calcium. They are prescribed by homeopaths for conditions such as broken bones that are slow to heal, joint pain, and skin infections.

DATA FILE

Properties
- Prevents osteoporosis, and helps to treat the condition once symptoms manifest.
- Prevents cancer.
- Useful in the treatment of high blood pressure.
- Prevents heart disease.
- Useful in treating arthritis.
- Helps to keep skin healthy.
- Alleviates leg cramps.
- Encourages regular beating of the heart.
- Soothes insomnia.
- Helps the body to metabolize iron.
- Necessary for nerve-impulse transmission and muscular function.

Best Sources
Milk, cheese, dairy produce, leafy green vegetables, hard tap water, salmon, tinned fish, eggs, beans, nuts, tofu.

Dosages
Experts recommend that calcium be taken in a good multivitamin and mineral supplement, although extra doses may be given up to l,000mg. per day. More calcium is needed by women after the menopause, and while pregnant or breastfeeding.

For dosages of the homeopathic remedies Calc. carb., Calc. phos., and Hep. sulf., consult a practitioner.

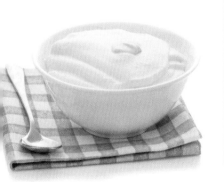

> **CAUTION**
> Doses over 2,000mg. per day may cause hypercalcemia (calcium deposits in the kidneys), but since excess calcium is excreted, it is unlikely to occur unless you are also taking excess quantities of vitamin D.

U.S. RDA none. E.U. RDA none.

CO COBALT

Cobalt is an essential trace mineral. It is a constituent of vitamin B12. The amount of cobalt in the body is dependent on the amount of cobalt in the soil, and therefore in the food we eat. Most of us are not deficient in cobalt, although deficiency is much more common in vegetarians.

DATA FILE

Properties
Cobalt is able, with vitamin B12, to:
- Prevent pernicious anemia.
- Help in the production of red blood cells.
- Aid in the synthesis of DNA and choline.
- Encourage a healthy nervous system.
- Reduce blood pressure.
- Maintain myelin, the fatty sheath protecting the nerves.

Best Sources
Fresh leafy green vegetables, meat, liver, milk, oysters, clams.

Dosages
Cobalt is rarely found in supplement form, but forms part of a good multivitamin and mineral supplement with the B-complex vitamins. An intake of 8mcg. daily appears to be adequate.

> **CAUTION**
> When used therapeutically, side-effects occur at doses of cobalt above 30mg. These include goiter, hyperthyroidism, and heart failure.

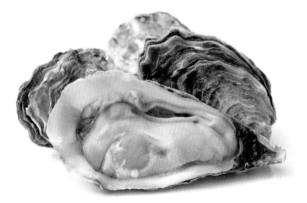

U.S. RDA none. E.U. RDA none.

CR CHROMIUM

Chromium is a trace mineral that was discovered in the body in the 1950s. It is an important regulator of blood sugar, and has been used successfully in the control and treatment of diabetes. It is involved in the metabolism of carbohydrates and fats, and is used in the production of insulin in the body.

High levels of sugars in the diet cause chromium to be excreted through the kidneys, so it is important to get enough in your diet if you eat sugary foods. The incidence of diabetes and heart disease decreases with increased levels of chromium in the body.

DATA FILE

Properties
- Aids in the control and production of insulin.
- Aids in the metabolism of carbohydrates and fats.
- Controls levels of cholesterol in the blood.
- Stimulates the synthesis of proteins in the body.
- Increases general resistance to infection.
- Suppresses hunger pains.

Best Sources
Wholegrain cereals, meat, cheese, brewer's yeast, molasses, egg yolk.

Dosages
There is no RDA, but it is suggested that 25mcg. per day is adequate. If necessary, supplements of up to 200mcg. per day can be taken.

> **CAUTION**
> There is no evidence that chromium is toxic, even in high doses, since any excess is excreted. However, it is suggested that you do not take more than 200mcg. daily unless supervised by a registered practitioner.

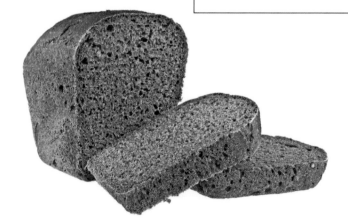

U.S. RDA 1.5–3mg. E.U. RDA 1.2mg.

CU COPPER

Copper is an essential trace mineral, and is necessary for respiration – iron and copper are required for oxygen to be synthesized in red blood cells. Copper is also important for the production of collagen, which is responsible for the health of our bones, cartilage, and skin. Copper is also one of the antioxidant minerals (see page 65), which may protect against free-radical damage. Arthritis sufferers report that copper bracelets reduce pain and inflammation associated with the condition, probably because traces of the mineral are absorbed by the skin and enter the bloodstream.

The homeopathic remedy Cuprum. met., used to treat complaints of the nervous system, contains copper. It should be used only under the care of a qualified practitioner.

DATA FILE

Properties
- May prevent cancer.
- Protects against cardiovascular disease.
- Useful mineral in the treatment of arthritis.
- Boosts the immune system.
- Acts as an antioxidant.

Best Sources
Animal livers, shellfish, nuts, fruit, oysters, kidneys, legumes.

Dosages
Copper appears in good multivitamin and mineral supplements, and can be taken alone up to 3mg. daily.

> **CAUTION**
> Excess intake can cause vomiting, diarrhea, muscular pain, and dementia.

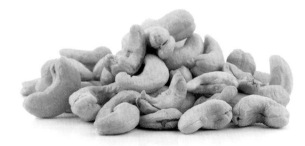

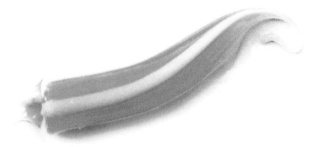

*U.S. RDA 1mg. fluoride, 3.6mg.
sodium fluoride. E.U. RDA none.*

F FLUORINE

Fluorine is a trace mineral found naturally in soil, water, plants, and animal tissues. Its electrically charged form is "fluoride," which is how we usually refer to it. Although it has not yet been officially recognized as an essential nutrient, studies show that it is important in many processes, and may play a major role in the prevention of many 21st-century killers, like heart disease.

The major source of fluorine is drinking water, which is sometimes fluoridated, or has enough naturally occurring fluoride to make fluoridation unnecessary. Fluoride supplements should always be taken with calcium.

DATA FILE

Properties
- Fluorine protects against dental caries.
- Protects against, and also treats, osteoporosis.
- It may help to prevent heart disease.
- May help to prevent calcification of organs and musculoskeletal structures.

Best Sources
Seafood, animal meat, fluoridated drinking water, toothpaste, tea.

Dosages
A major source is drinking water, if your area has a fluoridated supply, and the typical daily intake is 1–2mg. Tablets and drops are available from pharmacies, but should be limited to 1 mg. daily in adults, and 0.25–0.5mg. for children.

> **CAUTION**
> An excess of fluoride causes fluorosis, characterized by irregular patches on tooth enamel, and depresses the appetite. Eventually the spine calcifies. Fluorosis is rare and occurs at levels far above 10mg. per day. Do not supplement fluoride without the advice of your dentist.

*U.S. RDA 10–18mg., pregnant women 30mg.
E.U. RDA 14mg.*

FE IRON

Iron is a trace mineral that is essential for human health. Iron-deficiency anemia, which is the condition most commonly associated with deficiency, was described by Egyptian physicists as long ago as 1500 B.C.E. Today, 10 percent of all women in the Western world suffer from iron-deficiency anemia.

We now know that iron is present in our bodies as hemoglobin, which is the red pigment of blood. Iron is required for muscle protein and is stored in the liver, spleen, bone marrow, and muscles. Efficient absorption of iron is highest in childhood, and reduces as we age. Our bodies need vitamin C in order to assimilate iron in an effective fashion.

The homeopathic remedy Ferr. phos. is made from iron phosphate. It is prescribed for inflammation, coughs, colds, and chills.

DATA FILE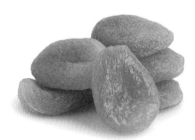

Properties
- Improves physical performance.
- Anticarcinogenic.
- Prevents learning problems in children.
- Prevents and cures iron-deficiency anemia.
- Improves immunity.
- Boosts energy levels.
- Encourages restful sleep and maintains energy levels.

Best Sources
Shellfish, brewer's yeast, wheat bran, offal, cocoa powder, dried fruit, cereals.

Dosages
Pregnant, breastfeeding, and menstruating women, infants, children, athletes, and vegetarians may require increased levels of iron. Your general physician will prescribe iron supplements if they are necessary. Maximum dosage is around 15mg. daily, unless under medical supervision.

> **CAUTION**
> Excess iron can cause constipation, diarrhea, and, rarely, in high doses, death. Be very cautious when giving children iron supplements — even doses as little as 3g. can cause death.

GE GERMANIUM

Germanium is a mineral that is abundant in the surface of the Earth. Almost all foods commonly eaten contain some germanium. Some conditions have been reported to respond favorably to germanium given at therapeutic doses, including arthritis, angina, stroke, Raynaud's disease, burns, and pain associated with cancer.

Germanium is believed to function by boosting the action of oxygen in generating energy. Because it maintains an equilibrium within the body, germanium is said to reduce high blood pressure, lower cholesterol levels, and generally to exert a good effect on the immune system. Germanium is now considered to be one of the antioxidant minerals (see page 65).

DATA FILE

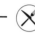

Properties

- Maintains the homeostasis in the body, and therefore may reduce high blood pressure and cholesterol levels.
- Germanium boosts the immune system.
- May be analgesic.
- May have antiviral, antibacterial, and antitumor activity.
- Useful as part of a cancer treatment program.
- Helps chronic Epstein-Barr virus syndrome.
- Useful in the treatment of HIV/AIDS.

Best Sources

Bran, wholewheat flour, vegetables, garlic, seeds, meats, dairy products.

Dosages

Germanium supplementation is not recommended without a physician's supervision.

> **CAUTION**
> Germanium is safe up to quite a high level, although skin eruptions and diarrhea have been reported in some patients taking therapeutic doses. Only use the supplement under the supervision of a physician or nutritionist.

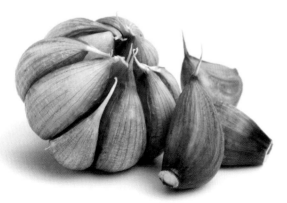

I IODINE

Iodine is a mineral that was first discovered in 1812 in bladderwrack. Iodine was extracted and given its name because of its violet color. It occurs naturally and is a crucial constituent of the thyroid hormones, which monitor our energy levels.

Iodine deficiency is one of the key world health problems, and at least 200 million people suffer from conditions linked to inadequate iodine in the diet. Lack of iodine can cause goiter, underactive thyroid, cretinism, and can eventually lead to myxedema.

DATA FILE

Properties

- Determines the level of metabolism and energy in the body.
- Relieves the pain of fibrocystic breasts.
- Protects against the toxic effects of exposure to radioactive materials.
- Prevents goiter.
- Prevents thyroid disorders.
- Loosens mucus in the respiratory tract.
- Natural antiseptic.

Best Sources

Seafood and seaweed. Most table salt is fortified with iodine.

Dosages

Iodine is best taken as potassium iodide. Take only up to 150mcg. under the supervision of your physician or nutritionist.

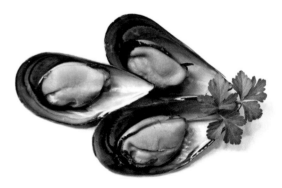

> **CAUTION**
> Iodine is toxic in high doses and may aggravate or cause acne. Large doses may interfere with hormone activity. Cruciferous foods like cabbage, brussels sprouts, cauliflower, and broccoli contain substances which can cause hypothyroidism by antagonizing iodine. Anyone who eats large quantities of these vegetables should consider an iodine supplement.

U.S. RDA 3,500mg. E.U. RDA 3,500mg.

K POTASSIUM

Potassium is one of the most important minerals in our body, working with sodium and chloride to form "electrolytes," the essential body salts that make up our body fluids. Potassium is crucial in order for the body to function. It plays a role in nerve conduction, the beating of the heart, energy production, the synthesis of nucleic acids and proteins, and the contraction of muscles.

Sweating can cause a loss of potassium, as do chronic diarrhea and diuretics. People taking certain drugs, including corticosteroids, high-dose penicillin, and laxatives, may suffer from potassium deficiency. Symptoms of this can include vomiting, abdominal distension, muscular weakness, loss of appetite, low blood pressure, and intense thirst.

The homeopathic remedy Kali. phos. is prepared by adding a dilute phosphoric acid to a solution of potassium carbonate (also known as potash), and is used to treat conditions affecting the nervous system, and for exhaustion.

DATA FILE

Properties
• Activates enzymes that control energy production.
• Prevents and treats high blood pressure.
• May help to protect against stroke.
• Improves athletic performance.
• May help treat and prevent cancer.
• Maintains water balance within cells.
• Stabilizes the internal structure of cells.
• Acts with sodium to conduct nerve impulses.

Best Sources
Fresh fruit and vegetables, particularly bananas, plus dried fruit.

Dosages
Eat more fresh fruit and vegetables to increase potassium intake. Diuretic users and those in a hot climate may need up to 1.5g. in supplementary potassium daily. Take with zinc and magnesium for best effect.

> **CAUTION**
> In excess (doses above 3,500mg.), potassium may cause muscular weakness and mental apathy, eventually stopping the heart.

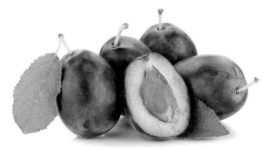

U.S. RDA 300–400mg. E.U. RDA 300mg.

MG MAGNESIUM

Magnesium is a mineral that is absolutely essential for every biochemical process taking place in our bodies, including metabolism and the synthesis of nucleic acids and protein.

Magnesium deficiency is very common, particularly in the elderly, heavy drinkers, pregnant women, and regular, strenuous exercisers, and it has been proved that even a very slight deficiency can cause a disruption of the heartbeat. Other symptoms of magnesium deficiency include weakness, fatigue, vertigo, nervousness, muscle cramps, and hyperactivity in children.

Taken under the care of a registered practitioner, the homeopathic remedy Mag. phos. is said to have an anti-spasmodic effect.

DATA FILE

Properties
• Magnesium is necessary for many body functions, including energy production and cell replication.
• Essential for transmission of nerve impulses.
• Helps to prevent kidney stones and gallstones.
• Useful in the treatment of prostate problems.
• Repairs and maintains body cells.
• Required for hormonal activity.
• Required for most body processes, including production of energy.
• Useful in the treatment of high blood pressure.
• Protects against cardiovascular disease.
• Helps to treat the symptoms of premenstrual syndrome.

Best Sources
Brown rice, soybeans, nuts, brewer's yeast, wholewheat flour, legumes.

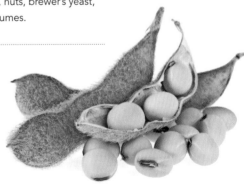

Dosages
Intake may be inadequate in the average Western diet, so supplements of 200–400mg. are recommended.

> **CAUTION**
> Magnesium is toxic to people with renal problems or atrioventricular blocks. High doses are believed to cause flushing of the skin, thirst, low blood pressure, and loss of reflexes in some people, although this is rare.

U.S. RDA 2.5–7mg. E.U. RDA none.

MN MANGANESE

Manganese is an essential trace element that is necessary for the normal functioning of the brain, and effective in the treatment of many nervous disorders, including Alzheimer's disease and schizophrenia. Deficiency is usually related to a poor diet, particularly one where there is a high intake of foods that are processed and refined.

Our understanding of manganese is still incomplete, but it may prove to be one of the most important nutrients in human pathology. It appears likely that manganese is one of the antioxidant minerals (see page 65). There is some evidence that diseases such as diabetes, heart disease, and schizophrenia are linked to manganese deficiency.

DATA FILE

Properties
- Manganese maintains the healthy functioning of the nervous system.
- Necessary for female sex hormones.
- Necessary for the synthesis of the structural proteins of body cells.
- Necessary for normal bone structure.
- Important in the formation of thyroxin in the thyroid gland.
- Necessary for the functioning of the brain.
- Used in the treatment of some nervous disorders.
- Necessary for metabolism of glucose.

Best Sources
Cereals, tea, green leafy vegetables, wholewheat bread, pulses, nuts.

Dosages
2–5mg. is adequate, but doses up to 10mg. are thought to be safe.

> **CAUTION**
> Toxic levels are usually quite rare, but symptoms of excess manganese may include lethargy, involuntary movements, posture problems, and coma.

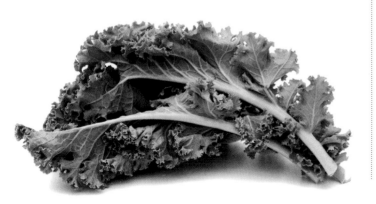

> **CAUTION**
> Molybdenum is toxic in doses higher than 10–15mg., which cause gout (a build-up of uric acid around the joints).

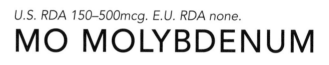

U.S. RDA 150–500mcg. E.U. RDA none.

MO MOLYBDENUM

Molybdenum is an essential trace element, and a vital part of the enzyme that is responsible for the utilization of iron in our bodies. Molybdenum may also be an antioxidant, and research indicates that it is necessary for optimum health.

Molybdenum can help to prevent anemia and is known to promote a feeling of wellbeing. A deficiency may result in dental caries, sexual impotence in men, and cancer of the gullet. Deficiency is usually the result of eating foods from molybdenum-deficient soils, or a diet that is high in refined and processed foods.

DATA FILE

Properties
- For utilization of iron, fats, and carbohydrates; and the excretion of uric acid.
- Prevents impotence.
- Protects against cancer, anemia, and dental caries.

Best Sources
Wheat, canned beans, wheat germ, liver, pulses, whole grains, offal, eggs.

Dosages
Optimal intake is not decided, but 0.075–0.25mg. per day is adequate, and experts suggest 50–100mcg. per day as a preventive measure. It is toxic in doses higher than 10–15mg., causing gout.

U.S. RDA 800–1,200mg. E.U. RDA 800mg.

P PHOSPHORUS

Phosphorus is a mineral that is essential to the structure and function of the body. It is present in the body as phosphates, and in this form aids the process of bone mineralization and helps to create the structure of the bone.

Phosphorus is also essential for communication between cells, and for energy production. Phosphorus appears in many foods, and deficiency is rare. Because of its role in strengthening our bones, we should eat twice as much calcium as phosphorus.

In homeopathy, the remedy Phos. is given to those suffering from anxiety and digestive disorders.

DATA FILE

Properties
- Forms bones and teeth.
- Produces energy.
- Cofactor for many enzymes and activates B-complex vitamins.
- Increases endurance, and fights fatigue.
- Forms RNA and DNA.

Best Sources
Yeast, dried milk and milk products, wheat germ, hard cheeses, canned fish, nuts, cereals, eggs.

Dosages
Phosphorus deficiency usually accompanies deficiency in potassium, magnesium, and zinc, so take a supplement containing all four. Take under medical supervision only.

> **CAUTION**
> Phosphorus can be toxic at dosages or intake above 200mg. per day, in some cases causing diarrhea, the calcification of organs and soft tissues, and making the body unable to absorb iron, calcium, magnesium, and zinc.

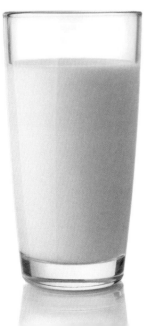

U.S. RDA 50–100mcg. E.U. RDA 10–75mcg.

SE SELENIUM

Selenium is an essential trace element that has recently been recognized as one of the most important nutrients in our diet. It is an antioxidant (see page 65) and is vitally important in human metabolism. Selenium has been proved to provide protection against a number of cancers, and other diseases.

Selenium is necessary for the body's manufacture of proteins, and helps the liver to function efficiently. It also forms part of the male sperm, which means that deficiency can be linked to infertility in men. Other symptoms of deficiency include reduced immune activity, hair loss, and chest pains.

DATA FILE

Properties
- Maintains healthy eyes and eyesight.
- Maintains good skin and healthy hair.
- Stimulates immune system.
- Prevents many cancers.
- Improves liver function.
- Protects against heart and circulatory diseases.
- May work to impede the aging process.
- Can detoxify alcohol, many drugs, smoking, and some fats.
- Increases male potency and sex drive.
- Useful addition to the treatment of arthritis.
- Alleviates hot flushes and symptoms of menopause.
- Helps treat dandruff.

Best Sources
Wheat germ, bran, tuna, onions, tomatoes, broccoli, kidneys, wholewheat bread.

Dosages
It has been suggested that men take 75mcg. of supplementary selenium and women take 60mcg. Selenium supplementation should be taken with 90–120mcg. of vitamin E to ensure that selenium works most efficiently.

> **CAUTION**
> Selenium can be toxic in very small doses. Symptoms of excess include blackened fingernails and a garlic-like odor on the breath and skin. Take no more than 500mcg. daily unless supervised by a registered practitioner.

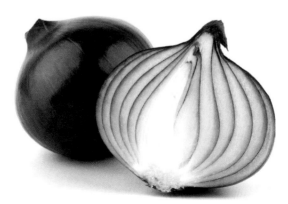

U.S. RDA none. E.U. RDA none.

SI SILICON

Silicon is a trace element that is only just starting to be understood. It has been proved to be essential to animals, and it is thought that it is crucial to human life as well. Scientists believe that silicon plays some part in the make-up of our connective tissues, bones, skin, and fingernails. Silicon is also known to play a role in preventing osteoporosis, by assisting the utilization of calcium within the bones. It also improves the strength of hair and nails by improving the production of keratin and collagen. Silicon is available as a supplement in the form of silicon dioxide.

Silicea is a homeopathic remedy for disorders of the bones, joints, and skin.

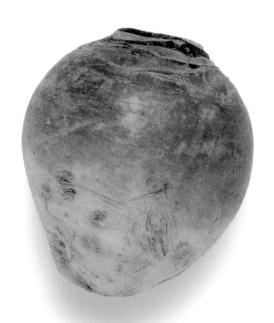

DATA FILE

Properties

• Helps guard against certain heart and circulatory diseases.
• Helps to prevent osteoporosis.
• Believed to help prevent falling hair.
• Involved in maintaining the health of bones, skin, and fingernails.

Best Sources

Found in whole grains, vegetables, hard drinking water, seafood.

Dosages

There is no official RDA, but we need 20–30mg. each day. Most of us get about 200mg. in our diet.

CAUTION
Excess silicon can cause kidney stones, but only at very high doses.

U.S. RDA none. E.U. RDA none.

V VANADIUM

Vanadium is a trace mineral that has only recently been proved necessary for human life. At the turn of the 20th century, French physicians believed that vanadium was a miracle cure for a variety of illnesses, but it proved to be toxic at the levels they were prescribing, and it became less popular.

Today, it is believed that elevated levels of vanadium may cause manic depression, which is perhaps a clue to a little-understood disease. Normal doses are thought to reduce appetite, and to reduce blood fat and cholesterol levels.

DATA FILE

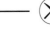

Properties
- Reduces high blood sugar by mimicking the effect of insulin on the cells.
- Prevents dental caries.
- Aids in the production of red blood cells.
- Encourages normal tissue growth and fat metabolism.
- Slows down cholesterol formation in blood vessels.
- Prevents heart disease and heart attacks.

Best Sources
Found in fish, parsley, radishes, strawberries, lettuce, cucumber.

Dosages
Vanadium supplements are not available, although some newer multivitamin and mineral supplements may contain low levels of it.

CAUTION

Vanadium is very toxic and is linked to manic depression in high quantities. Excess vitamin C can cause deficiency in some individuals.

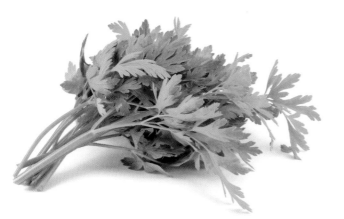

U.S. RDA 15mg. E.U. RDA 15mg.

ZN ZINC

Zinc is one of the most important trace elements in our diet, and it is required for more than 200 enzyme activities within the body. It is the principal protector of the immune system, and is crucial for regulating our genetic information. Zinc is also vital for the structure and function of cell membranes.

Zinc is an antioxidant (see page 65) and can help to detoxify the body. A zinc deficiency can cause growth failure, infertility, impotence, and, in some cases, an impaired sense of taste. Eczema is commonly linked to zinc deficiency, and new research points to the fact that postnatal illness may be attributable to insufficient zinc in the diet. A weakened immune system and a poor ability to heal may also indicate deficiency.

DATA FILE

Properties
- Boosts the immune system.
- Prevents cancer.
- Prevents and treats colds.
- Maintains senses of taste, smell, and sight.
- May help to prevent age-related degenerative effects.
- Prevents hair loss.
- Treats acne and various other skin problems.
- Useful in treatment of rheumatoid arthritis.
- Prevents blindness associated with aging.
- Increases male potency and sex drive.
- Used to treat infertility.

Best Sources
Offal, meat, mushrooms, oysters, eggs, wholegrain products, brewer's yeast.

Dosages
Take 15–30mg. daily, and increase copper and selenium intake if taking more zinc.

CAUTION

Very high doses (above 150mg. per day) may cause some nausea, vomiting, and diarrhea.

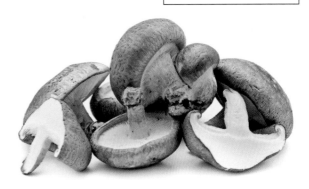

L-ARGININE

L-arginine is one of the most important and most useful of the amino acids, with a significant role to play in the function of the muscles, growth, and healing, helping to regulate and support key components of the immune system. It is also extremely important for male fertility.

For adults, L-arginine is a nonessential amino acid, which means that it is capable of being synthesized in the body and it is therefore not essential that we get additional amounts in our daily diet. For children, however, L-arginine is essential.

DATA FILE

Properties
- Boosts immunity.
- Inhibits the growth of a number of tumors.
- Builds muscle and burns fat, by stimulating the pituitary glands to increase growth hormone secretion.
- Helps to promote the healing of burns and other wounds.
- Helps to protect the liver and to detoxify harmful substances.
- Increases sperm count in men with a low count.

Best Sources
Raw cereals, chocolate, nuts.

Dosages
The optimal intake is unknown, but doses up to 1.5g. appear to be safe. Take L-arginine with lysine, which inhibits herpes attacks in carriers.

> **CAUTION**
> Take on an empty stomach, and do not take in excess. This could cause mental and metabolic disturbances, as well as nausea and diarrhea. Prolonged high doses may be dangerous to children, and to anyone with liver or kidney problems.

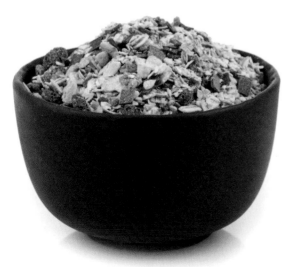

L-ASPARTIC ACID

L-aspartic acid is a nonessential amino acid which has been used for many years in the treatment of chronic fatigue. Studies confirm the efficiency of this amino acid in raising energy levels, and in helping to overcome the side-effects of drug withdrawal.

DATA FILE

Properties
- Disposes of ammonia, helping to protect the central nervous system.
- Helps treat fatigue.
- May improve stamina and endurance.

Best Sources
Oysters, meat, oat flakes, sprouting seeds, avocado, asparagus.

Dosages
Supplements are available in 250–500mg. tablets; take 3 times daily with juice or water.

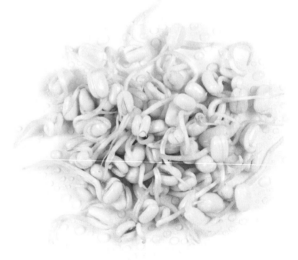

> **CAUTION**
> Do not take supplements with protein, such as milk. Do not take more than 1g. without the supervision of your physician.

W.H.O. RDA cysteine and methionone 15mg. total per kg. body weight.

L-CYSTEINE

Cysteine contains sulfur, which is said to work as an antioxidant, protecting and preserving the cells in the body. It is also believed to protect the body against pollutants, but much work has still to be done to understand the effects of this amino acid.

DATA FILE

Properties
- May protect against copper toxicity.
- Protects the body against damage by free radicals (see page 65).
- May help to reverse damage done by smoking and alcohol abuse.
- Offers protection against X-rays and nuclear radiation.
- May help to treat arthritis.
- Helps to repair DNA, thereby preventing the effects of aging.

Best Sources
Eggs, meat, dairy products, some cereals.

Dosages
Take with vitamin C for best effect (three times as much vitamin C as L-cysteine). Doses up to 1g. are considered to be safe, but consult your physician first.

> **CAUTION**
> Diabetics should not take L-cysteine supplements unless supervised by a physician. L-cysteine may also cause kidney stones, but a high vitamin C intake should prevent this from occurring.

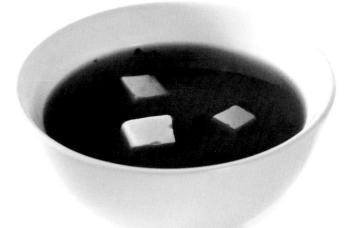

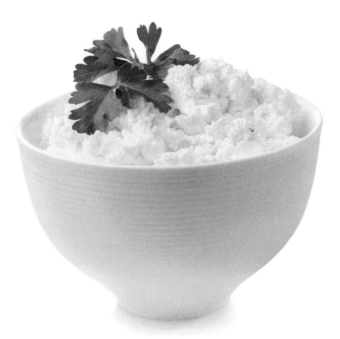

L-GLUTAMINE

L-glutamine is a derivative of glutamic acid, which is believed to help reduce cravings for alcohol. Studies are inconclusive as to the real benefits of taking this amino acid, and it is recommended that you do not take more than 1g. daily unless you are supervised by your physician.

DATA FILE

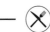

Properties
- Believed to help reduce craving for alcohol.
- May help to speed the healing of peptic ulcers.
- May help to counter attacks of depression.
- May energize the mind.
- May help to treat and prevent colitis.

Best Sources
Meat, dairy products, eggs, beans, vegetables, wheat, papaya, fermented foods such as miso.

Dosages
Up to 1g. daily is believed to be safe, but supplement only under the supervision of your physician.

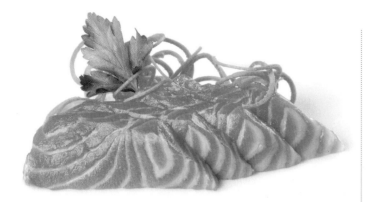

L-GLYCINE

Glycine is considered to be the simplest of the amino acids, with a variety of properties that are still being studied by scientists. It is a nonessential amino acid, which means your body can produce it on its own if not enough glycine is in your diet.

DATA FILE

Properties
- May help to treat low pituitary gland function.
- May be used in the treatment of spastic movement, particularly in patients suffering from multiple sclerosis.
- May help treat progressive muscular dystrophy.
- Used in the treatment of hypoglycemia, since it stimulates the release of glucagon, which mobilizes glycogen, which can then be released into the bloodstream as glucose.

Best Sources
Animal products, including meat, fish, poultry, and dairy.

Dosages
Doses below 1g. are thought to be safe, but research is ongoing.

CAUTION
It is recommended that you do not take this amino acid as a supplement unless supervised by your physician.

W.H.O. RDA 10mg. per kg. body weight.
L-HISTIDINE

L-histidine is one of the essential amino acids, for both adults and children. Lack of histidine may be linked with eczema in children.

DATA FILE

Properties
- Used in the treatment of arthritis sufferers, who have an abnormally low level of this amino acid in their blood.
- May boost the activity of suppressor T-cells, which could be useful in the fight against HIV/AIDS and autoimmune conditions.

Best Sources
Meat, fish, seafood, dairy, rice, wheat, rye, cauliflower, mushrooms, bananas, citrus fruits.

Dosages
Do not take more than 150mg. daily unless supervised by your physician.

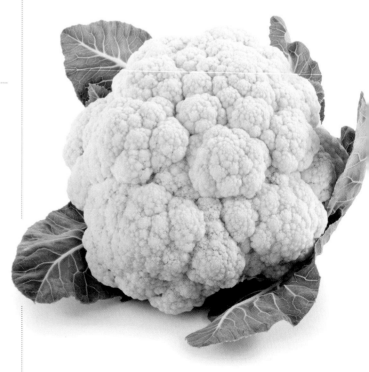

W.H.O. RDA 30mg. per kg. body weight.

L-LYSINE

L-lysine is an essential amino acid, which means that it is necessary for life. It is needed for growth, tissue repair, and for the production of antibodies, hormones, and enzymes. Lysine should be obtained from eating foods such as fish, milk, cheese, and eggs, although it is possible to purchase lysine supplements.

DATA FILE

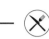

Properties
- Inhibits herpes – high doses are now believed to be effective in reducing the recurrence of outbreaks.
- May assist in building muscle mass.
- Helps to prevent fertility problems.
- Improves concentration.

Best Sources
Found in fish, milk, lima beans, meat, cheese, yeast, eggs, and all proteins.

Dosages
Up to 500mg. daily is believed to be safe. Some experts recommend 1,000mg. daily at mealtimes. It is usually advised that amino acids are taken on an empty stomach, with some juice or water. Take L-lysine with an equal quantity of arginine if an increase in muscle mass is the desired goal.

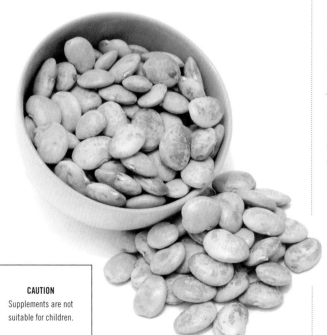

> **CAUTION**
> Supplements are not suitable for children.

W.H.O. RDA cysteine and methionine 15mg. total per kg. body weight.

L-METHIONINE

Methionine is a sulfur-containing amino acid that is very important in numerous processes in the body. Research shows that it may help to prevent clogging of the arteries by eliminating fatty substances.

DATA FILE

Properties
- May help to eliminate fatty substances from the blood, lowering the risk of heart attack.
- May help to regulate the nervous system.
- In conjunction with choline and folic acid, it may prevent some tumors.
- Necessary for the biosynthesis of taurine and cysteine.

Best Sources
Eggs, milk, liver, fish, sesame seeds.

Dosages
It is best to obtain this amino acid through a healthy, balanced diet.

> **CAUTION**
> Supplementation is not advised, although some physicians may suggest it in specific circumstances.

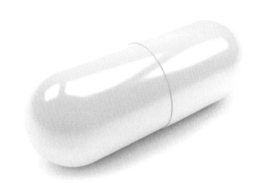

DL-PHENYLALANINE (DLPA)

DLPA is a form of the amino acid phenylalanine created from equal parts of D (synthetic) phenylalanine and L (natural) phenylalanine. DLPA has a unique role of activating and producing endorphins, which are the body's natural painkillers. Many people who do not respond to conventional painkillers respond successfully to DLPA, and its painkilling action increases over time. Do not confuse DLPA with L-phenylalanine.

DATA FILE

Properties
• A natural painkiller, useful for chronic pain and conditions like migraine, neuralgia, and leg cramps.
• Antidepressant.

Dosages
Tablets are generally available in 375mg. doses, and can be taken up to six times daily (a maximum dose of 1.5g.). Higher doses should only be taken under the supervision of your physician. Take two or three times daily, before meals.

> **CAUTION**
> Not suitable for pregnant women or for those who suffer from phenylketonuria (PKU). DLPA may elevate blood pressure, so check with your physician if you suffer from any circulatory disorder.

W.H.O. RDA phenylalanine and tyrosine 25mg. total per kg. body weight.

L-PHENYLALANINE

L-phenylalanine is an essential amino acid that is necessary for a number of biochemical processes, including the synthesis of neurotransmitters in the brain. It is said to promote sexual arousal and to release hormones that help to control appetite.

DATA FILE

Properties
• May help to alleviate a bout of depression.
• May help to control addictive behavior.
• Encourages mental alertness.
• Promotes sexual arousal.
• Reduces hunger and cravings for food.

Best Sources
Proteins, cheese, almonds, peanuts, sesame seeds, and soybeans.

Dosages
L-phenylalanine is usually available in 500mg. doses. Take on an empty stomach for best effect, and do not take with protein.

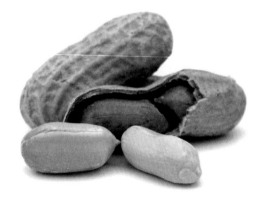

> **CAUTION**
> If you suffer from skin cancer, do not take L-phenylalanine. People with high blood pressure should only take supplementary L-phenylalanine under the supervision of their physician. Not suitable for use with MAOI antidepressants. Pregnant women should not take this amino acid.

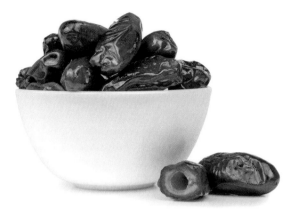

W.H.O. RDA 4mg. per kg. body weight.

L-TRYPTOPHAN

This essential amino acid is used by the brain, along with several vitamins and minerals, to produce serotonin, a neurotransmitter. Serotonin, which regulates and induces sleep, is also said to reduce sensitivity to pain. It was one of the first amino acids to be produced for sale as a supplement, and it is useful as a natural sleeping aid.

DATA FILE

Properties
• May help to encourage sleep and to prevent jet lag.
• Reduces sensitivity to pain.
• Lessens a craving for alcohol.
• Natural antidepressant, and may help to reduce anxiety and panic attacks.

Best Sources
Chocolate, dried dates, cottage cheese, milk, meat, fish, turkey, bananas, and other protein sources.

Dosages
Used to prevent panic attacks and depression, L-tryptophan should be taken between meals with juice or water (no proteins). To help induce sleep, take 500mg. along with vitamin B6, niacinamide, and magnesium an hour or so before bedtime.

> **CAUTION**
> There is some evidence that L-tryptophan may cause liver problems in high doses, and although studies vary, it is now believed that it can be toxic in very high doses. Take only on the advice of your physician.

W.H.O. RDA phenylalanine and tyrosine 25mg. total per kg. body weight.

L-TYROSINE

L-tyrosine is not an essential amino acid, which means that it is synthesized in the body, from phenylalanine. Tyrosine is involved with important neurotransmitters in the brain, and it is said to energize and help to relieve the effects of stress.

DATA FILE

Properties
• Helps to relieve stress, and encourages alertness and fewer physical symptoms of tension and stress.
• May act as an antidepressant.
• May be used to treat the emotional symptoms of premenstrual syndrome.
• May help to aid in the treatment of addiction to and withdrawal from cocaine and other addictive drugs.

Best Sources
Chicken, turkey, fish, dairy products, peanuts, almonds, pumpkin seeds, sesame seeds, soybeans, lima beans, avocados, bananas.

Dosages
Take supplements with juice or water on an empty stomach (do not take with proteins, such as milk). Some experts suggest that it is more effective when taken in conjunction with up to 25mg. of vitamin B6.

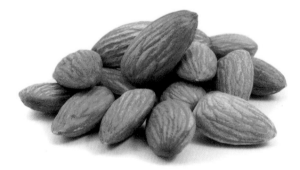

> **CAUTION**
> Do not take tyrosine supplements if you suffer from migraine headaches, or if you take MAOI antidepressants. People suffering from high blood pressure or skin cancer should not take supplementary tyrosine without the approval of a physician.

BEE AND FLOWER POLLEN

In flowering plants, the pollen-producing spores are located in the stamens of flowers. Flower pollen is said to be purer than bee pollen. Bee pollen is found in the hives themselves. It is rich in protein and amino acids, and forms, with honey, the basic diet of all the bees in the hive, except for the queen (see Royal Jelly, page 234). Pollen has been used as medicine around the world for thousands of years.

DATA FILE

Properties
- Rich in both amino acids and protein.
- Helps to suppress appetite and cravings.
- May help to improve skin problems and retard the aging process.
- May help to treat problems of the prostate.
- Energizes the body.
- Regulates the bowels.
- May boost immunity and diminish allergies.

Best Sources
Unpasteurized honey contains small amounts of bee pollen.

Dosages
Taken daily, 400mg. doses appear to be safe. Take pollen with food.

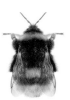

> **CAUTION**
> If you suffer from hay fever or an allergy to bee stings, you may suffer a reaction to bee pollen. See your physician or practitioner before taking this supplement.

BIOFLAVONOIDS

Bioflavonoids were originally called vitamin P, and are also known as flavones. They accompany vitamin C in natural foods, and are responsible for the color in the leaves, flowers, and stems of food plants. Their primary job in the body is to protect the capillaries, to keep them strong, and to prevent bleeding. Bioflavonoids are also anti-inflammatory. Many of the medicinally active substances contained in herbs are bioflavonoids.

DATA FILE

Properties
- Reduces bruising in susceptible individuals.
- Protects capillaries.
- Protects against cerebral and other hemorrhaging.
- Reduces bleeding during menstruation.
- Antioxidant (see page 65), and encourages the antioxidant qualities of vitamin C.
- Antiviral, anti-inflammatory, and antiallergy.
- May help to cure colds.

Best Sources
Citrus fruits, apricots, cherries, green peppers, broccoli, lemons. The central white core of citrus fruits is the richest source.

Dosages
Bioflavonoids are not toxic, and should be taken together with vitamin C for best effect.

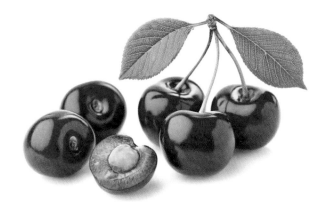

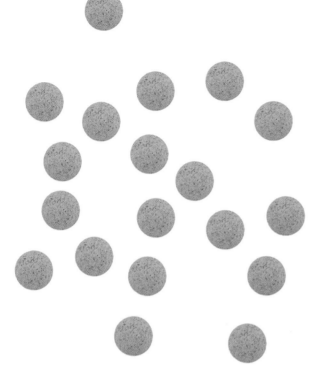

BREWER'S YEAST

Brewer's yeast is the same type of yeast that is used in the brewing process, and is quite different from the yeast that causes thrush. It is a rich source of B vitamins and amino acids, as well as some minerals, in particular chromium and selenium. It also contains naturally occurring nucleic acids, which are said to enhance the immune system.

DATA FILE

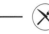

Properties
- May reduce wrinkling and help treat skin problems.
- Works as an effective wound-healing agent.
- Encourages the healing of burns.
- Rich source of B vitamins, which can help to relieve stress and nervous disorders.
- Encourages the activity of the immune system.
- Increases energy.
- Used externally, to detoxify skin.

Best Sources
Brewer's yeast is most commonly taken in its powdered form, but it is also found in Vegemite and Marmite.

Dosages
Brewer's yeast comes in tablets, or as a powder that can be sprinkled on food or drink.

CAUTION
Brewer's yeast is not toxic and can be taken daily without any side-effects. Some experts suggest that it may cause yeast infections and chronic fatigue syndrome, but this has largely been disclaimed.

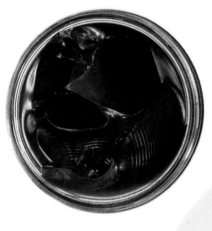

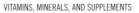

CHARCOAL

Charcoal is a porous, solid product obtained when materials such as cellulose, wood, peat, bituminous coal, or bone are partially burned in the absence of air. Charcoal has always been popular for dealing with flatulence, bloating, and irritable bowel syndrome, by soaking up gas. Charcoal can also be useful in the long-term management of kidney patients.

In homeopathy, charcoal from beech, poplar, and silver birch trees are the ingredients for the remedy Carb. veg., which is used to treat fatigue, poor circulation, and digestive problems, such as indigestion and flatulence.

DATA FILE

Properties
- Reduces cholesterol in the blood.
- Reduces the risk of atherosclerosis.
- Absorbs gas and so acts as an antacid.
- Binds with cholesterol, toxins, and waste in the intestine, which has a cleansing effect.

Best Sources
Charcoal is available in tablet, powder, and capsule form.

Dosages
High doses (more than 50g. per day) should be supplemented with a well-balanced vitamin and mineral supplement. For dosages of the homeopathic remedy Carb. veg., consult a registered practitioner.

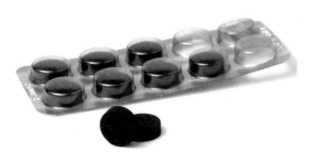

CAUTION
Activated charcoal can bind with and inactivate some therapeutic drugs and supplemental nutrients, and should be taken at least one hour before or after drugs or supplements are taken. If you are on prescription drugs, take charcoal only with your physician's advice.

CO-ENZYME Q10

Co-enzyme Q10 is a vitamin-like substance found in all cells of the body. It is biologically important, since it forms part of the system across which electrons flow in the cells during the process of energy production. When there is a Q10 deficiency, the cell cannot function effectively, and the rate at which the muscle cells work is adversely affected.

DATA FILE

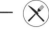

Properties
- Enhances immunity.
- Improves the heart-muscle metabolism.
- May help to prevent coronary inefficiency and heart failure.
- Anti-aging.
- Important for the efficient functioning of muscle cells.
- Necessary for healthy functioning of the nervous system and the brain cells.

Best Sources
Meat (it is also made within the body).

Dosages
Taken as a supplement 3 times a day, 10mg. has a therapeutic effect within the body.

CAUTION
Co-enzyme Q10 is fat soluble, and therefore may be toxic in high doses.

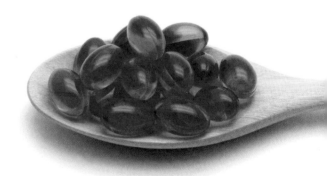

EVENING PRIMROSE (GLA)

Native Americans were the first to recognize the potential of evening primrose oil as a healer, and they decocted (boiled) the seeds to make a liquid for healing wounds. Evening primrose oil is a rich source of gamma-linoleic acid, which is better known as GLA. The body makes GLA from essential fatty acids (EFAs). EFAs have numerous functions in the body, one of which is to manufacture hormone-like substances called "prostaglandins," which have very important effects on the body, such as toning blood vessels, balancing our water levels, and improving the action of the digestive system, and brain functioning. Prostaglandins also have a beneficial effect on the immune system.

DATA FILE

Properties
- Reduces scaling and redness, prevents itching, and encourages healing in cases of eczema. Also used in the treatment of psoriasis.
- Discourages dry skin, and ensures that the cellular membranes that make up the skin are stable and strong. There is some evidence that the oil retards the aging process.
- May help to prevent multiple sclerosis, and appears to be particularly useful for children suffering from the condition.
- May help in cases of liver damage caused by alcohol (cirrhosis of the liver), hyperactivity in children, and cystic fibrosis.
- May have a stimulating effect on the body, encouraging it to convert fat into energy, which would make it an excellent treatment for obesity.
- Hormonal imbalances, perhaps causing conditions like premenstrual syndrome, and symptoms of the menopause, may be eased by evening primrose oil, reducing bloating, water retention, irritability, and depression.
- Reduces the inflammation of rheumatoid arthritis.
- May have an immunosuppressive effect on the body.

Best Sources
Evening primrose oil is most often taken in the form of capsules, but it is also available as an oil (sometimes flavored), and it can be applied to the skin to treat skin conditions.

Dosages
Take 500mg. each day for two months, and then for the 10 days preceding menstruation if you suffer from premenstrual syndrome. During the menopause, 2,000–4,000mg. should be taken daily for four weeks, and then 500–1,000mg. daily thereafter.

For asthma, take two 500mg. tablets three times daily for three to four months; then one tablet three times daily. If you are taking steroids, this treatment will not work because steroids interfere with evening primrose oil's action.

> **CAUTION**
> Do not use if you suffer from temporal-lobe epilepsy or manic depression.

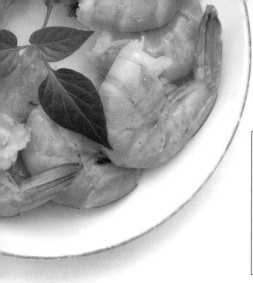

INOSITOL

Inositol is not a true vitamin, as it can be synthesized by the body, but it forms part of the B-complex family of vitamins, and is present in cereals and vegetables as phytic acid. There is a high concentration in the brain, stomach, spleen, liver, and heart.

DATA FILE

Properties
- Helps to dissolve fat.
- May help to prevent anxiety and tension.
- Ensures healthy hair and strong nails.
- Controls levels of cholesterol in the blood.
- Helps to encourage natural sleep.
- May help to treat schizophrenia and other nervous disorders.

Best Sources
Liver, wheat germ, brown rice, citrus fruits, nuts, cereals.

Dosages
Natural sources are best, but if you are prescribed supplements, take in the form of myo-inositol to a maximum of 1,000mg. daily.

> **CAUTION**
> Fish oils may be harmful in diabetics, causing increases in blood sugar and a decline in insulin secretion.

FISH OILS

Fish oils contain two long-chain fatty acids called eicosopentaenoic acid (EPA) and docosahexaenoic acid (DHA) that affect the synthesis of prostaglandins, which have a regulatory effect on the body. There are numerous claims for fish oils, which are now believed to improve overall health and treat many health conditions.

DATA FILE

Properties
- May be useful in the treatment of kidney disease, and can counteract the effects of some immunosuppressive drugs.
- May help to prevent cancer, in particular the onset of breast cancer.
- Stops progression of arthritis symptoms.
- May help to protect against high blood pressure.
- Helps to prevent cardiovascular disease.
- May help to prevent and treat psoriasis.

Best Sources
Fish, in particular herring, salmon, tuna, cod, prawns.

Dosages
People suffering from arthritis or psoriasis can take up to 4g. daily, but for most people it is more appropriate to increase your intake of fish and seafood in order to achieve the benefits of the fish oils in their natural form. The maximum suggested dosage for supplements, taken without the supervision of your physician, is 900mg. per day.

> **CAUTION**
> Diabetics should only take inositol under the supervision of their physician.

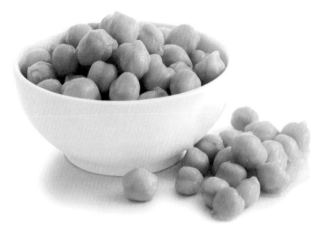
LECITHIN

Lecithin has for some time been a popular supplement, used for a variety of health conditions. It is comprised of choline, inositol, fatty acids, and phosphorus, and is available as a liquid or as dry granules. It is widely used in foods to maintain consistency, and is probably one of the few nutritious food additives.

DATA FILE

Properties
- Protects against cardiovascular disease.
- Helps to reduce high blood pressure.
- Used to treat memory loss and conditions of the nervous system such as dementia and Alzheimer's.
- May help in the treatment of mental disorders such as bipolar disorder.
- Lecithin has some action against viruses.
- May prevent and also treat gallstones.
- May help to treat viral hepatitis, repairing the membranes of the liver cells.

Best Sources
Found in egg yolks, soybeans, chickpeas, liver, meats, fish, cauliflower, cabbage.

Dosages
Doses of up to 1g. daily are acceptable, but see your physician to discuss your individual needs. Lecithin appears in a wide range of foods, and it is probably best to increase your intake of these rather than supplementing.

PROPOLIS

Propolis is a sticky material collected by bees from buds or tree bark and used to seal the inside of the hive. It is a mixture of wax, resin, balsam oil, and pollen. It is said to act as an antibiotic and bactericide, and may be used to help wounds to heal. Propolis is rich in bioflavonoids.

DATA FILE

Properties
- Enhances immunity.
- Helps wounds to heal.
- Boosts energy.
- Naturally anesthetic and antibiotic.
- Reduces cholesterol levels in the blood.
- Helps to reduce the incidence and duration of colds.

Best Sources
Propolis is available in tablet and liquid form.

Dosages
Propolis does not appear to have any toxic levels, but see your practitioner for details of suitable dosage.

CAUTION

Because this product contains pollen, it may cause an allergic reaction in susceptible individuals.

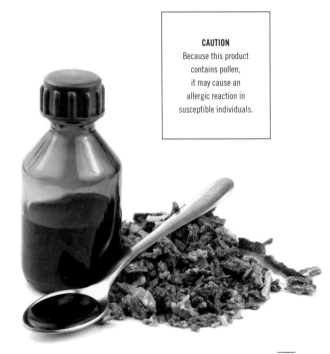

ROYAL JELLY

Royal jelly has been used for centuries for its health-giving and rejuvenating properties, and it is rich in vitamins, amino acids, and minerals. It is also the prime source of fatty acid, which is said to increase alertness and act as a natural tranquilizer (when necessary). Royal jelly is secreted by the salivary glands of the worker bees to feed and stimulate the growth and development of the queen bee.

DATA FILE

Properties

- Antibacterial.
- May prevent the development of leukemia.
- Has a yeast-inhibiting function, preventing conditions such as thrush and athlete's foot.
- Contains the male sex hormone testosterone, which may increase libido.
- Used to treat subfertility.
- May be useful in the treatment of myalgic encephalomyelitis (ME) and muscular dystrophy.
- Helps to reduce allergies.
- Boosts the body's resistance to the harmful side-effects of chemotherapy and radiotherapy.
- Controls cholesterol levels.
- Boosts the immune system.
- Treats skin problems, including eczema, psoriasis, and acne.
- Combined with pantothenic acid, royal jelly provides relief from the symptoms of arthritis.

Best Sources

Fresh royal jelly is better, although more expensive than tablets.

Dosages

Most tablets contain 100–500mg. of royal jelly. Optimum dosage is about 150mg. per day.

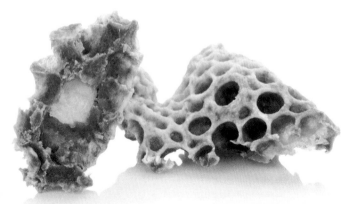

SEAWEEDS

Seaweeds are not plants, but part of the Protista kingdom. They are better known as "algae," and there are four main types. Seaweeds appear in many foods, medicines, and cosmetics, and have been used therapeutically for thousands of years. Seaweeds are an excellent source of protein and also the richest natural source of iodine, which makes them useful in the treatment of goiter.

DATA FILE

Properties

- Antiviral activity.
- May prevent cancer.
- Used in the prevention and treatment of goiter.
- May help to reduce the effects of carcinogens, as well as radioactive material.
- Helps to counter the side-effects of radiotherapy and chemotherapy treatment.
- Naturally antacid.
- Used in the treatment of intestinal disorders.
- Used in the treatment of exudative wounds.

Best Sources

Take seaweeds in their natural form, available from health food stores and many grocery stores (particularly oriental food stores).

Dosages

There is no recommended dosage for supplements, so consult a registered practitioner.

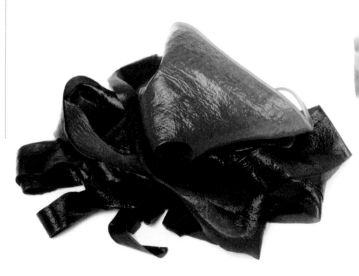

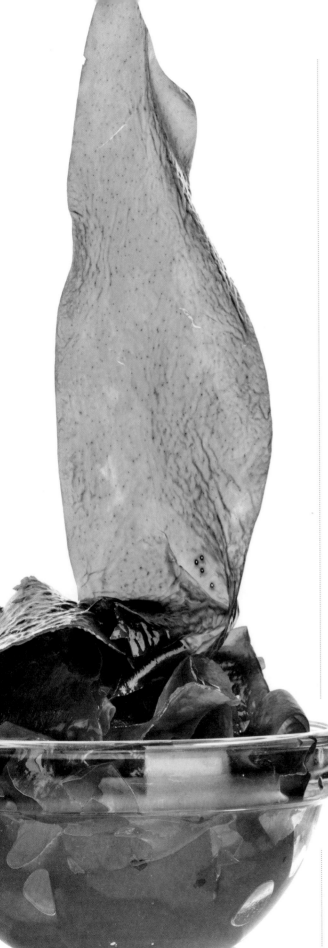

SPIRULINA

Spirulina are blue-green bacteria or algae, which are rich in GLA (gamma-linoleic acid; see page 231) and a wide variety of nutrients, including beta-carotene, inositol, calcium, vitamin E, magnesium, and phosphorus. In ancient times, spirulina was used as a staple food by the Aztecs of Mexico. It is now marketed in health food stores as a high-protein food supplement.

DATA FILE

Properties

- Rich in nutrients and high in protein (particularly useful for vegetarians).
- May suppress appetite.
- Maintains skin health, keeping it blemish-free, and treats skin disorders.
- May contribute to healthy functioning of the intestines.
- General tonic properties.
- May be rejuvenating.
- Many spirulina have anti-cancer properties.

Best Sources

Fresh or freeze-dried spirulina.

Dosages

There is no recommended dosage for spirulina, so consult a registered practitioner.

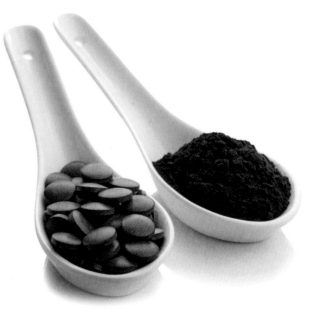

TREATING COMMON AILMENTS

CHAPTER THREE

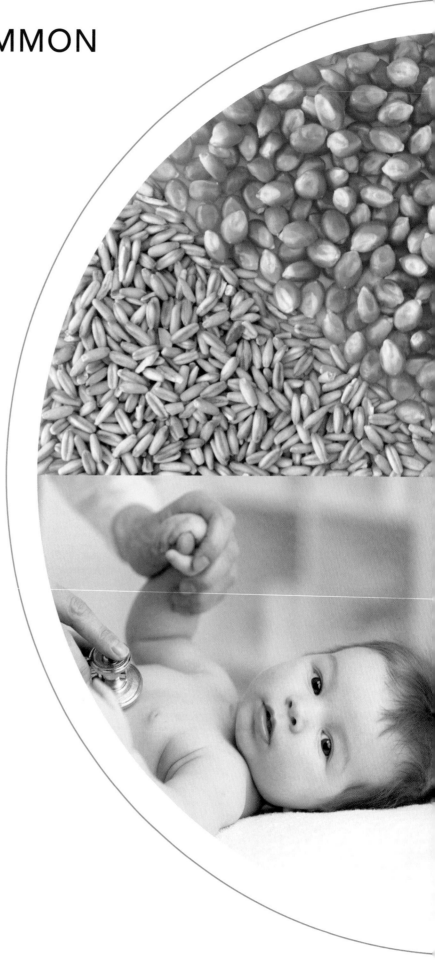

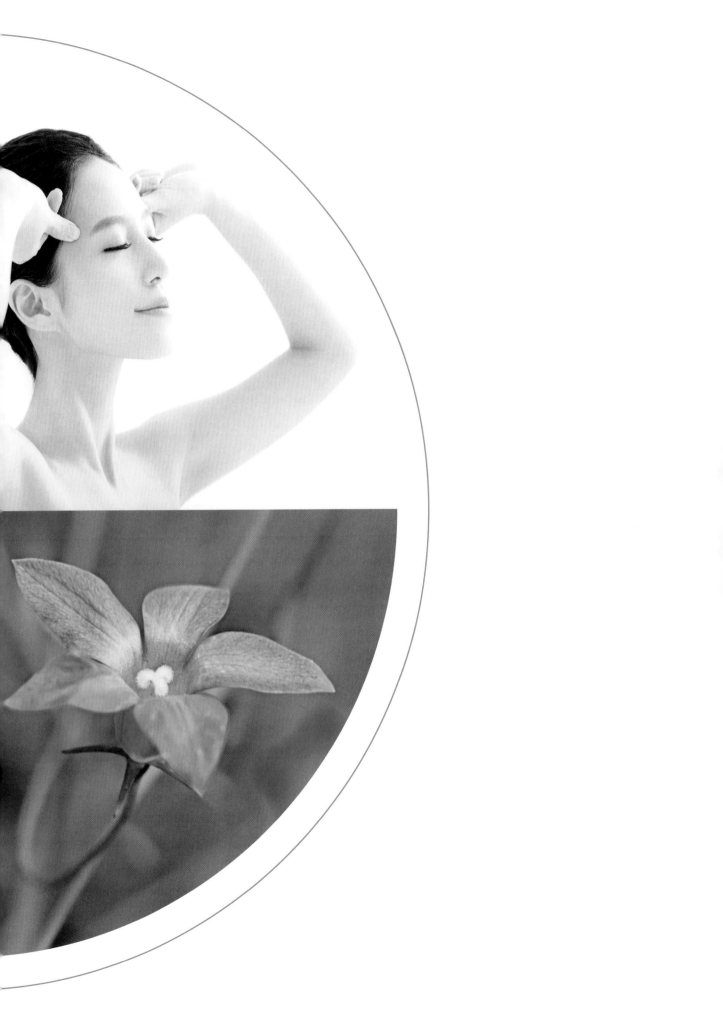

A GUIDE TO TREATMENT

Before using healing remedies, you first need to know the ailment or health condition you are treating. While some ailments might be obvious from the outset, such as a cough, feeling nauseous, or having a small cut on your arm, others can be harder to identify. As keen as you may be to treat everything yourself, it is important to recognize when you need to seek the advice of a trained and qualified medical practitioner for an accurate diagnosis.

HOW TO DIAGNOSE MINOR AILMENTS
—

Some health conditions are relatively easy to identify. Symptoms such as sneezing and coughing may be due to a cold, particularly if you know germs are going around or you have been in recent contact with someone else who has a cold. The sudden appearance of a rash or hives (urticaria) might be linked to an allergy you already know you have. If you come up in bruises when you know you knocked your leg recently, then that is likely to be the cause.

Sometimes your ailment might not be instantly obvious, or could be caused by one or more factors. Before you rush in and assume you know what the cause must be, it helps to carefully consider all your symptoms. This will help you make a more discerning diagnosis and reduce the risk of your treating an ailment with the wrong remedy.

When making an assessment and diagnosing your minor ailments, it helps to consider factors such as:

• What symptoms you have
• When your symptoms started
• If anything makes your symptoms better
• If anything makes your symptoms worse
• What conditions you have had in the past
• How you are feeling
• If your symptoms could be linked to anything you have done, eaten, or experienced recently
• Any medication or herbal remedies you are currently taking
• Any allergies you have.

These are the types of questions a health practitioner will ask you when you go to see them, so they are a good starting point for you to think about.

Some forms of healing therapies, such as traditional Chinese medicine (TCM), also look at the state of your tongue and your pulse rate to help with diagnosing ailments, but without professional training, these observations are unlikely to offer you much assistance for diagnosing minor ailments.

If you are at all unsure about your personal diagnosis, or if your healing remedies do not have any effect, always go to consult a qualified medical practitioner.

WHEN TO SEE A QUALIFIED MEDICAL PRACTITIONER
—

As good as natural medicine is for many minor ailments, there are times when you should see a qualified medical practitioner for advice and treatment.

If you have any concerns about your baby's health, take them for a check-up with a qualified medical practitioner.

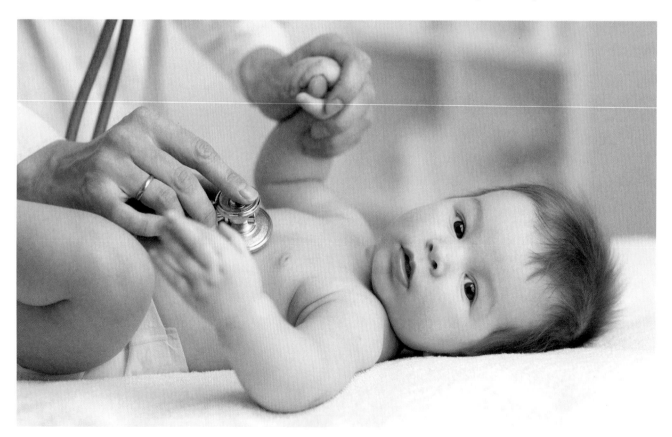

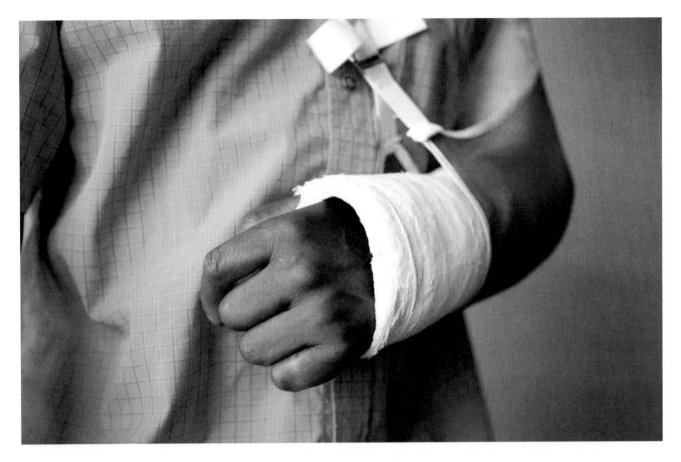

Some health symptoms can be signs of underlying illness and getting a diagnosis as soon as possible can often be crucial for treatment.

Other symptoms might be linked to existing medical conditions, or even caused by prescription medicines that you are taking, so a proper medical review is helpful.

Some situations require medical treatment immediately. Examples of when to call the emergency medical services include if someone:

- Loses consciousness, or is suddenly confused
- Has persistent chest pain
- Has seizures (fits) that do not stop
- Has difficulty breathing
- Has severe bleeding that cannot be stopped
- Has a severe allergic reaction
- Has severe burns or scalds.

There are many other symptoms where it is important to be assessed by a medical practitioner, rather than trying to diagnose or treat them yourself. These include:

- A temperature or fever of 100.4°F (38°C) or above
- Coughing up blood
- A cough or hoarse voice that lasts for more than three weeks
- Severe pain that is increasing
- Unusual bruising for no apparent reason
- A severe headache or migraine that has lasted longer than 24 hours
- Blood in your stools
- Blood in your urine
- A rash that is worsening and spreading
- A rash that does not fade when you press a glass on it
- Sore, broken skin that has become red, inflamed, and oozing
- A mole that suddenly changes color, shape, or size or starts bleeding
- Diarrhea that lasts for three days or more
- Drowsiness or confusion
- Feeling generally unwell for no apparent reason
- Losing weight without trying
- Finding a new lump or bump somewhere on your body.

Seek advice from a qualified medical practitioner if you have been involved in an accident or you suspect broken bones.

Other situations where you should seek medical assistance include:

- If you have been involved in an accident
- If you have had a blow to the head
- If you think you could have broken bones
- If you have a large or deep burn, if a burn is very blistered and painful, or if the burn is on your hands or face
- If you have been bitten by a person or an animal.

These lists do not cover every important symptom. If you feel unwell, or have any concerns about a medical condition, always see a health practitioner for advice. Even if it is a false alarm and nothing serious, it will offer reassurance that nothing major is wrong. Extra care should be taken with babies, children, the elderly, and pregnant women. Your family's health is important, so do not put yourself or others at risk by trying to diagnose or treat symptoms you do not fully understand.

USING NATURAL REMEDIES SAFELY

WHETHER TO SELF-TREAT
—

Herbal remedies are often regarded as natural and safe because they are derived from plants. However, in the same way that orthodox prescription medications and drugs can have side-effects, so too can herbal remedies, especially if taken at the same time as certain prescription medications. Healing plants and other natural remedies can be powerful and need to be treated with respect – both in terms of knowing how and when you use them, and when not to use them.

For minor ailments and easily identifiable health concerns, treating yourself with natural healing remedies may make sense.

If you are at all unsure what health ailment you are dealing with, or whether or not a particular remedy is suitable, it is best to be cautious and not try to treat it yourself. Herbal remedies can be powerful and it is not worth putting yourself or anyone else at risk.

There are also particular groups of people and various circumstances in which you need to take particular care and not try to self-treat.

**IF YOU ARE PREGNANT
OR BREASTFEEDING**
—

In the same way that a lot of prescription medications are not advised to be used while you are pregnant or breastfeeding, so too are natural healing remedies. During pregnancy, not only is your body going through huge changes, but you are also carrying your unborn baby. Although there might be times when you are tempted to try natural remedies to ease pregnancy ailments, it is best to err on the side of caution and avoid using anything without first checking with the medical team looking after your pregnancy. In addition, always tell the medical team about any herbal remedies you have been taking.

Consuming black cohosh (*Actaea racemosa*) can put pregnant women at risk of premature labor.

The effects of using certain herbal remedies during pregnancy could be major. Angelica, for example, may cause womb contractions, while using black cohosh can put you at risk from premature labor.

The same note of caution applies when you are in labor, too. Herbal remedies could potentially interact with any drugs given to you to help you during birth. Plus certain herbal remedies are linked to blood thinning, which could pose problems if you need a cesarean section and put you at risk of extra bleeding.

When your baby has arrived and you are breastfeeding, it is wise to continue avoiding herbal remedies for a while, unless your medical team says it is safe, as what you consume can be passed on to your baby through your milk.

BABIES AND CHILDREN
—

Babies and children can react differently to natural remedies than adults, due to their size and age. Remedies that may be safe for adults are not always suitable for use at all in infants and children, so it is best not to give them any herbal remedies without expert advice and checking with a medical practitioner.

THE ELDERLY
—

As people get older, the way the body works naturally undergoes changes, and the risk of experiencing side-effects due to taking medication – both herbal remedies, prescribed, and over-the-counter medication – increases.

The kidneys become less able to excrete medication into urine and the liver is not able to break down, or metabolize, medications in the way it used to. Due to this, any medications taken may remain in the body for longer and affect people in different ways.

Always consult a medical practitioner before taking a herbal remedy, especially if you are on any other drugs.

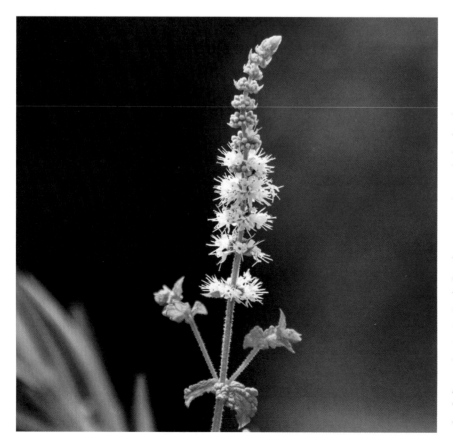

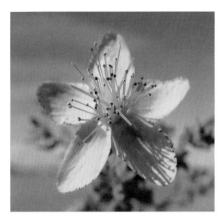

Although widely used, St. John's wort (*Hypericum perforatum*) can cause side-effects when taken alongside prescription medications.

IF YOU ARE TAKING
OTHER MEDICATIONS
—

If you are already taking any over-the-counter or prescribed medications, check first with a medical practitioner or pharmacist before taking any herbal or natural remedies. Some ingredients can react badly with conventional medications, affecting their effectiveness and causing unexpected side-effects.

For example, taking the herbal medicine St. John's wort, which is often used for low moods, can cause side-effects if you are also taking various prescribed medicines, including medication for depression.

Even a seemingly innocuous ingredient such as grapefruit can react with certain prescription medications. Grapefruit contains a chemical called furanocoumarin, which can affect drug metabolism, or the amount of time it takes for a medication to be broken down by the body. As a result, if you have grapefruit, or grapefruit juice, while taking some medications it can cause more of the active drug to be present in your body, leading to some very unpleasant and potentially serious side-effects.

IF YOU ARE HAVING SURGERY
—

If you have got a planned surgical operation coming up, it is important to inform your medical practitioner in advance if you are taking any herbal medicines. They may need you to stop taking the medicines in the weeks leading up to your operation.

Some herbal medicines can affect anesthetics and other medications used before, during, and after operations. Others can interfere with your blood clotting and blood pressure, and could increase your risk of experiencing bleeding during or after you have had surgery.

IF YOU ARE HAVING
TREATMENT FOR CANCER
—

Natural remedies, especially herbal medicine, can interact with conventional cancer treatments, such as radiotherapy, chemotherapy, biological therapy, or hormone treatment. They may make certain cancer drugs less effective or increase the risk of suffering from side-effects. There is still a lot to be learnt about the interaction between cancer treatments and natural remedies, so before using any type of healing remedy, talk to your medical practitioner or cancer doctor first.

People with cancer should avoid deep massage. Massage techniques may need to be adapted if you are having cancer treatment, and avoid massage on any areas of the body where you are receiving radiotherapy. Always talk to your doctor or specialist nurse before massage.

Valerian (*Valeriana officinalis*) is one of many herbal remedies that should not be used in conjunction with anesthetics.

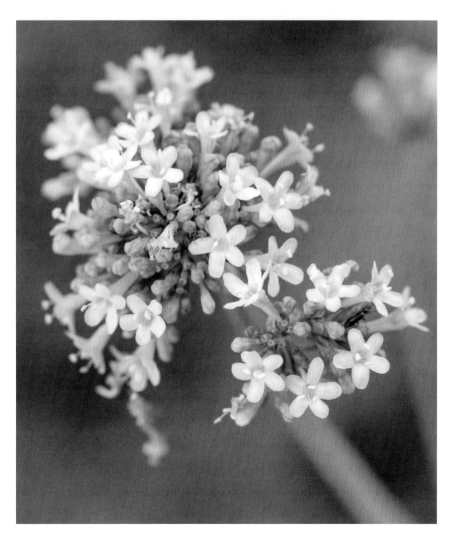

DISORDERS OF THE MIND AND EMOTIONS
ADDICTIONS

An addiction is an overwhelming craving for or dependence on a substance, usually a drug, alcohol, or nicotine. The addiction may be limited to mental dependence, but it can become physiological if the way in which the body functions has changed through prolonged use of a substance. In such cases the addict will experience physical "withdrawal" symptoms without the substance in question.

SYMPTOMS
In drug addiction:
• Loss of control over use of the drug or other substance
• Mood swings and irrational behavior • Sore or red eyes with dilated or constricted pupils • Irregular breathing • Trembling hands • Itchy or runny nose • Nausea
In drug withdrawal:
• Craving • Depression • Restlessness • Yawning • Sweating
• Abdominal pain • Vomiting • Diarrhea • Loss of appetite
• Gooseflesh

TREATMENT
Ayurveda
This has proved very successful in treating addictions of all types, which it sees as fundamental imbalance within the body. Treatment will be tailored to your specific constitution and personal characteristics. (See page 20.)

Chinese Herbalism
For alcoholism, heat would be cleared from the lung and liver, with Xi Gua (watermelon) or Ge Gen (kudzu vine) to detoxify blood. Strong green tea is used to cool the liver. (See page 94.)

Herbalism
To calm the nervous system and reduce symptoms during withdrawal, take skullcap and valerian daily as a tea. (See pages 181 and 195.) Cramp bark helps nervous tension and jitters. (See page 197.)

Aromatherapy
Antidepressant oils include chamomile, clary sage, and ylang ylang. Use in the bath, and in a vaporizer by your bedside. (See page 47.) Try massage with detoxifying oils such as juniper. (See page 142.) Bergamot is extremely useful in cases of food addiction. (See page 107 Aromatherapists suggest changing oils at regular intervals, so you do not come to regard a particular oil as a prop.

Flower Essences
Crab apple, for anyone who needs purification. (See page 148.) Gorse, when you are stuck in a negative pattern. (See page 192.)

Nutrition
Treatment would ensure that deficiencies caused by addictions (such as vitamin B in alcoholics) are righted. Alcoholics are often deficient in GLA (gamma-linolenic acid), and it is recommended that you take evening primrose (a rich source) to help prevent mood swings. (See page 231.)

Mind–Body Healing
Meditation, massage, and yoga can help maintain a positive mental attitude. Talking or art therapies may form part of an ongoing treatment program. (See pages 68–71.)

> **CAUTION**
> Addictions to physical substances should always be treated by a registered practitioner. Do not discontinue any prescription drugs unless you are under supervision.

Massage with detoxifying oils such as juniper can help both body and mind.

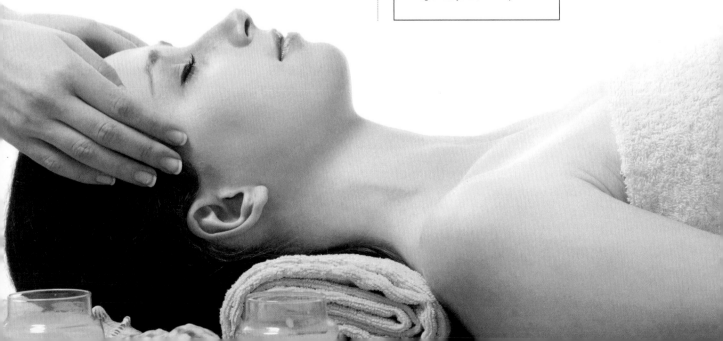

OBSESSIONS AND COMPULSIONS

An obsession is a persistent, recurring thought or idea, while a compulsion is an overwhelming drive to perform a particular act. When a person becomes dominated by these intrusions, despite knowing that they are irrational, he or she is said to be suffering from an obsessive-compulsive disorder. This may take the form of a hand-washing ritual, for example, or repeated checking that doors and windows are locked. The problem is often triggered by a stressful life event, but can also be due to subtle brain damage (usually the result of illnesses affecting the brain), especially when due to encephalitis. Obsessive-compulsive disorder is rare, although minor obsessional symptoms probably occur in about 15 percent of the population. At least two-thirds of all people who have obsessive-compulsive disorder respond well to therapy. Symptoms may recur under stress but can usually be controlled.

SYMPTOMS
- Fear of contamination • Dermatitis caused by repeated washing
- Inefficiency caused by repeated and meticulous checking
- Aggressive thoughts and behavior • Possible depression

TREATMENT

Herbalism
Drink certain infused herbs which act on the nervous system, including hops (*Humulus lupulus*), valerian, vervain, chamomile, and passiflora (*Passiflora incarnata*). Taken on a regular basis, these herbs may help to ease tension and restrict various behavioral problems. (See pages 149, 195, and 196.)

Aromatherapy
Relaxing oils, such as Roman chamomile or marjoram, may help to achieve balance. Use regularly in the bath or on a burner in your room. (See pages 149 and 157.)
Ylang ylang and clary sage may also help. (See pages 95 and 178.)

Homeopathy
Aurum is useful for feelings of worthlessness and overwhelming thoughts of death and dying.
Silicea for unshakable feelings of inadequacy, and an overwhelming urge to count small objects. (See page 220.)
Take Anacardium when you feel that your mind is not your own and is being controlled by an external force. (See page 182.)

Flower Essences
Cherry plum, for the fear of losing your mind, and to deal with irrational thoughts or behavior. (See page 170.)
Crab apple, for those who feel unclean on any level. (See page 148.)
Vervain, for those who need space for reflection. (See page 196.)
White chestnut, for an overactive mind, full of unwanted patterns of thought. (See page 76.)

Nutrition
Ensure you have a well-balanced diet, including plenty of nutritious and calming foods, such as wholegrain oats. (See page 89.)

Mind–Body Healing
To ease stress and help to calm an overactive mind, consider relaxation therapies such as meditation and breathing techniques. (See pages 68–69.)
For obsessive-compulsive disorder, contact your physician to be referred to a specially trained therapist, who may use techniques such as cognitive behavioral therapy. (See page 69.)

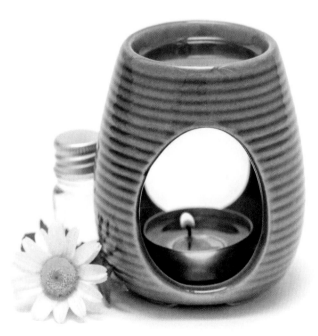

Add Roman chamomile oil to a burner or your bath.

PHOBIAS

A phobia is an irrational fear that the sufferer finds impossible to overcome. Some of the most common fears are claustrophobia (fear of enclosed spaces), agoraphobia (fear of open spaces), and acrophobia (fear of heights). A phobia can, however, relate to just about any object, person, or situation, and is probably caused by a subconscious reflex to avoid repeating an unpleasant experience. For the sufferer it may cause little more than mild embarrassment, or it may be totally debilitating and disruptive to everyday life. An estimated 10 percent of people in the U.K., and slightly more in the U.S., suffer from phobias of some description. Recent research indicates that most sufferers can cure themselves.

SYMPTOMS
• Rapid pulse • Profuse sweating • High blood pressure
• Trembling • Nausea

TREATMENT

Ayurveda
Lemon or lime may be suggested for dizziness, and individual treatment would be prescribed according to your specific needs. (See page 20.)

Chinese Herbalism
A herbalist may suggest cooling herbs, and the formula Gui Pi Wan, which addresses emotional problems.
Ren Shen (ginseng), Dang Gui (Chinese angelica), and Yuan Zhi (senega root) may also be useful. (See pages 82, 160, and 166.)

Valerian tea can help
to relieve tension.

Herbalism
Valerian tea can help to reduce tension. Drink an infusion as required. (See page 195.)

Aromatherapy
Essential oils can be very useful in the treatment of phobias. The effect of certain smells can help to release tension and induce a feeling of calm. Some of the best oils to try are: bergamot, chamomile, clary sage, geranium, jasmine, juniper, lavender, marjoram, melissa, and ylang ylang, which are sedative. They can be used in the bath, in massage with a light carrier oil (such as sweet almond), or in a vaporizer. Carry a bottle of diluted oils with you – perhaps in a small sprayer – and apply them to the temples or pulse points in times of fear. (See page 47.)

Homeopathy
There are dozens of homeopathic remedies that can be used to treat phobias, but they will be prescribed constitutionally, that is, the treatment would be tailored to your exact needs. Some to try may be:
Phosphorus, for fear of the dark. (See page 219.)
Arnica, for fears that are brought on by an accident. (See page 86.)

Flower Essences
Treatment would be based on your individual state of mind, but some of the following may help:
Mimulus, for the everyday fears of known things, spiders, being late for work, flying, and being ill. (See page 153.)
Aspen is for unknown fears, the vague and dark fears which hover and play on the imagination. (See page 168.)
Rock rose should be added when the fear is turning into terror and perhaps even panic. (See page 135.)
Cherry plum is for the fear that everything will fall apart. (See page 170.)
Red chestnut is for fear for another's safety. (See page 76.)
The most important Bach Flower Remedy for fear, anxiety, and phobias, Rescue Remedy, is made up of five essences: cherry plum, rock rose, impatiens, clematis, and star of Bethlehem. It works to treat fear, loneliness, despondency, and loss of focus. It rebalances the sufferer after an emotional upset and is particularly useful in panic attacks. Apply a few drops of the remedy to your tongue or pulse points. (See page 158.)

Nutrition
Vitamin B-complex and C are important for nerve functioning. Ensure that you eat regular meals, since low blood sugar can exacerbate the problem.

Mind–Body Healing
Phobias respond well to talking therapies as well as to cognitive behavioral therapy. (See page 69.)
For an immediate response to a stressful situation or panic attack, relaxation techniques, visualization, and breathing techniques will all be beneficial. (See page 68.)

DEPRESSION

Depression is a prolonged feeling of unhappiness and despondency, often magnified by a major life event such as bereavement, divorce, or retirement. Many women experience depression after childbirth. Clinical depression is a genuine illness that overwhelms the sufferer so that he or she feels a hopelessness, dejection, and fear out of all proportion to any cause. Someone who is depressed may contemplate or attempt suicide.

SYMPTOMS
- Slow speech • Poor concentration • Confusion and irritability
- Self-accusation and loss of self-esteem • Insomnia and early-morning waking • Emptiness and despair
- Loss of appetite • Loss of sexual drive

TREATMENT
Ayurveda
Detoxification treatment would be followed by specific oral medication to balance the three doshas. Treatment is always individual. (See page 20.)

Chinese Herbalism
Depression is believed to be caused by stagnation of the liver qi, and may be treated with Dang Gui (Chinese angelica), Bai Shao (peony root), and Gan Cao (licorice). (See pages 82, 132, and 159.)

Herbalism
The best antidepressant and nervine (with a specific action for nerves) herbs include: lemon balm, borage, linden, oats, rosemary, and vervain. These can be taken as herbal teas, added to the bath, or taken as tablets, or in tincture form (herbs suspended in alcohol). (See pages 89, 152, 175, 191, and 196.)

Aromatherapy
There are a number of antidepressant oils, which can be used in the bath, in a vaporizer, on a light bulb and in massage. They include: neroli, jasmine, geranium, melissa, and rose. Ylang ylang, lavender, clary sage, and chamomile are sedative and antidepressant. (See page 47.)

> **CAUTION**
> If symptoms persist or are severe, seek advice from a qualified physician.

Homeopathy
It will be necessary to see a homeopath to receive treatment that is suited to you, and which addresses the cause of your depression. Specific remedies include Aurum, for feelings of worthlessness, suicidal feelings, and self-disgust.

Flower Essences
Cherry plum, for "fear of the mind being over strained, of doing dreaded things," and of being violent to oneself or others. (See page 170.)
Agrimony, for deeply held emotional tensions that are hidden from others. (See page 77.)
Gorse helps to combat feelings of hopelessness. (See page 192.)
Gentian will help to improve a mild depression and despondency caused by a setback. (See page 130.)
Wild mustard is for blacker and deeper feelings when there is no apparent cause. (See page 184.)
Sweet chestnut should be taken if you feel anguished and stretched beyond endurance. (See page 100.)

Nutrition
Depression that occurs just before menstruation (PMS) may be caused by a vitamin B6 deficiency; postnatal depression may be caused by a deficiency of vitamin B12 and folic acid. Nutritional supplements and allergy tests may be suggested by a practitioner. Ensure you have an adequate intake of vitamin C. Some therapists may recommend supplementing the amino acid tryptophan. (See pages 208, 209, 210, and 227.)

Mind–Body Healing
Mind–body therapies are proven to be particularly effective for alleviating depression, from regular exercise to talking or music therapies. (See pages 68–71.)

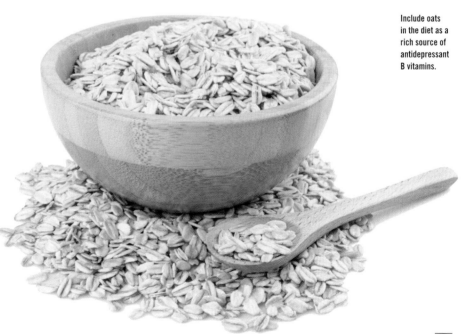

Include oats in the diet as a rich source of antidepressant B vitamins.

STRESS

Each individual is able to cope with a different amount of stress in life, and while some seem to draw on endless reserves to keep going, others succumb. A certain amount of stress provides stimulation, but prolonged stress can cause mental and physical damage. Most of us think of tense situations and worries as being the cause of stress. In reality, stresses are wide-ranging. They include environmental stresses, such as pollution, noise, housing problems, cold, or overheating; physical stresses, such as illnesses, injuries, an inadequate diet; and mental stresses, such as relationship problems, financial strains, bereavement, and job difficulties. All these factors affect the body, causing it to make a series of rapid physiological changes, called "adaptive responses," to deal with threatening or demanding situations. In the first stage of stress, hormones are poured into the bloodstream. The pulse quickens, the lungs take in more oxygen to fuel the muscles, blood sugar increases to supply added energy, digestion slows, and perspiration increases. In the second stage of stress, the body begins to repair the damage caused by the first stage. If the stressful situation is resolved, the stress symptoms vanish. If the situation continues, however, exhaustion sets in, and the body's energy gives out.

SYMPTOMS
- Insomnia • Depression • High blood pressure • Hair loss
- Allergies • Ulcers • Heart disease • Digestive disorders
- Menstrual problems • Palpitations • Impotence
- Premature ejaculation

TREATMENT
Ayurveda
An Ayurvedic practitioner would prescribe supportive herbs, and use a balancing treatment specific to your needs. (See page 20.)

Chinese Herbalism
Chinese medicine takes the view that it is not stress that causes illness, but how we deal with it. Herbs would be prescribed according to your specific needs, in order to support you throughout stressful periods, and tonify. (See page 24.)
Treatment may be aimed particularly at the kidneys, which have become exhausted through overwork, and to support the blood and qi, which need to circulate harmoniously in the body. (See pages 22–23.)

Traditional Home and Folk Remedies
Pumpkin seeds, which contain high quantities of zinc, iron, and calcium, as well as B vitamins and proteins, which are necessary for brain function, will help you to deal with the effects of stress.
Oats are vital for a healthy nervous system. In periods of stress, start the day with oatmeal, which will help to keep you calm, and prevent depression and general debility. (See page 89.)

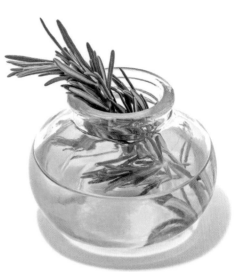

A massage blend that includes rosemary essential oil strengthens the adrenal system.

Herbalism
Herbs that encourage relaxation and act as a tonic to the nervous system include lemon balm, lavender, chamomile, passiflora (*Passiflora incarnata*) and oats. These can be drunk as an infusion when in a stressful situation. (See pages 89, 143, 149, and 152.)
Ginseng is an "adaptogenic" herb, which means that it lifts you when you are tired and relaxes you when you are stressed. It also works on the immune system and energizes. Some therapists recommend a daily dose at stressful times. (See page 160.)

Aromatherapy
Massage with aromatherapy oils is very comforting, particularly the element of touch, and a few drops of essential oil in the bath can offer an opportunity to "wash away" the problems of the day while experiencing the benefits of the oil. Suitable oils include basil, chamomile, geranium, lavender, neroli, and rose. (See pages 106, 143, 149, 156, 161, and 174.)
Oils that strengthen the adrenal system, which is weakened by stress, include rosemary, ginger, and lemongrass. (See page 47.)

Nutrition
Eating a good, balanced diet will make your body stronger and able to cope more efficiently with stress. (See page 58.)
B vitamins are often depleted by stress, so ensure that you are getting enough in your diet, or take a good supplement. (See pages 206–209.)
There is some evidence that bee and flower pollen can boost immunity and energize the body. Do not eat if you are allergic to honey or bee stings. (See page 228.)
An amino acid called L-tyrosine appears to energize, and studies show that people taking this supplement react better to stressful situations, staying more alert and less anxious, and have fewer complaints about physical discomforts. (See page 227.)
Vitamin C is a great stress reliever, and boosts immunity, making you fitter and healthier. (See page 210.)

Mind–Body Healing
During times of intense stress, breathing techniques and visualization may calm the mind. (See page 68.)
For longer-term relief for a continuing stressful situation, regular exercise, including yoga, as well as talking or behavioral therapies, are beneficial. (See pages 69–71.)

ANXIETY

Anxiety is an element of many psychological disorders, including phobias, panic attacks, obsessive-compulsive disorders, and post-traumatic stress disorder. Anxiety is a state of fear or apprehension in the face of threat or danger. It is a natural, healthy response since it allows the body to prepare itself (through adrenaline) to cope with the danger. Anxiety can, however, take a person over – a condition known as anxiety neurosis – and the person is then said to be in an anxiety state. This may be chronic anxiety, with a constant feeling of worry, associated with depression, or an acute anxiety attack, when the sufferer will be suddenly overwhelmed by fear and feelings of dread. When we are faced with a frightening or threatening situation, our body goes into a "fight or flight" response, when adrenaline pours into the system and the body prepares itself for action. When no action follows, and nervous energy is not discharged, there is physiological confusion, otherwise known as a panic attack. Symptoms may include dizziness, visual disturbance, clammy hands, racing heart, dry mouth, and overbreathing.

SYMPTOMS
• Dry mouth • Sweaty palms • Rapid pulse • Palpitations
In anxiety neurosis:
• Breathlessness • Headaches • Weakness • Fatigue • Tightness in the chest • High blood pressure • Abdominal pain • Diarrhea • Insomnia • Loss of appetite

TREATMENT
Ayurveda
An Ayurvedic medical practitioner would balance the tridoshas, and use panchakarma for balancing the vátha. (See page 20.)

Chinese Herbalism
A Chinese herbalist might suggest Ren Shen (ginseng), Dang Gui (Chinese angelica), and Bai Shao (white peony root) with Chai Hu (thorowax root) for relaxation. Treatment would strengthen the spleen and enliven liver qi. (See pages 82, 159, and 160.)

Traditional Home and Folk Remedies
Oats contain thiamine and pantothenic acid, which act as gentle nerve tonics (See page 89.)

Herbalism
Herbal remedies would be used to calm the nervous system and to relax.
Skullcap and valerian are useful herbs, blended together for best effect. Drink this as a tea three times daily while suffering anxiety symptoms. (See pages 181 and 195.)
Lady's slipper and linden may ease anxiety and tension. (See page 191.)

Aromatherapy
A relaxing blend of essential oils of lavender, geranium, and bergamot in sweet almond oil or peach kernel oil may be used in the bath at times of great stress and anxiety. (See page 47.)

Homeopathy
Constitutional treatment will be appropriate for chronic conditions, and there are a number of remedies that will prove useful for relieving acute attacks. These include:
Nat. mur. may be useful if you have a tendency to dwell on morbid topics and generally hate fuss. (See page 154.)
Calcarea, if you fear for your sanity, forget things, and feel the cold. (See page 213.)

Flower Essences
Remedies are prescribed according to the personal characteristics of the sufferer, and the cause and nature of the anxiety.
Try elm for anxiety accompanying a feeling of being unable to cope, or red chestnut for anxiety over the welfare of others. (See pages 76 and 193.)
Try aspen, for anxiety brought on for no apparent reason. (See page 168.)
Rescue Remedy is useful during attacks. (See page 158.)

Nutrition
Increase your intake of B vitamins, which work on the nervous system, and avoid caffeine in any form. (See pages 206–209.)

Mind–Body Healing
For relief during moments of intense anxiety, practice breathing and visualization. For help with anxiety neurosis or panic attacks, consult a registered practitioner, who may suggest talking therapies as part of a long-term strategy. (See pages 68–69.)

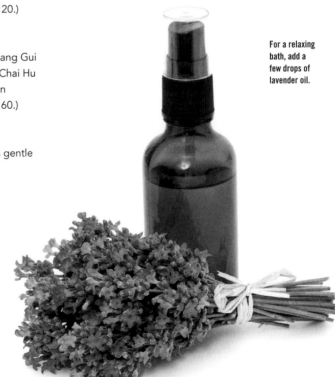

For a relaxing bath, add a few drops of lavender oil.

INSECURITY

Insecurity is a feeling that affects everybody at one time or another. It can be triggered by physical, social, financial, or emotional factors, and can often induce anxiety and its associated symptoms. Whatever the initial cause, when a person feels insecure that person's entire perception of his or her own competence and self-worth are thrown into question. Chronic insecurity, which can manifest itself as depression, shyness, lack of confidence, or an inability to form stable relationships, has less to do with external events than with unrealistic expectations and a poor self-image.

SYMPTOMS
• Dry mouth • Sweaty palms • Rapid pulse • Palpitations
In anxiety neurosis:
• Breathlessness • Headaches • Weakness • Fatigue • Tightness in the chest • High blood pressure • Abdominal pain • Diarrhea
• Insomnia • Loss of appetite

TREATMENT
Chinese Herbalism
Try herbs that work to balance the nervous system, including Ye Jiao Teng (fleeceflower stem), Fu Ling (poria), and Suan Zao Ren (wild jujube seeds). (See pages 167, 168, and 201.)

Herbalism
Use uplifting herbs such as rosemary, lavender, ginseng, damiana, or valerian. They can be drunk as infusions 3 times daily. (See pages 143, 160, 175, 192, and 195.)

Aromatherapy
Jasmine lifts the spirits and improves mental outlook: add a few drops to a vaporizer or your bath (not at bedtime). (See page 141.)
Marjoram and thyme are cheering and can boost self-image. (See pages 157 and 190.)

Homeopathy
Seek advice from a registered practitioner for remedies to address anxiety stemming from particular causes, such as a traumatic experience or bereavement. Other remedies may help for more generalized anxiety that results in tearfulness.

Flower Essences
Mimulus is appropriate for fear of known things, timidity, and shyness. (See page 153.)
Crab apple, for poor self-image. (See page 148.)
Elm, for those who are usually confident but are experiencing a temporary crisis of confidence because they are overwhelmed by responsibility. (See page 193.)

Mind–Body Healing
Practice any mind–body therapy that encourages you to relax, including yoga and meditation. (See pages 68–71.)

Sunflower oil contains lecithin, which enhances functioning of the brain.

MEMORY LOSS

A total or partial loss of memory is known as amnesia. It occurs as a result of physical or mental disease (such as senile dementia), or physical trauma (such as a blow to the head or a fractured skull). It can also occur in some forms of psychiatric illness in which there is no apparent physical damage to the brain. Amnesia can be a complication of alcoholism, and can result from depression, stress, poor nutrition, inadequate sleep, or lack of stimulation.

SYMPTOMS
• Loss of immediate, short-term, or long-term memories
• Distress as a result of failure to remember

TREATMENT
Chinese Herbalism
Herbs to aid memory include Ye Jiao Teng (fleeceflower root) and black ginger seed. (See page 167.)
Memory loss caused by stress or fatigue may be treated with Gou Qi Zi (Chinese wolfberry). (See page 147.)

Herbalism
Ginseng powder can act as a memory aid. (See page 160.)
Add gotu kola to your food for several days. (See page 101.)
Rosemary is said to comfort the brain and refresh the memory, and sage is also useful. (See pages 175 and 177.)

Flower Essences
Use star of Bethlehem, when memory is affected by an accident, bad news, or trauma. (See page 158.)

Nutrition
Your diet should be rich in B vitamins and protein, as amino acids are necessary for the brain to function efficiently. An amino acid supplement (containing all 22 acids) may be useful. Acetylcholine, which is formed in the body from lecithin, may help. Increase your intake of lecithin (found in sunflower oil and eggs) or take it as a supplement. (See pages 206–209, 222–227, and 233.)

Mind–Body Healing
Relaxation techniques may help with the distress and anxiety caused by memory loss. (See pages 68–69.)

INSOMNIA

A common complaint, insomnia is the inability to sleep or the disturbance of normal sleep patterns. It is difficult to qualify, because everyone has different sleep requirements, and sleeplessness is, in fact, a natural feature of aging. Insomnia is often caused by worry, emotional stress, and exhaustion. Other causes include pain; excess caffeine, alcohol, and drugs; food allergy; or sleeping in a stuffy room. Insomnia can also be a symptom of depression. In recent years, sleep-disorders medicine has become virtually a new branch of medicine, with centers for diagnosis and treatment now located throughout the U.S.

SYMPTOMS
• Overactive mind • Nervousness • Restlessness • Nightmares
• Irritability • Mood swings involving hysterical behavior
• Fear of bedtime

TREATMENT

Chinese Herbalism
Useful herbs include Fu Ling (poria), Ye Jiao Teng (fleeceflower stem), and Suan Zao Ren (wild jujube). (See pages 167, 168, and 201.)
The herbalist may suggest that you sleep on a gypsum pillow, which contains crushed mineral gypsum, known as Shi Gao in traditional Chinese medicine.

Traditional Home and Folk Remedies
A hot foot bath before bed helps relaxation by drawing blood away from the head. Add a little mustard powder to the water to increase the effect. (See page 91.)
Lettuce is said to encourage sleep. Eat a large leaf about half an hour before bedtime.

Herbalism
A warm bath with an infusion of chamomile, catnip (*Nepeta cataria*), lavender, or linden may be recommended. (See pages 143, 149, and 191.)
A cup of warm herb tea just before bed will soothe and help you relax. Try chamomile, catnip, lemon balm, and linden. (See pages 149, 152, and 191.)
Place a lavender pillow under your usual pillow. (See page 143.)

Aromatherapy
A few drops of chamomile oil, clary sage, or lavender can be added to the bath. (See pages 143, 149, and 178.)
Try a gentle massage just before bedtime, with a few drops of chamomile, lavender, rose, or neroli blended into a light carrier oil. (See pages 106, 143, 149, and 174.)
Place a few drops of lavender oil on your bedroom light bulb, just before bed, or place a few drops on a handkerchief and tie it to the bed. (See page 143.)

Flower Essences
Worrying thoughts and mental arguments might respond to white chestnut. (See page 76.)
Indecision can be treated with scleranthus. (See page 180.)
Stress, strain, frustration, and inability to relax might respond to vervain or rock water, vine, elm, beech, or impatiens. (See pages 126, 140, 193, 196, 198, and 205.)

Nutrition
Increase your intake of vitamins B, C, folic acid, zinc and calcium. Try a calcium supplement just before bedtime. (See page 213.)

Mind–Body Healing
Relax for at least 1 hour before going to bed, by meditating, reading, or taking a warm bath. Take regular exercise during the day, but not within 4 hours of going to bed.

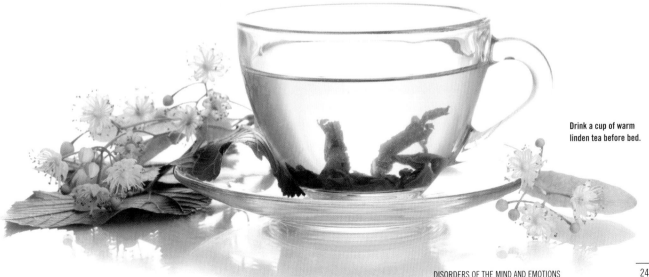

Drink a cup of warm linden tea before bed.

DISORDERS OF THE BRAIN AND NERVES

MULTIPLE SCLEROSIS

Multiple sclerosis (MS) is a chronic disease of the nervous system in which the protective sheaths that cover the nerves become inflamed and scarred, resulting in loss of nerve function. The initial attack is usually followed by recovery, but sufferers inevitably experience a cycle of remission (sometimes for years) and relapse with steadily increasing neurological damage and disability. The degree of improvement after each attack decreases and the physical disability is usually progressive. Eventually there may also be intellectual impairment. The cause of MS is unknown.

SYMPTOMS
• Limb weakness • Visual deterioration, particularly in the center of the visual field • Double vision • Loss of sensation • Staggering • Impaired speech • Facial paralysis

TREATMENT
Flower Essences
Rescue Remedy may help to ease the symptoms and control shaking and anxiety. (See page 158.)

Nutrition
Eat plenty of foods that contain gamma-linoleic acid, which is found in sunflower and safflower oil, as well as evening primrose products. (See page 231.) Get plenty of vitamins B3, B6, B12, folic acid, C, and E, and the minerals zinc and magnesium. (See pages 207–211, 217, and 221.)

Mind–Body Healing
Regular activity or exercise is extremely beneficial for those with MS. Relaxation techniques, therapies, and support groups may help those suffering anxiety or depression as a result of their diagnosis. (See pages 68–71.)

Eating foods that contain safflower oil can benefit those with MS.

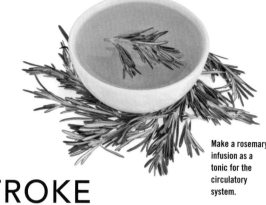

Make a rosemary infusion as a tonic for the circulatory system.

STROKE

A stroke (cerebrovascular accident, or CVA) results from an interruption of the blood supply to any part of the brain. This may be caused by bleeding into or around the brain (cerebral hemorrhage), a clot which blocks an already damaged artery (cerebral thrombosis), or a small clot elsewhere in the bloodstream that eventually causes obstruction in an artery to the brain (cerebral embolism). Smoking, diabetes, high blood pressure, and atherosclerosis are all risk factors.

SYMPTOMS
• Sudden numbness or weakness in the face, arm, or leg, especially on one side of the body • Sudden confusion • Trouble speaking • Difficulty understanding speech • Sudden trouble seeing in one or both eyes • Sudden trouble walking • Sudden dizziness, loss of balance, or lack of coordination • Sudden severe headache

TREATMENT
Ayurveda
Ayurveda is a very popular method for rehabilitation of paralysis, including the special panchakarma therapy for vátha. (See page 20.)

Chinese Herbalism
A Chinese herbalist is likely to offer herbs to regulate the blood condition after a stroke, such as Bai Shao (peony bark) and Gou Qi Zi (wolfberry). (See pages 147 and 159.)

Herbalism
Yarrow is recommended to improve circulation and tone the blood vessels after a stroke. Drink an infusion 3 times daily. (See page 74.) Rosemary can be drunk or eaten fresh as soon as possible to improve the health of the circulatory system. (See page 175.)

Flower Essences
Gorse and gentian could promote a positive mindset in those who are frightened or depressed. (See pages 130 and 192.)

Nutrition
A good intake of oily fish and vitamin E with a wholefood diet is the best prevention against the small blood clots in the brain that can cause strokes. (See pages 58–59 and 211.)
Nutritional therapists may use ginkgo biloba after a stroke to improve circulation and prevent further strokes. (See page 131.)

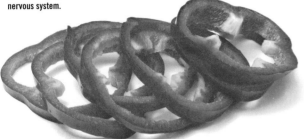

Include foods rich in vitamin C, such as red pepper, in your diet to help the nervous system.

PARKINSON'S DISEASE

Parkinson's is a progressive disease in which degeneration of the nervous system, particularly the nerve cells in the brain, causes loss of control over voluntary movement. The damage is irreversible and the exact cause as yet unknown. It occurs most commonly among the elderly, and affects men more than women. Parkinson's involves the central gray matter of the brain (basal ganglia), resulting in deficiency of a neurotransmitter known as dopamine. The common form of this disease is caused by a premature degeneration of certain basal nuclei.

SYMPTOMS
• Difficulty in walking, tending to stoop and shuffle • Involuntary head movements • Stiffness of facial muscles, resulting in a fixed expression • Stiffness of tongue muscles, causing impaired speech • Worsening tremors, making it difficult to write, use cutlery or drink from a cup • Eventually, in some cases, senile dementia

TREATMENT
Chinese Herbalism
The cause is believed to be deficient blood and kidney yang, which may be helped by Tian Ma (gastrodia), Bai Shao (peony root), and Gou Qi Zi (wolfberry). (See pages 130, 147, and 159.)

Herbalism
Herbs that boost the nervous system and brain function include ginseng, wild oats, astragalus and Chinese angelica. (See pages 82, 87, 89, and 160.)

Nutrition
Take vitamin B6 and C for nervous function. (See pages 208 and 210.)

Mind–Body Healing
Exercise will help to reduce muscle stiffness: sports such as tennis or cycling may be helpful, or gentler activities like walking, gardening, and yoga. Support groups and talking, art and music therapies are also recommended. (See pages 69–71.)

EPILEPSY

Epilepsy is an indication of an abnormality in brain function. Generalized epilepsy (grand mal and petit mal) is the most common form and is caused by a great electrical discharge across the surface of the brain on both sides. Partial-seizure epilepsy (simple and complex) is confined to a localized area of the brain, often, but not always, the temporal lobe.

SYMPTOMS
In a grand mal seizure:
• Seizure may begin with a shout • Loss of consciousness
• Foaming at the mouth • Loss of bladder and bowel control
• Rhythmic contraction of all the body's muscles • The sufferer may end the seizure in a deep sleep
In a petit mal seizure (particularly common among children):
• Momentary loss of consciousness • Possibly jerky contractions of facial and finger muscles
In a simple partial seizure:
• Hallucinations of smell, vision, or taste • Twitching movements ·
In a complex partial seizure, as for a simple partial seizure, plus:
• Fear • Anger • A period of unresponsiveness • Behaving in a robot-like way • May be violent if interfered with

TREATMENT
Herbalism
Herbs to relax the nervous system, including vervain and valerian, may be useful in reducing attacks. (See pages 195 and 196.)

Aromatherapy
Extremely small doses of rosemary might be helpful in treating epilepsy, but this must only be done under the supervision of an aromatherapist with a medical qualification. (See page 175.)

Flower Essences
Take a few drops of Rescue Remedy if you feel an attack coming on. This will calm you and could possibly abort an attack. (See page 158.)

Nutrition
Extra vitamin B5, magnesium, calcium, and zinc may help to prevent attacks. (See pages 208, 213, 217, and 221.)
Vitamin D and B6 deficiency can prompt attacks. (See pages 208 and 210.)

CAUTION
Always seek advice from a physician before taking herbal remedies. Never attempt to open the mouth or force anything between the teeth of somebody who is suffering an epileptic seizure. Loosen the person's clothing and ensure that he or she is not in any danger, and then wait until the seizure has run its course. Prolonged, repeated grand mal attacks, with no recovery of consciousness, require urgent medical attention. Avoid certain aromatherapy oils, including sage, fennel, hyssop, and wormwood.

SHINGLES

Shingles is an extremely painful disease caused by the herpes zoster virus (which is also the chicken pox virus). Following an attack of chicken pox the virus remains dormant in the body. Many years later a drop in the efficiency of the immune system may cause reactivation of the virus, this time in the form of shingles, causing acute inflammation in the ganglia near the spinal cord. Shingles occurs most often in people over the age of 50 and may be activated through surgery or X-ray therapy to the spinal cord and its roots. In younger people, it is often associated with a weakening of the immune system. The pain, which can be disabling, may continue for a few months after the blisters heal.

SYMPTOMS
• First sign of shingles is sensitivity in the area to be affected, then pain • Fever • Sickness • Rash of small blisters develops on the fourth or fifth day, which turn yellow within a few days, form scabs, then drop off, sometimes leaving scars

TREATMENT
Traditional Home and Folk Remedies
Grind cinnamon, cloves, and nutmeg in a pestle and mortar. Add water to make a thick paste. Apply to spots to numb the pain. (See pages 104, 125, and 153.)
Celery juice or celery tea can alleviate the pain and help to tone up the nervous system. (See page 84.)
Apply bruised juniper berries to the spots for effective pain relief. (See page 142.)
Fresh lemon can be cut and applied to the affected areas to relieve the pain. (See page 108.)

Herbalism
Make an infusion of the following nervine herbs and drink three times daily: oats, skullcap, St. John's wort, and vervain. (See pages 89, 138, 181, and 196.)
Diluted tinctures or cold infusion of marigold, plantain, and St. John's wort can be used to bathe the affected area. (See pages 93, 138, and 165.)

Aromatherapy
Essential oils can combine analgesics with antiviral properties, and can be applied as a compress, added to the bath, or massaged into the skin. Try combining two or more of bergamot, chamomile, geranium, eucalyptus, melissa, lavender, and tea tree.
Dab the sores with lemon or geranium oil diluted in a little water. (See pages 108 and 161.)

Nutrition
Supplementation with vitamin E reduces the long-term symptoms of shingles. Take up to 1 mg. daily, in 3 doses, with food. (See page 211.)

> **CAUTION**
> Shingles of the face may affect the eyes and should receive appropriate specialist medical attention.

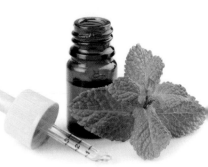

Peppermint oil, rubbed into the inflamed area, is a traditional remedy for neuralgic pain.

NEURALGIA

Neuralgia is the term used to describe any pain originating in a nerve. If there is damage at any point along the route of a nerve, pain will then be referred to the area served by the affected nerve. Infection causing inflammation in a nerve can also cause neuralgia. The pain may be intermittent or continuous. Neuralgia has different causes, which give rise to certain specific types of neuralgic pain. In trigeminal neuralgia, the facial nerve is affected, causing severe one-sided facial pain. In sciatica, spinal nerves are trapped between vertebrae, causing pain of varying severity in the back, sometimes extending down to the foot. Post-herpetic neuralgia is caused by a previous attack of shingles, resulting in a burning pain at the site of the rash. In glossopharyngeal neuralgia, pain is felt in the ear, the throat, and at the back of the tongue.

SYMPTOMS
• Pain of varying severity and location, as described above

TREATMENT
Traditional Home and Folk Remedies
Celery juice or celery tea will help to ease pain. (See page 84.)
Warm chamomile compresses applied to the affected area will ease inflammation and pain. (See page 149.)
Rub lemons or peppermint oil on the affected area for pain relief. (See pages 108 and 152.)
Clove oil can be used to ease pain in the mouth. (See page 125.)

Herbalism
Drink infusions of lemon balm, meadowsweet, rosemary, and skullcap. (See pages 127, 152, 175, and 181.)

Aromatherapy
Massage eucalyptus, lavender, or chamomile into the area, or add the infused herbs to the bath. (See pages 124, 143, and 149.)
A compress of rosemary essential oil will improve the circulation in the area, which will encourage healing. (See page 175.)
Blend one drop of mustard and pepper oils in some grapeseed oil, and massage into the affected area. (See pages 91 and 164.)

Nutrition
Vitamins B1, B2, and biotin help nerve health. (See pages 206, 207, and 212.)
Take extra vitamin E and chromium. (See pages 211 and 214.)

MIGRAINE

The classic feature of a migraine is a throbbing headache, usually on one side of the head only. This is caused by the narrowing and dilating of the blood vessels in a part of one side of the brain. An attack may last for up to two days. There are two main types of migraine, common and the comparatively rare classical. Migraine can be hereditary, and may be triggered by many factors, including stress, hormonal changes (around menopause, menstruation, and occasionally pregnancy), oral contraceptives, and food that contains tyramine, an amino acid that affects the blood vessels. Foods rich in tyramine include bananas, cheese, chocolate, eggs, oranges, spinach, tomatoes, and wine. Other triggers include changes or extremes in temperature, lighting, or noise level. Migraine occurs in about 10 percent of the population, and is more common in women. Children may suffer from migraine, but this often manifests itself as an abdominal pain rather than a headache. About 60 percent of all migraine sufferers are women, and most patients first develop symptoms between the ages of 10 and 30.

Inhalations, baths, or massages of sweet marjoram, melissa, or rosemary essential oils can relieve the pain of migraines.

SYMPTOMS

In common migraine:
• Slowly developing severe headache, lasting from a few hours to two days • Pain is made worse by the smallest movement or noise • Nausea • Sometimes vomiting

In classical migraine:
• Headache preceded by an aura which generally takes the form of a visual disturbance such as temporary loss of vision, focusing problems, blind spots, and flashing lights • Possible speech problems • Occasional weakness or temporary paralysis of the limbs or extremities • Nausea and vomiting • Sensitivity to light

TREATMENT

Ayurveda
Treatment would be aimed at Ayurvedic oral formulas, and panchakarma shirovirechana. (See page 20.)
Vilwadi lehya, an Ayurvedic product, can help with nausea.

Chinese Herbalism
In TCM, the cause of migraines is believed to be excess liver qi stagnation, weakness in the stomach, and an imbalance of stomach and liver. Useful herbs include Jue Ming Ji (*Cassia tora*) and Ju Hua (chrysanthemum). (See page 268.)

Herbalism
Feverfew is an effective remedy for reducing the frequency of migraine. Take 2 or 3 small leaves between a little fresh bread, daily. Feverfew tablets are also available. (See page 187.)
Apply a warm compress of Jamaican dogwood (*Piscidia piscipula*) to the temples and forehead during an attack. Jamaican dogwood can be toxic if taken internally and should be used under the guidance of a registered medical herbalist.

Aromatherapy
Peppermint and lavender oils, applied to a cool compress, will help to relieve symptoms. (See pages 143 and 152.)
Inhalations, baths, or massage of lemon balm, rosemary, or sweet marjoram can relieve the pain and shorten the duration of attacks. Used regularly, these methods can be preventive. (See pages 152, 157, and 175.)
A dab of lavender oil at the base of the nostrils can be used at the first signs of an attack. (See page 143.)

Homeopathy
Treatment is constitutional, but the following remedies may be helpful in the event of an attack:
Silicea, for pain that begins in the back of the head, settling above an eye. This is alleviated by wrapping the head. (See page 220.)
Lycopodium, for pain that is worse on the right side of the body, painful temples, and dizziness. (See page 147.)
Nat. mur., for headache which is blinding and throbs, and which is worsened by warmth and movement, and where the attack is preceded by numbness around the mouth and nose. (See page 154.)

Nutrition
Take extra vitamins B5, C, and E, and also evening primrose oil. (See pages 208, 210, 211, and 231.)
Add fresh root ginger to food. (See page 200.)

HEADACHE

Headaches are usually due to muscular tension in the head, neck, or shoulders, or to congestion of the blood vessels supplying blood to the brain and muscles. In some cases, a headache may be a symptom of a more serious underlying disorder, but often headaches are caused by stress, tiredness, poor posture, caffeine, alcohol, drugs, food allergy, eyestrain, sinusitis, or low blood sugar. They can also be the result of a head injury. There are many different types of headache, and the degree and intensity of pain vary accordingly. Cluster headaches produce short, severe attacks of pain centered over one eye. They are so called because they occur in clusters, many times a day, for several months. Spontaneous remissions often take place, but the pain usually returns some months or years later. Cluster headaches are suffered most often by males. Researchers suspect that cluster headaches may be caused by a disorder in histamine metabolism, since they are usually accompanied by allergy symptoms such as tearing, nasal congestion, and a runny nose.

SYMPTOMS
• Sensation of a tight band around the head • Feeling of pressure at the top of the head • Bursting or throbbing sensation • Eye and neck pain • Dizziness

TREATMENT

Ayurveda
An Ayurvedic treatment for sinus-related headaches is the steam inhalation of coriander seeds. Put the coriander seeds into a small bowl. Pour on some boiling water, drape a towel over your head and the bowl, and inhale the steam. (See page 113.)
Heat 3 tablespoons of mustard oil, soak a cloth in the solution, and apply to the forehead. (See page 91.)

Chinese Herbalism
Eat a small piece of fresh ginger root or make ginger tea from the fresh root or tea bags. If you prefer, mix a large pinch of powdered ginger into a glass of cool water and drink it, or try powdered ginger in capsules. (See page 200.)
Ren Shen (ginseng) may also be helpful for headaches. (See page 160.)

Traditional Home and Folk Remedies
A ginger or mustard foot bath may ease pain and warm the body. (See pages 91 and 200.)
Chamomile tea soothes headache symptoms. (See page 149.)
A few grains of cayenne pepper, added to tea, ease a headache. (See page 98.)
Fresh garlic bulbs will clear headaches that have a feeling of congestion. (See page 79.)
Parsley and peppermint teas will clear the head. (See pages 152 and 162.)

Herbalism
Sitting with a cup of mild herbal tea is often good for a tension headache. Try peppermint, spearmint, chamomile, rosehip, meadowsweet, or lemon balm. (See pages 127, 149, 152, and 174.)
Valerian root tea can also be helpful, but it may induce sleep, so use it with caution. (See page 195.)
Studies suggest that patients who eat a few fresh feverfew leaves or take an extract of the leaves every day have fewer and less severe migraines. (See page 187.)

Aromatherapy
The relaxing qualities of lavender oil make it a good treatment for a tension headache. This essential oil is very gentle, so you can massage a few drops of neat oil into your temples and the base of your neck. (See page 143.)
Try mixing a drop or two of peppermint oil in a bowl of hot water and inhaling the steam, then lie down with a warm compress soaked in sweet marjoram oil on your forehead. (See pages 152 and 157.)
Try taking a bath with relaxing oils such as chamomile or ylang ylang to soothe and relieve pain. (See pages 95 and 149.)

Nutrition
Frequent headaches could be a signal that you are low on some important vitamins and minerals. Low levels of niacin and vitamin B6 can cause headaches, for example, and all the B vitamins are needed to help combat stress and avoid tension headaches. Protein-rich foods such as chicken, fish, beans and peas, milk, cheese, nuts, and peanut butter are all good dietary sources of both niacin and vitamin B6. (See pages 206–209.)
The minerals calcium and magnesium work together to help prevent headaches, especially those related to a woman's menstrual cycle. (See pages 213 and 217.)

Mind–Body Healing
Regular exercise and relaxation techniques may help with stress headaches. When headaches are caused by poor posture, yoga or the Alexander technique may be helpful. (See pages 68–71.)

> **CAUTION**
> Headaches with associated features such as double vision, projectile vomiting, weakness, paralysis, vertigo, or one-sided deafness require urgent medical attention. Headaches are very occasionally an indication of a serious disorder, such as a brain tumor.

Heat 3 tablespoons of mustard oil, pour on to a cloth, and apply to the forehead to ease throbbing.

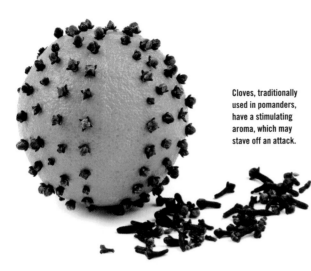

Cloves, traditionally used in pomanders, have a stimulating aroma, which may stave off an attack.

FAINTING

Fainting (or a vasovagal attack) is a brief loss of consciousness, usually brought on by shock, distress, or pain, and is most likely to occur in warm, crowded places. Other causes include prolonged coughing, straining to defecate, or blowing an instrument. Fainting may also result from postural hypotension (see "Dizziness"). Fainting is caused by a temporary shortage of blood supply to the brain, and there is also a slowing of the heart rate. Fainting acts as a type of safety mechanism in that the fall restores the blood supply to the brain by gravity.

SYMPTOMS
The characteristic loss of consciousness may be preceded by:
• Yawning • Sweating • Nausea • Rapid breathing and a weak pulse
• Impaired vision • Ringing in the ears • Weakness • Confusion

TREATMENT
Traditional Home and Folk Remedies
Eat fresh or grated apple when you start to feel faint, as it is both restorative and calming. (See page 148.)
Chew dried cloves, which are stimulating. (See page 125.)

Herbalism
Small sips of ginger tea, or root ginger chewed, will help to restore, and prevent an attack. (See page 200.)
A hot drink of honey and peppermint will help to prevent loss of consciousness. (See page 152 and 203.)

Aromatherapy
Hold a tissue with a few drops of peppermint or neroli oil, which can help when you feel faint or are in a state of shock. (See pages 106 and 152.)
A few drops of rosemary oil, massaged into the temples, prevents loss of consciousness. (See page 175.)

Flower Essences
Rescue Remedy placed on the tongue or temples may help to prevent fainting. (See page 158.)

DIZZINESS

Dizziness is the sensation that everything around the sufferer is spinning, or that the brain is moving within the skull. In severe cases the sufferer may lose his or her balance and fall to the ground. Dizziness can be caused by a fault in the inner ear's balancing mechanism, or it may be due to a neurological disturbance. It can also be brought on by travel sickness, hyperventilation, anxiety, alcohol, drugs, and standing up suddenly from a sitting or lying position (postural hypotension). Postural hypotension is more common in the elderly and in people taking antihypertensive (high blood pressure) drugs.

SYMPTOMS
• Spinning sensation • Cold sweats • Nausea • Vomiting • Pallor

TREATMENT
Ayurveda
Add the juice of a lime or lemon to half a glass of soda water and sip in small doses. (See pages 105 and 108.)

Chinese Herbalism
Fresh ginger, Gui Zhi (cinnamon), and peppermint may help. (See pages 104, 152, and 200.)

Herbalism
Small sips of fresh ginger tea, made with root ginger, will help to ease the symptoms. (See page 200.)
Take teas of rock rose flowers or wild rose flowers, with a little honey. (See pages 135 and 174.)

Flower Essences
If dizziness is associated with panic, stress, or anxiety, Rescue Remedy will be calming and restorative; take as required. (See page 158.)

Nutrition
Eat foods that contain vitamins B2 and B3, or take them as supplements. Consume extra salt if you are sweating a great deal. (See page 207.)

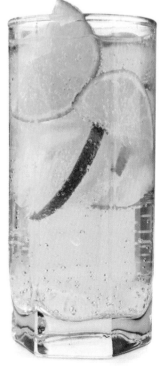

> **CAUTION**
> Severe or prolonged dizziness should be reported to your physician.

Ayurveda recommends drinking soda water with the juice of a lime or lemon.

SKIN AND HAIR PROBLEMS

DERMATITIS

Dermatitis is a very loose term (often used interchangeably with eczema) used to describe an inflammation of the skin from any cause. Exogenous dermatitis is caused by external factors (irritants such as washing powder), and tends to occur around infected wounds or ulcers. Endogenous forms are due to internal problems, including metabolic disorders. Scratching always aggravates dermatitis and may also cause infection. Types of dermatitis include: diaper rash, caused by the ammonia in urine; atopic dermatitis, complicated by allergies such as hay fever; infantile eczema; seborrheic dermatitis (see "Dandruff," page 261); dermatitis artefacta, caused by unnecessary scratching (it is self-inflicted and usually indicates an underlying emotional problem). The symptoms of dermatitis vary in severity and appearance according to the cause. Dermatitis can occur in single episodes, or may be chronic.

SYMPTOMS
• Redness • Blistering • Swelling, weeping, and crusting of skin
• Itching with a strong impulse to scratch • Burning sensation

TREATMENT

Chinese Herbalism
Dittany bark and puncture vine fruit may help with itching.

Traditional Home and Folk Remedies
For dermatitis on the hands, rub them with the cold wet coffee grounds left after you have brewed a pot of coffee, to soothe.

Herbalism
Apply compresses of vervain or thyme tea to the area to soothe and cool. (See pages 190 and 196.)

Aromatherapy
Dilute and massage a few drops of aspic, cedarwood, niaouli, or chamomile into the affected area to ease itching. (See page 47.) For contact dermatitis, try calendula or chamomile oil. (See pages 93 and 149.)

Homeopathy
For a nettle rash-type itchiness, try Urtica Urens cream. (See page 194.)

Flower Essences
Crab apple is the cleansing remedy. It works well when added to water for washing and baths. (See page 148.)
Impatiens is very useful for people whose rashes are associated with feelings of irritability and impatience. Take internally or mix into a neutral cream. (See page 140.)
Rescue Remedy, taken internally or used externally in a cream or wash, is useful for treating most skin problems. (See page 158.)

USEFUL FACTS
• Skin-contact dermatitis includes primary irritant dermatitis, allergic dermatitis, and photochemical dermatitis.
• Primary irritant dermatitis is the most common type and is caused by the direct toxicity of certain chemicals that come in contact with the skin.
• Allergic dermatitis involves the immune mechanism and requires prior sensitization of an individual to agents such as cosmetics, chemicals, plants, drugs, or costume jewelry.
• Photochemical dermatitis occurs when an individual with photosensitizing chemicals on his or her skin is exposed to light.

After brewing fresh coffee, save the grounds and rub them on your hands to relieve symptoms.

ECZEMA

Eczema (also called dermatitis) is an inflammation of the skin that causes itching and redness. It is a feature of many different skin disorders arising from many different causes. It can also be hereditary. Eczema is only infectious if it becomes secondarily infected. Types of eczema include: contact eczema (caused by allergens such as plants, metals, detergents, and chemical irritants); atopic eczema (associated with allergies such as hay fever); pomphylox eczema (triggered by emotional stress); and varicose eczema (occurring in the region of varicose veins).

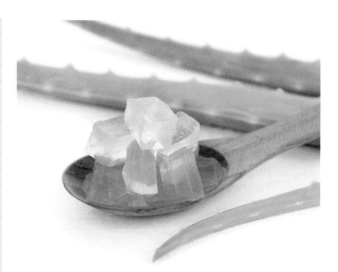

Smooth aloe vera gel into patches of dermatitis to relieve itchiness and aid healing.

SYMPTOMS
• Red, scaly, cracked patches of skin, particularly on the hands, ears, feet, and legs • Burning and itching with a strong urge to scratch, possibly leading to infection, particularly in children
• Small fluid-filled blisters which may burst to form sores

TREATMENT

Ayurveda
Senna pods and aloe vera may be used. (See pages 80 and 99.) Treatment might consist of a number of related therapies, including herbalism, diet and lifestyle changes, cleansing routines, and treatment to balance the body systems so that they work more efficiently. (See page 20.)

Chinese Herbalism
Chinese herbs will be prescribed according to the specific cause and symptoms of your eczema, but some possible herbs are: Qing Hao (wormwood), Bai Shao (peony root), and Long Dan Cao (Chinese gentian). (See page 159.)

Traditional Home and Folk Remedies
An oatmeal bath will soothe irritation and reduce annoying itching. (See page 84.)
Bathe sore patches with an infusion of witch hazel diluted in warm water. (See page 134.)

Herbalism
Try drinking an infusion of burdock, chamomile, heartsease (*Viola tricolor*), marigold, and red clover (*Trifolium pratense*), all of which are anti-inflammatory herbs. (See pages 85, 93, and 149.)
Chickweed ointment (*Stellaria media*) can be applied directly to the affected area, and calendula oil may also be useful.
(See page 93.)
Blackberry leaf tea can be used topically.
Aloe vera gel, from the leaf of the plant, will encourage healing. (See page 80.)

Aromatherapy
Massage the affected areas with essential oils of chamomile, sage, geranium, and lavender, all blended together with a little carrier oil. (See pages 143, 149, 161, and 178.)

Homeopathy
Eczema requires constitutional treatment, which means that treatment is tailored to your specific needs. Urtica Urens cream may be useful in the meantime. (See page 194.)

Flower Essences
Impatiens is very useful for people whose rashes are associated with feelings of irritability and impatience. Take internally or mix into a neutral cream. (See page 140.)
Rescue Remedy, taken internally or used externally in a cream or wash, is useful for skin troubles. (See page 158.)

Nutrition
Increase your intake of vitamin A, found in liver, eggs, butter, milk, and red and orange vegetables. (See page 206.)
Take a B-complex supplement each day, and make sure your tablet contains good levels of niacin (B3), which is also found naturally in peanuts, meat, fish, and pulses. (See pages 206–209.)
Vitamin C and bioflavonoids (which are often contained in a good vitamin C supplement) act as a natural antihistamine. (See pages 210 and 228.)
Evening primrose oil has been used successfully in the treatment of eczema, reducing itching and encouraging healing. (See page 231.)

USEFUL FACTS
• A person may contract eczema at any age and at any place on the body, but the ailment occurs chiefly on the ears, hands, feet, and legs.
• In infants, eczema is often caused by allergy to certain proteins in wheat, milk, and eggs.
• Emotional problems and severe mental stress are suspected of causing eczema in adults.
• Often, a family history of eczema exists, implying that heredity is also involved in some way.

PSORIASIS

Psoriasis may affect any part of the body, but most often the elbows, knees, shins, scalp, and lower back. The characteristic bright pink or red plaques covered with silvery scaling are caused by a thickening of the outer skin layers. Psoriasis tends to run in families and usually begins in adolescence. Cold damp conditions, stress, anxiety, or an acute illness may all be triggers.

SYMPTOMS
• Pain (rather than itching) • Cracks in dry areas of the hands and feet
• Pustules on the palms or foot soles (pustular psoriasis) • Glazed but not scaly plaques in moist areas of the body (flexural psoriasis)
• Distortion and pitting of the nails in some cases

TREATMENT
Chinese Herbalism
Dittany bark and puncture vine fruit may help with itching.

Traditional Home and Folk Remedies
Take at least 1 tablespoonful of olive oil a day and at least one raw vegetable salad. (See page 156.)
Garlic is cleansing, and may ease the symptoms and prevent attacks. (See page 79.)

Herbalism
Licorice may help with inflammation. (See page 132.)
Yarrow used twice weekly in bath water has proved beneficial in some cases. (See page 74.)
Nettle tea and products based on nettles may be helpful. (See page 194.)

Aromatherapy
Sedative and antidepressant oils such as lavender and chamomile can help to reduce the stress that exacerbates the condition. Use in the bath, massage, and skin creams. (See pages 143 and 149.)
Bergamot essential oil, cajeput, and Roman chamomile can all be used as a beneficial massage oil. They may also be added to a bath, or placed in a vaporizer. (See pages 107, 149, and 151.)

Nutrition
Increase your intake of protein, vitamin A (as beta-carotene), vitamin C, vitamin E, selenium, and B-complex vitamins as part of a balanced diet or a good supplement. (See pages 206–219.)

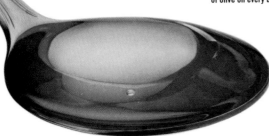
Take at least 1 tablespoon of olive oil every day.

URTICARIA

Urticaria is an allergic condition also known as hives or nettle rash. The rash of raised, whitish-yellow areas of skin surrounded by red inflammation is caused by the release of histamine into the tissues in response to triggers which may include heat, cold, sunlight, scabies, bites and stings, contact with plants, food additives, sensitivity to certain foods, and stress or anxiety. Acute urticaria typically develops very quickly, and usually disappears just as quickly; chronic urticaria is more persistent.

SYMPTOMS
• Rash of weals, especially on limbs and trunk • Intense itching
• Swelling of the tongue and larynx may occur, possibly interfering with breathing • A feverish feeling • Possibly nausea

TREATMENT
Ayurveda
Aloe vera can be used topically to soothe the rash. (See page 80.)

Chinese Herbalism
The source of urticaria is considered to be heat and wind when red; and heat, cold and wind for a cold white rash. Treatment may include Fang Feng (ledebouriella). (See page 144.)

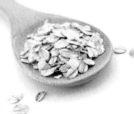
An oatmeal bath will soothe urticaria.

Traditional Home and Folk Remedies
Add a few tablespoons of baking soda to the bath to relieve itching. (See page 202.)
An oatmeal bath will soothe the rash. (See page 84.)
Add a cupful of vinegar to the bath water to restore the balance of the skin. (See page 204.)

Herbalism
An infusion of chickweed (*Stellaria media*) and chamomile can be used to bathe the affected area. (See page 149.)
Lemon balm and heartsease (*Viola tricolor*) can be drunk 3 times daily to soothe and reduce inflammation. (See page 152.)
For urticaria brought on by anxiety and stress, drink an infusion of valerian twice daily. (See page 195.)
Urtica Urens, or nettle, cream will soothe and promote healing. (See page 194.)

Aromatherapy
A warm bath with essential oil of chamomile or lemon balm will soothe the skin and help to prevent stress-related attacks. (See pages 149 and 152.)

Flower Essences
Impatiens is very useful for people whose rashes are associated with feelings of irritability and impatience. Take internally or mix into a neutral cream. (See page 140.)

PRICKLY HEAT

Prickly heat, or heat rash, occurs as a result of sweat duct blockage (probably due to excessive dampness of the skin) in particularly hot and humid weather. It produces a rash of red spots on the face and/or body, which usually disappears within hours of the sufferer moving into the shade, or his or her acclimatization. The rash is a result of salt crystals forming in the sweat gland ducts. Occasionally, prickly heat may develop into patches of eczema. Children, the elderly, and the obese are all particularly susceptible.

SYMPTOMS
• Constant prickling or itching sensation • Tiny blisters may form in severe cases

TREATMENT
Herbalism 🌿
Chickweed infusions (*Stellaria media*) can be made into cool compresses and applied to the affected area. Chickweed ointment can be applied as needed.

Aromatherapy 🜄
Add a few drops of lavender and sandalwood oils to a little calendula oil, and massage into the affected area. (See pages 93, 143, and 179.)

Homeopathy 🜖
Apis, taken every 2 hours for up to 10 doses. (See page 203.)

Flower Essences ⚘
Impatiens is very useful for itching. Take internally or mix into a neutral cream. (See page 140.)
Rescue Remedy, taken internally or applied externally in a cream or wash, helps most skin troubles. (See page 158.)

Nutrition ✕
Consume plenty of vitamin C, which will help to discourage itching and the rash. (See page 210.)

Citrus fruit is a good source of vitamin C, needed to alleviate skin problems.

To help sweaty feet, rub a little cypress oil into the skin.

PERSPIRATION

Perspiration is generally stimulated by heat and is the body's way of regulating temperature. Excessive sweating (or hyperhidrosis) is caused by overactive sweat glands. It may be confined to specific areas such as the palms of the hands, armpits, groin and feet, or it may occur all over the body. When perspiration exceeds the bounds of what is considered normal, it may be due to an overactive thyroid gland, the menopause, prolonged fever, or stress or other psychological factors.

SYMPTOMS
• Body odor may occur if perspiration contacts bacteria on the skin • In severe cases, skin may become damp and damaged

TREATMENT
Chinese Herbalism 🥣
Excess sweating is thought to be caused by a deficiency of qi or yin. (See pages 22–23.)
For yin deficiency, use Mai Men Dong (ophiopogon), Huang Bai (cork tree bark), and Bai Shao (peony root). (See pages 157, 159, and 162.)
Try Fang Feng (ledebouriella) and Huang Qi (astragalus) for deficient qi. (See pages 87 and 144.)

Herbalism 🌿
Marigold infusion can be drunk to produce a perspiration increase, when necessary. (See page 93.)
A herbal deodorant would include cloves, myrrh, coriander seeds, senna, lavender, and thyme, in equal amounts and ground to a powder. Use in the bath, or under the arms. This may cause a rash in sensitive people. (See pages 99, 112, 113, 125, 143, and 190.)

Aromatherapy 🜄
Cypress oil is astringent and refreshing, and can be massaged into the feet for excess perspiration, or combined with lavender oil in a light massage oil and massaged under the arms. (See page 117.)
Oils with deodorizing properties are bergamot, clary sage, eucalyptus, neroli, petitgrain, and rosewood. (See page 47.)
Detoxifying oils include fennel, garlic, juniper, and rose. (See pages 79, 128, 142, and 174.)
Basil, chamomile, juniper, peppermint, and tea tree oils promote sweating, if there is a lack of it. (See page 47.)

SUNBURN

Sunburn occurs on exposure to bright sunlight and is caused by the effects of ultraviolet light. It is most likely to affect people with pale complexions or those who are unused to being in the sun.

SYMPTOMS
• Reddened skin • Extreme soreness • A sensation of heat in burned areas • Blistering in severe cases

TREATMENT
Ayurveda
Aloe vera can be used on burned areas to soothe and to heal. (See page 80.)

Traditional Home and Folk Remedies
Rub a little vitamin E oil into the affected area, soon after the burning, to help the healing process and prevent peels and scarring. (See page 211.)

Herbalism
Urtica Urens (nettle) ointment eases the pain and helps to prevent skin damage. (See page 194.)

Aromatherapy
Add a few drops of lavender and chamomile oils to a tub of live yogurt, and apply to affected areas to soothe, encourage healing, and reduce inflammation. (See pages 142, 143, and 149.)

Flower Essences
Rescue Remedy cream heals damaged tissue and reduces discomfort. (See page 158.)

Vitamin E oil encourages the sunburned skin to repair itself. Rub it in as an aftersun treatment.

WARTS

A wart is a small, hard growth, usually brown or flesh-colored, on the skin. It may be caused by any one of 30 strains of the human papilloma virus. Warts are highly contagious, but not dangerous, and can occur more frequently when the immune system is compromised.

SYMPTOMS
• Small, hard growth on the skin • Verrucas may be painful if they are on a weight-bearing part of the foot

TREATMENT
Traditional Home and Folk Remedies
Rub fresh lemon into the wart daily, and keep moist (with a plaster), paring back any hardened skin. (See page 108.)
Rub fresh garlic into the wart to fight the fungal infection, and eat lots of garlic to boost immunity. (See page 79.)
Mix castor oil and baking soda into a paste, and apply at night with a plaster, leaving it exposed during the day. (See page 202.)

Herbalism
Squeeze the fresh sap of a dandelion stalk onto the wart every day until it disappears. (See page 188.)

Aromatherapy
Apply a little lemon oil directly to the wart; continue treatment until the wart disappears. (See page 108.)
When the wart disappears, add a few drops of lavender oil to vitamin E oil and apply to the area for a week, to encourage healing and prevent scarring and further infection. (See page 143.)
Body massage with rosemary, juniper, or geranium helps to strengthen the immune system. (See pages 142, 161, and 175.)

USEFUL FACTS
• The common wart, verruca vulgaris, may occur anywhere.
• Verruca plana is a round, yellowish, flat-topped wart found mainly on the backs of the hands.
• Verruca filiformis is a long, thin wart found on the eyelids, armpits, and neck.
• The venereal wart, a pink, cauliflower-like growth, is found on the genitals and is sexually transmitted.

Rub fresh lemon juice into a wart.

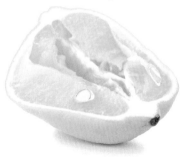

CAUTION
Genital warts must be treated in an STD or GU (genitourinary) clinic. Treatment can be complemented by healing remedies, but only under the care of a registered practitioner.

Massage tea tree oil
into the scalp.

DANDRUFF

Dandruff occurs when the fine cells of the outer layer of skin on the scalp are shed at a faster rate than normal, causing the characteristic flakes of dead skin. This is caused by a disorder of the sebaceous glands. If too little sebum is secreted the hair is dry and dandruff appears as white flakes; if too much sebum is produced the hair is greasy, and the dandruff yellow. The flakes are usually most obvious after brushing or combing the hair, which loosens them. Certain types of seborrheic dermatitis are also responsible for dandruff, which will cause inflammation and itchiness in addition to flaking.

SYMPTOMS
• Flaking scalp • In seborrheic dermatitis, inflammation and itchiness

TREATMENT
Herbalism
To improve circulation to the scalp, rosemary is the herb of choice, taken internally as a tea and used as an application:
For dry hair, rub rosemary-infused oil into the scalp before washing. For greasy hair, add rosemary vinegar or a few drops of rosemary essential oil to the rinsing water. (See page 175.)
Take a combination of the herbs burdock, bladderwrack, and heartsease (*Viola tricolor*) internally to improve the general condition of the scalp. (See pages 85 and 129.)

Aromatherapy
Rosemary, cedarwood, tea tree, or patchouli can be massaged into the scalp, added to unscented shampoos, and used in the final rinse when washing your hair. (See pages 100, 150, 166, and 175.)
Dilute lavender oil in a little almond or coconut oil and massage into the scalp to eliminate dandruff. (See page 143.)

Nutrition
Increase your intake of selenium, vitamin E, vitamin C, B-complex vitamins, and zinc. (See pages 206–209, 210, 211, 219, and 221.)

HAIR LOSS

Baldness, or alopecia, may be temporary or permanent. It is normal to shed about 150 hairs a day, but sometimes this number may be increased by stresses on the body. Hereditary hair loss, often called pattern baldness, affects men far more than women, because it depends on the influence of the male hormone testosterone. Other causes of hair loss include severe illness with high fever, severe nutritional deficiency, pregnancy and childbirth, shock, stress, damage to the skin (from burns, infection, radiation), skin cancer, chemotherapy, excess of vitamin A, hypothyroidism, and syphilis.

SYMPTOMS
• Partial or total loss of scalp hair

TREATMENT
Chinese Herbalism
Hair loss is attributed to deficient liver and kidneys, and specific herbs to address this include Gou Qi Zi (wolfberry) and Ye Jiao Teng (fleeceflower vine). (See pages 147 and 167.)

Traditional Home and Folk Remedies
Sage tea, drunk and applied externally, will stimulate hair growth. (See page 177.)
Nettle tea helps to cleanse the system, and encourages the growth of hair. (See page 194.)

Herbalism
Improve circulation to the head with daily intake of rosemary tea and shoulder stands. (See page 175.)
Massage the scalp with infused oil of fenugreek or ginger. (See pages 191 and 200.)
Rinse with nettle vinegar. (See page 194.)

Aromatherapy
Lavender, rosemary, clary sage, cedarwood, patchouli, or ylang ylang can be massaged into the scalp and added to mild unfragranced shampoos. (See page 47.)

Nutrition
Increase your intake of vitamin B-complex (high-dosage tablet, twice daily), choline, inositol, calcium, magnesium, vitamins, and minerals in a good supplement. (See pages 206–232.)

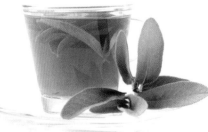

If you suffer from hair loss, try drinking sage tea to stimulate growth. Make it by pouring a cup of boiling water on 1–2 teaspoonfuls of leaves.

BOILS

A boil is a swollen, pus-filled area occurring on the site of an infected hair follicle. The staphylococcus bacterium is usually responsible, but other causes may include eczema, scabies, diabetes, poor personal hygiene, or obesity. A boil begins as a painful red lump, then hardens and forms a yellow head. The most common areas for boils to appear are the back of the neck, the groin, and the armpits. A boil on an eyelash is known as a stye, and where a group of adjacent hair follicles are affected the resultant boil is known as a carbuncle.

SYMPTOMS
• Burning, throbbing sensation in and around the affected area
• Sensitivity to the slightest touch once pus has formed

TREATMENT
Traditional Home and Folk Remedies
Apply a warm poultice made with figs or honey to the affected area. (See pages 126 and 203.)
Soak a sterile cloth with hot thyme tea and hold it over the boil for a time. (See page 190.)
A hot cabbage leaf poultice, applied to the area, will help to draw out the infection. (See page 92.)
Eat plenty of garlic if you are prone to boils; garlic is cleansing and chronic boils indicate that you may have a high level of toxins in your body. (See page 79.)

Herbalism
Drink infusions of thyme or red clover (*Trifolium pratense*) 3 times daily during attacks. (See page 190.)
Drink echinacea 2 or 3 times daily to boost the immune system and purify the blood. (See page 122.)

Aromatherapy
A warm compress with essential oil of chamomile, lemon, lavender, or thyme will help to bring the boil out. (See page 47.)

Homeopathy
Hep. sulf., for boils that are sensitive and weep easily. This will also bring the boil to a head. (See page 213.)

Draw out the infection with a warm cabbage leaf.

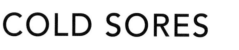

A healthy diet, including plenty of whole grains, prevents many health problems by keeping the immune system at optimum efficiency.

COLD SORES

Cold sores are painful fluid-filled blisters which crust over after bursting. They usually appear on the mouth and around the lips or nose, sometimes in clusters. They are caused by viral infection (herpes simplex). The virus is harbored by most people, most of the time, but is most likely to cause problems when the immune system is compromised, dealing with other viral infections (such as a cold), or when one is run down. Cold sores are highly contagious.

SYMPTOMS
• Pain and soreness from the crusting blister • Cracking and weeping may occur, particularly if sores are in the corners of the mouth

TREATMENT
Herbalism
St. John's wort tincture, applied immediately, should prevent development of a sore. (See page 138.)
Once the cold sore is established, myrrh tincture can be applied sparingly to help dry it up. (See page 112.)

Aromatherapy
Bergamot, eucalyptus, and tea tree oils will help to treat the blisters, and should be applied at the first sign of a sore. (See pages 107, 124, and 150.)
Lavender oil will help to heal blisters that erupt. (See page 143.)

Nutrition
Cold sores crop up when you are run down, so eat healthily and get plenty of the following nutrients, which boost immunity: Wholegrain cereals like brown rice and wholewheat bread, fruit, pulses (beans and lentils), and nuts and seeds for their vital oils.
A daily multivitamin and multimineral preparation – especially one containing antioxidant nutrients. (See page 65.)
Vitamin C stimulates immunity and is antiviral as well as being antifungal. (See page 210.)
Acidophilus will encourage the healthy bacteria in your gut, which will help to fight off infections. (See page 142.)
Zinc stimulates the immune system, and acts as an antiviral and antifungal agent. (See page 221.)

CAUTION
Cold sores are infectious, so wash hands carefully after applying any lotion, and use a personal towel.

ABSCESS

An abscess is a pocket of pus that may occur in any bacterially infected area of the body. White blood cells are sent by the body's defense system to attack the bacteria in question and they do so by engulfing them, thereby creating the pus-filled swelling. Dental abscesses (usually around the root of a tooth) are particularly common, and very painful.

SYMPTOMS
- Swelling, pain, and discomfort in the affected area
- The abscess and surrounding area may feel hot to the touch
- Fever • Nausea • Sweating

TREATMENT
Chinese Herbalism
Treatment would address heat and fire-poison in the blood.
Externally, use Bai Shao (peony root) or Da Huang (rhubarb) ointment. (See pages 159 and 173.)
Internally, Ju Hua (chrysanthemum), dandelion, and Huang Lian (golden thread) are useful. (See pages 113, 188, and 268.)

Traditional Home and Folk Remedies
Apply a warm fig or honey poultice. (See pages 126 and 203.)
Soak a sterile cloth with hot thyme tea and apply. (See page 190.)
A hot poultice, made with cabbage leaves, will help to draw out infection. (See page 92.)

Herbalism
Drink infusions of thyme or red clover (*Trifolium pratense*) 3 times daily during attacks. (See page 190.)
Drink echinacea tea 2 or 3 times daily to boost the immune system and purify the blood. (See page 122.)

Aromatherapy
A warm compress with essential oil of chamomile, lemon, lavender, or thyme will help to bring the abscess out. (See page 47.)

To make a warm fig poultice, use either lightly roasted fresh figs, or dried figs. Split the fig and mash up the interior. Place the mixture on a clean piece of linen, gauze, or cotton. Warm by placing on a hot water bottle.

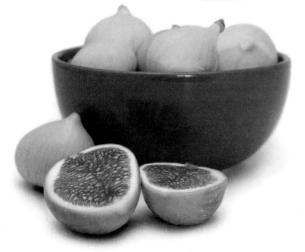

ACNE

Acne is a skin disorder most common among adolescents, although the condition is not confined to adolescence. It is caused by the hormonal changes at puberty, which lead to an increase in the activity of the sebaceous (oil-producing) glands. Sebaceous glands secrete through pores and hair follicles – which are most abundant on the face and scalp – a fatty lubricant known as sebum. Acne occurs when the pores become clogged with sebum. Blackheads – external plugs formed of sebum and dead cells – may be invaded by bacteria, which cause pus-filled inflammations, or pimples. Certain foods may increase irritation in susceptible persons.

SYMPTOMS
- Red spots • Spots may become inflamed, infected, and painful

TREATMENT
Chinese Herbalism
Contact a registered practitioner to discuss Cai Feng Zhen Zhu and Chuang Wan/Margarite acne pills.
Treatments to clear excess heat in the blood and stomach include Ju Hua (chrysanthemum), dandelion, and Jin Yin Hua (honeysuckle), with cucumber and watermelon juice applied externally. (See pages 116, 146, 188, and 268.)

Herbalism
A facial steam with chickweed (*Stellaria media*), elderflower, and marigold may draw out infection. (See pages 93 and 178.)
Take echinacea, burdock root, or yellow dock, sipped 3 times daily as a decoction, to cleanse the system and fight infection. (See pages 85, 122, and 176.)
Massage comfrey ointment into any old spots to reduce scarring. (See page 186.)

Flower Essences
Gorse is useful for people who have given up hope of finding a cure. (See page 192.)

Nutrition
Eliminate processed foods.
Try a multivitamin supplement low in iodine. (See page 60.)
Increase intake of vitamin E, vitamin A, and zinc. (See pages 206, 211, and 221.)

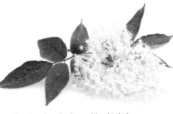
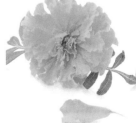

Try steaming the face with a herbal infusion. Put chickweed (top right), elderflower (above), and marigold (right) in a bowl, and pour on boiling water.

IMPETIGO

Impetigo is a highly contagious skin infection caused by bacteria such as streptococci and staphylococci. Infection may follow a break in the skin or occur secondarily to dermatitis, insect bites, and fungus infections. The skin reddens and small, fluid-filled blisters appear on the surface. In severe cases there may be swelling of the lymph nodes in the face or neck, accompanied by fever. Itching is common and scratching can spread the infection. It usually first appears around the mouth and nose, but can spread rapidly if other parts of the body are touched after touching a blister. It can be passed on to others by direct contact or by sharing towels. Impetigo occurs most commonly (although not exclusively) in children, particularly in hot, humid climates.

SYMPTOMS
• Reddening of affected areas • Small fluid-filled blisters which often burst, then dry out to form a yellow crust • Itching • Very rarely, a kidney inflammation or blood poisoning may develop

TREATMENT
Traditional Home and Folk Remedies
Dab the area with cider vinegar, as often as possible throughout the day. (See page 204.)
Clean the area with fresh cabbage juice 2 or 3 times daily. (See page 92.)
Honey is a strong antibiotic and can be applied directly to the sores, and taken internally to boost the immune system. (See page 203.)

Aromatherapy
A few drops of tea tree oil, applied neat to the affected area, will encourage healing and prevent the infection from spreading; it also has immuno-stimulant properties to help your body fight infection. (See page 150.)

Nutrition
Vitamin A is necessary for healthy skin. (See page 206.)
Ensure that you get enough of the B-complex vitamins in your diet. (See pages 206–209.)
Vitamin C will help the body to fight infection. (See page 210.)

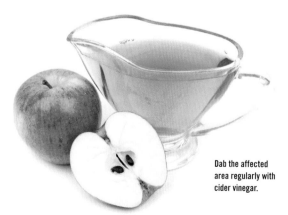
Dab the affected area regularly with cider vinegar.

A rosemary oil blend can be massaged into the base of the nails to help improve circulation.

NAIL PROBLEMS

Nails are subject to several possible problems. Onycholysis is the term for detachment of the nail from its bed. This may occur as a result of a collection of blood (a hematoma) forming underneath it, most commonly caused by injury. Other possible causes of onycholysis include psoriasis, thyrotoxicosis, and fungus infection. Paronychia is an infection of the soft tissue around the nail. It is usually the result of repeated minor injury, causing pain, swelling, and inflammation. Pus may sometimes appear at the nail edge. Horizontal ridges usually indicate an infection in the skin around the nail. Nail thickening is a feature of psoriasis and fungus infection. Nail-biting is an anxiety- or boredom-related habit which, in severe cases, may cause damage to the cuticles and even infection.

SYMPTOMS
• Shedding of the nail • Ridges in the nail • Thickening of the nail • Pus around the nail edges

TREATMENT
Chinese Herbalism
Brittle nails are attributed to the kidneys, and watermelon and nori (seaweed) would be advised. (See page 234.)

Aromatherapy
Add a little rosemary oil to a light carrier oil and massage into the base of the finger and toenails to improve circulation to the area. (See page 175.)
Use tea tree oil on the affected area for bacterial or fungal infections. (See page 150.)

Homeopathy
Silicea, for deformed nails with white spots. (See page 220.)

Nutrition
Take zinc, vitamin C, and vitamin B-complex for fungal infections. (See pages 208–209, 210, and 221.)
White spots are often a sign of a deficiency of zinc or vitamin A. (See pages 206 and 221.)
Deformed nails can be caused by deficiency of vitamins A, B-complex, and C, calcium, magnesium, zinc, and essential fatty acids. (See pages 206–210, 213, 217, 221, and 231.)
Iron deficiency can lead to nail problems. (See page 215.)
Fungal infections can be improved by eating live yogurt each day, or taking acidophilus supplements. (See page 142.)

EDEMA

Edema is swelling or puffiness of tissues due to fluid retention. It is an obvious physical symptom of a number of disorders including kidney disease, heart failure, and cirrhosis of the liver. Edema may also occur as a result of injury (where the injured blood vessels are made more water-permeable) and changes in hormonal levels (before menstruation, during pregnancy, or through the use of oral contraceptives).

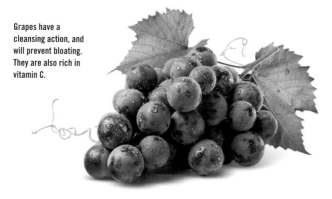

Grapes have a cleansing action, and will prevent bloating. They are also rich in vitamin C.

SYMPTOMS
• Swelling of tissues • May be accompanied by weight gain and breathing difficulties

TREATMENT
Chinese Herbalism
The problem is thought to be excess water and kidney deficiency; useful herbs include Ren Shen (ginseng), Fu Ling (poria), and Gui Zhi (cinnamon twigs). (See pages 104, 160, and 168.)
Wu Ling San pills tonify the spleen yang to move water and resolve edema, particularly edema of the lower abdomen.
Jin Gui Shen Qi Wan formula tonifies the kidney yang to resolve edema, particularly of the lower legs.

Traditional Home and Folk Remedies
Evening primrose oil, taken in capsule form daily, can help to prevent water retention. (See page 231.)
Swelling can be relieved by eating fresh apples. (See page 148.)
Celery is also a good diuretic, and acts on the kidneys to encourage their action. (See page 84.)
Eat fresh grapes to prevent bloating.

Herbalism
Yarrow, dandelion, and uva ursi are diuretics, and they can be drunk three times daily, as required. (See pages 74, 85, and 188.)

Aromatherapy
Essential oils of rosemary, lavender, and geranium will help to reduce bloating and discourage depression. (See page 47.)
Rub a little cedarwood, fennel, rosemary, or sandalwood oils, blended in a light carrier oil, into the areas most affected. (See pages 100, 128, 175, and 179.)

SCABIES

Scabies is an infestation of the skin by the mite *Sarcoptes scabiei*, or itch mite. The mites burrow in the skin to lay eggs, particularly in the sides of the fingers, the elbows, groin, buttocks, nipples, and penis. The newly hatched mites reach adulthood within 14 days, and they, in turn, mate on the skin, thus perpetuating the infestation. Scabies is extremely infectious and can be transmitted by direct or indirect contact.

SYMPTOMS
• Intense itching, particularly at night • Rash, which may become infected as a result of scratching

TREATMENT
Aromatherapy
Use tea tree or lavender oil on the sores, to heal and prevent itching and inflammation. (See pages 143 and 150.)
Rub the whole body with neat lavender oil, then make a solution of lavender, aspic, and juniper in 4 teaspoons of vodka, and use that daily until symptoms improve. (See pages 142 and 143.)

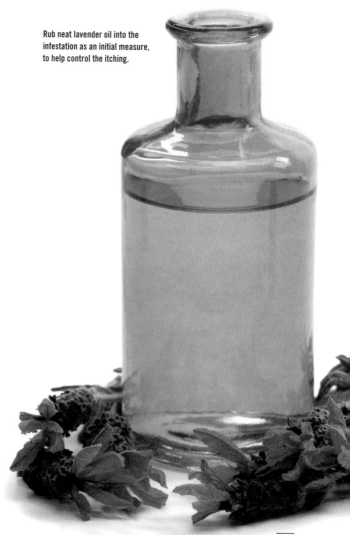

Rub neat lavender oil into the infestation as an initial measure, to help control the itching.

CELLULITE

Cellulite, believed to be accumulations of fat under the skin, is far more prevalent among women than men, and is thought to have some links with female hormones. Possible triggers are poor circulation, alcohol, refined sugars, and caffeine, which contribute to the build-up of toxins in the body.

SYMPTOMS
• Areas of skin with a dimpled orange peel appearance which may be slightly tender • Occurs predominantly on the buttocks, hips, thighs, and upper arms

TREATMENT
Traditional Home and Folk Remedies
Eat fresh parsley, which is a good detoxificant and diuretic. (See page 162.)

Herbalism
Massage with juniper-infused oil and take a cleansing tea with herbs such as marigold. (See pages 93 and 142.)
Fresh ginger improves circulation in the body; drink an infusion, or chew fresh ginger daily. (See page 200.)
Juniper berries are cleansing and detoxifying, and chewing them can help prevent and treat cellulite. (See page 142.)

Aromatherapy
A blend of geranium and rosemary or grapefruit, juniper or cypress, can be used in massage and skin lotion, or added to the bath while using a loofa to stimulate tissues. (See page 47.)
Rose oil soothes tissues, and affects liver function, to encourage cleansing. It also strengthens the veins, which helps circulation. Add a little to the bath, or massage into the area. (See page 174.)

Nutrition
Avoid cigarettes, caffeine, alcohol, and other toxins, which are believed to build up in the body, and drink plenty of fresh water to flush the system.

Mind–Body Healing
Regular cardiovascular exercise is beneficial for toning muscles and reducing body fat, which can improve the appearance of cellulite. (See page 70.)

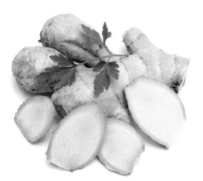

Parsley is a diuretic; it is also high in vitamin C. Fresh ginger stimulates body processes such as circulation.

> **CAUTION**
> Do not use juniper berries in herbal preparations if you have diabetes, as they lower the blood sugar. Do not eat fresh parsley in pregnancy.

CORNS AND CALLUSES

A callus is a hardened and thickened area of skin occurring as a result of constant friction. The skin cells respond to the friction by reproducing, which results in the characteristic hardening of skin. Calluses generally appear on the fingers and toes, knees, palms of the hands, and soles of the feet. When a callus on a toe joint becomes painful, it is known as a corn. The pain is caused by pressure on nerve endings. Soft corns can appear between the toes. Manual laborers are prone to calluses, which can be permanent, while ill-fitting shoes and high heels can be responsible for calluses on the feet or corns.

SYMPTOMS
• Hardened and thickened area of skin • Possibly pain

TREATMENT
Ayurveda
Place your feet in a basin with 4 tablespoons of mustard seeds and some boiling water to soothe. (See page 91.)

Traditional Home and Folk Remedies
Corns can be softened and treated by painting them with fresh lemon juice or vinegar. (See pages 108 and 204.)
Apply compresses of fresh garlic to the area. (See page 79.)

Aromatherapy
Tea tree is a good oil for skin problems, and has mild analgesic and anti-inflammatory properties, which will help to ease the discomfort of corns and calluses. (See page 150.)
Pare the thickening skin away, and apply an emollient cream with rose oil. (See page 174.)

Nutrition
Increased intake of vitamins A and E can help to encourage the health of the skin. (See pages 206 and 211.)

Prepare a compress of fresh garlic, which is a traditional antiseptic treatment for dispersing hard swellings.

ATHLETE'S FOOT

Ahlete's foot (or tinea pedis) is a fungal infection that attacks the warm, moist areas between the toes, most commonly between the fourth and fifth toes. It is highly infectious, spreading through close physical contact, notoriously in the changing facilities at public swimming baths. Once acquired, athlete's foot is very persistent. It usually affects people with particularly sweaty feet, and those whose personal hygiene is inadequate.

SYMPTOMS
• Discomfort and itching • Painful cracks in the skin • Peeling skin
• Dry and scaly or damp and blistered skin • Unpleasant odor
• In severe cases the toenails may crumble

TREATMENT
Traditional Home and Folk Remedies
Apply a little live yogurt to the area daily, for its antifungal properties. (See page 142.)

Herbalism
Echinacea, marigold, and myrrh tinctures, which are antifungal, can be dabbed on the affected area as often as required. (See pages 93, 112, and 122.)

Aromatherapy
A foot bath with tea tree oil, eucalyptus, patchouli, myrrh, and/or lavender is effective as all the oils are soothing and antifungal. Also add to unscented skin lotion. (See page 47.)

Homeopathy
Treatment would be constitutional to boost the immune system, but Silicea might be useful. (See page 220.)

Nutrition
Take extra vitamin C and zinc, to boost immune activity and help fight infection. (See pages 210 and 221.)
Take acidophilus tablets daily to help restore natural bacteria in the body that help to fight fungal infections. (See page 142.)

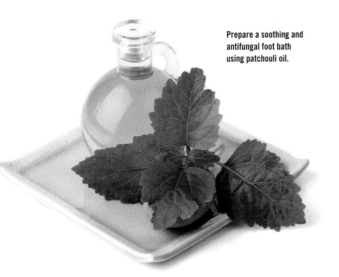

Prepare a soothing and antifungal foot bath using patchouli oil.

CHILBLAINS

A chilblain is a circular, raised, red swelling appearing on the fingers or toes during cold weather. It is caused by the narrowing of small arteries in the cold, which restricts the flow of blood. This leads to tissue damage in the area concerned from shortage of oxygen and glucose fuel, and bacteria may also accumulate there.

SYMPTOMS
• Round red swelling on fingers or toes • Pain and itching

TREATMENT
Chinese Herbalism
Treatment would be aimed at deficient yang qi, and useful herbs include Gui Zhi (cinnamon twigs), red sage, Dang Gui (angelica), and dried ginger. (See pages 82, 104, 177, and 200.)

Traditional Home and Folk Remedies
Ginger, taken internally as a tea or chewed, or externally (in the bath), will warm the body, and both prevent and treat chilblains. (See page 200.)
A roasted onion poultice can be applied to chilblains to draw the heat to the surface and encourage healing. (See page 78.)
A poultice of mustard can be applied to chilblains to warm the area. (See page 91.)

Herbalism
Nettle creams and ointments can be applied to the affected area. Drink nettle tea. (See page 194.)
Improve the general circulation of the body by taking rosemary tea with a pinch of cayenne. (See pages 98 and 175.)
Rub a hot oil made with cayenne, pepper, or mustard over the chilblain. Do not apply this if the skin is broken: use calendula ointment instead. (See pages 91, 93, 98, and 164.)

Aromatherapy
Lemon, lavender, chamomile, cypress, peppermint, or black pepper essential oil can be used in massage, in a bath or foot bath, or dabbed on the affected area. (See page 47.)

Nutrition
Eat plenty of garlic, and brewer's yeast, which will encourage the healthy functioning of the circulatory system. (See pages 79 and 229.)
Increase your intake of oily fish, which are rich in vitamins D and B3.

Add a pinch of cayenne pepper to rosemary tea to improve circulation, or rub a cayenne hot oil over an unbroken chilblain.

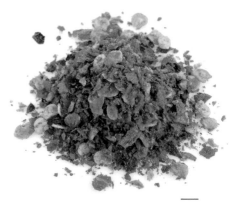

EYE PROBLEMS
GLAUCOMA

Glaucoma results from the pressure of fluid in the eyeball becoming too high. This causes compression and obstruction of the blood vessels that feed the optic nerve, resulting in optic nerve fiber damage and visual disturbances. Untreated, glaucoma leads to blindness, but is usually only found if looked for in routine eye checks. It tends to run in families, and its incidence increases with age. A warning sign of acute glaucoma may be a sub-acute attack, usually at night. In chronic simple glaucoma, the progressive loss of peripheral vision can go unnoticed until the damage is irreversible.

SYMPTOMS
In acute glaucoma:
• Painful, red eye, hard to touch • Possibly dilated pupil • Misting of vision, then severe visual impairment • Nausea and/or vomiting
• Possibly abdominal pain
In sub-acute glaucoma:
• Visual disturbances such as seeing concentric rings around lights
• Fogginess of vision • Dull aching pain in the eye
In chronic simple glaucoma:
• Slow loss of peripheral vision • Loss of central vision follows

TREATMENT
Flower Essences
When symptoms begin, take Rescue Remedy, which will calm you and help you to deal with the pain. (See page 158.)

Nutrition
Avoid excessive quantities of protein in your diet, which can exacerbate or contribute to glaucoma.
Ensure you have an adequate intake of vitamins A, B1, B12, C, and the minerals chromium and zinc, which can contribute to the health of the eyes. (See pages 206, 209, 210, 214, and 221.)

> **CAUTION**
> Symptoms of acute or sub-acute glaucoma require urgent medical attention.

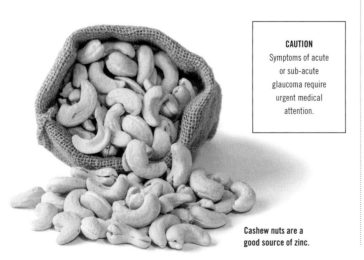

Cashew nuts are a good source of zinc.

CATARACT

A cataract is an opacification of the edges of the lens of the eye which has spread inward to reach the part of the lens that is directly behind the pupil. It is caused by a coagulation of the proteins of the lens. Cataracts are often hereditary or a part of aging, but may also be a feature of Down's syndrome, diabetes, nutritional deficiencies, severe skin problems, or long-term use of steroids. Radiation or injury to the eye can also cause cataracts, and they may be present at birth as a result of German measles during pregnancy.

A Chinese herbalist may prescribe chrysanthemum flowers.

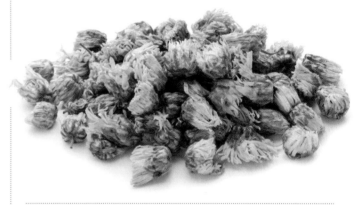

SYMPTOMS
• Progressive loss of image clarity and blurring • Change in the perception of colors • Scattering of light rays, which can make night driving difficult or dangerous • A person with a fully formed cataract may only distinguish light and dark

TREATMENT
Chinese Herbalism
Treatment would address weak liver and kidneys resulting from deficient blood. Herbal remedies include Gou Qi Zi (wolfberry) and Ju Hua (chrysanthemum). (See page 147.)

Homeopathy
Silicea, if your cataract has begun to affect your sight. (See page 220.)
Phosphorus, for a misting sensation. (See page 219.)
Calcarea, when circular lines are evident on the lens. (See page 213.)

Nutrition
Increase your intake of antioxidants, including vitamins A, C, and E, and also selenium, which prevent the growth of cataracts in the eyes. (See pages 206, 210, 211, and 219.)
Bioflavonoids will help in prevention and treatment, and these can be taken separately or in conjunction with vitamin C. (See pages 210 and 228.)

> **CAUTION**
> Always seek advice from a qualified physician.

BLACK EYE

A "black eye" (known medically as a periorbital hematoma) is the result of blood being released from veins in the eyelids and surrounding area into the tissues around the eye. This produces the characteristic blackish-blue bruising.

SYMPTOMS
• Soreness in and around the eye • Pain on pressure • Swelling, which may make it difficult to open the eye

TREATMENT
Herbalism 🌸
Make an infusion of fresh lavender leaves, and wrap it in a fine handkerchief. Place it on the bruised area when the leaves have cooled. (See page 143.)

Traditional Home and Folk Remedies 🖐
Bruise caraway seeds, and heat them with hot, soft bread. Cool slightly and apply to the bruised area. (See pages 97 and 202.)
A cool witch hazel compress can be applied to the area to encourage healing. (See page 134.)
Place a cold compress on the area, which will reduce swelling and allow fluid to circulate, which will facilitate healing.

Aromatherapy 💧
A few drops of calendula, lavender, and marjoram oil can be placed on a cool cloth and applied to the bruise. Avoid the eyelids and the corner of the eye. (See pages 93, 143, and 157.)

Homeopathy 💊
Arnica should be taken as soon as possible after the injury, and continued until the bruising disappears. (See page 86.)

Flower Essences 🌷
Lightly dab Rescue Remedy cream over the affected area to help the healing process. (See page 158.)
Rescue Remedy can be taken internally after the trauma to help you cope with pain and encourage healing. (See page 158.)

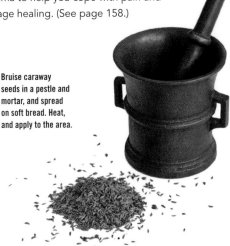

Bruise caraway seeds in a pestle and mortar, and spread on soft bread. Heat, and apply to the area.

CONJUNCTIVITIS

Conjunctivitis is an inflammation of the conjunctiva (the mucous membrane that covers the outer layer of the eyeball and lines the eyelids). It is generally caused by either viral or bacterial infection, or by an allergic reaction to substances such as pollen, cosmetics, and solutions used for contact lenses. Either one or both eyes may be affected. Viral conjunctivitis is a common ailment which sometimes occurs in epidemic proportions, spreading rapidly. It produces only minimal discharge. Bacterial conjunctivitis produces a yellow discharge which hardens during sleep, causing stickiness in and around the eye. Allergic conjunctivitis causes swollen and puffy eyelids, but no discharge.

SYMPTOMS
• Redness of the eyes • Soreness, irritation, and grittiness
• Possibly slightly blurred vision • Possibly discharge

TREATMENT
Ayurveda ⬟
Treatment would consist of panchakarma treatment (detoxification), and nasya, together with inhalations and an eyewash. Treatment would be specific to your needs. (See page 20.)

Chinese Herbalism ✍
The source of the problem is believed to be wind heat in the liver meridians, and herbal treatment might include bamboo leaves, violets, and chrysanthemum flowers. Boil these together, strain, and use the cool water to bathe the eyes. (See page 268.)

Traditional Home and Folk Remedies 🖐
Apply cold bread to closed eyes to reduce the inflammation of conjunctivitis, and soothe itching. (See page 202.)
Boil fennel seeds to make an eyewash for conjunctivitis and sore, inflamed eyes. (See page 128.)
Honey water can be used to cleanse the eye; it acts to destroy any infection, soothe, and encourage healing. (See page 203.)

Herbalism 🌸
Infusions of the following herbs can be taken internally to ease the condition: echinacea (which boosts the immune system and acts as a natural antibiotic), eyebright (also known as euphrasia), golden seal (*Hydrastis canadensis*), and sage. (See pages 122, 125, and 177.)
Infusions of chamomile, elderflower, eyebright (or euphrasia), and golden seal can be applied externally. A tincture of some of these herbs can also be used to make an eyewash. (See pages 125, 149, and 178.)

Aromatherapy 💧
Make a warm compress with a few drops of lavender, chamomile, or rose oil, and apply to the affected area to encourage healing and draw out infection. (See pages 143, 149, and 174.)

EYESTRAIN

Eyestrain is used to describe any discomfort or distress related to the eyes or seeing. It is not, however, a medical term. The body's response to visual difficulty is to contract the muscles around the eye, and it is this that may cause the sensation of strain. Prolonged and constant use of smartphones, computers and tablets, intense periods of reading, wearing incorrectly prescribed glasses, and working in bad light can all lead to eyestrain, but these things do not necessarily damage the eyes as is popularly believed.

SYMPTOMS
• Feeling of tightness around the eyes • Focusing difficulties
• Recurrent headaches, particularly across the forehead and behind the eyes

TREATMENT
Chinese Herbalism
Chinese practitioners believe that eye problems may be due to exhausted blood. Gou Qi Zi (wolfberry) and Ju Hua (chrysanthemum) may be useful. (See pages 147 and 268.)

Traditional Home and Folk Remedies
A slice of cucumber over tired, strained eyes is invigorating and soothing. (See page 116.)
Drink fresh lemon juice, which is restorative. (See page 108.)
Roast an apple and apply the pulp to the eye area to relieve inflamed or tired eyes.
(See page 148.)

The ancient Greeks used fresh white cabbage juice, mixed with a small amount of honey, to relieve sore or inflamed eyes. (See page 92.)

Herbalism
Cool compresses of chickweed (*Stellaria media*), eyebright (also known as euphrasia), or marigold should be placed over the eyes and left for 10–15 minutes. (See pages 93 and 125.)

Aromatherapy
A few drops of fennel oil, on a cool compress laid over the eye area, will soothe puffy, inflamed eyes. (See page 128.)
Add 1 drop of lemon or rose aromatherapy oil to 2 tablespoons of carrier oil, and massage into the temples and the bony areas around the eyes (avoid the immediate eye area). (See pages 108 and 174.)

Homeopathy
The following remedies can be taken up to 4 times per day for a week. If symptoms persist, see your homeopath.
Arnica, for tired eyes resulting from long periods of driving and looking into the distance. (See page 86.)
Nat. mur., when eyes are painful on looking up, down, or sideways. (See page 154.)

Nutrition
Vitamin A and vitamin B12 are useful if you suffer from periodic or chronic eyestrain. (See pages 206 and 209.)

Mind–Body Healing
Take regular breaks from staring at your screen to stretch, breathe, or even meditate for a few minutes. (See page 68.)

Massage the bony areas around the eyes with an aromatherapy oil blend.

STYE

A stye is an abscess occurring around the root of an eyelash, usually caused by staphylococcal bacteria. A collection of pus at the base of the eyelash produces the characteristic small, yellow head. Styes usually last for around seven days, but the infection may spread to adjacent follicles. They tend to occur when general resistance is low.

SYMPTOMS
• Pus at the base of an eyelash • Redness and swelling • Pain
• Irritation

TREATMENT
Chinese Herbalism
Anti-inflammatory herbs, and herbs to detoxify and boost the immune system will be appropriate, including the preparation Jin Yin Hua (honeysuckle flower), which acts as an antibiotic to help fight the bacterial infection. (See page 146.)

Traditional Home and Folk Remedies
A warm bread poultice applied directly to the stye will help bring out the infection. (See page 202.)

Herbalism
Echinacea will boost the immune system, which is particularly useful if you suffer from recurrent styes. (See page 122.)
Chamomile or eyebright (also called euphrasia) can help to reduce swelling. (See pages 125 and 149.)
Marigold tincture can be applied directly to the stye, and taken internally to boost the immune system. (See page 93.)

Aromatherapy
A drop of lavender or tea tree oil, on a cotton swab, can be dabbed at the base of the stye. Take care not to let it enter your eyes. (See pages 143 and 150.)

> **CAUTION**
> Recurrent episodes of styes may be an indication of diabetes and should therefore be investigated.

Marigold treats all skin inflammations. Apply tincture to a stye.

TWITCHING EYELIDS

Twitching (fasciculation) of the eyelids is caused by a brief, involuntary contraction of the flat muscle around the eye. It is a very common phenomenon and is only a cause for concern if it is very persistent, as it may then be an indication of nerve disease. A twitch or tic commonly affecting adults is blepharospasm, in which there is spasmodic closure of one or both eyes. This is usually a feature of psychological disturbance and may be associated with other bodily tics.

SYMPTOMS
• Brief contractions of the muscles around the eye • Spasmodic closure of the eye

TREATMENT
Traditional Home and Folk Remedies
Place a slice of cucumber on the eyes to soothe and reduce irritation. (See page 116.)

Herbalism
Because most twitches are caused by tension or tiredness, relaxing herbs would be prescribed, including chamomile, lavender, and vervain. Drink as infusions. (See pages 143, 149, and 196.)

Aromatherapy
A few drops of lavender or marjoram oil added to the bath will relax and rejuvenate. (See pages 143 and 157.)
Try a few drops of chamomile or rose oil on a cool compress, placed over the eye area, and massage a drop in a light carrier oil into the muscles surrounding the eye area. Avoid the immediate eye area. (See pages 149 and 174.)

Flower Essences
Vervain is useful for those whose overenthusiasm is putting them under stress. (See page 196.)
Hornbeam, for exhaustion and the feeling of being in a rut. (See page 96.)
Impatiens, for irritability and a rushed lifestyle. (See page 140.)

Vervain is antispasmodic. The flower remedy is good for stress.

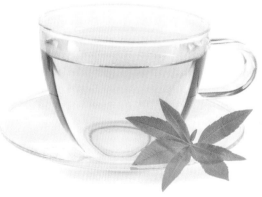

EAR PROBLEMS

MIDDLE EAR INFECTION

The most common ear infections are middle ear infections (otitis media). The middle ear is located behind the eardrum and connected to the throat by the Eustachian tube. Bacteria may therefore travel to the middle ear from the throat when infections occur there, or they may also enter through a perforation in the eardrum. The eardrum may be perforated, or ruptured, by shattering blasts or sharp objects, as well as by infection. Very loud noises, a change in pressure (such as when flying), and violent sneezing while suffering an ear infection may also, in some cases, cause perforation. Young children, with shorter and straighter Eustachian tubes than adults, are especially prone to middle ear infections. The tendency is also apparently inherited. Chronic infections may also be associated with allergies, tuberculosis, measles, and other diseases. In severe cases of otitis media, pressure in the middle ear builds up to such an extent that the eardrum perforates in order to release the discharge. This may lead to external ear infection and a degree of temporary or permanent hearing loss.

SYMPTOMS
• Intense pain • Fever • Discharge
• Sometimes, hearing loss

TREATMENT
Ayurveda
Purified and concentrated extracts of garlic might be used to control and treat infection. (See page 79.)
Panchakarma would be appropriate. (See page 22.)

Traditional Home and Folk Remedies
Peel the skin from a bud of garlic, and cut to fit the outside of the ear canal. Wrap in a piece of gauze, heat gently, and insert into the canal, making sure that the gauze continues to protrude from the ear and you do not push the garlic in too far. (See page 79.)

Herbalism
Mullein oil is a traditional herbal treatment. Place a few drops on a cotton ball and gently place in the ear canal. (See page 195.)
Anti-inflammatory and antibacterial herbs include chamomile, echinacea, golden rod (*Solidago virgaurea*), and golden seal (*Hydrastis canadensis*), and they can be taken internally or infused and dropped into the ear canal. (See pages 122 and 149.)
Steep yarrow and pour the warm liquid into the ear canal to soothe and reduce infection. (See page 74.)

Aromatherapy
Massage a blend of anti-infectious oils around the ear and down the neck. Suitable oils include lavender, chamomile, and tea tree. (See pages 143, 149, and 150.)
Mix a drop of clove oil in a little grapeseed carrier oil and massage around the neck and ear. (See page 125.)

Homeopathy
Chronic ear infections should be treated constitutionally. Acute attacks may respond to Hep. sulf., taken every half-hour for up to 10 doses. (See page 213.)

> **CAUTION**
> If symptoms persist or worsen, consult a physician. Always consult your physician if the eardrum "bursts" or perforates, as it can lead to serious complications, including deafness and, in some cases, meningitis.

Steep yarrow leaves in water, and pour the warm liquid into the ear.

OUTER EAR INFECTION

An inflammation or infection of the outer ear (otitis externa) can cause pain, discharge, and impaired hearing. Such symptoms may be due to infection by fungi or bacteria, or a foreign body in the ear. Boils or abscesses, resulting from infection by *staphylococcus* bacteria, lead to a build-up of pus which causes severe pain in the ear. Fungus infections are sometimes called "swimmer's ear" because dampness is favorable to fungal growth.

SYMPTOMS
• Severe pain • Impaired hearing • Possibly discharge
• Possibly swelling

TREATMENT
Traditional Home and Folk Remedies
A roasted onion can be applied to the outer ear canal (hot) to draw out infection and to ease the pain. (See page 78.)
A bread poultice (see "Earache," page 274) will reduce inflammation and pain. (See page 202.)
Warm a little garlic oil, saturate a cotton bud, and place in the entrance to the ear canal to draw out infection. (See page 79.)

Herbalism
Mullein oil will reduce external pain and encourage healing. St. John's wort oil exerts a similar beneficial effect. (See pages 138 and 195.)
Wash the ear canal with a warm infusion of herbs such as chamomile, elderflower, or golden seal (*Hydrastis canadensis*), which are antiseptic. (See pages 149 and 178.)

Aromatherapy
Apply a little tea tree oil to the end of a cotton bud and gently swab the outer ear canal, and the ear itself. (See page 150.)
Warm some marjoram oil in grapeseed oil, massage around the ear and dab a few drops into the ear canal. Apply a little more to a cotton ball and insert into the ear and leave overnight. This will reduce pain and encourage healing. (See page 157.)

Flower Essences
Take Rescue Remedy to ease symptoms and induce calm. (See page 158.)

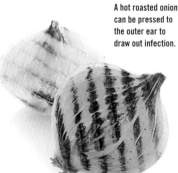

A hot roasted onion can be pressed to the outer ear to draw out infection.

> **CAUTION**
> Do not push any object deep inside the ear. If symptoms persist or worsen, consult a physician.

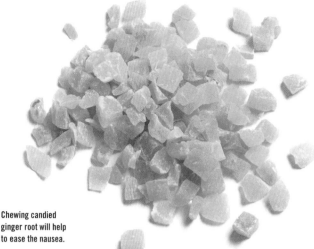

Chewing candied ginger root will help to ease the nausea.

LABYRINTHITIS

Labyrinthitis (otitis interna) is an inflammation of the part of the inner ear responsible for balance (the labyrinth). A viral infection is usually the cause of labyrinthitis (possibly in the course of mumps or flu), although it may be the result of infection spreading through the bone from middle ear infection. Infection may also reach the inner ear (via the bloodstream) from somewhere else in the body. Less commonly, a bacterial labyrinthitis results from a head injury. In labyrinthitis, inflammation of the fluid-filled chambers of the inner ear causes disruption of the individual's sense of balance.

SYMPTOMS
• Spinning sensation • Unsteadiness, faintness, and possibly falling
• Nausea • Vomiting • Partial deafness • Ringing or hissing in the ears (see "Tinnitus," page 275)

TREATMENT
Chinese Herbalism
Fresh ginger, Gui Zhi (cinnamon twigs), and peppermint will help with the dizziness. (See pages 104, 152, and 200.)
Sang Shen (mulberry fruit; *Morus alba*) can nourish the blood.

Herbalism
Treatment to boost the immune system, including echinacea, would be appropriate. (See page 122.)
Ginger root, candied or chewed raw, will help to ease the nausea. (See page 200.)
Chinese angelica can restore energy, and stimulate white blood cells and the formation of antibodies to fight infection. (See page 82.)

Homeopathy
Nat. mur., for symptoms accompanied by a headache and constipation. (See page 154.)
Phosphorus, when dizziness is made worse by looking down. (See page 219.)

> **CAUTION**
> Untreated bacterial inner ear infection may lead to permanent deafness, or spread to cause meningitis.

EARACHE

Earache is particularly common among children. It is usually (but not always) caused by a change in pressure in the middle ear as a result of a failure in the ear's pressure-equalizing mechanism. The failure occurs when the flow of air to and from the middle ear is impeded by a blockage in the Eustachian tube. The other most frequent causes of earache are acute infection of the middle ear or the ear canal (see pages 272 and 273). Pain in the ear area may be a feature of problems in other nearby parts of the body, such as the teeth, jaw, throat, or neck.

SYMPTOMS
• Pain in the ear • Young children may pull or rub on their ear
• Irritability

TREATMENT
Traditional Home and Folk Remedies
Warm a slice of bread with the crusts removed, and pound it with a handful of bruised caraway seeds. Add some hot brandy to make a paste, and apply as a hot poultice to the exterior of the ear to reduce inflammation. (See pages 97 and 202.)
Crush and simmer root ginger and make a poultice to apply to the exterior of the affected ear. (See page 200.)
Roast an onion, and then apply it hot (take care to test first) to the exterior of the ear for relief of pain. (See page 78.)

Herbalism
Apply a little St. John's wort oil to the exterior of the ear, and massage in gently. (See page 138.)
Massage a little warmed olive oil, with a few drops of chamomile or elderflower tincture, around the ear. (See pages 149 and 178.)

Aromatherapy
Make a hot compress, to apply directly to the ears and neck to ease the pain, using diluted chamomile, eucalyptus, lavender, or rosewood oils. When the poultice cools, warm it up by placing it on a hot water bottle. (See pages 83, 124, 143, and 149.)

Homeopathy
Take Chamomilla, which will help with severe pain and need of comfort. (See page 149.)
Try Hep. sulf., for throbbing pain made better by a warm compress. (See page 213.)

Flower Essences
Rescue Remedy can be applied to the temples or taken internally to soothe and reduce any panic. (See page 158.)

USEFUL FACTS
Earache may be a feature of:
• Enlarged adenoids causing Eustachian tube blockage.
• Infection of the middle ear in which the obstruction in the Eustachian tube interferes with fluid drainage.
• A boil or infection by viruses, bacteria, or fungi in the external ear passage.
• Teething in babies, and dental decay.
• Sinusitis.

> **CAUTION**
> Do not put anything inside the ear. Contact a physician if ear pain is accompanied by swelling of the ear, discharge from the ear, fever, vomiting, or hearing loss. Also contact a physician if symptoms persist.

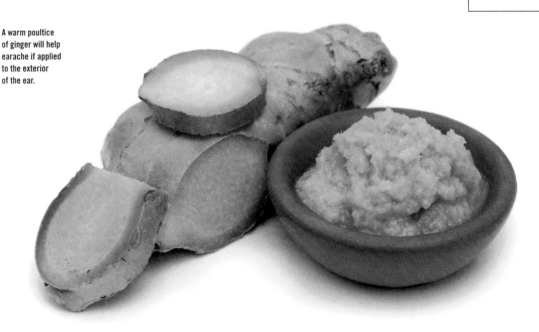

A warm poultice of ginger will help earache if applied to the exterior of the ear.

TINNITUS

Tinnitus is a hissing, buzzing, whistling, or ringing sound experienced in the ear (one or both). It is usually continuous, but the sufferer's awareness of it is intermittent. Tinnitus is related to damage to the hair cells of the inner ear. Persistent tinnitus is usually associated with a degree of hearing loss, and can be triggered by explosions or prolonged loud noise. It may also be a symptom of colds and flu, ear infections and excessive earwax, head injuries, Ménière's disease, otosclerosis, excessive smoking, and drugs such as quinine, antibiotics, aspirin, and alcohol.

SYMPTOMS
• Ringing, whistling, or hissing sound in one ear or both
• A degree of hearing loss

TREATMENT
Herbalism
For tinnitus caused by blood congestion or pressure in the head, try black cohosh (*Actaea racemosa*). Use 10–30 drops of tincture diluted in water, and drink it as often as necessary. (See page 75.)
Feverfew taken daily may prevent attacks. (See page 187.)
Tinnitus caused by poor circulation or high blood pressure may respond to treatment with hawthorn. (See page 114.)

Aromatherapy
Use oils that increase the circulation, including rosemary, cypress, lemon, and rose. Massage of the head, neck, and chest may help, as will one or more in a vaporizer or burner. (See page 47.)

Nutrition
Try increasing intake of magnesium, potassium, and manganese, as deficiency of these has been linked with tinnitus. (See pages 217 and 218.)

Mind–Body Healing
Sufferers find meditation, visualization, or breathing exercises to be useful. For trouble falling asleep, listening to calming music or sounds may help. A physician will pass on details of support groups, counselors with experience of working with tinnitus, occupational therapists, or cognitive behavioral therapists who offer sound therapy. (See pages 68–69.)

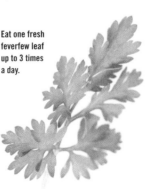

Eat one fresh feverfew leaf up to 3 times a day.

> **CAUTION**
> Tinnitus may be a sign of infection, brain injury, Ménière's disease, or otosclerosis

EARWAX

Earwax is a sticky, fatty secretion produced by the glands in the outer ear to protect the eardrum by trapping dust and small objects. Normal soft wax is disposed of naturally by the ear, but hard or dried wax accumulates. An excess of earwax obstructs the ear canal, and the blockage may be worsened by swimming or bathing since the wax absorbs water.

SYMPTOMS
• A sensation of fullness or aching in the ear • Partial hearing loss

TREATMENT
Chinese Herbalism
Drop a little warmed almond oil into the ear to soften the wax, making it easier to remove. (See page 169.)

Traditional Home and Folk Remedies
A little warmed garlic oil, dropped into the ear, will soften the wax and occasionally dislodge it. (See page 79.)
Use an ear candle (available from health stores) to heat and draw out excess wax.

Herbalism
Make a warm infusion of chamomile, elderflowers, or marigold, or put a few drops of the tincture into some warm water. Using a dropper, place the liquid in the ear canal and stop with a cotton ball. Repeat several nights running until the wax has softened and is absorbed by the cotton. (See pages 93, 149, and 178.)

Aromatherapy
Put a few drops of warm chamomile oil, blended in a light carrier oil, into the ear canal and block gently with a cotton ball. Repeat until wax has softened. (See page 149.)

> **CAUTION**
> Constant prodding or cleaning of the ear can lead to excessive earwax production. Never insert objects, such as cotton buds, into the ear.

A little almond oil dropped into the ear may soften earwax. Use an ear dropper, and lie with the head on a pillow. This allows the oil to penetrate the ear canal.

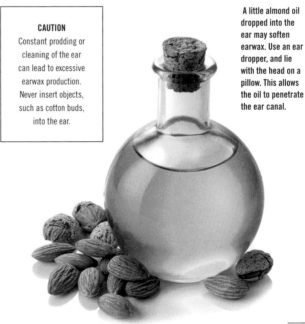

NASAL PROBLEMS
SINUSITIS

Sinusitis is an inflammation of the sinuses, the air-filled cavities located in the bones around the nose. When this occurs the lining of the sinuses swells, causing a blockage in the channel that drains them. A build-up of mucus discharge results, creating intense pressure and pain. Sinusitis usually develops as a complication of a viral infection such as a cold, but pollution or tobacco can also be triggers. Inflammation of the sinuses may also develop from an allergy or from bacteria introduced through the nasal channels, causing an infection accompanied by pain and tenderness. Chronic sinusitis may result from either form or a combination of both. Severe symptoms should be referred to your physician.

SYMPTOMS
• Nasal congestion with thick, stretchy mucus • Nosebleeds
• Sneezing • Loss of sense of smell • Headache with a sensation of pressure in and around the head • Severe pain around the eyes and cheeks (particularly on bending down), sometimes feeling like toothache

TREATMENT
Ayurveda
Treatment will involve the elimination of kapha with nasya (inhalation of oils). Detoxification will be appropriate. (See page 20.) Herbal treatment may be prescribed, including coriander for sinus problems and related headaches. (See page 113.)

Chinese Herbalism
Bi Van Pian pills are very good for sinusitis, especially with sticky yellow nasal discharge that is hard to get out.
A herbal prescription of Cang er Zi San, when there is lots of green nasal discharge, headache and pain.
Xin Yi San, when there is lots of clear or white nasal discharge, nasal congestion, and pain.
Peppermint, Jin Yin Hua (honeysuckle), and Chen Pi (mandarin peel) may be useful. (See pages 109, 146, and 152.)

Grate a freshly peeled horseradish root to a pulp and combine this with lemon juice. Taken between meals, it will help to clear the sinuses.

Traditional Home and Folk Remedies
Peppermint is antispasmodic and decongestant. Infuse some fresh or dried leaves in a bowl of boiling water, and inhale the steam. (See page 152.)
Combine the juice of a fresh peeled and pulped horseradish root with the juice of two or three lemons, and take a half-teaspoon between meals. Use for several months until the mucus in the sinus clears. (See pages 86 and 108.)

Herbalism
Elderflower is excellent for catarrh and sinusitis. Drink an infusion as required to reduce symptoms and encourage healing. (See page 178.)

Aromatherapy
Try steam inhalations of lavender, eucalyptus, and tea tree, which are anticatarrhal and antibacterial. Lavender in particular will act as an anti-inflammatory and ease any painful symptoms. (See pages 124, 143, and 150.)

Nutrition
Many sinusitis cases are caused by food allergy or intolerance. See a practitioner if you suspect this is the cause.

USEFUL FACTS
• More than 50 percent of sinusitis cases are caused by bacterial infection.
• In one U.S. study, 50 percent of sufferers had an immune-system problem.
• 10 percent of all cases are caused by dental problems.
• Maxillary sinusitis can result from a cold or can be caused by swimming in contaminated water.
• Rarely, extraction of a molar tooth will break the floor of the maxillary sinus, leaving an opening for bacteria to enter and cause infection.
• Frontal and ethmoid sinusitis share symptoms of localized headache, surface tenderness, and, occasionally, swelling of the eyelids.
• Sphenoid sinusitis can cause blurred vision because of the proximity of this sinus to the optic nerves.

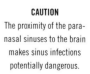

> **CAUTION**
> The proximity of the para-nasal sinuses to the brain makes sinus infections potentially dangerous.

CATARRH

Catarrh is the term used to describe the overproduction of thick phlegm by the mucous membranes of the air passages to the lungs, the larynx, the nose, and sinuses. Cells which produce and secrete a watery mucus are present in the mucous membranes, which line the passages, and they are composed of large, thin-walled veins whose blood supply serves to warm incoming air. Inflammation of the membranes as a result of a cold or flu is the usual cause, but other triggers include smoking, inhalation of dust, chronic sinusitis, upper respiratory tract infection, and allergy. A series of colds in close succession may lead to chronic catarrh. Complementary therapists believe that chronic catarrh that is not obviously due to viral or bacterial infection, allergy, chemical irritants, or dry air (all of which irritate or inflame the mucous membranes) is a symptom of general toxicity of the body catarrh and is the body's attempt to rid itself of toxins that are not being adequately dealt with by the liver, or properly excreted by the kidneys, bowels, and skin.

SYMPTOMS
• Blocked, possibly painful nose • Excessively runny nose • Cough with phlegm • Earache • Ulcers may develop on the septum (the bone that separates the nostrils) • Possibly nosebleeds

TREATMENT
Ayurveda
Coriander can help to relieve sinus problems and prevent the build-up of catarrh. Brown the seeds and boil them in water with root ginger. Boil until the liquid is reduced and drink (with a little honey) as required. (See pages 113 and 200.)

Chinese Herbalism
Drink ginger or sage tea, and drink onion water with a pinch of cayenne pepper. (See pages 78, 98, 177, and 200.)

Traditional Home and Folk Remedies
Peppercorns will help to clear catarrh. Chew one at a time, followed by a little hot water, and continue until the symptoms have gone. (See page 164.)
Eating either raw or cooked onions helps to purge stubborn catarrh. (See page 78.)
Try a drop of fresh lemon in each nostril. This is slightly painful, but enormously powerful! (See page 108.)
Mustard powder can be added to a foot bath to help decongest nasal passages and clear catarrh. (See page 91.)

Herbalism
Herbs such as golden rod (*Solidago virgaurea*), elderflower, and euphrasia are anticatarrhal and astringent. When catarrh is accompanied by infection, supplement with echinacea and garlic. (See pages 79, 122, 125, and 178.)

Aromatherapy
Thyme and eucalyptus oils may be inhaled to ease symptoms, and it is a good idea to keep niaouli by the bed, as it can help you to sleep. (See pages 124, 151, and 190.)
Many oils are decongestant and expectorant, including chamomile, hyssop, mint, niaouli, pine, and clary sage. Rub into the chest and temples in a light carrier oil, or place several drops in a bowl of boiling water and inhale. (See page 47.)

Homeopathy
Chronic catarrh should be treated constitutionally, but the following remedies may be helpful:
Nat. mur., for catarrh resembling raw egg white, with a dry nose and the loss of taste and smell. (See page 154.)
Calcarea, for yellow and smelly catarrh. (See page 213.)

Nutrition
Increase your intake of vitamin C and zinc, which help to reduce symptoms. (See pages 210 and 221.)
If you are prone to chronic catarrh, cut down on intake of dairy produce, which may exacerbate the condition. (See pages 59.)
Catarrh may also be caused by overconsumption of sugar and too many refined carbohydrates.
Ensure that your home is free of dust and avoid smoking.

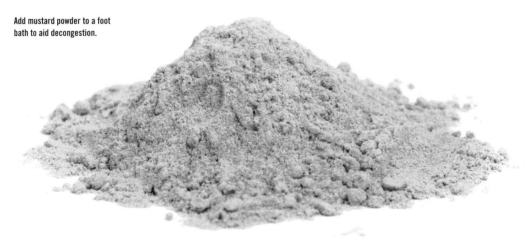

Add mustard powder to a foot bath to aid decongestion.

HAY FEVER

Hay fever (also known as allergic rhinitis) is an allergic reaction to airborne irritants such as grass, tree, or flower pollens. These allergens (and others including dust, animal fur, feathers, spores, plants, and chemicals) trigger a reaction that causes swelling of the nasal membrane and the production of the antibodies which release histamine. It is this chemical substance that is responsible for the characteristic allergic symptoms.

SYMPTOMS
• Runny nose and congestion • Sneezing • Red, itchy eyes
• Sore throat • Wheezing, which can develop into asthma

TREATMENT

Chinese Herbalism
Bi Van Pian, or "nose inflammation" pills, may be prescribed for wind cold or wind heat to the face: sneezing, itchy eyes, facial congestion and sinus pain, acute and chronic rhinitis, and nasal allergies.
A herbal prescription of Yu Ping Feng San, or "jade screen," helps prevent hay fever, and guards against allergies.
Cang er Zi Tang, or xanthium powder, is for allergic rhinitis with a thickened yellow catarrh or a blocked nose.

Traditional Home and Folk Remedies
A teaspoon of local honey, before and during the season, helps many people. (See page 203.)
Eat plenty of fresh garlic to boost the immune system, and to act as an anticatarrhal agent. (See page 79.)

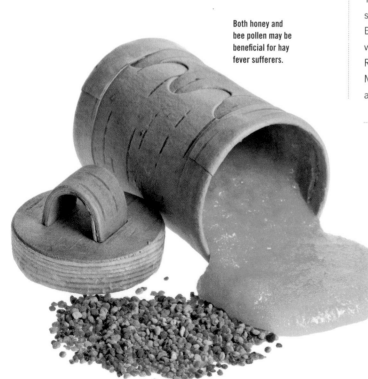

Both honey and bee pollen may be beneficial for hay fever sufferers.

Herbalism
Strengthen resistance with a tea of elderflowers and yarrow for some weeks before the pollen season starts. (See pages 74 and 178.)
Soothe itchy eyes with an elderflower, euphrasia, or chamomile compress. (See pages 125, 149, and 178.)
Euphrasia tea or capsules will relieve symptoms. (See page 125.)

Aromatherapy
Chamomile in the bath and in massage will help to ease symptoms. (See page 149.)
Steam or dry inhalations of lavender and/or eucalyptus can help for sneezing and runny nose. Also use in the bath. (See pages 124 and 143.)
Lemon balm may calm the allergic reaction. (See page 152.)

Homeopathy
Hay fever can be deep-seated and take some time to cure, and treatment should be constitutional. However, there are preventive remedies, including the following:
Allium, for hay fever where the sufferer has a burning nasal discharge. (See page 78.)
Euphrasia, when the eyes are itching and red. (See page 125.)

Flower Essences
Rescue Remedy will help to ease symptoms during an attack, and help to produce a more positive frame of mind. (See page 158.)

Nutrition
Vitamin C combined with bioflavonoids will act as a natural antihistamine to control symptoms. (See pages 210 and 228.)
Taking extra pantothenic acid may help to relieve hay fever symptoms. (See page 208.)
Bee pollen can help prevent allergies when taken for several weeks before the hay fever season. (See page 228.)
Royal jelly is also a useful hay fever treatment. (See page 234.)
Magnesium, found in bananas, may help to quell a hay fever attack. (See page 217.)

USEFUL FACTS
• The timing of hay fever symptoms will depend on the type of pollen at fault: tree pollen and grass pollen are released during spring and summer; weeds such as nettles, golden rod, and mugwort release their pollen in autumn. In the autumn, spores and mould are also likely to cause hay fever.
• Most cases involve some dermatitis (in the form of urticaria or hives), and temporary asthma is common during the hay fever seasons in susceptible people.
• Babies born in the spring, when more pollen is in the air, are more likely to develop hay fever later in life.

DISTURBED SENSE OF SMELL

The olfactory nerves in the nose have many hair-like nerve fibers or smell receptors. When we sniff, a waft of air passes over the receptors, allowing us to identify a smell. Loss of the sense of smell (or "anosmia"), whether temporary or permanent, can be debilitating. It may occur as a result of colds, or a head injury in which damage is sustained to the twigs of the olfactory nerve. Taste and smell are distinct. In the case of taste, chemicals that evoke sweet, sour, bitter, salty, and umami stimulate taste bud receptors in the throat and on the tongue and palate. This stimulation triggers nerve cells to send signals to the brain stem. Odors register in the brain when airborne chemicals stimulate receptors on the olfactory epithelium, high in the nose. However, the olfactory system is vitally important in determining food flavors. During chewing, odor-laden air is forced from the rear of the oral cavity to the olfactory receptors, evoking many flavor sensations that people usually associate with taste but which are almost completely dependent on the sense of smell.

SYMPTOMS
• Change in or loss of sense of smell • Decreased perception of taste

TREATMENT
Ayurveda
The senses are linked to the elements in Ayurvedic medicine, and any imbalance can be adjusted through balancing treatment. Treatment will be specific to the patient's needs. (See page 20.)

Nutrition
A zinc deficiency can cause problems with your sense of smell. Ensure that you have an adequate dietary intake, or take a daily supplement of zinc. (See page 221.)

> **CAUTION**
> Very rarely, cancer patients report specific smell and taste changes. If you suddenly develop an acute sense of smell, see your physician.

Oysters are an excellent source of zinc. Eat them raw or cooked in a tasty soup or chowder.

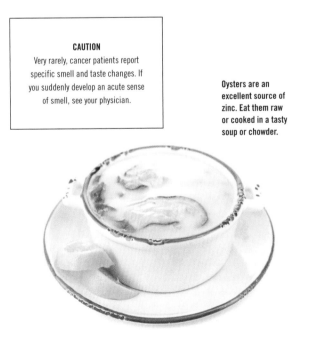

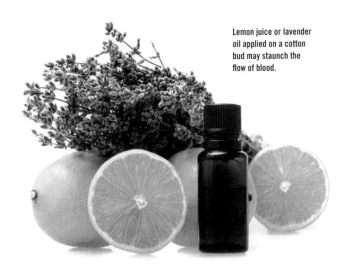

Lemon juice or lavender oil applied on a cotton bud may staunch the flow of blood.

NOSEBLEEDS

Nosebleeds are very common, resulting either from persistent probing, an injury, infection of the mucous membrane, or from drying and crusting. Injury or infection that damages the moist lining of the nose can quite easily rupture tiny local blood vessels and cause bleeding. More often, bleeding occurs for no apparent reason. There is some association between nosebleeds and high alcohol intake.

SYMPTOMS
• Intermittent bleeding from the nose • Possibly nasal soreness

TREATMENT
Traditional Home and Folk Remedies
Leaning forward and lightly pinching the sides of the nose can often stem a nosebleed.
Lemon is a natural styptic. Place a drop in the offending nostril, on the end of a cotton bud. (See page 108.)

Aromatherapy
Lavender oil, placed in the nostril on a cotton bud, will encourage healing and help staunch the blood. (See page 143.)

Homeopathy
Arnica, for a nosebleed brought on by injury or bruising. (See page 86.) Phosphorus, for a nosebleed brought on by blowing the nose violently. (See page 219.)

Flower Essences
A few drops of Rescue Remedy diluted in water and placed in the nostril may encourage the healing process. (See page 158.)

> **CAUTION**
> Nosebleeds that do not stop within a couple of hours should be checked by a physician. Do not stem the bleeding too quickly in those suffering from high blood pressure: allow the bleeding to continue for 10 minutes before taking action. Contrary to popular myth, nosebleeds are not always a sign of high blood pressure, but if you are over 40, or suspect high blood pressure, see your physician.

DENTAL PROBLEMS
GINGIVITIS

Gingivitis is inflammation of the gums. It may sometimes occur as a result of infection or ill-fitting dentures, but most usually it is caused by an accumulation of plaque and impacted food around and under the gums. Left untreated, gingivitis may lead to loosening of the affected tooth (periodontitis) through damage to the membrane securing it. It is a very common problem, particularly during pregnancy. Gingivitis may also result from systemic disorders such as vitamin C deficiency (scurvy) and endocrine disturbances (diabetes mellitus). Prevention and treatment include good oral hygiene and control or correction of local and systemic factors. The incidence of gingivitis appears to increase with age: at 10 years old, 15 percent of the U.S. population suffer; by the age of 50, more than 50 percent have gingivitis. A blood test can now detect gum disease six months before symptoms set in.

SYMPTOMS
- Swollen and tender gums which bleed easily after brushing
- Halitosis (bad breath) if areas of tissue death occur
- Possibly earache from referred pain

TREATMENT
Traditional Home and Folk Remedies
Peach pit tea is useful for mouth infections. Rinse your mouth with the hot tea three times a day. To make the tea, remove as much pulp as possible from the pits, soak them in boiling water for 5 minutes, then bake in a medium oven for 1 hour. Use one pit per cup of boiling water. Let steep for 10–15 minutes. (See page 170.)

Herbalism
Depending on the problem, some herbs, such as myrrh, are highly astringent and antiseptic, and may be useful locally. (See page 112.)
Comfrey mouthwash will help to heal mouth abrasions, and reduce swelling and bleeding. (See page 186.)

Aromatherapy
Dab on some clove oil, or suck a clove, for its antiseptic properties. (See page 125.)
Make a gargle containing a few drops of antiseptic oils, such as chamomile, clove, lemongrass, or niaouli. (See pages 118, 125, 149, and 151.)

Homeopathy
Gingivitis may be treated homeopathically. One of the following specific remedies may be taken every 4 hours for up to 3 days:
Nat. mur., when gums bleed easily, there are ulcers and a taste of pus in the mouth, accompanied by sensitive teeth. (See page 154.)
Phosphorus, for gums which bleed easily when touched, gaps between teeth and gums. (See page 219.)
Silicea, for painful, swollen gums, very sensitive to cold, and which bleed easily. (See page 220.)

Nutrition
Apart from a visit to a dental hygienist, followed by daily brushing and flossing, a healthy diet will promote healthy gums.
Vitamin C is important for the production of collagen. Most tissues in the body are made from this. (See page 210.)
Co-enzyme Q10 supplements have been found beneficial in some cases of gum disease. (See page 230.)

CAUTION
Gum inflammation can lead to periodontitis if not treated. This causes the teeth to loosen and fall out.

Bake peach stones, then steep in boiling water to make peach pit tea for gargling.

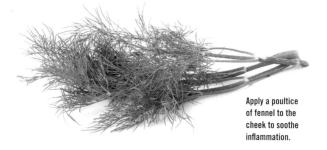

Apply a poultice of fennel to the cheek to soothe inflammation.

TOOTHACHE

Aching or pain in a tooth is generally a result of tooth decay (or "caries"). Dental caries is a bacterially caused destruction of the enamel and dentine of the tooth. When the hard enamel of the tooth is damaged, this allows infecting organisms to enter the tooth, which results in inflammation and pain. If a tooth is sensitive to heat, cold, or sweet things, nerves in the tooth may be inflamed due to advanced decay. If pain is absent, except when you bite, your tooth or filling may be broken. In either case, it is recommended that you see your dentist within 48 hours.

SYMPTOMS
• Aching or pain in a tooth • Sensitivity to heat, cold, or sweet things • Pain on biting

TREATMENT
Ayurveda
Crush a clove of garlic and apply to the tooth. (See page 79.)
Dip a small cotton ball into cinnamon oil and apply to the affected area. (See page 104.)

Chinese Herbalism
Treatment would address heat in the stomach, and decayed or damaged teeth.
Shi Gao (gypsum) and Ren Shen (ginseng) might be used to relieve heat. (See page 160.)

Herbalism
A herbalist might recommend tinctures of echinacea or myrrh to encourage healing and reduce the risk of infection. (See pages 112 and 122.)
Cayenne can act as a local anesthetic for painful teeth and gums. (See page 98.)
Fennel may be applied to the cheek in a poultice, which will reduce inflammation and ease symptoms. (See page 128.)

Aromatherapy
Peppermint or clove oils can be applied directly to the area as an analgesic. (See pages 125 and 152.)
Oil of coriander will reduce pain and inflammation. (See page 113.)
Rub a little lavender oil on the face and jaw to ease pain and distress. (See page 143.)

> **CAUTION**
> Toothache is an indication of an underlying problem, which should be investigated by a dentist immediately.

TOOTH ABSCESS

In cases of neglected tooth decay, infection may gain access to the root canal of the affected tooth or teeth. Inflammation of the tissues around the root causes tissue destruction and the collection of pus, forming an abscess. A tooth abscess may spread sideways under the gum to form what is known as a gumboil, which may open, giving relief from pain.

SYMPTOMS
• Intense pain, intermittent, or continuous and throbbing
• Increased pain on biting or chewing • Swelling and inflammation of the surrounding gum • In severe cases, fever

TREATMENT
Traditional Home and Folk Remedies
Break the large ridges of a cabbage, heat gently, and apply to the abscessed tooth. (See page 92.)
Split a fig, heat it, and apply to the abscess. (See page 126.)
Rinse your mouth with apple cider vinegar to reduce inflammation and infection. (See page 204.)
Chew fresh sage leaves or garlic, for antiseptic effect. (See pages 79 and 177.)

Herbalism
Comfrey mouthwash or ointment will help to heal and draw out the infection. (See page 186.)
Clove oil will reduce inflammation and ease pain. (See page 125.)
A hot garlic compress will draw out infection. (See page 79.)
A tincture of myrrh can be used as an antiseptic and healing mouthwash. (See page 112.)

Homeopathy
Try Hypericum and Calendula, used in solution as a mouthwash. (See pages 93 and 138.)
Take Hep. sulf., when the abscess is in place. (See page 213.)

Comfrey mouthwash or ointment will help with healing.

> **CAUTION**
> Symptoms of an abscess should be investigated by a dentist immediately.

DENTAL DISCOMFORT AFTER TREATMENT

Discomfort following dental treatment is usually caused by injury (perhaps to a nerve) or bruising around the tooth that has been worked on. This may occur immediately after treatment, or pain may follow initial discomfort after an anesthetic has worn off. There may also be some blood loss. Persistent pain following treatment may signal infection.

SYMPTOMS
• Dental soreness • Minimal blood loss

TREATMENT
Traditional Home and Folk Remedies
Oil of clove or macerated cloves can be applied to the area to prevent infection, reduce the inflammation, and prevent discomfort. (See page 125.)

Homeopathy
Arnica should be taken immediately after treatment, every hour for up to 10 doses. (See page 86.)
Phosphorus, for bleeding after a tooth has been extracted. Take every 10 minutes for 1 hour. (See page 219.)
Hypericum, for pain occurring after treatment. (See page 138.)

Flower Essences
Rescue Remedy will help to reduce the effects of trauma, and encourage the healing process. (See page 158.)

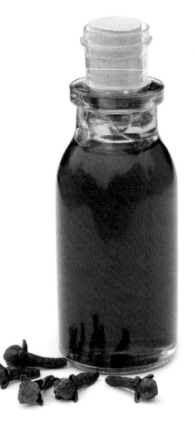

Apply oil of cloves to the site of dental treatment.

GRINDING OF TEETH

Habitual grinding or clenching of the teeth is known as bruxism. It is common among children and the elderly, and often occurs during sleep. In severe cases the enamel of the teeth may be worn away. There may be some links with anxiety.

Aspen may help to relieve anxiety.

SYMPTOMS
• Audible grinding or clenching of the teeth
• Wearing of tooth enamel

TREATMENT
Ayurveda
An Ayurvedic medical practitioner would balance the tridoshas, and use panchakarma for balancing the vátha. (See page 22.)

Chinese Herbalism
A Chinese herbalist might suggest Ren Shen (ginseng), Dang Gui (Chinese angelica), and Bai Shao (white peony root) with Chai Hu (thorowax root) for relaxation. Treatment would strengthen the spleen and enliven liver qi. (See pages 82, 159, and 160.)

Traditional Home and Folk Remedies
Oats contain thiamine and pantothenic acid, which are gentle nerve tonics. (See page 89.)

Herbalism
Herbal remedies would be used to calm the nervous system and to relax. Skullcap and valerian are useful herbs, blended together for best effect. Drink this as a tea 3 times daily while suffering the symptoms. (See pages 181 and 195.)
Linden may ease anxiety and tension that may exacerbate the condition. (See page 191.)

Aromatherapy
A relaxing blend of essential oils of lavender, geranium, and bergamot in sweet almond oil or peach kernel oil may be added to the bath to calm nerves and prevent attacks. (See pages 107, 143, and 161.)

Flower Essences
Rescue Remedy would be useful if there is an emotional cause underlying the condition. (See page 158.)
Elm, for anxiety accompanying a feeling of being unable to cope. (See page 193.)
Red chestnut, for anxiety over the welfare of others. (See page 76.)
Aspen, for anxiety for no apparent reason. (See page 168.)

FEAR OF DENTAL TREATMENT

Fear of dental treatment (dental phobia) is an extremely common phenomenon: some studies show that nearly 80 percent of the U.S. population suffer some feelings of fear about dental treatment. Full-scale phobia is one of the most common types of phobia in both the U.K. and the U.S. Sufferers develop intense feelings of anxiety and panic from an association between dentists and pain, despite the fact that modern dental technology has eliminated much of the pain of treatment. Both adults and children may be affected (children are particularly vulnerable if they sense that their parents are frightened). Most modern dentists are aware of the nervousness affecting many people, and may offer home visits or sedation, anesthetics, hypnosis, and other forms of relaxation. (See also "Phobias," page 244.)

SYMPTOMS
• Rapid pulse • Profuse sweating • High blood pressure
• Trembling • Nausea

TREATMENT

Ayurveda
Lemon or lime may help for dizziness, and individual treatment would be prescribed according to your needs. (See page 20.)

Chinese Herbalism
A herbalist may prescribe cooling herbs, and Gui Pi Wan formula, to help with emotional problems.
Ren Shen (ginseng), Dang Gui (Chinese angelica), and Yuan Zhi (senega root) may also be useful. (See pages 82, 160, and 166.)

Herbalism
Valerian tea can help to reduce tension. Drink an infusion as required. (See page 195.)

Aromatherapy
The effect of certain smells can help to release tension and induce a feeling of calm. Some of the best oils to try are bergamot, chamomile, clary sage, geranium, jasmine, juniper, lavender, marjoram, melissa, and ylang ylang, which are sedative. They can be used in the bath, in massage with a light carrier oil (such as sweet almond), or in a vaporizer. Carry a bottle of diluted oils with you and apply to the temples or pulse points before dental treatment. (See pages 95, 107, 141, 142, 143, 149, 152, 157, 161, and 178.)

Homeopathy
Aconite, for intense fear. Take before and after treatment. Chamomilla, for a child who throws a tantrum about seeing the dentist. (See page 149.)

Flower Essences
Mimulus, for fear of known things. Make a personal remedy, and take a few drops every time you think of the dentist. Take hourly before going for treatment. (See page 153.)
Rescue Remedy will help to reduce feelings of fear and panic. Take hourly before treatment, and also during treatment. (See page 158.)

Mind–Body Healing
Techniques such as meditation, positive visualization, self-hypnosis, and breathing are all ideal for overcoming the anxiety experienced in the dentist's waiting room. Contact a therapist for advice on what would work best for you. (See pages 68–69.)

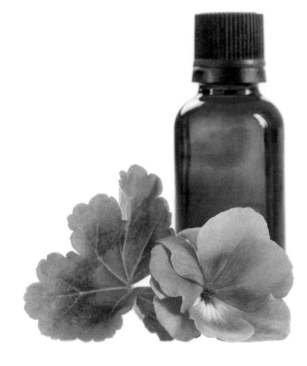

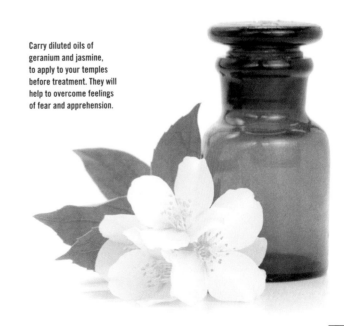

Carry diluted oils of geranium and jasmine, to apply to your temples before treatment. They will help to overcome feelings of fear and apprehension.

MOUTH AND THROAT PROBLEMS
SORE THROAT

A sore throat (or pharyngitis) is an inflammation of the pharynx, the area of the throat between the back of the nose and the beginning of the trachea and vocal cords. It is usually caused by infection, which can be viral or bacterial in origin. A sore throat is a feature of illnesses such as tonsillitis and may also signal the onset of glandular fever, flu, or scarlet fever. If scarlet fever is not treated with antibiotics it may lead to rheumatic flu or kidney failure. Inflammation of the throat can also be caused by heavy smoking or drinking, abuse of gargles or mouthwashes, general vitamin deficiency, or food allergy; it can also be a symptom of blood disorders such as anemia. A sore throat will usually resolve itself in a few days, but infection, accompanied by high fever and malaise, may take up to three weeks. Streptococcal sore throat, or strep throat, is an inflammation of the throat and tonsils caused by bacteria and is the most common type of strep infection. Onset is usually sudden and is accompanied by pain, redness, and swelling in throat tissues, pus on the tonsils, fever, headache, and malaise. If left untreated, strep throat can lead to rheumatic fever.

SYMPTOMS
- Hoarseness • Thirst • Pain, causing difficulty swallowing
- Possibly a burning sensation • Slight fever • Enlarged and tender lymph nodes in the neck • Possibly earache

TREATMENT
Ayurveda
Dasamoola rasayna, an oral syrup, will treat a sore throat.
Crush a piece of root ginger to extract the juice, and add to a tablespoon of honey and 3 tablespoons of lime. Sip 4 times a day.

A blend of crushed root ginger, honey and lemon or lime can be sipped.

Chinese Herbalism
Yin Qiao Jie du Pian pills, for a sore throat accompanied by flu symptoms, swollen lymph nodes, and headaches.
Sang Ju Gan Mao Pian or Sang Ju Yin Pian, for a sore throat with symptoms of cold.
Liu Wei di Huang Wan, for kidney yin-deficient sore throat.
Also for chronic dry sore throat, with hot palms and soles, and night sweats.
Jin Yin Hua (honeysuckle) tea may be useful. (See page 146.)

Traditional Home and Folk Remedies
Gargle with salt water to ease symptoms and reduce inflammation. (See page 205.)
Apply an apple cider vinegar compress to the throat to ease symptoms. (See page 204.)
Gargle with honey water, which acts to encourage healing and deal with infection. (See page 203.)
White cabbage juice is anti-inflammatory and will draw out infection. (See page 92.)
A hot honey and lemon drink will reduce symptoms and encourage healing. (See pages 108 and 203.)

Herbalism
Eat fresh garlic whenever possible, to absorb its antibacterial and antiviral properties. (See page 79.)
A gargle of red sage will help to soothe a sore throat. (See page 177.)
Tincture of calendula can be added to a cup of boiled water for a mouthwash to encourage healing and treat infection. (See page 93.)
Burdock or comfrey teas will ease the pain. (See pages 85 and 186.)

Aromatherapy
A steam inhalation of benzoin, lavender, or thyme will ease the discomfort and help to treat the infection. (See page 47.)
Massage a little lavender oil, blended in a light carrier oil, into the neck. (See page 143.)
Dab the throat with diluted tea tree oil on a cotton bud: it is analgesic and fights infection, which will help to ease symptoms and treat the cause. (See page 150.)

Homeopathy
Apis, when the pain is worse on the right side of the body, and improves after cold drinks. (See page 203.)

Nutrition
Increase vitamin C intake, with plenty of citrus fruits. (See page 210.)
Suck a zinc lozenge. (See page 221.)

TONSILLITIS

Tonsillitis is an inflammation of the tonsils located at the back of the throat. It is generally due to either viral or bacterial infection (often by the streptococcal bacteria), and causes swelling and redness of the tonsils, possibly with white or yellow spots of pus. The adenoids may also become inflamed and infected. Tonsillitis can occur at any time but is particularly common during childhood. In rare cases complications such as quinsy (an abscess behind the tonsil), kidney inflammation, or rheumatic fever may develop. In chronic tonsillitis the tonsils tend to flare up in episodes of acute infection, causing scarring that makes them difficult to treat in subsequent attacks.

SYMPTOMS
• Swelling and redness of the tonsils, possibly with white or yellow spots of pus • Swelling and tenderness of the lymph nodes in the neck • Sore throat with pain on swallowing • Headache • Earache • Weakness and malaise • Fever • Bad breath • Constipation

TREATMENT

Ayurveda
Apply a cloth with mustard oil to the forehead to ease the pain and reduce fever. (See page 91.)
Root ginger can be chewed, and mixed with honey and lemon to make a soothing drink. (See pages 108, 200, and 203.)

Chinese Herbalism
Treatment would be aimed at fire, poison, wind, and heat. Avoid spicy food and drink Jin Yin Hua (honeysuckle) tea. (See page 146.)

Traditional Home and Folk Remedies
Blackcurrant tea or juice (hot) will treat infection and relieve the sore throat.
Drink plenty of hot honey and lemon, or honey and apple cider vinegar, to fight infection and boost immunity. (See pages 108, 203, and 204.)

Herbalism
A red sage gargle will address infection and reduce symptoms. (See page 177.)
Herbs to boost the immune system include echinacea, garlic, myrrh, and sage. (See pages 79, 112, 122, and 177.)
Marigold will help the lymphatic system. (See page 93.)
Herbs to reduce fever by inducing sweating are chamomile, elderflowers, yarrow, and linden. (See pages 74, 149, 178, and 191.)
Agrimony, elderflowers, plantain, and raspberry leaves tone the mucous membranes, and clear the catarrh and inflammation. (See pages 77, 165, 176, and 178.)
Herbs to soothe painful tonsils include comfrey, marshmallow, and mullein. (See pages 114, 186, and 195.)

Aromatherapy
Thyme oil is a powerful antiseptic and has a local anesthetic effect to reduce the discomfort. Use in a vaporizer, and add to a light carrier oil and massage into the neck. (See page 190.)
Lavender and benzoin can be added to a cup of cooled, boiled water and gargled. (See pages 143 and 186.)
Tea tree oil, applied neat to the tonsils on the end of a cotton bud, fights infection and discomfort. (See page 150.)

Homeopathy
Chronic tonsillitis must be treated constitutionally, but for acute conditions try:
Hep. sulf., for a feeling that there is a fishbone caught in the throat, and when pain is alleviated by warm drinks, the breath is foul, and there is yellow pus. (See page 213.)
Lycopodium, for a throat sore on the right side, and where the tongue is dry and puffy but not coated, the throat is better after cold drinks, and worse between 4 and 8 a.m. or p.m. (See page 147.)

Nutrition
Cod liver oil tablets, along with vitamin C and garlic, will speed up the healing process. (See pages 79, 210, and 232.)

> **CAUTION**
> Contact your physician if tonsillitis is suspected.

Drinking blackcurrant tea or, for children, hot blackcurrant juice is a pleasant way to treat the infection causing tonsillitis.

LARYNGITIS

Laryngitis is an inflammation of the voice box (the larynx) in which the larynx and vocal cords become swollen and sore, distorting the vocal apparatus. Acute laryngitis is usually a complication of a sore throat, cold, or other upper respiratory tract infection, and should last for only a few days. It can also be an allergic reaction to inhaled pollen. Chronic laryngitis is more persistent and may be caused by long-term irritation from smoking, overuse of the voice, or excessive coughing. It can be an occupational hazard for singers and teachers.

SYMPTOMS
• Throat is inflamed and mucus-coated in acute laryngitis • Larynx is dry and inflamed in chronic laryngitis • Hoarseness • Difficulty in raising the voice above a whisper • Dry, irritating cough

TREATMENT
Chinese Herbalism
Treatment would address poisoned heat in the lungs, and the following herbs may be appropriate: peppermint, Jin Yin Hua (honeysuckle flowers), Bai He (lily), and Gan Cao (licorice). (See pages 132, 146, and 152.)

Traditional Home and Folk Remedies
Drink a glass of honey and lemon, or honey and apple cider vinegar, in hot water as required to reduce any inflammation and infection, and encourage healing. (See pages 108, 203, and 204.)

Herbalism
Drink an infusion of red sage, or gargle, to reduce inflammation. (See page 177.)
Echinacea both treats and prevents laryngitis. Drink an infusion 3 times daily. (See page 122.)

Aromatherapy
Gargle with a drop of geranium, pepper, rosemary, or tea tree oil in a glass of boiled water, as required, to prevent and treat inflammation and infection. (See page 150, 161, 164, and 175.)
Massage the throat area with a drop of lavender or tea tree oil in a light carrier oil. (See pages 143 and 150.)
Try a steam inhalation of sandalwood or thyme to ease inflammation and reduce infection. (See pages 179 and 190.)

Homeopathy
Spongia, for a dry, barking cough – particularly useful for croup. (See page 185.)
Apis, where the problem has been caused or exacerbated by allergy, and there is redness and swelling. (See page 203.)

Nutrition
Eat a diet rich in vitamin C to increase resistance to infection. (See page 210.)
Avoid alcohol.

Eating bananas encourages the growth of healthy bacteria in the body.

ORAL THRUSH

Oral thrush is a fungal infection that appears as raised creamy spots on the lining of the mouth, lips, and throat. The *Candida albicans* fungus occurs naturally in the mouth and other moist, warm areas of the body, but if excessive growth takes place infection can result. This may occur if the bacteria that usually keep it in check are themselves under attack by antibiotics, or if the immune system is compromised for any other reason.

SYMPTOMS
• Pain, soreness, and irritation in the affected area • Raised creamy spots in the mouth

TREATMENT
Chinese Herbalism
Qin Jiao (Chinese gentian) and Qing Hao (wormwood) may be prescribed to treat fungal infections of the mouth.

Traditional Home and Folk Remedies
Eat fresh live yogurt, and dab onto the affected patches, as required. (See page 142.)
Olive oil prevents yeast becoming fungus in the body, and should be drunk or used in cooking, as often as possible. (See page 156.)
Rub raw garlic onto the affected areas, and incorporate plenty of raw garlic into your diet. (See page 79.)
Lemon will help to soothe discomfort and encourage healing. Drink a cup of hot lemon and honey in water 3 times daily. (See pages 108 and 203.)

Herbalism
Aloe vera mouthwash has an antifungal effect. (See page 80.)
Barberry prevents the growth of fungus, and stimulates the immune system. Take 3 times daily. (See page 90.)
Chew fresh juniper berries to reduce inflammation and attack the *Candida* fungus. (See page 142.)

Aromatherapy
Add a few drops of myrrh, tea tree, or lavender oil to a cup of boiled water and rinse the mouth several times daily to destroy fungal infection. (See pages 112, 143, and 150.)

Nutrition
Take acidophilus tablets, and eat plenty of ripe bananas to encourage the growth of healthy bacteria in the body, which will reduce the severity of attacks and act to prevent them. (See page 142.)

MOUTH ULCERS

Mouth ulcers are white, gray, or yellow open sores with an outer ring of red inflammation, and occur when the mucous membrane or skin surface becomes pitted, resulting from an erosion or disintegration of the tissues. They appear on the inside of the lips, cheeks, or floor of the mouth, and may occur as a result of aggressive tooth brushing, ill-fitting dentures, accidentally biting the side of the mouth, or eating very hot food. They can also be triggered by stress or being run down, and can be a feature of Crohn's disease, ulcerative colitis, and celiac disease, or food allergy. Women may be particularly prone to mouth ulcers around menstruation. In children, contact with the herpes simplex virus that causes cold sores may manifest itself as mouth ulcers. Mouth ulcers are common, affecting one in five U.S. adults.

SYMPTOMS
• Pain and stinging in affected area, particularly when eating acidic or spicy foods • Dry mouth

TREATMENT
Ayurveda
Rub the tongue with a piece of ginger, and chew fresh root ginger to treat fungal infections of the mouth. (See page 200.)
Aloe vera is useful for mouth ulcers associated with the herpes virus. (See page 80.)

Herbalism
Tincture of myrrh can be added to a cup of boiled water and used as a mouth rinse to destroy infection or infestation. Use the tincture neat and apply to sores in the mouth with a cotton bud. (See page 112.)
Rub a little aloe vera gel into the affected area. (See page 80.)

Aromatherapy
Mix a drop of geranium and lavender oil in a cup of boiled water and gargle as required. (See pages 143 and 161.)

Nutrition
Take supplements of vitamin A, E, and B2. (See pages 206, 207, and 211.)
Vitamin E oil can be applied directly to the ulcers. (See page 211.)

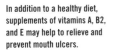

In addition to a healthy diet, supplements of vitamins A, B2, and E may help to relieve and prevent mouth ulcers.

BAD BREATH

Bad breath (or halitosis) is often caused by accumulated food debris as a result of poor dental hygiene, smoking, and alcohol consumption. It may be accompanied by dribbling during sleep and a yellowish, thickly coated tongue. Bad breath can also be a symptom of many disorders including gingivitis, tonsillitis, sinusitis, oral thrush, diabetes, acute bronchitis, liver failure, chronic gastritis, underproduction of saliva, constipation, and cancer of the mouth, throat, larynx, lungs, or esophagus.

SYMPTOMS
• Unpleasant odor on the breath • Bad-smelling saliva: lick your wrist then allow it to dry to test

TREATMENT
Ayurveda
Chew fresh coriander or cardamom seeds after meals. They act as a digestive and discourage bad breath. (See pages 113 and 122.)

Chinese Herbalism
Treatment would be aimed at stomach damp heat, using Huang Lian (golden thread), peppermint tea, Huo Xiang (giant hyssop), and radish seeds. (See pages 77, 113, and 152.)

Traditional Home and Folk Remedies
Drink a combination of carrot, celery, watercress, and cucumber juice with some paprika. (See pages 84, 116, 120, and 154.)
Store your toothbrush in grapefruit seed extract to destroy bacteria which may be encouraging bad breath. (See page 109.)

Herbalism
Chew fresh rosemary leaves, or make a mouthwash with a pinch of cloves, cinnamon, anise seed, and rosemary. Steep in a cup of sherry for a week, and then strain. Use daily as required. (See pages 104, 125, and 175.)
Chew fresh watercress, which is rich in chlorophyll and vitamin C. (See page 154.)
Chew walnut bark, then gargle with lemon water. (See page 141.)
Chew fresh parsley or mint. (See pages 152 and 162.)

Aromatherapy
Add a drop of myrrh essential oil to a cup of cool, boiled water, and rinse the mouth daily. (See page 112.)
Thyme or fennel oil will be equally effective. (See pages 128 and 190.)

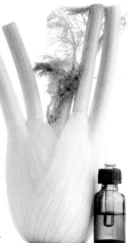

Fennel oil can be added to a cup of cool, boiled water. Rinse the mouth with it daily.

LUNG AND RESPIRATORY DISORDERS

ASTHMA

Asthma is a condition in which the muscles of the bronchi (the air tubes of the lung) contract in spasm, obstructing the flow of air and making breathing out, in particular, very difficult. Asthma is becoming increasingly common, especially among children, and may be triggered by a number of factors, including allergens (such as house dust or pets), pollution, infection, emotional trauma, or physical exertion. Asthma is divided into two categories: intrinsic, for which there is no identifiable cause for attacks, and extrinsic, which is caused by something, usually inhaled, that triggers an attack. In many asthma patients, inflammation of the lining of the airways leads to increased sensitivity to a variety of environmental triggers that can cause narrowing of the airways, resulting in obstruction of airflow and breathing difficulty. In some patients, the mucous glands in the airways produce excessive thick mucus, further obstructing airflow. An asthma attack may be brief or last for several days. Typically, an attack begins within minutes after exposure to a triggering agent. Some patients have only occasional or "seasonal" symptoms, while others have daily symptoms.

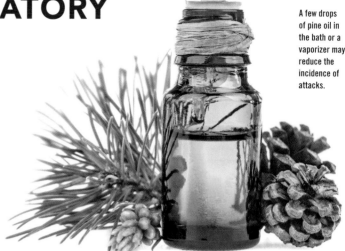

A few drops of pine oil in the bath or a vaporizer may reduce the incidence of attacks.

SYMPTOMS
• Difficulty in breathing • Increase in pulse rate • Wheezing, especially on breathing out • Persistent dry cough • Sensation of tightness around the chest

TREATMENT

Ayurveda
Common ginger and stramonium (*Datura stramonium*) may be used to treat asthma. However, stramonium is toxic in large doses, so consult a registered Ayurvedic practitioner and your physician before use. (See page 200.)

Chinese Herbalism
The cause of the illness is considered to be phlegm produced by weakness of the spleen and kidneys. Almond may be prescribed to open the lungs. (See page 169.)

Herbalism
Any of the herbs suggested for stress (see page 284) will help you to relax, which should decrease the incidence of attacks. Wild sunflower (elecampane) can be infused to treat asthma. Drink daily if you are prone to attacks. (See page 140.)
After a mild attack, hyssop, wild cherry bark (*Prunus serotina*), and motherwort will help. (See pages 139 and 144.)
Turmeric has a broncho-dilatory effect, and it can be sipped sprinkled in a cup of warm water. (See page 117.)

Aromatherapy
A steam inhalation of chamomile, eucalyptus, or lavender essential oils can be taken immediately after an attack to ease panic and to help open the airways. (See pages 124, 143, and 149.)
Pine oil in the bath or a vaporizer will reduce the incidence of attacks. (See page 163.)
Bergamot, clary sage, neroli, chamomile, and rose are antispasmodic, as well as being relaxant, and they will be particularly useful at preventing attacks brought on by stress. (See pages 106, 107, 149, 174, and 178.)

Flower Essences
Take Rescue Remedy when you feel symptoms coming on, in addition to any medications prescribed by your physician. This may ease symptoms and prevent a full-blown attack. (See page 158.)

Nutrition
As well as maintaining a healthy diet, increase your intake of vitamin B6, which is said to reduce the frequency and severity of attacks. (See page 208.)

Mind–Body Healing
Regular, moderate aerobic exercise is as important for people with asthma as for everyone else. If exercise triggers attacks, ensure that medication is always at hand. For children, ensure that teachers and coaches know what to do in the event of an attack.

CAUTION

Asthma is a serious medical condition, so consult a physician if it is suspected. Always consult a physician before taking herbal remedies for asthma. Do not discontinue use of medications prescribed for asthma, as they must be taken regularly to be effective. A prolonged attack of severe asthma that does not respond to simple remedies requires immediate medical attention. If a cough lasts for more than 10 days, or is accompanied by fever, difficult breathing, blue lips, drowsiness, or difficulty in speaking, contact your physician.

COUGHS

Coughs are necessary to expel foreign bodies and mucus from the trachea and airways of the lungs. Coughing is a symptom rather than an illness, and can indicate sinusitis, croup, bronchitis, pneumonia, flu, viruses, the early stages of measles, asthma, whooping cough, or an excess of catarrh from the nose or sinuses, due to irritation or infection. A dry cough may be caused by mucus from infections or colds, chemicals in the atmosphere, a foreign object, or nervousness which constricts the throat. A loose, wetter cough is caused by inflammation of the bronchial tubes produced by an infection or allergy. A constant nighttime cough, or one that recurs with each cold and is hard to get rid of, may indicate asthma.

SYMPTOMS
• Coughing, dry and tickly or producing mucus • Constant nighttime coughing may cause insomnia

TREATMENT
Ayurveda
Brown 4 tablespoons of coriander seeds in a frying pan, then boil with 4 cups of water and 4 slices of root ginger. Reduce to 2 cups of liquid, strain, and drink. (See page 200.)
Sunflower may also be helpful. (See page 140.)

Traditional Home and Folk Remedies
A tincture of garlic (place several garlic cloves in brandy and leave for 2 or 3 weeks, then strain) or garlic syrup (tincture, or fresh garlic mixed with a little honey) will help the body to fight infection. It also works to cleanse the blood. (See page 79.)
Ginseng in hot herbal tea warms the body and eases symptoms. (See page 160.)
Honey and lemon will ease coughs. (See pages 108 and 203.)
Mustard powder, mixed with a little water, can be made into a poultice and applied to the chest area. (See page 91.)
Apply a warm roasted onion poultice to the chest, or drink a warm onion broth to cleanse and reduce congestion. (See page 78.)

Herbalism
Peppermint tea can be drunk to soothe. (See page 152.)
Add lightly macerated licorice root sticks to your herbal drink to ease. (See page 132.)
Aniseed (*Pimpinella anisum*), marshmallow, and wild cherry bark (*Prunus serotina*) are good for unproductive coughs. (See page 81.)
Use golden seal (*Hydrastis canadensis*), plantain, and thyme if infection is present. (See pages 165 and 190.)

Aromatherapy
Inhale the steam from a few drops of eucalyptus oil in boiling water, as it is expectorant and decongestant. (See page 124.)
Pine oil, in a vaporizer, will ease coughing and act to restore the lungs. (See page 163.)
Massage frankincense or sandalwood into the chest and back. (See pages 90 and 179.)
Essential oil of myrrh reduces mucus and phlegm. (See page 112.)

Homeopathy
Phosphorus, for a tickling cough in delicate people with weak chests. (See page 219.)
Chamomilla, for a dry, irritating cough with wheezing, and which is worse at night and makes you feel irritable. (See page 149.)

USEFUL FACTS
• An acute cough starts suddenly, and is usually resolved within a day or two.
• A chronic cough persists, sometimes for many weeks.
• A productive cough brings up lots of catarrh or mucus.
• A nonproductive cough brings up very little or no mucus, and usually sounds harsh and hard.

CAUTION
If a cough lasts for more than 10 days, or is accompanied by fever, difficult breathing, blue lips, drowsiness, or difficulty speaking, contact your physician.

Drink warm onion soup to ease congestion.

FLU

More properly known as influenza, flu is a viral disease of the upper respiratory tract, spread by the contaminated droplets (via coughing and sneezing) of other sufferers. The three main types of flu are caused by three types of Orthomyxovirus virus: A, B, and C. Type C, once caught, confers immunity. Types A and B, however, are constantly mutating so that our bodies cannot build up resistance against them. Approximately every 10 years, influenza pandemics have been caused by new strains of type-A virus. Epidemics, or regional outbreaks, have appeared every 2 to 3 years for influenza A, and every 4 to 5 years for influenza B. Incubation of the virus is generally one or two days, during which time it is highly infectious, and therefore notoriously impossible to contain. The incidence of infection is highest among school-age children, partly because of their lack of previous exposure to various strains. Vaccines have been developed that have been found to be 70–90 percent effective for at least six months against either A or B types. Vaccination is considered especially important for older people, patients with cardiac or respiratory diseases, and pregnant women.

SYMPTOMS
• High fever, possibly accompanied by shivering • Sore throat, and possibly a dry, unproductive cough • Runny nose • Sneezing • Breathlessness • Weakness • Headache • Stiff and aching joints • Muscular pain • Nausea • Loss of appetite • Possibly insomnia and depression

TREATMENT
Ayurveda
Heat mustard oil and apply as a compress to the head to reduce fever. (See page 91.)
Crush root ginger, add to a little honey and lime, and drink as required. (See page 200.)
Bitter orange, sunflower, and coriander may be useful in treating flu. (See pages 106, 113, and 140.)

Traditional Home and Folk Remedies
Some warmed apple juice (preferably fresh) can ease the fever. (See page 148.)
Barley water is a traditional remedy for high fever, particularly one caused by infection and inflammation. (See page 136.)
Ginseng powder can be added to herbal teas to restore. (See page 160.)
Drink hot lemon and honey in a cup of warm water to ease inflammation and fever. (See pages 108 and 203.)
Gargle with lemon juice to kill germs. (See page 108.)

Herbalism
Drink an infusion of boneset (*Eupatorium perfoliatum*) to relieve aches and pains and clear congestion.
Fenugreek with lemon and honey will help to bring down fever and soothe aching limbs. (See pages 108, 191, and 203.)
Ginseng is a great all-round restorer and will help to bring down body temperature to normal. (See page 160.)
Use sage and licorice to prevent flu. (See pages 132 and 177.)

Aromatherapy
Gargle with tea tree oil to prevent the spread of infection. (See page 150.)
Use a eucalyptus or peppermint inhalation to unblock sinuses and the chest. (See pages 124 and 152.)
Massage tea tree and geranium oil into the chest and head to reduce symptoms and fight infection. (See pages 150 and 161.)
Oils that act to bring down fever include bergamot, chamomile, melissa, and tea tree. (See pages 107, 149, 150, and 152.)

Nutrition
Eat plenty of foods rich in vitamin C, bioflavonoids, and zinc, which will encourage healing, help to fight infection, and boost the action of the immune system. (See pages 210, 221, and 228.)
Royal jelly acts as a tonic and an antiviral agent. (See page 234.)

CAUTION
Flu victims 50 years old or older, children, and immune-deficient people are at risk of developing pneumonia and other secondary infections. Over the age of 65, pneumonia and flu are the fifth leading cause of death.

Freshly made apple juice is a good home remedy, providing vitamin C to help to combat injection. Using a juice extractor enables this to be made quickly and easily. The apple juice can be poured into a pan and gently warmed, but it must not be boiled or overheated or the vitamin content will be severely reduced.

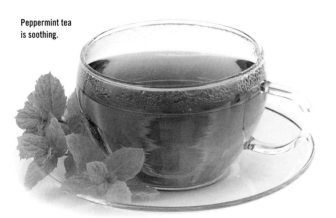
Peppermint tea is soothing.

EMPHYSEMA

Emphysema is a progressive disease in which the tiny air sacs in the lungs (alveoli) break down, reducing the area available for gas exchange. This means that insufficient oxygen reaches the vital organs, and too much carbon dioxide enters the bloodstream. Emphysema is particularly common among heavy smokers and sufferers of asthma and chronic bronchitis. Industrial pollutants may also be a cause, as well as hereditary factors. The exact cause of pulmonary emphysema is unknown. Cigarette smoking is closely associated with the disease, and in some cases a genetic link is suspected, in that a significant number of people with emphysema lack a gene that controls the liver's production of a protein called alpha-1 antitrypsin, or AAT. Emphysema rarely occurs before the age of 40, and women appear to be less prone.

SYMPTOMS
• Breathlessness, especially on exertion • Cough, producing sputum • Chest may become barrel-shaped as the disease progresses • Blue tinge to the skin (cyanosis) • Respiratory failure may eventually occur

TREATMENT
Ayurveda
Boil 2 or 3 cloves of garlic in 2 cups of water until tender. Crush into the water and drink to relieve chest pain. (See page 79.)
Stramonium (*Datura stramonium*) may be useful.

Herbalism
Peppermint tea will soothe inflammation and help to open lungs. (See page 152.)
Slippery elm bark soothes the chest and lungs, and can be added to any herbal tea. (See page 193.)

Aromatherapy
Massage oils of cedarwood, peppermint, or eucalyptus into the chest daily, to open lungs and reduce coughing. (See page 47.)
Make an inhalation of eucalyptus, and use as required to expel phlegm. (See page 124.)

> **CAUTION**
> If emphysema is suspected, consult a physician.

BRONCHITIS

Bronchitis is an inflammation of the lining of the bronchi (the air tubes of the lungs). Acute bronchitis, in which mucus infected with bacteria is expelled from the lungs, often follows a viral illness such as a cold or flu. Chronic bronchitis results from prolonged irritation of the bronchial membrane, causing coughing and the excessive secretion of mucus for extended periods. By far the most common cause of chronic bronchitis is cigarette smoking, but air pollution, industrial fumes, and dust are also recognized lung irritants.

SYMPTOMS
• Cough, dry at first but with gradually increasing sputum
• Possibly chest pain • Fever • Shortness of breath and wheezing
• In chronic bronchitis, symptoms may begin in winter but persist

TREATMENT
Ayurveda
Heat mustard oil and apply as a compress to the head to reduce fever. (See page 91.)
Crush root ginger, add to a little honey and lime, and drink as required. (See page 200.)

Chinese Herbalism
Acute conditions will respond to Zhe Bei Mu (fritillaria bulb), Che Qian Zi (plantain seed), and Jie Geng (balloon flower root). (See pages 129 and 165.)
Chronic conditions respond to Jin Yin Hua (honeysuckle), Sang Ye (mulberry leaves), and Zhi Zi (gardenia fruit). (See page 146.)

Traditional Home and Folk Remedies
Honey and lemon work to fight infection and ease coughs. (See pages 108 and 203.)
Combine mustard seed powder and water to make a poultice to decongest the chest. (See page 91.)
Onions will soothe inflamed membranes and induce perspiration. (See page 78.)

Herbalism
Rub garlic oil into the chest to fight infection and encourage healing. (See page 79.)
Drink ginseng in hot water, as it will help to eliminate infection and ease coughing fits. (See page 160.)
Peppermint tea will soothe the cough and bring out the infection. (See page 152.)

Aromatherapy
Oils to help clear the congestion include eucalyptus and thyme, which can be inhaled as required. (See pages 124 and 190.)
Ginger oil can be diluted and rubbed into the chest for chronic bronchitis, to dispel mucus. (See page 200.)

> **CAUTION**
> If your temperature rises above 39 degrees, or if you cough blood, call your physician.

HYPERVENTILATION

Hyperventilation is the term used to describe the act of breathing more quickly and deeply than normal, which causes excessive loss of carbon dioxide from the blood. This can lead to an increase in blood alkalinity. It can occur at high altitudes, as a result of heavy exercise, during panic attacks, or as a response to poisoning (as in aspirin overdose). Hyperventilation associated with diabetes or kidney failure represents the body's efforts to eliminate excess carbon dioxide in dealing with acidosis.

SYMPTOMS
• A feeling of not getting enough air • Muscles of the forearms and calves may go into spasm, causing involuntary bending and extension of the wrists and ankles

TREATMENT
Chinese Herbalism
A Chinese herbalist might suggest Ren Shen (ginseng), Dang Gui (Chinese angelica), and Bai Shao (white peony root) with Chai Hu (thorowax root) for relaxation. (See pages 82, 159, and 160.)

Traditional Home and Folk Remedies
Oats contain thiamine and pantothenic acid, which act as gentle nerve tonics. (See page 89.)

Herbalism
Herbal remedies would be used to calm the nervous system and to relax. Skullcap and valerian are useful herbs, blended together for best effect. Drink this as a tea three times daily while suffering symptoms. (See pages 181 and 195.)
Linden may also work to ease factors that may be causing the condition. (See page 191.)

Aromatherapy
A relaxing blend of essential oils of lavender, geranium, and bergamot in sweet almond oil or peach kernel oil may be used in the bath at times of great stress and anxiety. (See page 47.)

Flower Essences
Rescue Remedy will help to calm down during an attack. (See page 158.)
Elm, for an attack linked to anxiety accompanying a feeling of being unable to cope. (See page 193.)

Nutrition
Avoid caffeine and increase your intake of B vitamins, which work on the nervous system. (See pages 206–209.)

Mind–Body Healing
To ease hyperventilation caused by stress or emotional trauma, breathe through pursed lips, or pinch one nostril and breathe through your nose. Slow your breathing to 1 breath every 5 seconds, which may gradually ease symptoms.

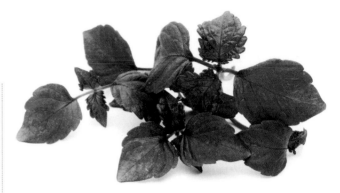

In Chinese medicine, perilla may be used to ease hiccups.

HICCUPS

A hiccup is a common irritation of the diaphragmatic nerves which causes involuntary inhalation of air. A lowering of the diaphragm and the sudden closure of the vocal cords result in the characteristic hiccup sound. Hiccups may be brought on by indigestion and drinking carbonated drinks, and can also occur during pregnancy and as a result of alcoholism. Most attacks last only a few minutes, usually with a brief interval in between attacks. Frequent, prolonged attacks of hiccups, which are extremely rare, may lead to severe exhaustion.

SYMPTOMS
• Prolonged episodes of hiccups may be accompanied by chest pain • If persistent, hiccups can be exhausting

TREATMENT
Chinese Herbalism
The cause is thought to be heat, cold, or food stagnation. Zi Su Geng (perilla stems), Da Huang (rhubarb), and ginger will be used to treat hiccups. (See pages 173 and 200.)

Traditional Home and Folk Remedies
Squirt some lemon juice to the back of your throat, or suck a piece of fresh lemon. (See page 108.)
Give young children a sip of water with honey. (See page 203.)

Aromatherapy
Inhalation or massage with mandarin oil may ease hiccups and other digestive spasms. (See page 109.)

Homeopathy
For a sore chest and retching, take Mag. phos. every 15 minutes for up to 6 doses. (See page 217.)

CAUTION
While hiccups are usually quite innocuous, they may be a feature of more serious disorders such as pleurisy, hiatus hernia, and pneumonia.

COMMON COLD

A cold is an infection of the upper respiratory tract which may be caused by any one of up to 200 strains of virus. These are spread either by inhaling droplets coughed or sneezed by others, or, more probably, by direct hand-to-hand contact with sufferers. When infection occurs, the walls of the respiratory tract swell and produce excess mucus, giving rise to a stuffy or runny nose, throat discomfort, malaise, and occasional coughing. Colds can produce fevers of up to 39°C (102°F) in infants and children, but such fevers in adults indicate that the infection is probably influenza. The incubation period is 1–3 days, after which symptoms occur, and most colds run their course in 3–10 days. Infants and elderly people are susceptible to complications such as sinusitis, ear inflammations, and pneumonia. In conventional medicine, colds are treated with rest and fluids, in addition to decongestants as needed. Aspirin is recommended only when symptoms are severe, because it increases viral shedding and makes the sufferer more contagious.

SYMPTOMS
• Sneezing • Runny nose • Mild fever • Headache • Coughing
• Sore throat • Catarrh

TREATMENT
Ayurveda
Brown 4 tablespoons of coriander seeds in a frying pan, then boil with 4 cups of water and 4 slices of root ginger. Reduce to 2 cups of liquid, strain, and drink. (See page 200.)
Sunflower may be useful. (See page 140.)

Chinese Herbalism
Che Qian Zi (plantain seed), peppermint, Sang Shen (mulberry), Jin Yin Hua (honeysuckle), and Huang Qin (skullcap) for weakness of the lung, cold, and wind. (See pages 146, 152, and 181.)

Traditional Home and Folk Remedies
Barley water with lemon and honey will shorten the duration of a cold. (See page 136.)
Cinnamon is an excellent warming herb, and can be added to food and drinks, or as an oil to a vaporizer, to treat and prevent colds and flu. (See page 104.)

Fresh garlic, eaten daily, will discourage the onset of a cold. Garlic will also work to reduce fever. (See page 79.)
Honey, eaten fresh or added to herbal teas, will encourage healing and prevent secondary infections occurring. (See page 203.)
Steep lemons in hot water, and a little honey. Drink regularly in the cold season, or during a cold, to restore yourself and prevent infection. This will also treat coughs. (See pages 108 and 203.)
A mustard poultice on the chest or mustard added to a foot bath will act as a decongestant. (See page 91.)

Herbalism
Ginger promotes perspiration and helps soothe the throat. (See page 200.)
Echinacea will encourage immune response, and acts as a natural antibiotic. (See page 122.)
Peppermint helps to reduce the symptoms of a cold. (See page 152.)
Ginseng powder, added to any warming herbal tea, will boost the immune system and help the body fight infection. (See page 160.)

Aromatherapy
Tea tree and lemon oils help to fight infection. Massage, in a light carrier oil, into the chest and head, or place in the bath or a burner. (See pages 108 and 150.)
Lavender oil in the bath will help you sleep, to aid recovery, which is particularly useful if there is a cough. (See page 143.)
Eucalyptus oil can kill bacteria and soothe inflamed mucous membranes. (See page 124.)

Homeopathy
Allium, for streaming nose and eyes where the discharge makes the nose red raw. (See page 78.)
Nat. mur., for colds with a crop of cold sores, sneezing, and watery eyes. (See page 154.)

Nutrition
Citrus fruit is rich in vitamin C, which will help the body to fight infection. (See page 210.)
Zinc is known to reduce the duration of a cold. Suck a zinc lozenge at the first signs. (See page 221.)
Royal jelly acts as a tonic and an antiviral agent. (See page 234.)

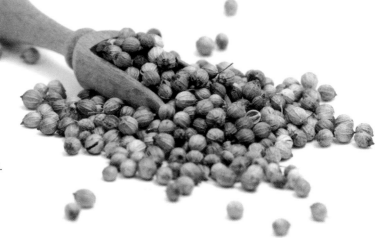

Coriander is useful in treating colds. To make a decoction, brown 4 tablespoons of coriander seeds. Add 4 cups of water and bring to the boil. Add 4 slices of root ginger, reduce the liquid to 2 cups, then strain. Drink to reduce a fever.

HEART, BLOOD, AND CIRCULATORY DISORDERS

HIGH BLOOD PRESSURE

Blood pressure is the force with which the blood presses against the arterial walls as it circulates. In a person with high blood pressure, or hypertension, this force is greater than normal and causes the arterial walls to narrow and thicken, putting extra strain on the heart. Blood pressure fluctuates even in healthy individuals. It tends to increase with physical activity, excitement, fear, or emotional stress, but such elevations are usually transient. Most physicians will not make the diagnosis of hypertension unless the pressure is high on at least three separate occasions. Obesity, alcohol and sugar intake, and hereditary and ethnic factors all contribute, as will diabetes, kidney disease, and pregnancy.

SYMPTOMS
• Mild hypertension has no symptoms; in severe hypertension: Headaches • Shortness of breath • Visual disturbances • Giddiness

TREATMENT
Ayurveda
The Ayurvedic products Dashamoola and Sarpaganda are used for treating high blood pressure.

Chinese Herbalism
Internal wind is believed to be the cause, and treatment will calm liver yang and blood wind. The herbs used might include Ju Hua (chrysanthemum flowers), Bai Shao (peony root), and Huang Qi (astragalus). (See pages 87, 159, and 268.)

Traditional Home and Folk Remedies
Eat plenty of fresh raw garlic, which acts as a tonic to the circulatory system and maintains its health. (See page 79.)

Herbalism
Hawthorn berries, infused, are a good heart tonic. (See page 114.)
Cramp bark can be used to encourage the arteries to dilate. (See page 197.)
Linden and yarrow are also useful in the treatment of high blood pressure. (See pages 74 and 191.)

Aromatherapy
Lavender will soothe and relax. (See page 143.)
Regular massage with oils of lavender, marjoram, and ylang ylang can have a beneficial effect. (See pages 95, 143, and 157.)

Nutrition
In societies that consume little or no salt, the incidence of hypertension is extremely low. Reduce the amount of salt you eat. Eat a healthy, low-fat diet.
Increase your intake of dietary fiber, and of potassium, calcium, and magnesium, which encourage the action of the heart. (See pages 58, 213, and 217.)
Cut back on alcohol and caffeine, and stop smoking.

Mind–Body Healing
Regular exercise, and the loss of any excess weight, will help hypertension. Talk to your physician about forms of exercise that are right for you. (See page 70.)
Try to get at least six hours' sleep per night.

USEFUL FACTS
• Blood pressure is conventionally written as two numbers, systolic pressure over diastolic pressure. Systolic pressure is the maximum blood pressure that occurs during the contraction of the heart; diastolic pressure is the lowest pressure measured during the interbeat period.
• Hypertension is usually described as being a systolic pressure greater than 139, or a diastolic pressure greater than 89, or both. The World Health Organization defines it as being consistently above 160mm. Hg. systolic, and 95mm. Hg. diastolic.

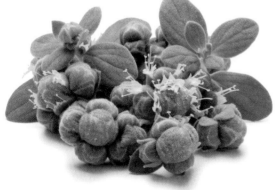

A relaxing massage with aromatherapy essential oils, such as marjoram, may be of benefit in cases of hypertension.

> **CAUTION**
> Routine blood pressure checks should be undertaken by everyone as a matter of course. Sustained high blood pressure can cause severe damage to the heart, kidneys, and eyes, and should not be ignored. Do not take herbal remedies while taking conventional medication without consulting your physician.

Tea made from hawthorn tops may be beneficial for hypotension.

LOW BLOOD PRESSURE

Low blood pressure, or hypotension, is an abrupt fall in blood pressure due possibly to the heart's failure to maintain it or to severe loss of fluid from the circulation. It is perhaps most commonly noticed on standing up suddenly, but can also result from severe hemorrhage, burns, gastroenteritis, or dehydration. Hypotension may result in fainting. Older people in particular and those taking drugs against hypertension may experience fainting episodes.

SYMPTOMS
• Fainting • Paleness • Weak pulse • Dilated pupils

TREATMENT
Chinese Herbalism
Treatment would be aimed at deficient qi in the blood and heart. Ren Shen (ginseng) and Dang Gui (Chinese angelica) might be used. (See pages 82 and 160.)

Herbalism
Ginger, hawthorn tops, and rosemary will also be useful as they are stimulating and work to encourage circulation. (See pages 114, 175, and 200.)

Aromatherapy
Regular massage with oils of black pepper, lemon, sage, or rosemary, which stimulate and warm, will be useful. (See pages 108, 164, 175, and 178.)

Homeopathy
Treatment would be constitutional, but Coffea may help if you feel a tendency to faint. (See page 111.)

CAUTION
Hypotension can be fatal, and must be given urgent medical attention.

LEUKEMIA

Leukemia is the name given to a group of diseases in which certain white blood cells reproduce arbitrarily, replacing and interfering with the blood's normal components. Untreated, this disorder will lead to a fatal shortage of red blood cells, bleeding, or infection. Acute leukemia is rapid in onset, affecting children in particular, while chronic leukemia is slower in onset, with a much greater life expectancy for sufferers. Only conventional medicine offers effective treatments for leukemia. Aromatherapy and flower remedies, used with care, can offer much needed support to those undergoing conventional treatment.

SYMPTOMS
In acute leukemias:
• General aching • Tiredness • Susceptibility to infection
• Bleeding gums • Sore throat • Swelling of glands in the neck, groin, and armpits • Appetite and weight loss • Severe anemia
In chronic leukemias:
• Slow onset of fatigue • Gradual enlargement of the spleen until it is big enough to cause a dragging sensation and pain in the upper left abdomen • Gradual weight loss • Nosebleeds • Painful and prolonged erections in men • Fever and night sweats

TREATMENT
Aromatherapy
Add a few drops of niaouli or bergamot to the bath, or place in a vaporizer. (See pages 107 and 151.)

Flower Essences
Mimulus, for fear and concern. (See page 153.)
Agrimony, for hiding true feelings of distress behind a cheerful face. (See page 77.)

Mind–Body Healing
Gentle yoga or meditation classes may help to calm the mind. Talking, music, or art therapies may offer a release for negative feelings. (See pages 68–71.)

CAUTION
Massage is not suitable for those suffering from leukemia.

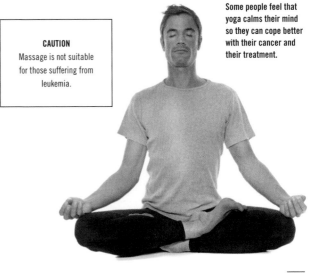

Some people feel that yoga calms their mind so they can cope better with their cancer and their treatment.

ANEMIA

Anemia is a deficiency of hemoglobin – the chemical that carries oxygen – in the red cells of the blood. The most common cause of anemia is iron deficiency resulting from excessive blood loss (through trauma, surgery, childbirth, or heavy menstrual bleeding), poor diet, or failure to absorb iron from food. Other causes of anemia include: excessive destruction of red blood cells (hemolytic anemia); vitamin B12 deficiency (pernicious anemia); and the inherited disorders of sickle cell anemia and thalassemia.

SYMPTOMS
• Weakness • Fatigue • Breathlessness on minimal exertion • Pale skin and lips • Headaches • Dizziness • Fainting in severe cases
In pernicious anemia:
• Nosebleeds • Sore tongue • "Pins and needles" in the hands and feet

TREATMENT

Ayurveda
A number of Ayurvedic products, including Kalyanaka ghritha (oral ghee), Kishor (oral pills), and Avipathi choorna (oral powder), would complement a treatment program.

Chinese Herbalism
The cause would be attributed to a spleen not transforming qi, and Gui Pi Wan (return spleen tablets) would be useful.

Traditional Home and Folk Remedies
Nettle tea is rich in iron; drink daily. (See page 194.)
Beet and carrot juice may be drunk to treat the condition. (See page 120.)

Herbalism
Chinese angelica root may be helpful. Take as tincture, decoction, or tea. (See page 82.)
Alfalfa, dandelion root, nettles, watercress, and yellow dock are rich in iron. (See pages 150, 154, 176, 188, and 194.)

Aromatherapy
Lavender essential oil is helpful where the anemia is associated with palpitations and dizzy spells. (See page 143.)
Massage with Roman chamomile essential oil. (See page 149.)

Homeopathy
Ferr. phos. helps assimilation of iron from food. (See page 215.)
Nat. mur., for anemia with constipation, headache, and a tendency to cold sores. (See page 154.)
Calc. phos., for anemia during a growth spurt, and irritability. (See page 213.)

Nutrition
Iron-rich foods include oats, egg yolks, pumpkin seeds, and watercress. (See page 215.)
Calcium, copper, vitamin C, and B vitamins must be present for the body to assimilate iron: ensure you have a sufficient intake in your diet. (See pages 206–209, 210, 213, and 214.)
Vegetarians should take extra vitamin B12. (See page 209.)
Avoid drinking tea at mealtimes as this makes iron absorption less efficient.

USEFUL FACTS
• Around 20 percent of anemia-sufferers are women, and 50 percent are children.
• The most common type of anemia is iron deficiency anemia, most often resulting from chronic blood loss; also from lack of iron in the diet, impaired absorption of iron from the intestine, or an increased need for iron, as occurs during pregnancy. Iron is an essential component of hemoglobin, which carries oxygen to the tissues in chemical combination with its iron atoms.
• Pernicious anemia is a chronic inherited disease of middle-aged and older people in which the stomach fails to produce a factor needed for the absorption of vitamin B12, which is essential for mature red blood cells.

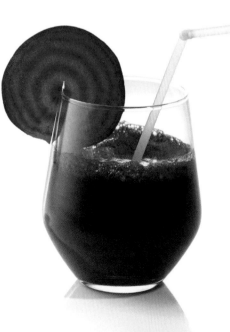

Beetroot juice and watercress may be beneficial for anemia.

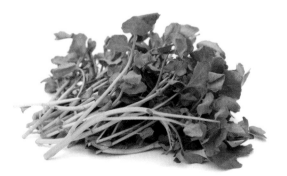

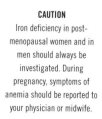

CAUTION
Iron deficiency in post-menopausal women and in men should always be investigated. During pregnancy, symptoms of anemia should be reported to your physician or midwife.

PALPITATIONS

The average heart beats about 72 times a minute and pumps about 3,600 gallons (13,640l.) of blood a day. During exercise, the pumping action automatically increases three- or fourfold, in response to the tissues' demand for increased oxygen. Palpitation refers to a fast or irregular heartbeat. Palpitations are quite common and usually harmless, often brought on by physical exertion or fright. Frequent or prolonged palpitations, however, may be an indication of heart disease, particularly if accompanied by dizziness, fainting, or chest pain. The sensation of a "missed" beat is due to a premature ectopic beat followed by a compensatory gap before the next beat. This can be induced by excitement, anxiety, or stimulants such as caffeine and nicotine.

SYMPTOMS
• Pounding in the chest following exercise • Uncomfortable awareness of a rapid heart rate when anxious

TREATMENT
Chinese Herbalism
Treatment would be aimed at addressing a heart blood deficiency, and may include the use of asparagus root and Suan Zao Ren (wild jujube seed). (See pages 87 and 201.)

Herbalism
Motherwort, drunk as an infusion, may help if palpitations are linked to anxiety or stress. (See page 144.)
Linden and valerian are useful herbs for treating palpitations. (See pages 191 and 195.)

Aromatherapy
If your palpitations are linked to emotional causes, calming oils such as ylang ylang, marjoram, lavender, and mandarin will help. Place a few drops in the bath, or use in regular massage. Carry a bottle with you, and sniff in times of distress. (See page 47.)
Peppermint, aniseed, lavender, lemon balm, rosemary, and neroli essential oils can be used separately or combined in a good massage oil to treat palpitations. (See page 47.)

Homeopathy
Nat. mur., for strong palpitations and chest constriction, made worse by heat. (See page 154.)

Carry a bottle of mandarin oil with you, so that you can sniff it during moments of stress.

ATHEROSCLEROSIS

Atherosclerosis is a degenerative disease of the arteries in which a fatty patch (atheroma) consisting mainly of cholesterol builds up on the wall of an artery. This eventually hardens and partially blocks the artery, causing the formation of a blood clot behind it. It is a progressive condition, generally worsening with age, and is most dangerous when the arteries supplying blood to the heart and brain are affected. Contributing factors to the development of atherosclerosis include smoking, high blood pressure, high blood cholesterol, heredity, and diabetes.

SYMPTOMS
• No symptoms at first, but it can cause life-threatening problems such as heart attacks and strokes if untreated

TREATMENT
Traditional Home and Folk Remedies
Increase your intake of olive oil, which breaks down cholesterol and fatty deposits in the blood. (See page 156.)
Drink barley water daily for a healthy heart. (See page 136.)
Garlic, onions, and yogurt all have a beneficial effect on the heart. (See pages 78, 79, and 142.)

Herbalism
Lavender oil helps to regulate the heart. Use the herb in the bath, or the oil in a vaporizer or gentle massage. (See page 143.)
Rosemary – fresh, dried, or as an oil – can be used to stimulate the circulatory system. (See page 175.)
Hawthorn berries and tops, and linden are both useful herbs for arterial diseases. (See pages 114 and 191.)

Aromatherapy
Regular massage with juniper and lemon can help to break down fatty deposits in the body. (See pages 108 and 142.)

Nutrition
Eat more fiber, fruits, and vegetables, and reduce your intake of salt, sugar, and saturated fats. (See page 58.)
Increase your intake of foods with bioflavonoids, to improve artery health. (See page 228.)
Stop smoking and cut down alcohol.

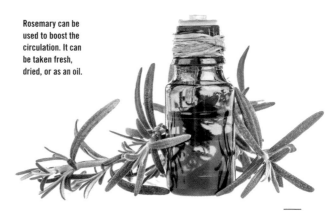

Rosemary can be used to boost the circulation. It can be taken fresh, dried, or as an oil.

VARICOSE VEINS

Varicose veins are swollen and twisted veins, most commonly found in the legs but also in the rectum (where they are known as hemorrhoids), the scrotum, and the esophagus. The swelling is caused by a weakness in the valves of the veins, which leads to increased pressure on the vein walls. This can be the result of deep vein thrombosis, obesity, pregnancy, prolonged sitting or standing, constipation, prolapse, or it may be hereditary.

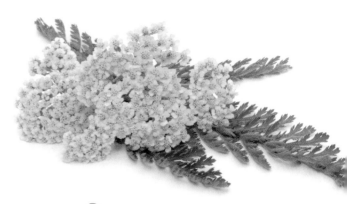

SYMPTOMS
• Extremely sore, swollen, and tender veins • Swelling of the legs
• Bruising and discoloration • Burning sensation • Aching calves
• Irritated and flaky skin • Ulcers • In severe cases, a vein may rupture and bleed

TREATMENT
Chinese Herbalism
The source of the problem is bad circulation, stagnant qi, and stagnant blood, and the following herbs would be used: Dang Gui (angelica), Gui Zhi (cinnamon twigs), and Huang Qi (astragalus). (See pages 82, 87, and 104.)
Honey might be used externally. (See page 203.)

Traditional Home and Folk Remedies
Raw beetroot should be eaten daily, for its healing and strengthening action.
A mustard poultice may help to encourage circulation in the area. (See page 91.)

Herbalism
Calendula oil, or marigold tea as a compress, can be applied. (See page 93.)
Herbs to repair and tone the veins include hawthorn berries, horse chestnut, prickly ash (*Zanthoxylum americanum*), and yarrow, all of which can be infused and drunk. (See pages 74, 76, and 114.)

Aromatherapy
Rosemary oil, blended with a light carrier oil, can be massaged into the legs. (See page 175.)
Essential oils of juniper and lavender can be diluted and massaged into the surrounding area, or used in the bath. (See pages 142 and 143.)

Homeopathy
Hamamelis, for bruised, sore veins, and piles. (See page 134.)
Carb. veg., for mottled and marbled skin. (See page 230.)
Ferr. phos., for pale legs that redden easily, but are better on walking. (See page 215.)

Nutrition
Increase your intake of vitamins E and C, and bioflavonoids, which improve blood vessel health. (See pages 210, 211, and 228.)
Increase your intake of dietary fiber, which will prevent constipation. (See page 58.)
Rutin helps to keep the vein walls in good shape.

Mind–Body Healing
Regular exercise will help with circulation in the legs. Contact your physician or a personal trainer to work out an exercise program that is right for you. (See page 70.)
Avoid standing for long periods, and elevate the affected area when resting.

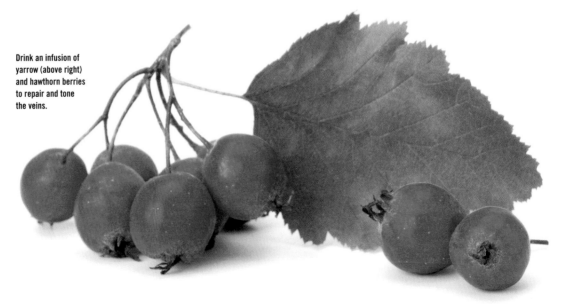

Drink an infusion of yarrow (above right) and hawthorn berries to repair and tone the veins.

RAYNAUD'S DISEASE

Raynaud's disease is a disorder in which the arteries of the fingers and (less often) the toes go into spasm on exposure to cold. Raynaud's disease is more common in women than men, and its onset usually occurs in young adulthood. It affects mainly young women, has no known cause, and is rarely serious. Raynaud's phenomenon, however, caused by disease or occupational hazard, is more problematic: inflammation of the arteries of the fingers and toes occurs, sometimes leading to the formation of a blood clot.

SYMPTOMS
• Tingling sensation, burning, and numbness in fingers or toes
• Affected areas turn white, then blue, then red • Painful ulcers or even tissue death (gangrene) can occur in cases where the disease persists for years

TREATMENT

Ayurveda
Massage hands and feet with a mixture of warm mustard and sesame seed oils. (See page 91.)

Chinese Herbalism
Dang Gui (angelica) and Gui Zhi (cinnamon twigs) may be useful. (See pages 82 and 104.)

Traditional Home and Folk Remedies
Keep fingers and toes warm in cold weather.

Herbalism
Cayenne pepper can be added to any herbal tea to stimulate the circulation and warm the body. (See page 98.)
Fresh ginger can be chewed, and the juices swallowed, to improve circulation and act as a tonic to the heart. (See page 200.)

Aromatherapy
Rubefacient oils such as black pepper, lemon, and rosemary can be massaged into the affected area to increase circulation and warmth. (See pages 108, 164, and 175.)

Nutrition
Increase your intake of iron, and ensure that you take plenty of foods rich in vitamin C alongside, which helps the absorption of iron. (See pages 210 and 215.)
Stop smoking, and see if avoiding caffeine helps.

Mind–Body Healing
Try to minimize your stress levels. Relaxation techniques such as breathing and yoga will be beneficial. (See pages 68 and 71.)
Regular cardiovascular exercise will improve the circulation. (See page 70.)

BRUISING

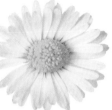

Bruising (or ecchymosis) results from the release of blood from the capillaries into the tissues under the skin. The characteristic bluish-black mark on the skin lightens in color and eventually fades as the blood is absorbed by the tissues and carried away. Bruising usually occurs as a result of an injury, but can occasionally be spontaneous and an indication of an allergic reaction, or more serious diseases such as leukemia and hemophilia.

SYMPTOMS
• Pain on pressure • In severe cases, pain on attempting to move the affected area

TREATMENT

Traditional Home and Folk Remedies
Macerated and heated cabbage leaves can be applied to the affected area. (See page 92.)
A mustard poultice or black pepper oil draws the blood away from the bruise. (See pages 91 and 164.)
A vinegar compress can be used for all bruises or swelling. Avoid the eye area. (See page 204.)
Use roasted onions in a poultice to help heal bruising. (See page 78.)

Herbalism
Bathe the area in witch hazel, which disperses the blood and encourages healing. (See page 134.)

Flower Essences
Rescue Remedy can be applied to the bruised area, to encourage healing and prevent the negative effects of trauma. (See page 158.)
Crushed agrimony roots and leaves can be used as a compress for bruises or taken internally. (See page 77.)
Comfrey is exceptional for healing, and can be applied as a compress or poultice on the bruise. (See page 186.)
Daisy (*Bellis perennis*) is also known as bruisewort. Bruise the leaves and flowers and add them to wheatgerm oil.
Crushed yarrow can be placed on fresh cuts or bruises. (See page 74.)

Nutrition
Increase your intake of vitamin C and bioflavonoids to help capillary health. (See pages 210 and 228.)

CAUTION
A case of bruising without any obvious cause requires medical investigation as it may be an outward symptom of a more serious condition.

Bruise the leaves and flowers of the common daisy, add to wheatgerm oil, then rub over a bruise.

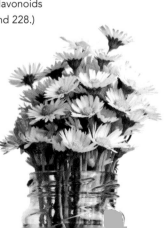

DISORDERS OF THE DIGESTIVE SYSTEM

JAUNDICE

Jaundice refers to a yellowing of the whites of the eyes and of the skin caused by bilirubin, a natural coloring substance. Under normal circumstances, bilirubin is released by red blood cells and passed to the intestine in bile, via the liver. If the liver is diseased, however, or if there is bile duct blockage, it accumulates in the blood, causing the characteristic yellow staining of tissue. Newborn infants frequently develop mild jaundice, which lasts several days until a normal excess of red blood cells is destroyed. This condition is not normally considered to be serious, although hospital care may be required for a few hours or days. However, erythroblastosis fetalis, a serious form of jaundice in infants, generally is due to an Rh factor incompatibility. Adolescents and young adults who have a viral inflammation of the liver often develop jaundice; jaundice in middle-aged adults is commonly due to gallstones. In older adults, jaundice may signal cancer of the liver or the bile ducts. It is often the first symptom of liver damage in heavy drinkers.

SYMPTOMS
• Yellowing of the skin and the whites of the eyes
• Darkened urine • Pale-colored stools

TREATMENT
Chinese Herbalism
Treatment would be aimed at dampness in the gall bladder and liver, and useful herbs may include Zhi Zi (gardenia fruit), Qing Hao (oriental wormwood), and Huang Bai (cork tree bark). (See page 162.)

Herbalism
These herbs can be used to tonify the liver: golden seal (*Hydrastis canadensis*), vervain, barberry, dandelion, and wild yam. (See pages 90, 121, 188, and 196.)

Aromatherapy
Oils that strengthen the liver include chamomile, cypress, lemon, peppermint, rosemary, and thyme. Use one or a blend of these oils in massage, or in a vaporizer in your room. (See page 47.)

Nutrition
Drink fresh carrot and lemon juice daily. (See pages 108 and 120.)
Avoid alcohol and caffeine.
Eat plenty of fresh fruit and vegetables, as well as whole grains and cereals. (See pages 58–59.)

> **CAUTION**
> Jaundice is not a disease in itself, but is an indication of an underlying disorder such as hepatitis, gallstones, hemolytic anemia, cirrhosis of the liver, pancreatitis, or pancreatic cancer. The cause of jaundice should always be investigated immediately. Jaundice in a newborn baby always requires medical attention, although it is rarely serious.

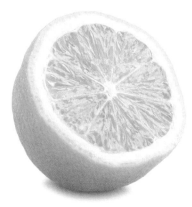

Drink a glass of carrot and lemon juice daily.

NAUSEA AND VOMITING

Nausea and vomiting are symptoms of various disorders, which include gastroenteritis, inner ear infection, migraine, excessive food or alcohol intake, hiatus hernia, pancreatitis, indigestion, food poisoning, gallstones, or liver disease. They may also be caused by hormonal changes in pregnancy and menstruation, travel, or by certain smells and sights. A constant feeling of nausea with no vomiting, but with a headache and abdominal pain, is most likely to be stress- or anxiety-related.

TREATMENT
Herbalism
Drinking ginger tea or chewing a piece of crystallized ginger warms the stomach and allays cold nausea. This can be used for relief of sickness in pregnancy or during travel. (See page 200.) Persistent nausea may indicate liver trouble: seek advice. Take decoction or coffee made of dandelion root. (See page 188.)

Flower Essences
Rescue Remedy be useful for prolonged or distressing vomiting: it will help to reduce panic and calm the mind and body. (See page 158.)

Nutrition
Take vitamin B6 for morning sickness (consult your physician first) and for travel sickness. It is appropriate for children if given in half-doses. (See page 208.)

Dandelion root is a liver stimulant and tonic. Drink dandelion coffee when nausea may be a result of liver problems.

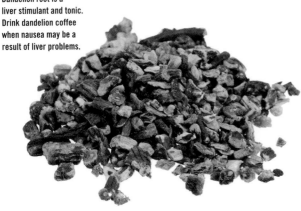

> **CAUTION**
> If nausea or vomiting are accompanied by severe pain lasting for more than one hour, or if vomit is blood-stained, seek urgent medical advice. If constant vomiting leads to dehydration, characterized by dark yellow and strong-smelling urine, dizziness or lightheadedness, tiredness or lack of responsiveness, and dry mouth, lips and eyes, seek medical advice.

GASTROENTERITIS

Gastroenteritis is an acute inflammation of the stomach and intestine, causing violent upset. It may be due to bowel organisms such as salmonella or other bacterial toxins or viruses that may contaminate food or water; food intolerance; or excessive alcohol intake. It can also be a side-effect of certain drugs. Gastroenteritis is most serious in the elderly and in babies because of the danger of dehydration.

SYMPTOMS
• Fever • Abdominal pain • Nausea and vomiting • Diarrhea
• In severe cases, shock and collapse

TREATMENT
Traditional Home and Folk Remedies
Very ripe bananas will ease nausea, act as a gentle constipant, and help to restore the healthy bacteria in the intestines.
Live yogurt, taken by the teaspoon throughout the day, can help to restore bacteria to the stomach and digestive tracts. (See page 142.)
Honey is a natural antibiotic and anti-inflammatory. Mix a few teaspoonfuls in a cup of warm water and sip. Freeze into ice cubes if you find hot drinks difficult to manage. (See page 203.)

Herbalism
Make an infusion of comfrey root and meadowsweet to treat the infection and relieve symptoms. (See pages 127 and 186.) Arrowroot or slippery elm tea can be sipped during the worst symptoms to soothe the digestive tract, and afterward to help restore bowel health. (See page 193.)

Aromatherapy
Massage chamomile and geranium essential oils into the abdomen to bring relief from pain and discomfort. (See pages 149 and 161.)

Gently massage chamomile essential oil into the abdomen to relieve discomfort.

> **CAUTION**
> If symptoms persist for more than 48 hours, or are accompanied by severe pain, call for emergency help. In young children and the elderly, gastroenteritis requires prompt medical advice.

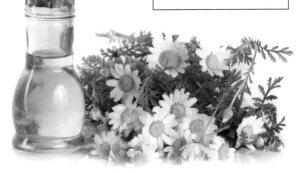

STOMACH ULCERS

Peptic ulcers, commonly called "stomach ulcers," occur most commonly in the duodenum (called duodenal ulcers), near the junction with the stomach, and in the stomach wall (properly called stomach or gastric ulcers). They usually occur singly as round or oval wounds. The erosions are usually shallow, but can penetrate the entire wall, leading to hemorrhage and possibly death. When gastric juices (consisting of hydrochloric acid, mucus, and a digestive enzyme called pepsin) act upon the walls of the digestive tract, a peptic ulcer results. Peptic ulcers tend to become chronic. The peptic ulcer develops when there is imbalance between the normal "aggressive" factors, the acid-peptic secretions, and the normal "resistance" factors, such as mucus and rapid cellular replacement. Physical and mental stress are thought to be triggers, as are hereditary factors, smoking, excessive alcohol intake, and non-steroidal anti-inflammatory drugs (NSAIDs). Gastric ulcers affect both men and women, usually over the age of 40, while duodenal ulcers are more common in men. Ulcers in the lower esophagus are relatively rare and are usually associated with hiatus hernia and esophagitis.

SYMPTOMS

• Ulcers may bleed, causing blood in vomit and dark, blackish stools
• Occasionally an ulcer perforates, causing severe pain and shock
In gastric ulcers:
• Gnawing, burning pain, which is worse during or after eating
• Nausea • Vomiting
In duodenal ulcers:
• Intermittent upper abdominal pain characteristically relieved by eating • Pain usually begins mid-morning and sufferers are often woken by it at night

TREATMENT

Ayurveda
Suitable herbs that might be suggested include bitter orange, coriander, and kalanchoe. (See pages 106 and 113.)

Chinese Herbalism
Treatment would be aimed at unblocking stagnant stomach qi, excess heat, and a weak spleen. Suitable herbs may include dandelion, Ren Shen (ginseng), and Yan Hu Suo (corydalis tuber). (See pages 160 and 188.)

Herbalism
Licorice has a soothing effect on the stomach and the mucous membranes, and a decoction can be drunk three or four times each day to ease symptoms. (See page 132.)
A decoction of marshmallow root is healing. (See page 81.)
Comfrey or slippery elm may also be of help. (See pages 186 and 193.)

Aromatherapy
Oils of chamomile, frankincense, geranium, and marjoram can be diluted and massaged into the abdomen. (See page 47.)

Homeopathy
Treatment would be constitutional, but the following remedies may be appropriate:
Anacardium, when pain is relieved by eating. (See page 182.)
Phosphorus, for burning pains and vomiting which are better for cold drinks. (See page 219.)

Nutrition
Talk with a nutritionist about maintaining a healthy diet. Smoking and alcohol may worsen ulcers.

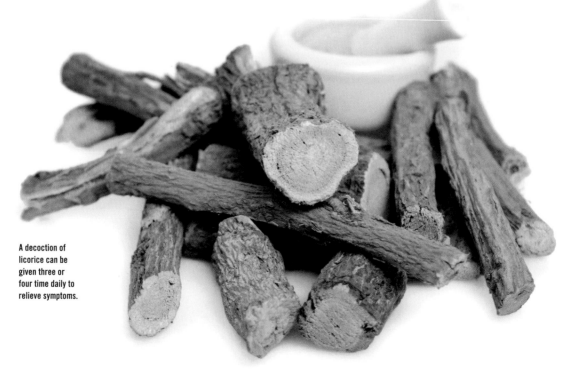

A decoction of licorice can be given three or four time daily to relieve symptoms.

INDIGESTION

Indigestion (or dyspepsia) is a general term that usually refers to abdominal discomfort, nausea, heartburn (burning sensation or pain behind the breastbone), hiccups, and flatulence. Indigestion refers to discomfort in the upper abdomen – gastric distress – often brought on by eating too much, by eating too quickly, or by eating very rich, spicy, or fatty foods. Nervous indigestion is a common effect of stress. Indigestion is also commonly caused by excessive smoking, excessive alcohol or caffeine consumption, pregnancy, or anxiety. It can also be a feature of several diseases, including esophagitis (inflammation of the lining of the esophagus), gastroenteritis (see page 301), peptic ulcer (see page 302), and gallstones (see page 305).

SYMPTOMS
• Abdominal discomfort • Nausea • Heartburn (burning sensation or pain behind the breastbone) • Hiccups • Flatulence

TREATMENT
Ayurveda
Crush fresh root ginger to extract the juice. Mix with the juice of a lime and a lemon, add a pinch of salt, and drink. (See page 200.)

Chinese Herbalism
Treatment would address a weakness of the spleen and stomach. Rice and wheat sprouts would be used. (See page 159.)

Traditional Home and Folk Remedies
Eat a slice of fresh pineapple after meals to ease symptoms. Clove tea and cinnamon tea are both digestive and will soothe away the symptoms. (See pages 104 and 125.)
Fennel, eaten raw or cooked, or the bruised seeds infused and drunk, acts as a digestive. (See page 128.)
Peppermint leaves can be infused and drunk to relieve indigestion, and to soothe any gas pains. Peppermint oil can be rubbed into the abdomen for instant relief. (See page 152.)
Drink a little warmed vinegar and honey in a cup of hot water to ease digestive complaints. (See pages 203 and 204.)

Herbalism
Try an infusion of peppermint or fennel tea after meals or when feeling full and windy. (See pages 128 and 152.)
Improve the general tone of the digestive tract with bitter aperient herbs such as dandelion and gentian (*Gentiana lutea*), taken 20 minutes before food. (See page 188.)
A cold stomach can be warmed by eating 3 cardamom pods, or a pinch of ginger or cayenne. (See pages 98, 122, and 200.)
Fresh dill (*Anethum graveolens*), added to boiling water and steeped, will reduce flatulence and gas pains.

Homeopathy
Chronic indigestion should be treated constitutionally, but the following remedies may be useful during an attack:
Carb. veg., after rich foods, with gas and belching. (See page 230.)
China, for windy stomach, and a bloated and sluggish feeling, and where stools have the appearance of chopped egg. (See page 103.)
Lycopodium, for a bloated stomach with heartburn, and a full feeling even when hungry, especially where food causes instant discomfort. (See page 147.)

Nutrition
If you feel the cause of your indigestion may be dietary, try cutting out common triggers such as alcohol, caffeine, raw onions, spicy foods, and chocolate. Foods known to cause excess wind include: beans and other pulses, bran, dried fruit, and vegetables such as cabbage, broccoli and Brussels sprouts. If you suspect a food intolerance, discuss the problem with your physician. Milk and dairy products, as well as gluten, are common culprits.

Mind–Body Healing
If indigestion is linked to stress, relaxation techniques and yoga will be helpful. (See pages 68–71.)

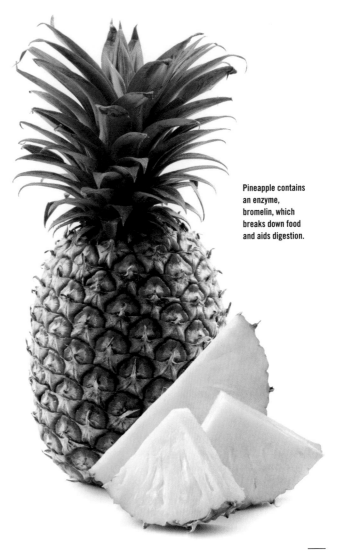

Pineapple contains an enzyme, bromelin, which breaks down food and aids digestion.

TRAVEL SICKNESS

Travel or motion sickness is a sensitivity to the constant passive movement of the body while in a car, boat, airplane, train, or bus. Some people may even experience it in lifts. Why only some people experience travel sickness is unclear. The syndrome appears to arise from sensory mismatch, when the information coming to the brain from various sensory inputs does not add up, as when the eyes report a steady horizon, but the balancing (vestibular) system reports a rocking motion. Travel sickness appears to be more common in women, and children under the age of two. Elderly people do not seem to be so troubled by the problem. Severe travel sickness can cause a complete lack of coordination.

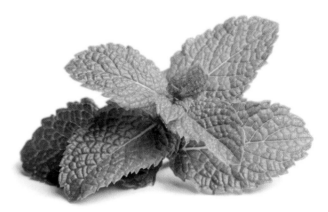

SYMPTOMS
• Progressive nausea • Vomiting • Pallor • Faintness • Dizziness
• Abdominal discomfort • Headache • Sweaty palms and face
• Increased salivation

TREATMENT

Ayurveda
Ginger, chewed fresh, may help symptoms. (See page 200.)
Oral syrup of Vilwadi Lehya will be useful.

Chinese Herbalism
Sipping a warm drink with grated root ginger may be helpful. (See page 200.)

Traditional Home and Folk Remedies
Look at a stable object, such as the horizon. Alternatively, close your eyes.
Do not read or look at a handheld screen, which may make your symptoms worse.
Open windows in the car or move to the top deck of a ship to get fresh air.

Herbalism
Chew fresh angelica leaves, and hang them in the car while traveling. (See page 82.)
Chew fresh or crystallized ginger to ease nausea. (See page 200.)
Fennel or chamomile tea will ease the symptoms. (See pages 128 and 149.)
Fresh peppermint leaves can be chewed, or drink an infusion to soothe and settle the stomach. (See page 152.)

Homeopathy
You could take the following remedies hourly when symptoms begin:
Arnica, when you are overtired and irritable. (See page 86.)
Sepia, when nausea is made worse by the smell of food and improved by eating. (See page 182.)

Nutrition
Do not eat a heavy meal before traveling. Stay hydrated by sipping cool water.

Mind–Body Healing
When symptoms occur, relax yourself by listening to music. Carry out breathing exercises, or count backwards from 1,000.

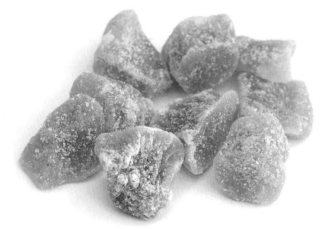

Take a store of crystallized ginger (left) and fresh peppermint leaves (above) on your travels.

GALLSTONES

Gallstones are hard stone-like masses occurring in the gall bladder or in the bile duct. They are usually about the size of a pebble, and most are composed of cholesterol, calcium, or both. Abnormal composition of bile (too much cholesterol, for example), blockage of bile outflow, infection, or hereditary factors may all cause gallstones. Risk factors include obesity, advancing age, a high-fat diet, and food intolerance.

SYMPTOMS
• Acute upper abdominal pain • Possibly high fever • Inflammation of the gall bladder (cholecystitis) • Some jaundice if the stones cause bile duct obstruction • Severe pain if a stone passes from the bile duct into the duodenum (biliary colic)

TREATMENT
Ayurveda
Kalanchoe can be used to treat gallstones.

Chinese Herbalism
Herbs such as lysimachia, pyrrosia leaf, and Da Huang (rhubarb) may break up and dissolve small stones. (See page 173.)

Herbalism
The following herbs will dissolve the gallstones, but it will take several months. Blend infusions of balmony, dandelion leaves, stone root, and fringetree bark. Take 2 or 3 times a day. (See page 188.)

Aromatherapy
Massage lavender and rosemary oils over the gall bladder area to relieve the pain. (See pages 143 and 175.)

Homeopathy
Treatment would always be constitutional, but China may help until you are able to seek advice. (See page 103.)

Nutrition
Reduce your intake of all fats, except olive oil, which may help to break up gallstones. (See page 156.)
Increase your intake of dietary fiber, and ensure that you drink plenty of water. (See page 58.)

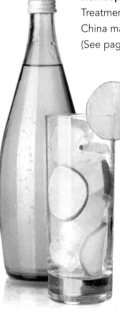

Increasing your intake of water is crucial to prevent gallstones.

> **CAUTION**
> If you suspect gallstones, take advice on treatment from your physician.

HEPATITIS

Hepatitis is a disorder involving inflammation of the liver. The acute form can subside after about two months or, rarely, can result in liver failure. Chronic hepatitis leads to cirrhosis and liver damage. Hepatitis A, once called infectious hepatitis, is the most common cause of acute hepatitis and is usually transmitted by food and water contaminated by human waste. Hepatitis B is spread mainly by blood or blood products, but can be transmitted from mother to fetus, and by intimate contact, including sexual intercourse. It often causes an initial episode of liver disease and occasionally leads to chronic hepatitis. Hepatitis C is the most common form of viral hepatitis. Type C is transmitted in blood and blood products (which are now screened for the virus), and it may be present in the body for many years before it damages the liver. Another strain of hepatitis C is uncommon in Europe and the U.S., but common in Mexico, Africa, and Asia, and usually contracted from contaminated water. Hepatitis C is a leading cause of chronic hepatitis and is considered a serious public health threat.

SYMPTOMS
• Loss of appetite • Dark urine • Fatigue • Sometimes fever • Liver may become enlarged • Jaundice may occur

TREATMENT
Chinese Herbalism
Hepatitis A would require treatment for excess liver and gall bladder damp heat. Suitable herbal remedies include Zhi Zi (gardenia fruit) and Qing Hao (oriental wormwood).
Hepatitis B would require treatment for deficient qi and a weakened liver. Suitable herbs include Bai Shao (peony root), Ren Shen (ginseng), Gan Cao (licorice), and Huang Qi (astragalus). (See pages 87, 132, 159, and 160.)

Traditional Home and Folk Remedies
Drink barley or rice water as an overall tonic. (See pages 136 and 159.)

Herbalism
Liver tonics may be taken daily to encourage healing and rejuvenation.
Any of the following herbs can be used: golden seal (*Hydrastis canadensis*), vervain, barberry, dandelion, and wild yam. (See pages 90, 121, 188, and 196.)

Aromatherapy
Oils that act as liver tonics include juniper, grapefruit, chamomile, and cypress. Massage them, in a little carrier oil, into the abdomen, or add drops to your bath. (See pages 109, 117, 142, and 149.)

Nutrition
Plenty of fluids are necessary to cleanse the system.
Extra vitamin C will help overcome the infection. (See page 210.)

> **CAUTION**
> If hepatitis is suspected, contact your physician.

CIRRHOSIS OF THE LIVER

The liver is a spongy gland that lies just below the diaphragm in the abdominal cavity, and it serves to metabolize carbohydrates and store them as glycogen; metabolize lipids (fats, including cholesterol and certain vitamins) and proteins; manufacture a digestive fluid, bile; filter impurities and toxic material from the blood; produce blood-clotting factors, and destroy old, worn-out red blood cells. The liver is able to regenerate itself after being injured or diseased; but if a disease progresses beyond the tissues' capacity to regenerate new cells, the body's entire metabolism is severely affected. Severely impaired livers are sometimes replaced. Cirrhosis of the liver is the replacement of normal tissue by nonfunctioning fibrous tissue, causing scarring (or fibrosis). Normal liver function is prevented and any remaining healthy liver cells are cut off from the blood supply they need. Cirrhosis occurs as the last stage in a range of liver disorders, and may be caused by hepatitis B, poisoning, and long-term alcohol abuse.

SYMPTOMS

• Appetite and weight loss • Continuous indigestion • Nausea and vomiting • General malaise • Loss of muscle power • Itching of the skin • Bad breath • Bleeding varicose veins (caused by the blood's attempt to use an alternative route from the liver back to the heart) • Vomiting blood

TREATMENT

Herbalism

Good liver tonics include barberry, dandelion root, golden seal (*Hydrastis canadensis*), vervain, wild yam, and yellow dock. Make an infusion of one or more and sip 2 or 3 times daily. (See pages 90, 121, 176, 188, and 196.)

Aromatherapy

Oils that work as a tonic to the liver and improve its function include chamomile, cypress, grapefruit, juniper, lemon, and orange. Mix a few drops in a warm carrier oil and massage into the abdomen, or add a few drops to your bath. (See page 47.)

Homeopathy

Constitutional treatment with an experienced homeopath will be necessary, but the following remedies may help until you have arranged treatment:

Phosphorus, when there is jaundice, a craving for cold water, and a tendency to bleed easily. (See page 219.)

China, when the liver is swollen and painful, and you feel chilly and full of wind. (See page 103.)

> **CAUTION**
> If cirrhosis of the liver is suspected, contact your physician. Consult with your physician before taking alternative remedies.

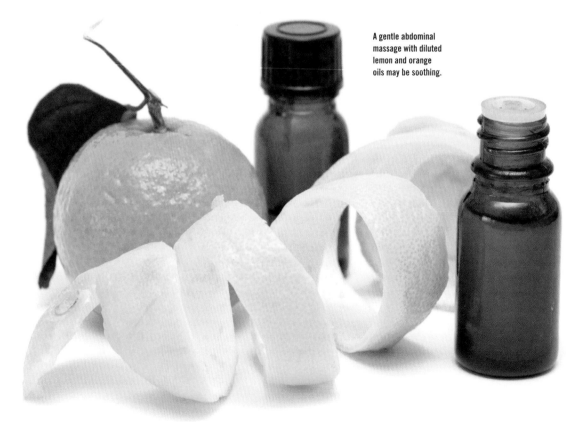

A gentle abdominal massage with diluted lemon and orange oils may be soothing.

PANCREATITIS

A long, thin organ, the pancreas has both digestive and endocrine functions, and for this reason contains two completely different types of cells. It measures about 5–6in. (12–15cm.) in length and is situated within the curve of the duodenum. Pancreatitis is an inflammation of the pancreas which can be either acute or chronic. Acute pancreatitis may be caused by interference (often from gallstones) with the outflow of digestive juices from the pancreas, as a result of which the pancreas begins to digest itself. Heavy drinking is another cause, and is almost always responsible for cases of chronic pancreatitis. Diagnosis of pancreatitis can be difficult since it closely resembles peptic ulcer and acute appendicitis.

An infusion of yellow dock root is recommended for an inflamed pancreas.

SYMPTOMS

In acute pancreatitis:
• Severe central abdominal pain, spreading to the back and shoulder, then the whole abdomen • Nausea • Vomiting • Shock
In chronic pancreatitis:
• Constant pain, often in the upper abdomen and back • Weight loss • Jaundice, if bile duct obstruction occurs

TREATMENT

Herbalism
Treatment would be individual, according to the cause of the illness.
Soothing herbs include licorice and yellow dock, drunk as an infusion in an attack. (See pages 122 and 176.)

Homeopathy
For chronic pancreatitis, constitutional treatment is necessary, but the following remedies may help in an attack:
Phosphorus, when there is jaundice and a craving for cold drinks that are then vomited. (See page 219.)
Iris, for watery stools, a burning sensation in the bowels, and cutting pains in the abdomen.

> **CAUTION**
> In the case of acute pancreatitis, ring for emergency medical attention.

CROHN'S DISEASE

For sufferers of Crohn's disease, segments of the bowel become inflamed, ulcerated, and thickened. Any part of the bowel may be affected, but usually it is the last part of the small intestine, the terminal ileum, that is involved. It is a chronic disease whose cause is unknown, although there may be a genetic and ethnic factor. Complications of Crohn's disease include arthritis, red swellings on the skin, mouth ulcers, eye inflammation, gallstones, urinary infections, and kidney stones. Bowel obstruction and various other complications may require surgical intervention.

SYMPTOMS
• Spasms of lower abdominal pain • Diarrhea • Appetite and weight loss • Anemia • Rectal bleeding in older sufferers

TREATMENT
Ayurveda
Coriander can help with diarrhea and the pain of Crohn's disease. It is an anti-inflammatory. (See page 113.)

Herbalism
An infusion of peppermint can help protect the gut lining from irritation, and help soothe griping. (See page 152.)
Hops have an antispasmodic action that reduces tension in the body, relieving colic and spasm in the gut. The bitters in hops also enhance the action of the digestive system. Hops are the flowers of the hop plant *Humulus lupulus*.

Aromatherapy
Lavender oil will help to reduce the effects of stress. Add it to your bath water, or use in body massage. (See page 143.)
Roman chamomile oil, rubbed into the abdomen, may help to soothe pain. (See page 149.)

Nutrition
You may need to take extra vitamin A, B, and D, and zinc supplement daily. (See pages 206–210 and 221.)
You may be allergic to some foods, such as dairy produce or wheat: see a nutritional therapist for advice. Avoid sugar and other refined carbohydrates.

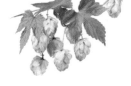

Hops are used herbally to relieve abdominal spasms and as a general aid to the digestive system.

> **CAUTION**
> Discuss all remedies with your physician.

CONSTIPATION

Constipation refers to unduly infrequent or irregular bowel movements, with difficulty, discomfort, and sometimes pain on passing dry, hard feces. It is usually harmless but may be an indication of an underlying disorder, especially in adults over the age of 40. Constipation may result from: insufficient fiber in the diet, immobility, hemorrhoids (see page 311), an anal fissure (see page 311), iron tablets, hypothyroidism (see page 338), or hormonal changes, such as those in pregnancy. Dietary causes include inadequate fluid intake; a lack of vitamin B1, B5, B6, potassium, magnesium, and zinc; too much animal protein; too many dairy products; and too much vinegar, pepper, salt, spices, and aluminum. If the diet is not at fault, the cause may be eating meals too fast, not taking enough exercise, tension, anxiety, depression, taking antibiotics, abusing laxatives, or abuse of certain over-the-counter drugs, such as cough mixtures.

SYMPTOMS

• Infrequent or irregular bowel movements • Pain during bowel movements • Dry, hard feces • Weight loss
Anxiety about constipation may cause:
• Headaches • Furred tongue • Loss of appetite • Nausea
• Fatigue • Depression

TREATMENT

Chinese Herbalism

Constipation is believed to be caused by heat, stagnation of qi, deficiency (of qi, yang, blood, or yin), or interior cold. Some suitable pills include:
Ma Ren Wan, for heat (dry stools, thirst, dark urine).
Run Chang Wan, for chronic constipation of any kind, especially in old age or after childbirth.
Mu Xiang Shun Qi Wan, for qi stagnation. (See page 88.)

Traditional Home and Folk Remedies

Dried apricots, prunes, and figs will have a laxative effect. (See page 126.)

Herbalism

Laxative herbs, which can be drunk as herbal infusions up to 3 times daily, include licorice, marshmallow root, rhubarb root, buckthorn (*Rhamnus purshiana*), and senna leaves. (See pages 81, 99, 132, and 173.)

Aromatherapy

Massage a few drops of marjoram, rosemary, or fennel oil, diluted in grapeseed oil, into the abdomen, to relieve constipation. (See pages 128, 157, and 175.)

Homeopathy

In homeopathy, constipation is regarded as a constitutional problem that requires consultations with a registered practitioner, but the following remedies may help with occasional symptoms:
Lycopodium, when there is flatulence but no need to open bowels for long periods of time; then stools are hard, and passed with pain. (See page 147.)
Sepia, when the belly feels full. (See page 182.)
Silicea, when there is a burning sensation after a bowel movement. (See page 220.)
Alumina, when there is no desire to open bowels until the rectum is full; the stool may be covered in mucus.

Nutrition

Increase your intake of dietary fiber, which will help to bulk out stools. (See page 58.)
Acidophilus will encourage the health of the intestines and make bowel movements more normal. (See page 142.)
Chronic constipation may respond to an increased intake of B-complex vitamins, particularly if it follows a course of antibiotics. Vitamin B1 is most effective. (See page 206.)

Mind–Body Healing

Regular exercise combined with relaxation techniques, such as meditation and deep breathing, when needed, will have a beneficial effect on constipation and the anxiety that can accompany it. (See pages 68–71.)

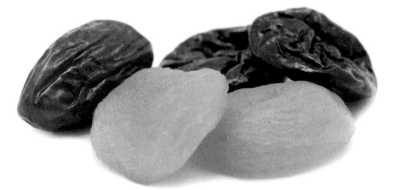

Dried fruits have a high fiber content, which will ease constipation.

DIARRHEA

Diarrhea occurs when normal reabsorption of water from the stools has not taken place, so that stools are loose and runny. The two basic mechanisms involved in diarrhea, which may operate independently or together, are excessive accumulation of fluid in the intestinal tract and excessive propulsive action in the intestines. Excessive fluid in the intestines can result from conditions that decrease the absorption of water from the colon, or from conditions that cause water to be secreted into the intestines, as in cholera and other infections. The body secretes excess water in order to "flush" disease and toxins. Excessive propulsive action may be caused by nervous and chemical factors or by partial obstruction of the intestine. Diarrhea is a feature of many conditions, including dysentery, food poisoning, cholera, typhoid, gastroenteritis, and parasitic infestation. It can also be brought on by stress or anxiety, and in babies it may be caused by lactose intolerance. Chronic diarrhea may be caused by Crohn's disease (see page 307), ulcerative colitis, or cancer of the colon.

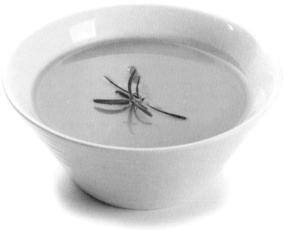

Make sure that you drink enough fluids as you are at risk of dehydration with diarrhea. If diarrhea is accompanied by other symptoms, restrict your food intake to soups, particularly carrot, as they are easily digestible.

SYMPTOMS
• Loose stools • Possibly abdominal cramps • Possibly wind
• Possibly vomiting

TREATMENT

Ayurveda
Senna pods and coriander can be used to treat diarrhea. (See pages 99 and 113.)

Chinese Herbalism
The full condition is caused by cold damp or damp heat; the empty condition is due to a spleen, stomach, or kidney yang deficiency. (See page 48.)
Huang Qin (skullcap root) may be suitable for acute diarrhea, as well as Huang Lian (golden thread), kapok flowers, and dandelion root. (See pages 113, 181, and 188.)
For chronic diarrhea, a treatment of Bu Gu Zhi (psoralea fruit), Dang Shen (codonopsis root), and Huang Qi (astragalus) may be given. (See pages 87 and 110.)
Huo Xiang Zheng Qi Wan, or agastache upright qi powder, for gastric flu. (See page 77.)
Mu Xiang Shun Qi Wan and Shen Ling Bai Zhu Wan, 2 pills taken together for alternating diarrhea and constipation (liver qi stagnation with spleen qi deficiency). The latter can be taken for chronic loose stools with poor appetite, tiredness, etc. (See page 88.)
Liu Jun Zi Pian, or Six Gentlemen Tablet, for loose stools, diarrhea, and indigestion resulting from spleen qi deficiency.
Xiang Sha Liu Jun Zi Wan, for loose stools, diarrhea, and indigestion, accompanied by nausea.

Traditional Home and Folk Remedies
Carrot juice or soup is very helpful, especially for infants. (See page 120.)

Herbalism
For acute diarrhea take a gentle laxative such as dock to clear away the cause of the irritant. (See page 176.)
A few drops of myrrh tincture in water will clear many infections. (See page 112.)
For chronic and nervous diarrhea, use chamomile or marigold mixed with a soothing, astringent herb such as raspberry leaf. (See pages 93, 149, and 176.)

Homeopathy
Chronic diarrhea should be treated constitutionally, but acute attacks may be treated with one of the following remedies:
Colocynthis, for diarrhea accompanied by griping pains, with yellowish, thin, and copious stools. (See page 105.)
China, for stools accompanied by wind, and made worse by fruit. (See page 103.)
Phosphoric acid, when stools contain undigested food and you feel better after passing them.

Nutrition
Increase your intake of potassium, which is easily lost in diarrhea and vomiting. (See page 217.)
Increase your intake of vitamins B1 and B3, which will address the digestive system. (See pages 206 and 207.)
Drink plenty of water, to flush the system.
Take a multivitamin and mineral supplement with food when you are able to eat properly again, to replace lost nutrients. (See page 60.)
Take plenty of fresh acidophilus for at least a month after an attack, to ensure the health of the bowels. (See page 142.)

Mind–Body Healing
When diarrhea is brought on by stress or anxiety, relaxation techniques such as visualization and meditation will be helpful. (See page 68.)

> **CAUTION**
> Consult a physician regarding episodes of diarrhea lasting more than 48 hours, particularly if there is fever and/or vomiting.

IRRITABLE BOWEL SYNDROME

Irritable bowel syndrome (IBS; or spastic colon) is a very common disorder with recurrent abdominal pain and intermittent diarrhea alternating with constipation. This may be caused by a disturbance in the muscle movement in the large intestine, triggered by anxiety, stress, or food intolerance. The vast majority of IBS sufferers are women, and the young to middle-aged are particularly vulnerable. In the Western world, 10–20 percent of the population suffers or has suffered from IBS. Up to half of all health cases dealt with by gastroenterologists are caused by IBS.

SYMPTOMS
• Intermittent diarrhea and constipation • Cramp-like abdominal pain, usually after eating, relieved by going to the toilet • Swelling of the abdomen • Excessive wind • Headache and back pain • General malaise • Sensation of fullness halfway through a meal • Undue awareness of bowel action • Anxiety

TREATMENT
Ayurveda
Coriander and hollyhock (*Alcea rosea*) are suitable herbs to treat IBS. (See page 113.)

Chinese Herbalism
Treatment would address weakness of the kidneys and spleen, excess damp in the intestines, and stagnation of liver qi. Some suitable herbs might include Da Huang (rhubarb), dandelion, magnolia, and Dang Gui (angelica). (See pages 82, 173, and 188.)

Herbalism
Slippery elm has a soothing action along the length of the gut. (See page 193.)
Try calming, antispasmodic teas such as chamomile, peppermint, and lemon balm. (See pages 149 and 152.)
Chew fresh ginger to help relieve spasms. (See page 200.)

Aromatherapy
Massage the abdomen with lavender or chamomile oils, which have antispasmodic qualities. (See pages 143 and 149.)
Detoxifying oils include juniper, garlic, fennel, and rose. Add to your bath water or use in massage. (See page 47.)

Homeopathy
Treatment must be constitutional, but Colocynthis may be suitable for griping pains brought on by anger. (See page 105.)

Flower Essences
Consider whether or not your condition is stress-related (see "Stress," page 246) and choose a remedy that fits your emotional symptoms. (See page 54.)
Rescue Remedy is useful during attacks, to calm. (See page 158.)
Mimulus will help if you are frightened by the thought of eating or of experiencing another attack. (See page 153.)

Nutrition
Vitamin A is necessary to keep the intestinal tract healthy. (See page 206.)
Take acidophilus to encourage the growth of healthy bacteria. (See page 142.)
A deficiency of zinc and vitamin B6 is indicated in many cases; ensure that your intake is adequate. (See pages 208 and 221.)
Dietary fiber helps to detoxify. (See page 58.)
If you suspect that food intolerance is causing your symptoms, contact a nutritionist for advice. Lactose intolerance is a common culprit.

Mind–Body Healing
Stress and anxiety may act as triggers for irritable bowel syndrome. If IBS worsens during periods of stress, relaxation techniques are likely to be beneficial. (See pages 68–69.)
In some cases, cognitive behavioral therapy and hypnotherapy have brought about dramatic improvements in IBS.

> **CAUTION**
> IBS shares symptoms with some more serious conditions, so take advice from a physician.

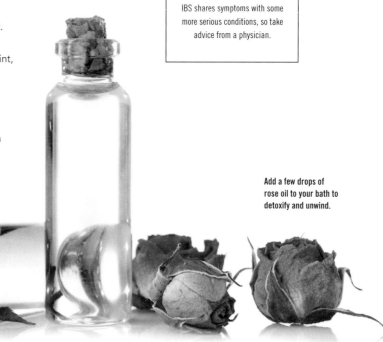

Add a few drops of rose oil to your bath to detoxify and unwind.

Eating fiber-rich foods, such as raw spinach, will prevent constipation, which is the major cause of anal fissures.

ANAL FISSURE

An anal fissure is a tear in the lower anal canal, close to the anal sphincter, and is often associated with internal hemorrhoids. When a stool is passed, the split is irritated, causing the sphincter muscles to go into painful spasm. Constipation is the root cause in most cases. Usually it heals quickly without complications but occasionally it may be chronic, spreading to the sphincter muscle and ending in infection.

SYMPTOMS
• Pain during bowel movements • Minor bleeding
• Irritation and discomfort

TREATMENT
Ayurveda
The following preparations may be helpful if the fissure is caused by constipation: Abhayarishta (an oral tonic), Gin (oral pills), or Sukumara Ghritha (oral ghee).

Traditional Home and Folk Remedies
Dab a little olive oil onto the fissure to encourage healing and relieve pain. (See page 156.)
Fresh lemon juice, applied to the fissure, will prevent infection and dull the pain. (See page 108.)

Herbalism
Dandelion coffee is a mild laxative, and can be drunk, as required, on a daily basis. (See page 188.)
Take a drink made of a cup of flaxseeds in a cup of water before bedtime to moisten stools. (See page 145.)
Slippery elm and cinnamon will lubricate. (See pages 104 and 193.)
Comfrey root can help to heal the sore and inflamed tissues. (See page 186.)

Aromatherapy
Apply a few drops of neat lavender or tea tree oil to the fissure to encourage healing and prevent infection. It may sting. (See pages 143 and 150.)

Nutrition
Acidophilus encourages the health of the bowels, and so should be taken daily as required. (See page 142.)
Eat plenty of foods that are high in dietary fibers, including whole grains, fresh, raw vegetables and fruits, and dried fruits.

PILES (HEMORRHOIDS)

Piles are swollen (or varicose) veins in the lining of the anus. The varicosity may be just above the anal canal, causing "internal" hemorrhoids, or at the lower end of the canal, causing "external" hemorrhoids. The latter may even protrude outside the anus ("prolapsed" hemorrhoids). Piles are caused by increased pressure on the veins of the anus, most commonly as a result of chronic constipation with straining, pregnancy, and childbirth. There may, however, be a congenital predisposition. Piles affect 50–75 percent of the U.S. population, and become more common with age.

SYMPTOMS
• Pain and bleeding during bowel movements • Soreness and itching around the anus • Possibly a mucus discharge from prolapsed hemorrhoids

TREATMENT
Ayurveda
There are several Ayurvedic preparations available from health food stores, including Abhayarishta, which is an oral tonic, and Dadimadi Ghritha (oral ghee).

Traditional Home and Folk Remedies
Red potato can be cut into a slim cigar shape and inserted into the anus to relieve symptoms. (See page 184.)
Sit on a cold bowl of water, or use a cold bidet, several times daily to reduce inflammation and swelling. (See page 205.)

Herbalism
Make a small witch hazel compress, and keep it on the affected area for as long as possible to reduce inflammation and encourage healing. (See page 134.)
Pilewort ointment, made from *Rananculus ficaria*, is useful, and should be applied 2 or 3 times daily.
Yellow dock is astringent and can be added to cocoa butter, which can be shaped into a suppository and placed in the anus. (See page 176.)
Internally, a course of dandelion root, horse chestnut, or yarrow can be helpful. (See pages 74, 76, and 188.)
Externally, horse chestnut can be applied. (See page 76.)
Clear congestion in the area with a good diet and teas of dock or dandelion root. (See pages 176 and 188.)

Aromatherapy
Apply a local compress of astringent essential oils of cypress, frankincense, lavender, or myrrh. (See page 47.)
Add a little rosemary oil to a warm bath to improve the circulation. (See page 175.)

Pilewort ointment may be soothing.

WIND

Wind (or flatulence) refers to the expulsion from the body of an excessive amount of air or gas, via the anus (breaking wind) or the mouth (belching or burping). Gas discharged via the anus is called flatus and comprises a number of gases, including hydrogen sulfide, which is responsible for the characteristic unpleasant smell. Wind can be caused by excessive swallowing of air (aerophagy), which may be a response to stress, or a consequence of eating too quickly. It is also a feature of disorders such as indigestion and irritable bowel syndrome. Certain foods such as pulses and beans produce more flatus than others. Gas is formed in the large intestine as a result of the action of bacteria on carbohydrates and amino acids in digested food: the gas consists of hydrogen, carbon dioxide, and methane. Gas formed in the intestine is passed only through the anus.

SYMPTOMS
• Besides its characteristic sounds, flatulence can cause abdominal discomfort

TREATMENT
Ayurveda
Ayurvedic preparations available include Digesic, which is an oral tablet, as well as Gasex and Ramabana.

Chinese Herbalism
Treatment would be aimed at stagnant stomach energy, and suitable herbs include Huo Po (magnolia bark), and orange or lemon peel. (See pages 106 and 108.)

Traditional Home and Folk Remedies
Charcoal is excellent for reducing gas in the stomach and intestines. (See page 230.)
Celery seeds can reduce flatulence. (See page 84.)

Herbalism
Fresh dill (*Anethum graveolens*), added to boiling water and steeped, will reduce flatulence and gas pains.
Try making an infusion of calamus root, also called sweet flag, drinking half a cup before meals. (See page 75.)

Homeopathy
Lycopodium, when gas feels stuck, is painful, and is made worse by onions, garlic, and fried foods. It can be taken every 30 minutes, for up to 6 doses. (See page 147.)

Nutrition
If excessive wind is causing a problem, try cutting down on foods that contain a lot of unabsorbable carbohydrates, including beans and pulses, apples, onions, dried fruits such as prunes and raisins, and vegetables such as broccoli, cabbage, cauliflower and Brussels sprouts.
If you suspect that a food intolerance is causing excessive wind, contact a nutritionist or your physician.
Excessive flatulence may also be caused by some medications and artificial sweeteners, such as sorbitol.

Mind–Body Healing
If episodes of excessive flatulence seem to be linked to stress, try relaxation techniques such as yoga, visualization, or meditation. (See pages 68–71.)

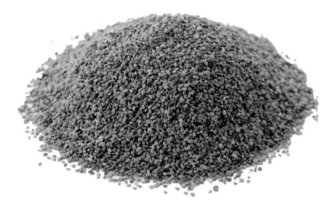

If you suffer from gas in the intestine, try taking celery seeds or an infusion of fresh dill.

> **CAUTION**
> Excessive flatulence accompanied by weight loss, severe abdominal pain, or bleeding during bowel movements requires medical attention.

CELIAC DISEASE

Celiac disease is a fairly common condition in which the small intestine becomes inflamed and is unable to absorb nutrients. The condition is caused by an adverse reaction to gluten, which is found in barley, rye, and wheat. Celiac disease is an auto-immune condition, which is when the body's immune system mistakenly attacks healthy tissue. In this case, the body mistakes substances found in gluten for a threat. The exact causes of the disease are unknown, but it may be related to both genetic and environmental factors. Although there is no cure for celiac disease, removing gluten from the diet will prevent long-term consequences of the condition. The possible consequences of continuing to eat gluten in the long term include bone-weakening (osteoporosis) and iron deficiency anemia.

SYMPTOMS

• Diarrhea • Abdominal pain • Bloating • Wind • Indigestion
• Constipation • Fatigue • Weight loss • Sometimes, an itchy rash
• Sometimes, menstrual problems or infertility

TREATMENT

Ayurveda

An Ayurvedic practitioner would view celiac disease as an imbalance within the immune system and treat it with balancing herbs, as well as advising on a gluten-free and nutritious diet.

Herbalism

In addition to advising on a gluten-free diet, a herbal practitioner may suggest anti-inflammatory agents, such as aloe vera supplements or paprika. (See page 80.)

Nutrition

Contact your physician, a qualified dietitian, or a celiac disease support group for advice on removing gluten from your diet. Sufferers should make sure that their gluten-free diet is healthy and balanced. Gluten is found in barley, rye, and wheat. These cereals find their way into pasta, baked goods, breakfast cereals, bread, and many pre-prepared meals and sauces. Gluten-free goods are often labeled on their packaging.

> **CAUTION**
> If you suspect celiac disease, contact your physician. In particular, pregnant women and children will need regular monitoring to ensure they do not suffer the effects of malnutrition.

Paprika may help to balance the immune system.

GASTRO-ESOPHAGEAL REFLUX

Gastro-esophageal reflux disease (GER) is characterized by acid leaking up from the stomach into the esophagus. It occurs when the ring of muscles at the bottom of the esophagus is weakened. In severe cases, surgery may be needed. GER may occur temporarily during pregnancy as a result of the growing womb pressing on the stomach, and the natural weakening of muscles.

SYMPTOMS

• Heartburn • Unpleasant taste • Inflamed esophagus • Bad breath
• Belching • Nausea or vomiting • Possibly, pain on swallowing

TREATMENT

Traditional Home and Folk Remedies

Drinking a glass of milk may calm reflux.
Drink cucumber juice or eat fresh cucumber to ease heartburn. (See page 116.)
Try eating walnuts to ease symptoms. (See page 141.)
During pregnancy, eating a portion of rice every day may ease heartburn. (See page 159.)
If reflux is a problem at night, try raising the head of your bed by about 8in. (20cm.) by placing blocks or books under the legs. Do not raise your pillows, as this can put strain on the stomach.

Herbalism

To reduce symptoms, take agrimony, marshmallow, or meadowsweet, as a tea or tincture. (See pages 77, 81, and 127.)
Licorice root may ease heartburn. (See page 132.)
Stir slippery elm powder into a glass of milk and drink before meals to ease digestion. (See page 193.)

Aromatherapy

Cardamom may ease heartburn, indigestion, and abdominal pain. (See page 122.)

Nutrition

It may help to eat smaller meals more frequently, and avoid eating within three hours of going to bed.
Avoid caffeine and spicy, rich, and fatty foods.
Drinking too much fruit juice or eating chocolate or tomatoes may worsen symptoms.
Stop smoking and reduce alcohol intake.

Mind–Body Healing

Stress can worsen GER, so try relaxation techniques such as yoga. (See page 71.)
Losing excess weight may help to control symptoms, so increase weekly exercise sessions.

> **CAUTION**
> Contact your physician if symptoms are severe or continual, you have difficulty swallowing, or you have symptoms such as vomiting blood, persistent vomiting, or severe weight loss. Consult with your healthcare practitioner before taking herbal remedies during pregnancy.

DISORDERS OF THE URINARY SYSTEM
KIDNEY STONES

Kidney stones (calculi) may occur anywhere in the kidneys or ureters and are the result of the crystallization of various substances in the urine, often when the body is dehydrated, causing the urine to be more concentrated. Dehydration alone, however, will not cause the formation of stones, and there is usually some other factor involved, such as kidney disease, infection, a bodily disturbance, or certain drugs. Most stones are combinations of calcium, magnesium, phosphorus, and oxalate. Collections of small kidney stones are known as "gravel," while much larger ones are called "staghorn" calculi. Differences in dietary and fluid intake may put certain people at higher risk for kidney stones. Recurrence of most stones can be prevented by therapy based on analysis of the stones, the urine, and the blood. If stones cause blockage of the urinary tract, this can cause a kidney infection, with fever and chills.

SYMPTOMS

Small stones may pass out undetected, but if a stone is lodged in the ureter:
• Agonizing pain (ureteric colic) • Pain may spread to the lower abdomen and groin • Blood in the urine • Nausea • Need to urinate more frequently than usual • Pain when urinating
• If infection occurs, fever and chill

TREATMENT
Chinese Herbalism
Herbs that may help with correcting kidney deficiency include Ren Shen (ginseng), Ze Xie (water plantain), Fu Ling (poria), Gui Zhi (cinnamon twigs), and Ma Huang (ephedra). (See pages 104, 160, and 168.)

Traditional Home and Folk Remedies
Include 2 tablespoons of extra virgin olive oil in your diet each day. (See page 156.)
Fresh lemon juice, drunk in a little hot water every morning, will help to flush the kidneys and break down stones. (See page 108.)

Herbalism
Herbs that can be used to dissolve the stones include celery seed, parsley, and stone root (*Collinsonia canadensis*). Sip a decoction 3 times daily. (See pages 84 and 162.)
During an acute attack, try infusions of corn silk (the tuft of thread-like fibers that protrude from the tip of an ear of corn), couch grass (*Elymus repens*) or yarrow. (See pages 74 and 200.)

Aromatherapy
Oils used to treat kidney stones include fennel, geranium, juniper, and lemon. These can be added to a light carrier oil and massaged into the bladder area, or used in the bath. (See page 47.)

Homeopathy
Treatment would be constitutional, but the following remedies may be useful for up to 10 doses:
Berberis, for stitching pain in the lower ribs and hips when urinating, which worsens if moving about. (See page 90.)
Lycopodium, for pain in the right side which stops at the bladder, and which is worse between 4 and 8 p.m. (See page 147.)

Nutrition
Drink plenty of water (about 6pt. [3l.] a day) to flush the kidneys. (See page 205.)
Avoid long-term use of vitamin C, calcium, or vitamin D supplements. (See pages 210 and 213.)
Extra magnesium and vitamin B6 will help. (See pages 208 and 217.)

USEFUL FACTS
• Kidney stones range in size from less than 1/5in. (5mm.) to over 1in. (2.5cm.) in diameter. The most common types of stones contain various combinations of calcium, magnesium, phosphorus, or oxalate. Up to 80 percent of stones are formed mainly of calcium.
• Less common types are due to inherited disorders characterized by excretion of abnormal amounts of cystine or xanthine.
• Kidney stones affect approximately 1 in 1,000 Americans. They are most common in the southeastern U.S., known as the "stone belt."
• Kidney stones tend to run in families, and four out of every five patients with kidney stones are male, usually between the ages of 20 and 30.

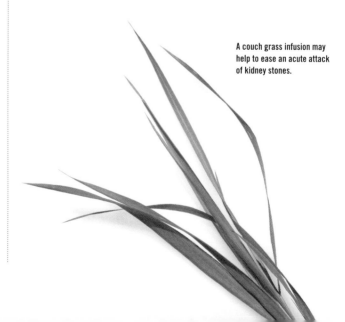

A couch grass infusion may help to ease an acute attack of kidney stones.

BLADDER STONES

Most bladder stones (calculi) are made up of crystals of calcium oxalate or uric acid. They are caused by the precipitation from solution of substances present in the urine. The stones may cause obstruction to urinary output, resulting in infection, although often they remain unrecognized. They occur with greater frequency in developing countries, and may be a result of a diet low in phosphate and protein. Bladder stones mainly affect men. Gout sufferers may experience bladder stones, and any disease which causes a high level of calcium in the blood and urine, such as hyperparathyroidism, may contribute to their formation.

SYMPTOMS
• Difficulty in passing urine • Stress incontinence
If infection develops, there may also be:
• Burning pain on urination • Small amounts of urine, cloudy and with an unpleasant smell • Fever • Dull ache in the lower abdomen

TREATMENT
Chinese Herbalism
Herbs that may correct kidney deficiency are Ren Shen (ginseng), Ze Xie (water plantain), Fu Ling (poria), Gui Zhi (cinnamon twigs), and Ma Huang (ephedra). (See pages 104, 160, and 168.)

Traditional Home and Folk Remedies
Fresh lemon juice, drunk in a little hot water every morning, will help to break down bladder stones. (See page 108.)
Barley or rice water will help to encourage the flow of urine and act as a tonic to the urinary system. (See pages 136 and 159.)

Herbalism
Herbs that can be used to dissolve the stones include celery seed, parsley, and stone root (*Collinsonia canadensis*). Sip a decoction 3 times daily. (See pages 84 and 162.)
During an acute attack, try infusions of corn silk (the tuft of thread-like fibers that protrude from the tip of an ear of corn), couch grass (*Elymus repens*), or yarrow. (See pages 74 and 200.)

Aromatherapy
A number of essential oils work on the urinary tract, including tea tree, sandalwood, juniper, and eucalyptus. Apply in hot compresses over the bladder area. (See page 47.)

Nutrition
Drink plenty of water (about 6pt. [3l.] a day) to flush the bladder.

Apply a hot compress of eucalyptus oil over the bladder area.

CYSTITIS

Cystitis is inflammation of the urinary bladder and/or urethra (the tube through which urine passes from the bladder out of the body). Inflammation usually occurs as a result of infection, bruising, or irritation. In the case of infection the bacteria involved are most often *Escherichia coli*, which will have traveled from the anus, via the urethra, to the bladder. Irritation and bruising can be caused by barrier contraceptives and sexual intercourse. Other causes of cystitis include chemical irritants (soap, bubble bath, bath oils), poor hygiene, insufficient drinking, food irritants, fruit juices, pregnancy, and the menopause. Drugs such as methenamine mandelate, nitrofurantoin, and cyclophosphamide may also cause cystitis. Cystitis is far more common in women than in men.

SYMPTOMS
• Burning pain on passing urine • Frequent and urgent need to pass urine, although little if any is passed • Dragging pain in lower abdomen and lower back • Nausea and possibly vomiting
• Possibly unpleasant smelling urine, which may contain blood

TREATMENT
Ayurveda
Boil 4 tablespoons of coriander seeds in 4 cups of water until the liquid is reduced to 2 cups. Strain and drink with a little honey. (See pages 113 and 203.)

Chinese Herbalism
Che Qian Zi (plantain seeds) would be used to address a problem with damp heat.

Traditional Home and Folk Remedies
Eat live yogurt; use as a douche to ease symptoms and prevent recurrence. (See page 142.)
Cranberry juice discourages bacteria from sticking to the walls of the bladder. (See page 194.)
Garlic tincture in food or drinks eases cystitis. (See page 79.)
Drink barley water and lemon juice daily.
(See pages 108 and 136.)

Herbalism
Herbs used to treat cystitis include urinary antiseptics and diuretics. Drink infusions of buchu (*Agathosma betulina*), corn silk, couch grass (*Elymus repens*), uva ursi, and yarrow. (See pages 74, 85, and 200.)

Cranberry juice is an excellent remedy for cystitis. Drink as much as possible to flush the urinary system.

URETHRITIS

Urethritis is an inflammation of the urethra (the tube through which urine passes out of the body). In women it is usually caused by a bladder infection, while in men it may be a symptom of other diseases, including gonorrhea and Reiter's syndrome. It may also result from damage to the urethra, from a catheter for example. Nonspecific urethritis (NSU) is a milder form thought to be caused in most cases by chlamydia, although the cause may not be established. NSU may be caused by a large number of different types of micro-organisms, including bacteria and yeasts. Other possible causes include exposure to irritant chemicals, such as antiseptics and some spermicidal preparations. Urethritis may be followed by scarring and the formation of a urethral stricture (narrowing of a section of the urethra), which can make the passing of urine difficult.

SYMPTOMS
- Burning sensation and sometimes severe pain on passing urine
- Blood in urine and possibly a pus-filled yellow discharge

In nonspecific urethritis, the symptoms are milder and the discharge in men is usually clear; in women there may be no symptoms, with occasionally increased discharge

TREATMENT

Ayurveda
Hollyhock (*Alcea rosea*) is a diuretic and can treat cystitis. However, some people may have an unusual reaction to the plant.
Boil 4 tablespoons of coriander seeds in 4 cups or water until the liquid is reduced to 2 cups. Strain and drink with a little honey. (See page 113.)

Traditional Home and Folk Remedies
Eat live yogurt, and use as a douche to ease the symptoms of infection and inflammation, and prevent recurrence of the urethritis. (See page 142.)
Cranberry juice, drunk daily, discourages bacteria from sticking to the urinary tract. It treats and prevents urethritis. (See page 194.)
Garlic tincture, added to food or warm drinks, will ease inflammation and fight infection. (See page 79.)
Drink barley water, several cups a day, with some lemon juice. (See pages 108 and 136.)

Herbalism
Herbs used to treat urethritis include urinary antiseptics and diuretics. You may drink infusions of any of the following herbs, alone or in combination: corn silk (the tuft of thread-like fibers that protrude from the tip of an ear of corn), couch grass (*Elymus repens*), uva ursi, and yarrow. (See pages 74, 85, and 200.)
Buchu (*Agathosma betulina*) will help to clear infection. Take as a tea, three times daily.

Aromatherapy
Bergamot, lavender, and sandalwood are soothing and antiseptic. Add them to the bath water every evening. (See page 47.)

Homeopathy
For NSU, antibiotics should be taken, as prescribed, but Apis may be helpful if it is not NSU. (See page 203.)

Nutrition
Drink plenty of water (6pt. [3l.] daily) to flush the urinary system. Take 1g. of vitamin C daily, which acts as a natural diuretic, boosts the immune system, and builds healthy mucous membranes. (See page 210.)
Take *acidophilus* after a course of antibiotics. (See page 142.)

CAUTION
All suspected cases of urethritis should be investigated by a physician, in case the cause is chlamydia or a similar infection.

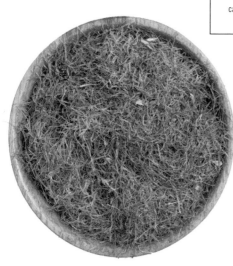

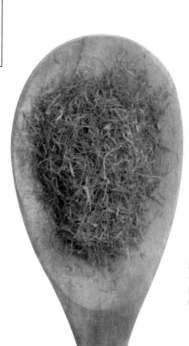

An infusion of corn silk may help to relieve urethritis.

INCONTINENCE

Incontinence is the inability to retain feces in the rectum, or an uncontrollable involuntary passing of urine. Incontinence, or involuntary urination, is extremely common. The most common form is stress incontinence, in which a small quantity of urine is "leaked" when there is increased pressure in the abdomen, as in laughing, sneezing, or coughing. Stress incontinence is often experienced after childbirth, as a result of injury or strain to the pelvic floor muscles, whose function it is to support the bladder and keep the urethra closed. Other causes include senile dementia, prostate enlargement, damage to nerve control as a result of stroke, multiple sclerosis, or local cancer, and bladder stones. Fecal incontinence (lack of normal control over passing feces) may occur in diarrhea, or if the controlling muscles have been damaged by disease or childbirth. Another cause is fecal impaction, which is often caused by long-standing constipation. (See "Constipation" on page 308 and "Diarrhea" on page 309 for treatment of fecal incontinence.)

SYMPTOMS

In stress incontinence:
• Urine leakage during laughing, sneezing, coughing, or running
In urge incontinence:
• Urine leaks during a sudden, intense urge to pass urine
In overflow incontinence:
• Inability to empty your bladder, which causes frequent leaking
Total incontinence:
• Bladder cannot store urine at all, which causes you to pass urine constantly

TREATMENT

Chinese Herbalism
Treatment would address kidney yang deficiency with internal cold, and the best herb to use is Jin Suo Gu Jing Wan, also called golden lock, taken as a tea.
If the condition accompanies prolapse, treatment will be given for deficient qi, using central qi pills. This will help with the control of fecal and urinary incontinence.

Herbalism
The seeds of the ginkgo biloba plant act as a tonic to the kidneys and bladder, and have been used for incontinence and excessive urination. However, these are toxic in large doses and should not be taken by children. (See page 131.)
Horsetail has toning and astringent properties, which make it useful both for incontinence and frequent urination. (See page 123.)

Homeopathy
Treatment would be based on the cause of the incontinence, but some of the following might be useful:
Ferr. phos., for an inability to control the bladder, with pain and a frequent urge to urinate. (See page 215.)
Sepia, for incontinence related to weak pelvic floor muscles, accompanied by the feeling that the abdomen is falling out of the vagina. (See page 182.)

Flower Essences
A number of remedies will help with negative emotions and distress. Some to try are:
Walnut, if incontinence is the result of change, such as pregnancy, a new baby, or menopause. (See page 141.)
Sweet chestnut, if you suffer from despair. (See page 100.)
Agrimony, if you hide behind a cheerful face. (See page 77.)
Crab apple if you feel unclean. (See page 148.)

Nutrition
Increase your intake of dietary fiber, which will prevent constipation and straining, a common cause of incontinence.
Drink plenty of water to ensure regular use of the bladder muscles.

Mind–Body Healing
If urinary incontinence occurs after childbirth, try regular exercise of your pelvic floor muscles. These are the muscles around your vagina and anus. They are the muscles that, if squeezed, can reduce or stop the flow of urine when you go to the toilet. To strengthen them, squeeze them 10 or 15 times in a row, while sitting comfortably and without tightening your stomach, thighs, or buttocks, and without holding your breath.

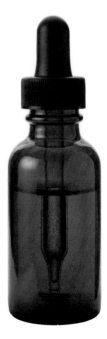

Walnut flower remedy may help if incontinence is a result of a new baby or the menopause.

DISORDERS OF THE REPRODUCTIVE SYSTEM: FEMALE

BREAST PROBLEMS

The female breast consists mainly of a round mass of glandular tissue comprising about 15–20 lobes, each having a duct leading to an opening on the nipple; the duct system and glandular tissue develop fully with pregnancy. The amount of fat sheathing the glandular tissue determines the size of the breast. Connective tissues, or stroma, form the foundation or framework of the breast. The layer of ligaments directly beneath the breast sends strands into the breast itself, providing the firm consistency of the organ. The deep layer of connective tissue sends strands in the opposite direction into the covering of the chest muscles. Common breast problems include tenderness, abscesses, tumors, cysts, blockages of the milk ducts, and breast cancer.

SYMPTOMS
• Tenderness • Swelling • Abscesses may produce swelling, redness, pain, and fever

TREATMENT

Ayurveda
Barberry can be applied externally for its antibiotic and antifungal action. (See page 90.)
Calamus oil will stimulate lymphatic drainage, and can be used for treating most breast problems. (See page 75.)
Celery seed is diuretic, and can be useful when breast problems are related to swellings, unless you are pregnant. (See page 84.)

Chinese Herbalism
A poultice made from powdered Da Huang (rhubarb root) can be applied to the breast to ease pain and swelling. (See page 173.)
Qian Cao Gen (madder root) and dandelion may also be useful. (See page 188.)

Traditional Home and Folk Remedies
Apply a bruised white cabbage leaf to the breast when there is infection, to heal and draw out the pus. (See page 92.)
Apply continuous compresses of strong peach tea to the affected area for infection. (See page 280.)
Bruised parsley leaf poultices can be used for hard and lumpy breasts. (See page 162.)

Herbalism
Herbs that encourage the lymphatic system are most useful for treating breast problems: marigold, marshmallow, nettles, and yellow dock. (See pages 81, 93, 176, and 194.)
As long as you are not pregnant, try taking the herb agnus castus for breast problems related to hormones (particularly premenstrually, and during the menopause). (See page 198.)

Aromatherapy
Geranium oil can be used in the bath for relief of tenderness and edema, or massage it, blended into a little carrier oil, into the affected area. Do not use if pregnant. (See page 161.)
Juniper, rosemary, lavender, and fennel oils will help to regulate hormone imbalance (but do not use during pregnancy) and relieve the symptoms of breast diseases. (See page 47.)

Homeopathy
For pain associated with premenstrual syndrome, try:
Nat. mur., when the breasts are retaining water. (See page 154.)
Calcarea, for heavy, pendulous breasts. (See page 213.)
For an abscess, try:
Hep. sulf., for localized pain with irritability. (See page 213.)
Silicea, for cracked, oozing nipples and feelings of exhaustion. (See page 220.)

Nutrition
Cut down on salty food to prevent water retention.
Supplements of evening primrose oil and vitamin B6 may be useful. (See pages 208 and 231.)
Cut down on caffeine, which can encourage the formation of cysts and lumps in the breast.
Breast pain and lumps may be alleviated by increasing your daily intake of vitamin A. (See page 206.)
Women with low levels of selenium may have a greater risk of suffering fibrocystic breast disease. (See page 219.)
Apply vitamin E cream to heal cracked nipples. (See page 211.)

> **CAUTION**
> Pregnant women should not take celery seed or agnus castus, or use geranium, fennel, juniper, or rosemary oils. Check your breasts once a month. Contact your physician if you notice any changes.

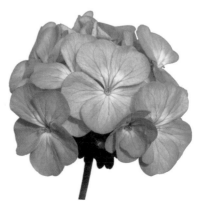

Add a few drops of geranium oil to the bath to ease premenstrual swelling and tenderness. It should be avoided during pregnancy.

BREASTFEEDING PROBLEMS

After the birth of a child, a mother's breast begins to produce milk, a natural process designed to provide complete nourishment for a baby for several months after its birth. Before milk is produced, the mother's breast produces colostrum, a deep-yellow liquid containing high levels of protein and antibodies. A newborn baby who feeds on colostrum in the first few days of life is better able to resist the bacteria and viruses that cause illness. The mother's milk, which begins to flow a few days after childbirth when the mother's hormones change, is a blue-white color with a very thin consistency. If the mother is well nourished the milk provides the baby with the proper balance of nutrition. The fat contained in human milk, compared with cow's milk, is more digestible for infants and allows for greater absorption of fat-soluble vitamins into the bloodstream from the baby's intestine. Calcium and other important nutrients in human milk are also better utilized by infants. Antigens in cow's milk can cause allergic reactions in a newborn child, whereas such reactions to human milk are rare. Human milk also promotes growth, largely due to the presence of certain hormones and growth factors. Breastfed babies have a very low risk of developing meningitis or severe blood infections, and have a 500–600 percent lower risk of getting childhood lymphoma. Breastfed babies also suffer 50 percent fewer middle ear infections.

SYMPTOMS
• Aching, swollen breasts • Blocked milk duct, possibly leading to mastitis • Cracked or sore nipples • Slow let-down of milk • Overproduction or underproduction of milk • Fussy baby during or after feeds

TREATMENT

Ayurveda
Cumin or fenugreek seeds can increase milk production. (See pages 116 and 191.)

Chinese Herbalism
Bai Shao (peony bark) and Qian Cao Gen (madder root) can be used for relieving mastitis. (See page 159.)

Traditional Home and Folk Remedies
Bruise parsley leaves, then apply them to hardened or knotty breasts during breastfeeding. (See page 162.)
Feed your baby a little diluted dill (*Anethum graveolens*) tea to prevent wind, which may be causing breastfeeding problems.

Herbalism
Calendula cream will soothe and encourage the healing of sore and cracked nipples, and is safe for the baby to swallow. (See page 93.)

Caraway, aniseed (*Pimpinella anisum*), dill (*Anethum graveolens*), and fennel promote the flow of breastmilk, and can be taken in the form of teas or infusions. (See pages 97 and 128.)
Compresses of marshmallow and slippery elm can often help with engorgement. (See pages 114 and 193.)
Red sage will dry up breast milk almost instantly, if necessary. (See page 177.)
Dilute tinctures of St. John's wort and marigold in boiled water and dab onto cracked nipples after each feed. (See pages 93 and 138.)
Take echinacea for any infection. (See page 122.)

Aromatherapy
Lavender oil, in the bath or in a vaporizer, can encourage the let-down reflex. Better still, try massaging your baby with 1 drop in a little light carrier oil before a feed, to relax you both. (See page 143.)
Caraway and vervain oils can be massaged into the breasts to stimulate the production of milk. (See pages 97 and 196.)
Calendula and chamomile oils can be applied to the breasts to ease inflammation. Wash before feeding. (See pages 93 and 149.)
Peppermint oil, in cold compresses, can reduce the flow of milk when there is engorgement. (See page 152.)

Flower Essences
Apply Rescue Remedy cream to the nipples when they are sore or cracked. (See page 158.)
Olive is useful for overwhelming fatigue. (See page 156.)
Walnut is useful for helping with change – in this case, the birth of your baby. (See page 141.)

Nutrition
Breastfeeding mothers need plenty of protein, vitamins, and iron. (See pages 58–60 and 215.)
Drink plenty of fluids while breastfeeding.
Apply vitamin E oil to sore and cracked nipples to help them heal. (See page 211.)

Mind–Body Healing
Breastfeeding problems can be stressful, upsetting, and exhausting. If possible, take advice from a breastfeeding counselor or lactation consultant. If problems feel overwhelming, chat with a counselor (sometimes available on breastfeeding helplines, such as those run by La Leche League).
To ease anxiety before or during feeding, try meditating, breathing exercises, and visualization. (See page 68.)

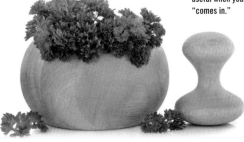

Bruise parsley leaves then apply to engorged breasts, which may be particularly useful when your milk "comes in."

MENSTRUAL PROBLEMS

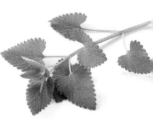

To ease the pain of menstruation, drink tea made from catnip twice daily.

The most common menstrual problems are dysmenorrhea (painful menstruation), menorrhagia (heavy menstrual bleeding), and amenorrhea (no menstrual bleeding). In primary dysmenorrhea there is either an increased level of or increased sensitivity to prostaglandin, the hormone-like substance that produces uterine contractions. Secondary dysmenorrhea (unusual menstrual cramps) begins at least three years after menstruation begins and may be caused by endometriosis, fibroids, a pelvic infection, stress, or a thyroid disorder. The symptoms for both include sharp pain or a dull ache in the lower abdomen and lower back, headaches, sweating, diarrhea. In severe cases, there may be vomiting and fainting. Menorrhagia is best described as bleeding that is so heavy that it interferes with normal life. It may be caused by fibroids, polyps, pelvic infection, endometriosis, hypothyroidism, blood-clotting disorders, stress, or use of an IUD or injectable contraceptive. Primary amenorrhea refers to menstruation not starting by the age of 18. This is usually due to low body weight or heredity. Secondary amenorrhea occurs when menstruation stops for more than six months due to pregnancy, weight loss, starting oral contraceptives, severe shock, stress, anemia, thyroid disorder, or a fibroid.

SYMPTOMS
• Painful menstruation • Heavy menstrual bleeding • No menstrual bleeding • Irregular menstruation

TREATMENT
Ayurveda
Aloe vera can induce menstruation. (See page 80.)
Basil can be used to promote menstruation. (See page 156.)
Caraway relaxes uterine tissue and is beneficial for menstrual cramps. (See page 97.)
Cardamom will help digestive problems associated with menstruation. (See page 122.)
Cedar stimulates the menstrual cycle, and celery seeds can treat irregular menstruation. (See pages 84 and 100.)

Chinese Herbalism
Excessive flow is considered to be caused by heat in the blood; scanty flow, late menstruation, and painful menstruation are due to cold in the blood.
Warming herbs, such as ginger, Ren Shen (ginseng), and Gui Zhi (cinnamon), may be used. (See pages 104, 160, and 200.)
Shan Zhu Yu (cornelian Asiatic cherry) can be used in the treatment of heavy menstrual bleeding. (See page 114.)

Traditional Home and Folk Remedies
Cinnamon bark will help to control menstrual flow. (See page 104.)
Diluted lemon juice cleanses the system and helps to control bleeding. (See page 108.)

Dried carrot powder taken daily may help to regulate the menstrual cycle. (See page 120.)
Cayenne pepper regulates bleeding. Add a few grains to any herbal tea. (See page 98.)
Beets help to regulate menstrual problems.
Strawberry leaves, taken over a long period, can help to regulate menstrual flow and ease pain.

Herbalism
Cramp bark is helpful for menstrual cramps. (See page 197.)
Lady's mantle is an astringent and is useful for heavy menstrual bleeding. Take 3 times daily, as required. (See page 78.)
Yarrow will help to regulate menstruation. (See page 74.)
Raspberry leaves can help to control an excessive flow of blood. (See page 176.)
Thyme tea, drunk each morning and evening, can control excessive flow. (See page 190.)
Angelica root can help to promote menstruation that is delayed. (See page 82.)
Catnip tea (*Nepeta cataria*), drunk each evening and morning during menstruation, will help to ease pain.
Peppermint tea will ease any bloating and pain during menstruation. (See page 152.)

Aromatherapy
Antispasmodic oils, such as clary sage, cypress, and lavender, will help to ease cramps. (See pages 117, 143, and 178.)
Clary sage and fennel oils, massaged into the lower back, can help to regulate hormone balance, and, through that, the menstrual cycle. (See pages 128 and 178.)
Heavy menstrual bleeding can be treated with geranium, rose, or cypress essential oils. Add to the bath water or use in a local massage. (See pages 117, 161, and 174.)

Nutrition
Vitamin B6, taken twice daily, can help prevent menstrual cramps. (See page 208.)
Iron and zinc will help in cases of heavy menstrual bleeding. (See pages 215 and 221.)
Take vitamin A and B6 for heavy bleeding. (See pages 206 and 208.)
Bioflavonoids can help to balance hormone levels and regulate the menstrual cycle. (See page 228.)
Deficiencies of zinc and vitamin B6 can result from absence of menstruation. (See pages 208 and 221.)

Mind–Body Healing
Regular exercise and relaxation can help with all aspects of menstruation problems. During a painful period, gentle exercise such as swimming or walking can ease pain, while yoga or pilates can both ease stress and act as a distraction. (See pages 70–71.)

PREMENSTRUAL SYNDROME

Premenstrual syndrome (PMS) is the term used to describe a huge range of symptoms, at least some of which are experienced by most women (especially those over 30) every month between ovulation and menstruation. The symptoms may be physical, emotional, or behavioral in character and are thought to be caused either by hormonal imbalance (possibly due to recent childbirth or a gynecological disorder) or by marginal (subclinical) nutritional deficiencies that can affect the fine hormone balance in the body. Interestingly, women who regularly consume caffeine are more likely to suffer from severe PMS, and there is sometimes a connection with a thyroid condition.

SYMPTOMS

• Breast enlargement and tenderness • Bloated abdomen • Headaches or migraines • Pelvic discomfort • Constipation or diarrhea • Greasy hair and skin • Tiredness • Emotional irritability and confusion • Anxiety • Disturbed sleep • Depression and, in severe cases, suicidal thoughts • Clumsiness and lack of coordination • Poor concentration • Violent or aggressive outbursts

TREATMENT

Ayurveda

Calamus root stimulates the adrenals, which will help PMS associated with stress. (See page 75.)
Caraway is useful for digestive problems associated with PMS, and is a natural diuretic. (See page 97.)
Myrrh is used for treating many conditions relating to menstruation. (See page 112.)
Angelica is specific for PMS. (See page 82.}

Chinese Herbalism

PMS is believed to be caused by an imbalance of spleen, kidneys, and liver, and can be treated with Dang Gui (angelica), Bai Shao (peony), Fu Ling (poria), and Huang Qin (skullcap). (See pages 82, 159, 168, and 181.)

Traditional Home and Folk Remedies

Swelling associated with PMS can be prevented by eating plenty of fresh, crunchy apples in the week prior to menstruation. (See page 148.)
Celery is also a good diuretic, and acts on the kidneys to encourage their action. (See page 84.)
Eat fresh grapes to prevent bloating.
Barley water, which is rich in B vitamins, can be drunk freely throughout your menstrual cycle to ease symptoms. (See page 136.)
To ease irritability and other emotional symptoms, eat plenty of oats. A bowl of warm porridge every morning may be helpful (See page 89.)

Herbalism

Try an infusion of agnus castus or false unicorn (*Chamaelirium luteum*), which balance the hormones. (See page 198.)
Herbs that help to reduce some of the symptoms of stress and anxiety include wild oats and vervain. (See pages 89 and 196.)
Water retention can be eased with couch grass (*Elymus repens*) or dandelion teas, drunk two or three times each day during the premenstrual phase. (See page 188.)
Rosemary, oats, cinnamon, and lemon balm will help to lift the spirits. (See pages 89, 104, 152, and 175.)
Skullcap, wood betony (*Stachys officinalis*), and vervain are good for addressing tension and depression. (See pages 181 and 196.)
Corn silk and burdock are useful for symptoms associated with bloating. (See pages 85 and 200.)
Take valerian for extreme tension. (See page 195.)
Chamomile, cinnamon, and peppermint will help with nausea and vomiting. (See pages 104, 149, and 152.)
Yellow dock will balance the blood sugar levels. (See page 176.)

Aromatherapy

Try essential oils of geranium and rosemary in your bath to relieve symptoms, including water retention and irritability. (See pages 161 and 175.)
Clary sage and rose may help with depression. (See pages 174 and 178.)
A light massage (whole body, or over the abdominal area) with lavender oil or clary sage will balance hormones and ease symptoms. (See pages 143 and 178.)

Flower Essences

Wild mustard, for depression. (See page 184.)
Scleranthus, for mood swings. (See page 180.)
Olive, for fatigue. (See page 156.)
Crab apple, for feeling repulsive and unliked. (See page 148.)

Nutrition

In addition to maintaining a healthy diet, take evening primrose oil, with the following supplements: vitamins C, E, and B6, magnesium, zinc, iron, and chromium. These should be taken continuously for one month, and subsequently during the fortnight preceding menstruation. (See pages 208, 210, 211, 214, 215, 217, 221, and 231.)

Mind–Body Healing

Regular sleep and exercise will improve the symptoms of PMS. Breathing exercises, meditation, yoga, and other techniques to relieve stress will be extremely beneficial. (See pages 68–71.)

Wood betony tea will help to relieve stress and anxiety. Use 1 teaspoon of dried betony leaves to 1 cup of boiling water, then steep for 5 minutes.

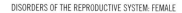

INFERTILITY

The term infertility, or failure to reproduce, is generally applied when failure to conceive follows regular, unprotected sex over an 18-month period. Infertility indicates a fault in the reproductive system and is very often treatable.

SYMPTOMS
• Failure to conceive after regular unprotected sex over an 18-month period

TREATMENT
Ayurveda
Cloves can tone the uterus, and garlic has a rejuvenating effect on the reproductive system. (See pages 79 and 125.)
Saffron is aphrodisiac, and can help when infertility is associated with sexual problems. (See page 115.)

Chinese Herbalism
Infertility is believed to be caused by damp heat and imbalance of yin and yang. Jin Suo Gu Jing Wan (golden lock) tea may be useful, but treatment is always individually prescribed.

Traditional Home and Folk Remedies
Oats are calming, and can help with the effects of stress, as well as toning the body. Eat as often as possible. (See page 89.)

Herbalism
Agnus castus is an excellent hormone regulator and will help if your menstruation is irregular, or you are not ovulating for hormonal reasons. (See page 198.)
Lemon balm and skullcap will help to reduce the effects of stress, which may be causing the condition. (See pages 152 and 181.)

Aromatherapy
Rose oil is said to increase sperm count and quality, as well as acting as a mild aphrodisiac. Add a few drops to your partner's bath, or perhaps engage in a little gentle massage, with 2 or 3 drops of rose essential oil in a mild carrier oil such as sweet almond oil. (See pages 169 and 174.)

Increasing your intake of essential fatty acids will help stimulate the production of your sex hormones.

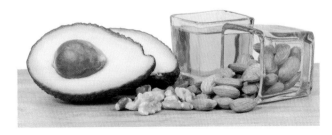

A few drops of geranium and melissa can be used neat in the bath, or diluted in a gentle carrier oil and massaged over the abdomen on a regular basis. (See pages 152 and 161.)
Tea tree and lavender oils can be used in abdominal massage, for treating any pelvic inflammation which may be preventing the woman conceiving. (See pages 143 and 150.)
If infertility is causing great anxiety, one of the relaxing oils, such as lavender, marjoram, or chamomile, can be used in the bath, or try it in a vaporizer. (See pages 143, 149, and 157.)
When repeated attempts to get pregnant have failed and you need a little encouragement to continue with love-making, ylang ylang is a lovely, relaxing oil that acts as an aphrodisiac. Use as a massage oil or in the bath. (See page 95.)

Flower Essences
White chestnut may be useful if you are extremely upset or tormented by the problem. (See page 76.)
For despondency, try gorse. (See page 192.)

Nutrition
Cut out alcohol, smoking, and drugs.
Eating plenty of whole foods rich in vitamins and minerals will not only ensure that sperm and egg are healthy, but that the woman's body is a welcoming home for the growing embryo.
Vitamin E and B6 may be supplemented, as low intake is often linked to a low sperm count. Vitamin E may regulate the production of cervical mucus in women. (See pages 208 and 211.)
Increase intake of EFAs (essential fatty acids) – in oily fish, fish liver oils, seeds, nuts, pulses, beans, evening primrose oil, unrefined vegetable oils) – to stimulate sex hormone production. (See pages 60, 231, and 232.)
Zinc deficiency has been linked to infertility. (See page 221.)

Mind–Body Healing
Regular exercise and the practice of relaxation techniques will encourage a healthy body and reduce stress. (See pages 68–71.)

USEFUL FACTS
Causes of infertility include:
• Age, as fertility declines in women over the age of 35.
• Cervical mucus may be too thick, or contain hostile antibodies.
• Endometriosis, when pieces of the womb lining migrate to the Fallopian tubes or the ovaries.
• Fibroids, which are benign growths of muscle.
• Narrowed or scarred cervix, perhaps resulting from surgery.
• Ovulation problems due to congenital abnormality, damage to the ovaries, or hormonal problems.
• Pelvic infections: scar tissue from infections can cause blockage of the fallopian tubes.
• Polycystic ovaries, which are repeated or multiple ovarian cysts.
• Smoking, which can cause constriction of blood vessels supplying the reproductive organs, which then inhibits their action.
• Stress, which may be linked to infertility.
• Womb problems such as adenomyosis, where scar tissue forms on the womb wall, an abnormal womb shape, and polyps.

MISCARRIAGE

Spontaneous abortion, or miscarriage, occurs when the embryo fails to develop, when there is complete or incomplete expulsion of the embryo or fetus, and placenta, or when the fetus dies prior to 20 weeks. If fetal death occurs at 20 weeks or more after the last period, it is termed a late fetal death or a stillbirth. Up to three-quarters of conceptions abort spontaneously. Most occur before the woman's pregnancy can be confirmed, prior to six weeks after her last period. In many cases, the womb sheds an embryo because it is not developing normally. Often, however, there is no explanation for miscarriage at all, although the following may be at greater risk: women over 40, pregnancies resulting from fertility treatment, twin or multiple pregnancies, and pregnancies where the placenta is faulty.

SYMPTOMS
In threatened miscarriage:
• Bleeding, clots, or a dark discharge from the vagina • Mucus in the vaginal blood • Abdominal pain, possibly cramp-like pain similar to menstrual cramps • Back pain
In inevitable miscarriage:
• Opening of the cervix and continuous bleeding (inevitable abortion) • Emptying of the uterus, after which the cervix closes and bleeding stops (complete abortion) • Partial emptying of the uterus, after which the cervix remains open and bleeding continues (incomplete abortion)

TREATMENT
Ayurveda
Herbs to tone the uterus and improve circulation may be useful, but treatment must be undertaken by a registered practitioner. (See page 20.)

Chinese Herbalism
Tu Su Zi (dodder seed) is used to help prevent miscarriages. (See page 118.)

Herbalism
Cramp bark may help to relax the uterus and prevent miscarriage. (See page 197.)
Tonic herbs to help prevent miscarriage include red raspberry leaves mixed with a little vervain. (See pages 176 and 196.)
Following miscarriage, you can use raspberry leaves to aid the healing of the uterus, and antiseptic herbs such as thyme or echinacea to help prevent infection. (See pages 122, 176, and 190.)
Rosemary and wild oats will help to support the nervous system following the trauma of miscarriage. (See pages 89 and 175.)

Aromatherapy
If you are concerned about miscarriage, use lavender oil in a vaporizer (not on the skin). It will also be useful following a miscarriage to help your body get back to normal. (See page 143.) Rose has an affinity with the reproductive system, and can be used in a vaporizer (not on the skin) to help prevent miscarriage. (See page 174.)

Flower Essences
Rock rose, for helplessness and terror. (See page 135.)
Mimulus, for gnawing fear of miscarriage. (See page 153.)
Star of Bethlehem, for shock. (See page 158.)
Gentian, for despondency following a very early miscarriage. (See page 130.)
Walnut, to help you adjust to the new situation. (See page 141.)

Mind–Body Healing
Miscarriage can have a profound effect on a woman, her partner, and family. Different people grieve in different ways. Some people come to terms with their loss in a few weeks, while others cannot face planning another pregnancy. When sadness, hopelessness, or anxiety is overwhelming, it may be helpful to find counseling, therapy, and support groups. Talk to your healthcare provider about what will suit you. (See pages 68–69.)

CAUTION

It is safest not to apply essential oils to the skin during the first trimester. Do not use oils, herbs, or other treatments during pregnancy without consulting with your healthcare provider. Always consult a registered healthcare provider if a threatened or inevitable miscarriage is suspected. Sudden, severe abdominal pain between the fifth and tenth weeks of pregnancy may indicate an ectopic pregnancy (one that develops in the Fallopian tube). This is a life-threatening condition requiring urgent medical attention.

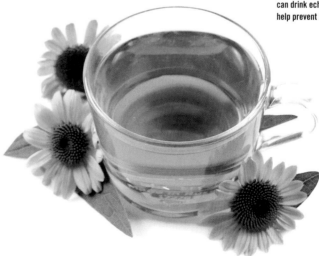

Following miscarriage, you can drink echinacea tea to help prevent infection.

PREGNANCY PROBLEMS

Women may experience problems during pregnancy, often as a result of hormonal changes. Some of the most common problems women experience are:

• Anemia (see page 296).
• Backache, due either to postural changes made to accommodate the extra weight, or to the position in which the baby is lying.
• Bleeding gums, caused by hormonal changes which lead to a thickening and softening of the gums.
• Constipation, when normal bowel action is slowed down by an increase of progesterone.
• Cramps, which occur mainly in the feet, calves, and thighs due to inefficient circulation (as a result of increased progesterone), and possibly calcium deficiency.
• Fainting, caused by a shortage of blood to the brain due to lowered blood pressure and an increased demand for blood to the womb.
• Flatulence, since digesting food is moved more slowly, which allows wind to build up.
• Fluid retention, when an upset in the balance of salt and potassium in the cells causes swelling in the hands, legs, and feet.
• Heartburn, a burning sensation in the upper chest, and possibly a sour taste in the mouth, which are caused by acidic juices rising back up the esophagus.
• Increased vaginal discharge, probably thickish and white.
• Insomnia, caused by general inevitable bodily discomfort toward the end of pregnancy.
• Morning sickness, which is nausea and/or vomiting usually in the first three months of pregnancy, but not necessarily confined to the morning or the first trimester.
• Pelvic pain, which is pain in the groin or inside of the thighs when walking, caused by pressure on the pelvic nerves.
• Piles (see page 311).
• Stretch marks, fine red lines (which eventually turn silver) appearing on the breasts, abdomen, and thighs, and caused by stretching of the skin.
• Tiredness, characterized by a desire to sleep a lot, particularly in the first three months.
• Varicose veins (see page 298).

TREATMENT

Ayurveda
Aloe vera can be applied externally to prevent stretch marks. (See page 80.)
Ginger can be taken for recurrent nausea in pregnancy. (See page 200.)
Eating caraway seeds deals with constipation and digestive problems. (See page 97.)
Cardamom suppresses vomiting when eaten with a banana. (See page 122.)

Cayenne, used externally, can ease muscle pain. (See page 98.)
Cloves tone muscles, so expectant mothers are recommended to eat them in the last month of pregnancy to strengthen the uterus. (See page 125.)
Long pepper, for muscle soreness, digestive problems, and constipation. (See page 164.)
Mustard can help with muscle and joint pain, and acts as a laxative. (See page 91.)

Chinese Herbalism
Xu Duan (teasel root), Ren Shen (ginseng), and Wu Jia Pi (acanthopanax root), for back pain. (See pages 74 and 160.)
Bai Shao (peony root) and Huang Qi (astragalus), for high blood pressure. (See pages 87 and 159.)
Ren Shen (ginseng), Gan Cao (licorice), and Chen Pi (mandarin peel), for an acid stomach. (See pages 109, 132, and 160.)
Huang Qi (astragalus), for overwhelming exhaustion. (See page 87.)
Suan Zao Ren (wild jujube) and Ye Jiao Teng (fleeceflower stem), for insomnia. (See pages 167 and 201.)
Ginger, for morning sickness. (See page 200.)
Fu Ling (poria) and Gui Zhi (cinnamon twigs), for edema. (See pages 104 and 168.)

Traditional Home and Folk Remedies
Eating yogurt will cool the pain of heartburn. (See page 142.)
Use a witch hazel compress on varicose veins, either in the legs or the vulva. A compress will also work on piles to reduce inflammation and encourage healing. (See page 134.)
For relief of varicose veins in the legs, apply neat lemon juice. (See page 108.)
Garlic helps the circulation, and can prevent cramping, varicose veins, and piles. (See page 79.)
Drink a glass of honey and apple cider vinegar in warm water before bed to help you sleep peacefully. (See pages 203 and 204.)
Celery juice can help you sleep when taken before bedtime. (See page 84.)
Chamomile, fennel, and thyme have antifungal properties, and can be used as a compress and pressed against the vagina to ease and treat thrush. (See pages 128, 149, and 190.)

Herbalism
Dandelion tea is a mild diuretic, and so will help with edema. (See page 188.)
Chamomile or peppermint tea will ease heartburn. (See pages 149 and 152.)
Dandelion leaves, nettles, chives, sorrel, and coriander leaves are iron-rich, which will help anemia. (See pages 113, 188, and 194.)
Chamomile, fennel, burdock, and ginger are gentle laxatives, safe for preventing constipation. (See pages 85, 128, 149, and 200.)
Lavender, vervain, and lemon balm will soothe the nerves and relax muscles. (See pages 143, 152, and 196.)
Lemon balm and chamomile tea can help prevent nausea, as can ginger and fennel. Take as infusions as required. (See pages 128, 149, 152, and 200.)
Slippery elm helps to soothe the digestive tract, and can help morning sickness and weak digestion. (See page 193.)

Hops (*Humulus lupulus*) can be used for treating severe vomiting. Calendula and marjoram are astringent and can be applied to the legs or vulva as required. (See pages 93 and 157.)

Peppermint can be drunk as an infusion to improve circulation and treat varicose veins. (See page 152.)

Chamomile, catnip (*Nepeta cataria*), and vervain can help insomnia, when taken before bedtime or during the night. (See pages 149 and 196.)

Chamomile, dandelion root, and nettle can be taken three times daily for piles. (See pages 149, 188, and 194.)

Marigold flowers can be infused, added to coconut oil, and rubbed into the skin to prevent stretch marks. (See page 93.)

Aromatherapy

It is best not to use essential oils during the first three months of pregnancy. After that, as long as your pregnancy is going well, use essential oils sparingly, after consulting with your healthcare provider.

Lavender oil can be rubbed into the temples for headaches, and into the back for muscle pains. (See page 143.)

Geranium, fennel, marjoram, and ylang ylang can be added to the bath to prevent constipation. (See page 47.)

Roman chamomile and marjoram are excellent in a full-body massage to ease the muscular pains of pregnancy. (See pages 149 and 157.)

Thyme, cypress, lavender, and lemon oils can be added to the bath water to strengthen the veins and increase circulation. (See pages 108, 117, 143, and 190.)

Essential oil of geranium can be added to the bath for piles. (See page 161.)

A gentle massage with lavender, chamomile, or lemon balm can relax and help you sleep. (See pages 143, 149, and 152.)

Add a few drops of tea tree or cinnamon oil to a cup of cool water and apply to the vaginal area on a clean cloth to treat thrush. (See pages 104 and 150.)

A light massage of lavender and neroli, in a carrier oil, can prevent stretch marks. (See pages 106 and 143.)

Massage lavender, geranium, or ginger oils into the lower back to ease pain and reduce tension. (See pages 143, 161, and 200.)

Homeopathy

Ferr. phos., for nausea a few hours after eating. (See page 215.)

Flower Essences

Olive is useful for dealing with general exhaustion. (See page 156.)

Crab apple may help with relief of nausea. (See page 148.)

Rescue Remedy may be useful for vomiting. (See page 158.)

Nutrition

In addition to following the advice about pregnancy diet given by your healthcare provider, ensure you get plenty of iron, to prevent and treat anemia. Take vitamin C together with iron, in order to aid iron absorption. (See pages 210 and 215.)

Folic acid is necessary during pregnancy for the healthy development of the fetus. (See page 209.)

Dietary fiber will help to prevent constipation. (See page 58.)

Eat plenty of foods rich in calcium to prevent cramp. (See page 213.)

Supplements of vitamin B6, zinc, and magnesium may help with nausea. (See pages 208, 217, and 221.)

Vitamins C and E, and bioflavonoids, zinc, and brewer's yeast will help to heal damaged blood vessels which are the cause of varicose veins. (See pages 210, 211, 221, 228, and 229.)

Take acidophilus for thrush. (See page 142.)

Ensure you have plenty of vitamins E, C, zinc, silica, and pantothenic acid, which can help to prevent stretch marks. (See pages 208, 210, 211, 220, and 221.)

Vitamin E oil can be applied neat to areas that are likely to become stretched, including the perineum. (See page 211.)

Mind–Body Healing

Consult with your healthcare provider about which exercise classes and activities are right for you during pregnancy. Tell your instructor that you are pregnant or take a class designed for pregnancy, such as pregnancy yoga. (See pages 70–71.)

> **CAUTION**
>
> It is safest not to apply essential oils to the skin during the first trimester. Do not use oils, herbs, or other remedies during pregnancy without consulting your healthcare provider. Many herbs, oils, and supplements are unsuitable for use during pregnancy, or may be unsuitable in your particular circumstances.

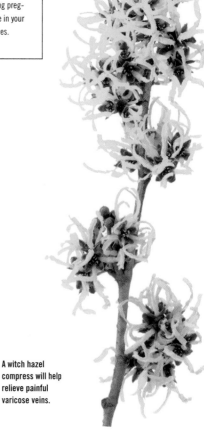

A witch hazel compress will help relieve painful varicose veins.

LABOR PAINS

Labor pains are caused by womb contractions. In the first stage of labor the contractions slowly dilate the cervix until it is wide enough to allow the baby's head to pass through. During the second stage, more powerful and more frequent contractions push the baby into the lower part of the birth canal and into the world. In the third stage, continued contractions help to expel the placenta. The pain itself varies at different stages. At first it may be no more than a dull discomfort eased by moving around. Later it may be likened to severe menstrual cramps which reach a peak then die out as the contraction ends. Pain may be felt in the lower abdomen, lower back, and the legs. The pain experienced appears to be different between women, and is related to their "pain threshold." Most women describe severe, in many cases almost unbearable, pain.

SYMPTOMS
• Pain in the lower abdomen, lower back, and legs • For some women, anxiety or distress

TREATMENT
Ayurveda
Basil is heating and can help to induce labor. (See page 156.)

Chinese Herbalism
Dang Gui (Chinese angelica) and Bai Shao (peony root), for abdominal pains experienced during and after childbirth. (See pages 82 and 159.)

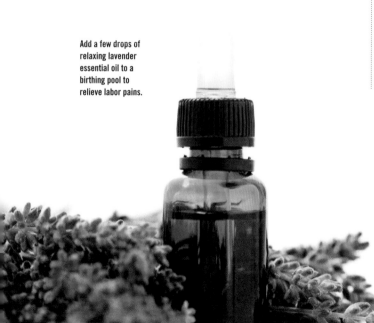

Add a few drops of relaxing lavender essential oil to a birthing pool to relieve labor pains.

Herbalism
Raspberry leaf, black cohosh (*Actaea racemosa*), and motherwort can help during the second stage of labor. These should not be taken earlier in pregnancy, and consult with your midwife that they are right for you. (See pages 75, 144, and 176.)
Angelica root and raspberry leaf can help with the delivery of the placenta. (See pages 82 and 176.)
Chamomile tea can be sipped to soothe and calm. (See page 149.)
Ginger may be used to speed up a slow labor. (See page 200.)

Aromatherapy
Clary sage, jasmine, and rose can be massaged into the lower back to relax the mother between contractions. (See page 47.)
Lemon balm oil can help to relieve the pain of childbirth, and should be used throughout the labor. (See page 152.)
Rub lavender oil into the lower back, or add it to the water of a birthing pool to ease pain. (See page 143.)

Homeopathy
Coffea, for violent, unbearable pain when the mother cries out and is understandably nervous between contractions. (See page 111.)
Carb. veg. is useful when the mother becomes exhausted during labor. (See page 230.)

Flower Essences
Rescue Remedy can be sipped for anxiety and tension. (See page 158.)
Olive, for overwhelming fatigue. (See page 156.)
For overstraining, use vervain. (See page 196.)
Sweet chestnut is good for utter despair, and for the feeling that the baby will never be born. (See page 100.)
Impatiens, when things do not seem to be happening fast enough. (See page 140.)

Mind–Body Healing
Breathing exercises, meditation, chanting, visualization and other relaxation techniques may be helpful during all stages of labor. (See page 68.)

POST-DELIVERY PROBLEMS

Almost all women suffer from problems of some kind following the trauma of childbirth, whether physical or emotional. These may include:

• Abdominal soreness, usually resulting from a cesarean section, from which it can take up to 12 weeks to recover.
• Anemia caused by blood loss during delivery (see page 296).
• Backache, which may relate to back strain during the birth process.
• Breastfeeding problems (see page 319).
• Exhaustion as a result of the birth, coupled with lack of sleep due to the needs of a crying baby.
• Hair loss caused by normal hormonal changes after the birth.
• Headache, which may be severe and last up to 48 hours after the delivery, for those who have an epidural injection.
• Piles (see page 311).
• Postnatal depression (see page 328).
• Prolapse (see page 330).
• Soreness in the genital area, caused by stitches from a tear or episiotomy, which may last for some days or weeks.

TREATMENT

Ayurveda
Aloe vera will encourage healing, and soothe spasm and inflammation. (See page 80.)
Vetiver is excellent for exhaustion and depression. (See page 197.)
Turmeric can be used for bruising. (See page 117.)
Saffron is a good overall herb for all postnatal problems. (See page 115.)

Chinese Herbalism
San Qi (notoginseng) will relieve swelling, stop hemorrhaging, and disperse bruising. (See page 160.)
Tian Ma (gastrodia rhizome) will help relieve headaches which come on after childbirth. (See page 130.)
Ren Shen (ginseng) will help to restore, boost energy levels, prevent infection, and encourage healing. (See page 160.)

Herbalism
Pain-relieving herbs include black cohosh (Actaea racemosa), lavender, and wild yam. (See pages 75, 121, and 143.)
St. John's wort and calendula will help healing.
An infusion of calendula can be used to assist in healing the perineum. (See pages 93 and 138.)
Witch hazel can be applied to the perineum to encourage healing and soothe pain. (See page 134.)
A comfrey compress can be applied to the perineum to speed healing. (See page 186.)

Golden seal (Hydrastis canadensis) will help with bleeding, as will beth root (Trillium erectum).
Golden seal and myrrh are excellent for dispelling uterine infections. (See page 112.)
Cramp bark will help with uterine infections, pain, and cramping. (See page 197.)
Beth root and horsetail can be added to the bath for incontinence and weak pelvic floor muscles. (See page 123.)
Nettles, chickweed (Stellaria media), and coriander will act as tonics for fatigue. (See pages 113 and 194.)

Aromatherapy
Geranium, rose, and clary sage act as uterine tonics and help the pelvic tissues to regain their elasticity after the birth. (See pages 161, 174, and 178.)
Lavender is useful for relief of afterpains. (See page 143.)
Chamomile, massaged into the abdomen, helps relieve pain and cramps. (See page 149.)
Jasmine has a tonic action on the womb. (See page 141.)
Apply lavender and chamomile, diluted in a little apricot kernel oil, to the affected area for sore stitches. (See pages 143 and 149.)

Homeopathy
Coffea, for sharp afterpains and exhaustion. (See page 111.)
China, for exhaustion following loss of blood. (See page 103.)
Carb. veg., for exhaustion with sweating. (See page 230.)
Sepia, for exhaustion with bearing-down pains. (See page 182.)
Arnica, to encourage healing and prevent bruising. (See page 86.)
Hypericum or Arnica tincture, diluted in water, to cleanse the perineum and any stitches. (See pages 86 and 138.)

Nutrition
Ensure that you are getting plenty of iron, which can help with fatigue. (See page 215.)
Vitamin B and chromium stabilize energy levels. (See pages 206–209 and 214.)
Vitamin E will encourage healing, and can be applied to stitches. (See page 211.)

In Ayurveda, saffron is traditionally prescribed for postnatal problems.

POSTNATAL ILLNESS

The term postnatal illness (PNI) covers the varying degrees of anxiety, fearfulness, and depression experienced by women after the birth of a baby. Its cause is thought to be the massive drop in pregnancy hormones, aggravated by general exhaustion and discomfort in the days following delivery. Mild "baby blues" usually begin three to four days after delivery, and last only a few days. Some women experience symptoms for several weeks. Many women suffer from baby blues, but in a few women the symptoms, initially a natural response to a new situation, last for much longer than a few weeks and seriously undermine their ability to cope. Postnatal depression (PND), also called postpartum depression (PPD), generally starts within weeks of the birth and may last for a year or more. In extreme cases there may be postnatal psychosis, characterized by virtual breakdown. Postnatal depression is most common in women with other stresses – marriage or relationship problems, anxiety about coping with a new baby, financial problems – as well as hormonal imbalances, blood sugar problems, and previous episodes of postnatal depression.

SYMPTOMS

In baby blues:
• Irritability • Tearfulness • Vulnerability • Mild depression
• Anxiety • Fears about responsibility
In postnatal depression:
• Constant sadness • Feeling unable to cope • Feelings of guilt and inadequacy • Loss of sex drive • Excessive worrying
In postnatal psychosis:
• Hyperactive, manic, and euphoric • Depressive • Panic attacks
• Insomnia • Almost schizophrenic behavior • Hallucinations

TREATMENT

Ayurveda
Camphor clears the mind and helps the nervous system. (See page 103.)
Cumin may be useful. (See page 116.)
Licorice strengthens the nerves. (See page 132.)
Individual treatment will be necessary to lift the spirits and to address any hormonal problems. (See page 22.)

Chinese Herbalism
Dang Gui (angelica), Bai Shao (peony root), Gan Cao (licorice), and Chai Hu (thorowax root) may be useful. (See pages 82, 132, and 159.)
Ren Shen (ginseng) will help to restore and to strengthen the whole person. (See page 160.)
Yuan Zhi (Chinese senega) can reduce insomnia and bouts of depression. (See page 166.)
Tu Su Zi (dodder seed) may help to restore hormone imbalances to normal. (See page 118.)

Herbalism
Agnus castus can help to restore the hormone balance in the body. (See page 198.)
St. John's wort and oats are nervine, and will help to reduce stress symptoms and anxiety. (See pages 89 and 138.)
Rosemary or lemon balm teas or tinctures will help the nervous system and lift depression. (See pages 152 and 175.)

Aromatherapy
Clary sage has a balancing effect on hormones, and so can help to treat and prevent postnatal illness. (See page 178.)
Jasmine and bergamot are tonics and relaxants, and can be used daily, either in the bath or in massage. (See pages 107 and 141.)
Ylang ylang and neroli are specific to PND, and can be used in a long, warm bath to ease symptoms. (See pages 95 and 106.)

Flower Essences
Gorse is good for feelings of hopelessness. (See page 192.)
Wild mustard, when you feel as if you are under a dark cloud for no apparent reason. (See page 184.)
Olive will help to address exhaustion. (See page 156.)
Sweet chestnut is for fits of utter despair. (See page 100.)

Nutrition
Eat regular, healthy meals and snacks to keep up your energy levels and boost your mood. Some experts believe that nutritional deficiencies are at the root of the problem: ensure you eat plenty of foods rich in vitamins C and B, calcium, iron, magnesium, and potassium. (See pages 206–209, 210, 213, 215, and 217.)
Tyrosine and tryptophan, amino acids, can help to ease postnatal depression. (See page 227.)

Mind–Body Healing
Regular exercise, and regular rest, help to boost mood. Both of these may be in short supply after the birth of a baby, so enlist what help you can. (See page 70.)
In the case of postnatal depression, therapy, including cognitive behavioral and interpersonal therapy, or a self-help course may be useful. Local support groups will be beneficial. (See pages 68–69.)

> **CAUTION**
> If postnatal depression or psychosis are suspected, take advice from your healthcare provider. Do not discontinue prescribed medication, or take herbal remedies alongside medication, until you have consulted with your phyisician.

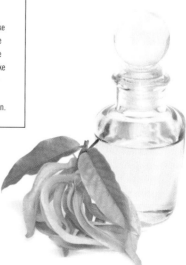

If you are suffering from baby blues or postnatal depression, relax in a warm bath with a few drops of ylang ylang.

MENOPAUSE SYMPTOMS

Menopause is the cessation of menstruation and a woman's reproductive capacity. It usually occurs around the age of 50, but may happen prematurely, or artificially after removal of the ovaries. Most symptoms that occur during menopause result directly from the estrogen deficiency produced by the failing ovaries. Interestingly, Japanese women suffer far fewer symptoms of the menopause because they eat more plant estrogens like tofu, soya, and miso.

SYMPTOMS

• Back pain • Dry, thinning hair and dry skin • Very heavy periods (flooding) • Very light periods • Hot flushes, mostly affecting the face and neck, and varying in frequency and duration • Incontinence through wear and tear, childbearing, and lack of estrogen • Osteoporosis • Psychological problems such as irritability, anxiety, insomnia, and poor memory • Increased hair growth on the face, stomach, or chest

TREATMENT

Ayurveda

Calamus root can be good for memory problems and mental stress. (See page 75.)

Celery seeds and cedar are balancing, and may help with menstrual problems. (See pages 84 and 100.)

Cinnamon is especially powerful during menopause, and is particularly useful for low libido and edema. (See page 104.)

Coriander is cooling, and acts as a diuretic and diaphoretic. It is also thought to be aphrodisiac. (See page 113.)

Aloe vera cools and cleanses the liver when taken internally, helping with any "hot" symptoms of menopause, including flushes, sweats, and swelling. (See page 80.)

Chinese Herbalism

Shan Zhu Yu (cornelian cherry) can be used for flooding, with Ren Shen (ginseng) for hot flushes. (See pages 114 and 160.)

Yuan Zhi (Chinese senega) may be useful for irritability, insomnia, and depression. (See page 166.)

Dang Gui (angelica), Bai Shao (peony root), and Chai Hu (thorowax root) will treat the symptoms of menopause, which is believed to be a weakness of kidneys, deficient blood, and a kidney–liver imbalance. (See pages 82 and 159.)

Herbalism

Valerian will help with anxiety and tension, and combined with skullcap relaxes the nervous system. (See pages 181 and 195.)

Ginseng will help with anxiety and irritability, increases mental alertness, and prevents feelings of fatigue. (See page 160.)

Dandelion cleanses the liver and helps the body to detoxify, which can reduce the risk of breast growths and other cell changes. (See page 188.)

Shepherd's purse (*Capsella bursa-pastoris*), lady's mantle, yarrow, golden seal (*Hydrastis canadensis*), beth root (*Trillium erectum*), and periwinkle (*Vinca* species) help with heavy bleeding. (See pages 74 and 78.)

Milk thistle can be used to treat painful breasts. (See page 183.)

Agnus castus can be used for breast tenderness. (See page 198.)

Black cohosh (*Actaea racemosa*) can restore female hormonal balance and help to prevent hot flushes. (See page 75.)

American ginseng can increase libido, as can agnus castus and black cohosh (*Actaea racemosa*). (See pages 75, 160, and 198.)

Ginkgo biloba can help with concentration. (See page 131.)

Cramp bark will help painful menstruation. (See page 197.)

Burdock root helps with dry and scaly skin, and licorice or chamomile, applied directly to the skin, will soothe and soften. (See pages 85, 132, and 149.)

Valerian can improve the quality of sleep. (See page 195.)

Motherwort can restore thickness and elasticity to the walls of the vagina. (See page 144.)

Dandelion is a natural diuretic and will help with any swelling associated with water retention. (See page 188.)

Aromatherapy

Clary sage will lift your mood and help to deal with fluctuating hormones. (See page 178.)

Chamomile, diluted in a little carrier oil, is adaptogenic, and will balance hormone levels causing night sweats, hot flushes, and other symptoms. (See page 149.)

Essential oils of damiana, and geranium or ylang ylang, are aphrodisiacs for low libido. (See pages 95, 161, and 192.)

Fennel can be massaged into the abdomen for water retention and symptoms of hormonal imbalance. (See page 128.)

Nutrition

Take magnesium and vitamin B-complex for anxiety and irritability. (See pages 206–209 and 217.)

Vitamin E, flaxseed oil, acidophilus, and vitamin B-complex will help with tender, lumpy breasts. (See pages 142, 145, 206–209, and 211.)

Co-enzyme Q10 will help lack of energy and fatigue; check that you are not anemic. (See page 230.)

Vitamin C can help regulate heavy bleeding (flooding) when combined with bioflavonoids. (See pages 210 and 228.)

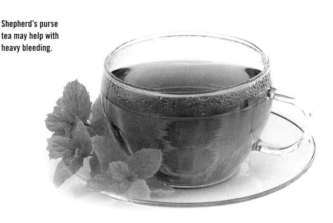

Shepherd's purse tea may help with heavy bleeding.

PROLAPSE

Prolapse occurs when the uterus and/or vagina slip downward due to a weakening or stretching of the muscles that would normally keep them in place. This may happen as a result of childbirth, allowing the uterus to bulge into the vagina and press on the bladder or rectum. If prolapse is complete, a large part of the vagina or uterus may actually protrude through the vaginal opening, causing soreness or ulceration, and encouraging infection. The risk of a prolapse may be heightened by a chronic cough, chronic constipation, or obesity. Neither prolapse is serious at first, but may become so if neglected. Surgery to tighten pelvic floor muscles may be necessary if exercises do not improve the muscle tone. A ring pessary, fitted behind the pubic bone, may be necessary in an elderly woman.

SYMPTOMS
• A sensation of something dropping down • Dragging feeling in lower abdomen • Backache • Fatigue • Possibly, frequent urge to urinate, stress incontinence, and urine infections

TREATMENT
Chinese Herbalism
Treatment would be aimed at deficient qi, and central qi pills would be useful. (See page 49.)

Herbalism
Motherwort and lady's mantle can help to restore the tone of the uterus and vagina. (See pages 78 and 144.)
Use astringent herbs such as horsetail, shepherd's purse (*Capsella bursa-pastoris*), and bay berry (*Myrica cerifera*). These can be taken as teas, tisanes, decoctions, and pills. They can also be used as a poultice and applied to the abdomen. (See page 123.)
Barberry stimulates the uterus to contract: do not use in pregnancy. (See page 90.)
For a prolapse after the menopause, try sage, calendula, ginseng, and wild yam: all estrogenic. (See pages 93, 121, 160, and 177.)
Chickweed (*Stellaria media*) ointment or douche can soothe and heal soreness of the vagina or cervix.
Pessaries with glycerin and golden seal (*Hydrastis canadensis*) can be helpful.

Aromatherapy
Massage the lower abdomen and back with diluted oils of rosemary and lemon to improve the circulation and tighten tissues. (See pages 108 and 175.)

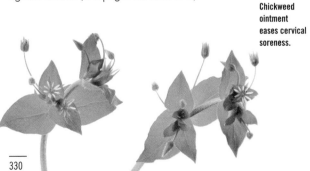

Chickweed ointment eases cervical soreness.

OVARIAN CYSTS

A cyst is an abnormal sac or cavity that contains liquid or semi-solid material enclosed by a membrane. Ovarian cysts most commonly occur in women between the ages of 35 and 55. Usually they are benign, but they can sometimes cause problems because of their size. Ovarian cysts may be caused by slight ovulation disorders, or by swelling of the lining of the ovary through fluid collection. The most common ovarian cyst is a follicular cyst that contains watery fluid. Pseudomucinous cysts contain a thick mucous fluid and can lead to complications if they rupture or become infected.

SYMPTOMS
• Pain, once the cyst has grown large enough to cause problems
• Abdominal discomfort • Possibly an increase in the size of the abdomen • Breathlessness • Varicose veins • Piles • Repeated or multiple cysts may affect fertility

TREATMENT
Chinese Herbalism
Tu Su Zi (dodder seeds) can balance the reproductive system. (See page 118.)
San Qi (notoginseng), for general relief of pain. (See page 160.)
Bai Shao (peony root) may be useful. (See page 159.)

Herbalism
Blue cohosh (*Caulophyllum thalictroides*) can help to restore the function of the reproductive system. Bladderwrack can be added to ensure normal thyroid function. (See page 129.)
Take dandelion root to help the liver metabolize estrogen. (See page 188.)
Agnus castus acts to restore estrogen levels. (See page 198.)

Aromatherapy
Basil, marjoram, and lavender can be massaged into the abdomen to ease pain and restore balance. (See pages 143, 156, and 157.)
Clary sage will help to balance hormones. (See page 178.)

Nutrition
Increase your intake of iodine, since thyroid problems may be at the root of the cysts. (See page 216.)
Vitamin E is helpful for preventing and treating cysts. (See page 211.)
The B-complex vitamins will help to re-establish hormone balance and the metabolism of estrogen by the liver. (See pages 206–209.)

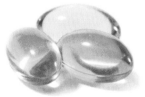

If you suffer from ovarian cysts, try taking vitamin E supplements.

PELVIC INFLAMMATORY DISEASE

Pelvic inflammatory disease (PID) is an umbrella term for infections and inflammations that have penetrated the reproductive system, i.e. the ovaries (ovaritis), Fallopian tubes (salpingitis), and uterus (see "Endometriosis"). Left untreated, these infections can develop and recur for years. Possible causes of PID are gonorrhoea and chlamydia cystitis (see page 315), various viruses, or the natural flora of the vagina. Triggers include anything that allows a lurking infection to travel, such as childbirth, abortion, surgery on the reproductive system or in the pelvic area, or an intrauterine device.

SYMPTOMS

In acute PID:
• Fever with shaking • Painful intercourse • Unusual vaginal discharge • Vaginal bleeding after sex or in mid-menstrual cycle • Severe lower abdominal pain • Back pain
In chronic PID:
• Weight loss • Backache and lower abdominal pain • Nausea • Diarrhea • Tiredness • Pain on urination • Reduced fertility

TREATMENT

Ayurveda
Aloe vera relieves inflammation, soothes muscle spasms, and purifies the blood. (See page 80.)
Angelica has antibacterial properties and eases pain. (See page 82.)
Gotu kola will help if the infection is linked to STDs. (See page 101.)

Chinese Herbalism
Bai Shao (peony root) can be used for abdominal pain. (See page 159.)
Gui Zhi (cinnamon) treats pain. (See page 104.)
San Qi (notoginseng) may be useful. (See page 160.)

Traditional Home and Folk Remedies
Peel a clove of garlic, wrap it in gauze, and tie a piece of string to one end. Place in the vagina and change daily. (See page 79.)

Herbalism
Echinacea will help to boost immunity as well as addressing the infection. (See page 122.)
Thyme and parsley will fight infection. (See pages 162 and 190.)

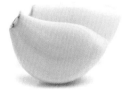

Place a piece of garlic wrapped in gauze inside the vagina. Its antibiotic and antiseptic actions may help to fight PID.

ENDOMETRIOSIS

Endometriosis is a condition where tissue that behaves like the lining of the womb (endometrium) is found in other parts of the body, including the ovaries, Fallopian tubes, stomach, bladder, or bowel. Endometrial tissue is still under the influence of the menstrual cycle's hormones, so it grows and bleeds each month, resulting in blood-filled cysts and scarring, wherever it is in the body. The condition can be extremely painful, or entirely painless, and it may cause infertility. Endometriosis mainly affects women of childbearing age. In severe cases, surgery may be advised. The exact cause of endometriosis is not known, but it may be caused by a problem with the immune system and there may be genetic factors. Some physicians think it is caused by retrograde menstruation, when blood containing endometrial cells flows backward into the abdominal cavity rather than out of the body.

SYMPTOMS

• Severe period pain • Extremely heavy periods • Pelvic pain • Pain during sex and when going to the toilet • Anal bleeding • Constant tiredness • Possibly, infertility

TREATMENT

Ayurveda
Angelica can help with pain. (See page 82.)
Include garlic and ginger in your diet. (See pages 79 and 200.)
Fry aloe vera gel with ghee, cumin, coriander seeds, and turmeric. Add honey to taste, then take twice daily to ease menstrual pain and soothe symptoms. (See pages 80, 113, 116, and 117.)

Chinese Herbalism
Bai Shao (peony root) and Gui Zhi (cinnamon) can be used for abdominal pain. (See pages 104 and 159.)

Traditional Home and Folk Remedies
Castor oil helps the body to rid itself of excess tissues and toxins. Take at the beginning of the menstrual cycle, when cramping is first noticed. Do not take during pregnancy.
Apart from during menstruation, try alternating hot and cold baths: hot water will ease cramping; cold will reduce inflammation.

Herbalism
Flaxseed helps to eliminate toxins from the body. Soak in water, strain, and drink. (See page 145.)
Turmeric has anti-inflammatory properties. (See page 117.)

Aromatherapy
Gently massage the pelvic area with lavender or sandalwood oils to relieve pain and relax. (See pages 143 and 179.)

Nutrition
Eat a healthy wholegrain and nutrient-rich diet to aid hormone balance. Include plenty of broccoli, cauliflower, Brussels sprouts, kale, cabbage, soy, and fiber. (See page 58.)

THRUSH

Thrush is caused by the yeast organism *Candida albicans*, which lives naturally in the vagina and also the mouth, bowel, and, to some extent, the skin. It only begins to cause problems when there is an overgrowth of it. Antibiotics, immunosuppressive drugs, a compromised immune system, periods of hormonal change and stress can all encourage *Candida* growth, and thrush as a result. Other aggravating factors include a high sugar intake, tight clothing, poor personal hygiene, and scented bath oils. Women seem to suffer more frequently from thrush, or candidiasis, than men.

SYMPTOMS
• Itchy, white vaginal discharge • Sore, red, dry, itchy vulva
• Stinging pain on urination • Soreness and discomfort during intercourse • Possibly a red rash extending down the thighs or to the anus

TREATMENT
Ayurveda
Garlic is a useful anti-infective agent, and works against fungi. Fresh garlic, taken as often as possible throughout the day, can act to fight infection and boost the immune system. (See page 79.) The following herbs may be used in internal and external preparations, for their antifungal properties: barberry, alfalfa, basil, cinnamon, coriander, myrrh, and wild sunflower (elecampane). (See pages 90, 104, 112, 113, 140, 150, and 156.)

Chinese Herbalism
Treatment would address excess damp and damp heat. Suitable herbs might include Long Dan Cao (Chinese gentian) and Qing Hao (*Artemisia annua*), also known as oriental wormwood. Dang Gui (angelica) or ginger will be useful when you feel generally depleted. (See pages 82 and 200.)

Traditional Home and Folk Remedies
Sit in a bowl of water to which a little vinegar or lemon juice has been added, to correct pH imbalance and maintain an acid environment. (See pages 108 and 204.)
A live yogurt douche will encourage the growth of healthy bacteria that will prevent fungal infection. Use regularly if you are prone to thrush. Apply to patches of oral thrush, and include live yogurt in your daily diet. (See page 142.)
Apple cider vinegar, added to a pint of warm water, can be used as a douche. (See page 204.)

Herbalism
Drink an infusion of echinacea or marigold to encourage healing, boost the immune system, and clear infection. (See pages 93 and 122.)
A douche of marigold or lavender flowers will ease symptoms. (See pages 93 and 143.)
Take echinacea 3 times daily for chronic cases of thrush, and every 2 hours in acute attacks, to boost the immune system. (See page 122.)
Useful antifungal herbs include marigold, cinnamon, and rosemary. (See pages 93, 104, and 175.)
Chamomile cream and chickweed (*Stellaria media*) ointment can be applied externally to soothe the itching and irritation. (See page 149.)
Soak a tampon in water with a few drops of golden seal (*Hydrastis canadensis*) tincture and insert; remove after one hour.

Aromatherapy
A tiny drop of tea tree oil, added to 2pt. (1.2l.) of warm, already boiled water, can be used as a douche. (See page 150.)
Massage with lavender or tea tree oil can boost the immune system and prevent further infections. (See pages 143 and 150.)

Nutrition
Take acidophilus tablets to restore the healthy bacteria in the body, which will help to fight the infection. (See page 142.)

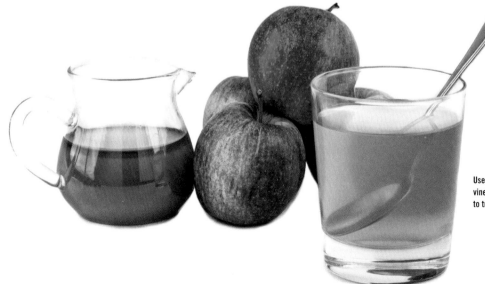

Use a douche of cider vinegar and warm water to treat vaginal thrush.

PAINFUL INTERCOURSE

Many women experience pain or discomfort during sexual intercourse (called dyspareunia) at different points in their lives, and it may be attributed to a number of causes, both physical and emotional:

• Childbirth, as the labor and delivery process can cause soreness and discomfort for some weeks, particularly if the woman has had an episiotomy (see pages 326 and 327).
• Endometriosis (see page 331).
• Fibroids, which are noncancerous growths in or on the walls of the uterus.
• Menopause (see page 329).
• Pelvic inflammatory disease (see page 331).
• Sexually transmitted diseases (STDs).
• Thrush (see opposite).

TREATMENT

Aromatherapy
Lavender and marjoram are relaxing, and can help you to get over the emotional trauma of painful sex. Try a relaxing full-body massage with your partner before intercourse. (See pages 143 and 157.)

Homeopathy
Treatment would be constitutional, and would depend on the cause of the pain. The following remedies may help while you are waiting for an appointment with a homeopath:
Calcarea Iod., for treating small fibroids with a yellow discharge. (See page 213.)
Sepia, when the problem is associated with prolapse. (See page 182.)

Flower Essences
Try mimulus, which will ease the fear of pain during sex. (See page 153.)
Rescue Remedy, taken before making love, will calm and reduce feelings of panic and anxiety. (See page 158.)

Nutrition
Take plenty of vitamins A and E, which will help restore the health of the reproductive system. (See pages 206 and 211.)
Acidophilus will help to maintain the balance of healthy flora in the body. (See page 142.)
Vitamin E capsules can be placed in the vagina to ease pain and dryness. (See page 211.)

Mind–Body Healing
Talking with a therapist may ease anxiety caused by painful intercourse, and may help to heal the scars of past emotional traumas. (See page 69.)

Marjoram is a warm, relaxing, and sedative herb. Use the essential oil in a massage or burn in a vaporizer.

DISORDERS OF THE REPRODUCTIVE SYSTEM: MALE

INFERTILITY

The term infertility is generally applied when failure to conceive follows an 18-month period of regular, unprotected sexual intercourse. It is usually a sign that something in the body is not working properly. The most common cause of infertility in men is a low sperm count (possibly due to environmental pollution). Poor sperm quality, inadequate mobility of sperm, no sperm at all, or an abnormality in the penis may also be responsible. In some cases the problem may be hormonal. Risk factors include smoking, excessive alcohol consumption, raised temperature around the testes (caused by tight trousers, or by varicose veins on the scrotum), certain prescription drugs, stress, or infection with mumps. A diet lacking in vitamins and minerals can also cause a man to be less fertile.

TREATMENT

Ayurveda

Saffron is used for the treatment of infertility. (See page 115.)
Sandalwood can help with impotence and acts as an aphrodisiac. (See page 179.)
Clove, ginger, cardamom, cinnamon, vetiver, and coriander are aphrodisiac. (See pages 104, 113, 122, 125, 197, and 200.)

Chinese Herbalism

Infertility is believed to be caused by damp heat, and an imbalance of yin and yang. The following combinations may be useful: Yi Zhi Ren (black cardamom), He Shou Wu (fleeceflower root), Gou Qi Zi (wolfberry), Du Zhong (eucommia bark), and Wu Wei Zi (schisandra), for problems associated with sperm. (See pages 81, 124, 147, 167, and 180.)

Herbalism

Remedies such as damiana and saw palmetto have hormonal effects, stimulating the male reproductive system while also acting as useful nerve restoratives. (See pages 183 and 192.)

Aromatherapy

Rose oil is said to increase sperm count and quality, as well as acting as a mild aphrodisiac. Add a few drops to your partner's bath, or perhaps engage in a little gentle massage, with 2 or 3 drops of rose essential oil in a mild carrier oil such as sweet almond oil. (See pages 169 and 174.)
If infertility is causing anxiety, any of the relaxing essential oils, such as lavender, marjoram, or chamomile, can be vaporized or used in a bath. (See pages 143, 149, and 157.)
When repeated attempts to get pregnant have failed and you need a little encouragement to continue with love-making, ylang ylang is a lovely, relaxing oil that will act as an aphrodisiac. (See page 95.)

Homeopathy

Treatment would be constitutional, but the following remedies may be helpful:
Lycopodium, for an increased desire for sex, but where intercourse is spoiled by anticipation of failure. (See page 147.)
Sepia, for a dragging sensation in the genitals, and no desire for sex. (See page 182.)

Flower Essences

Willow can be taken for resentment, bitterness, and self-pity about the problem. (See page 177.)
White chestnut, for worrying thoughts. (See page 76.)
Pine, for guilty feelings. (See page 163.)
Olive, for exhaustion and overwhelming fatigue. (See page 156.)

Nutrition

There is a possibility that a zinc deficiency might cause problems with male fertility. Studies in the U.S. have shown that zinc is essential for sperm formation, and men who have zinc deficiencies may produce zero or reduced sperm counts. Zinc is also linked to a man's sex drive. (See page 221.)
Cutting out alcohol, smoking, and drugs is suggested for both couples for the period before conception.
Vitamins E and B6 may be supplemented, as a deficiency is often linked to a low sperm count. (See pages 208 and 211.)
An increased intake of EFAs (essential fatty acids, found in oily fish, fish liver oils, seeds, nuts, pulses, beans, evening primrose oil, and unrefined vegetable oils) stimulates sex hormone production.

Mind–Body Healing

Massage and relaxation techniques such as meditation will help with the anxiety caused by infertility. (See pages 68–71.)

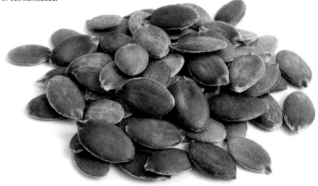

Foods that contain essential fatty acids, such as pumpkin seeds, are believed to stimulate the production of sex hormones.

PROSTATE PROBLEMS

The prostate is a small sex gland which surrounds the urethra (urine tube) under the bladder. Its function is to produce the fluid that transports and nourishes sperm as it is ejaculated. Common prostate problems include:

• Benign prostatic hyperplasia (BPH), a slow, noncancerous enlargement of the prostate, progressively constricts the urethra, causing obstruction in the flow of urine. Incomplete emptying of the bladder as a result causes a frequent urge to urinate at night as well as during the day.
• Prostatitis, inflammation of the prostate gland, is common in younger men and may be chronic or acute. Symptoms include a frequent urge to urinate, burning pain and difficulty in urinating, lower back pain, painful ejaculation, and inflamed testes.
• Prostate cancer is the second most common form of cancer in men. The prostate is enlarged, as in BPH, but is felt to be hard on examination. As well as an urge to urinate more frequently, there may be blood in the urine and pain on urinating. If the cancer is advanced there may also be bone pain and weight loss.

TREATMENT

Ayurveda
Gotu kola is cooling, rejuvenating, and diuretic. (See page 101.)
Cedar and celery seed are natural diuretics and will encourage urination. (See pages 84 and 100.)
Cinnamon is diuretic and analgesic, which will help ease the discomfort. (See page 104.)
Coriander is diuretic and aphrodisiac, which will help address the low libido that is associated with this condition. (See page 113.)

Chinese Herbalism
Prostate problems are believed to be caused by excess dampness and stagnant qi. The herbs Gui Zhi (cinnamon bark), Huang Bai (cork tree bark), and Ze Xie (water plantain) will be useful treatments. (See pages 104 and 162.)
Ren Shen (ginseng) is recommended for an enlarged prostate. (See page 160.)

Traditional Home and Folk Remedies
Watercress leaves are tonic and should be eaten as often as possible to help alleviate the problem. (See page 154.)
Sesame seeds have a beneficial effect in maintaining and enhancing sexual vigor.
Pumpkin seeds are a male sexual tonic, and are used in the treatment of prostate problems.

Herbalism
Saw palmetto is able to reduce inflammation of the prostate. (See page 183.)
Couch grass (*Elymus repens*) and horsetail can be given to help encourage urination, and can be drunk freely throughout the day as a natural diuretic. (See page 123.)

Aromatherapy
Clary sage and geranium, which have estrogen-like oils, can be used in whole-body massage or in the bath to treat the condition. (See pages 161 and 178.)
Bergamot, chamomile, and myrrh are anti-inflammatory, and will ease symptoms, particularly of prostatitis. (See pages 107, 112, and 149.)
Benzoin, sandalwood, frankincense, and cedarwood are all diuretic, and can be used both in the bath and for a full-body massage. (See pages 90, 100, 179, and 186.)

Nutrition
Lecithin, calcium, and magnesium may help treat prostate disorders. (See pages 213, 217, and 233.)
An increased intake of zinc can help to prevent and treat prostatitis. (See page 221.)
Evening primrose has been successfully used for prostate problems. (See page 231.)
Cold-pressed linseed oil can help if the condition is mild but recurrent. (See page 145.)
Flower pollen is widely used to treat problems of the prostate gland. (See page 228.)

Cinnamon, added to food or drinks, may ease the symptoms.

ERECTION PROBLEMS

Failure to achieve an erection that is firm enough, or sustained for long enough, to allow normal sexual intercourse is generally known as impotence. Its cause may be physical (organic), psychological, or a combination of both. Organic impotence may be due to an imperfect blood supply to the penis, an age-related loss of male sex hormones, diabetes, medicinal drugs, or various neurological conditions. Psychological factors such as lack of desire, depression, or fear of failure may be responsible for impotence, and alcohol, while enhancing sexual desire, can impede performance. Primary impotence is the case in which the male has never maintained an erection of long enough duration to engage in sexual intercourse. Secondary impotence is when a previously potent male loses the ability to maintain an erection during intercourse. Approximately 30 million men in the U.S. suffer from impotence.

TREATMENT

Ayurveda
Sandalwood is good for impotence, and accompanying anxiety and nervousness. (See page 179.)
Cinnamon tones the muscles and is noted for treating impotence. (See page 104.)
Ginger is warming and can help improve matters. (See page 200.)
Saffron is used for impotence and anxiety. (See page 115.)
Clove, ginger, cardamom, cinnamon, vetiver, and coriander are aphrodisiac. (See pages 104, 113, 122, 125, 197, and 200.)

Chinese Herbalism
Ren Shen (ginseng) can improve vitality and help to reduce feelings of anxiety. (See page 160.)
Impotence is believed to be caused by weakness of the kidneys and liver, with liver qi stagnation, and Gou Ji (cibot root) may be useful.
Dang Gui (Chinese angelica), Bai Shao (white peony root), and Chai Hu (thorowax) will help feelings of anxiety. (See pages 82 and 159.)

Traditional Home and Folk Remedies
Watercress leaves are tonic and should be eaten as often as possible to help alleviate the problem. (See page 154.)
Sesame and pumpkin seeds have a beneficial effect in maintaining and enhancing sexual vigor.
Avocado is excellent if you suffer from sexual problems. (See page 161.)

Herbalism
Peppermint leaves stimulate and warm the body, and will help to reduce feelings of anxiety. (See page 152.)
Anise is a powerful tonic: drink small amounts to treat impotence. Remedies like damiana and saw palmetto have dual hormonal effects, stimulating and toning the male reproductive system, and restoring nerves. (See pages 183 and 192.)

Aromatherapy
Essential oils of clary sage, sandalwood, and ylang ylang are natural aphrodisiacs and will help you to relax. Try a full-body massage, or a few drops in the bath. (See pages 95, 178, and 179.)

Homeopathy
Lycopodium, when you feel surges of desire, but anticipate failure. (See page 147.)
Caladium, for erections which occur during sleep, but disappear on waking, and a lack of erection even when sexually excited.

Flower Essences
Larch, for lack of sexual confidence and feelings of inadequacy. (See page 143.)
Gentian, for a sense of failure. (See page 130.)
Sweet chestnut, for despair and hopelessness. (See page 100.)
Crab apple, for feeling unclean on any level. (See page 148.)

Nutrition
Avoid alcohol, drugs, and caffeine, which constrict the blood vessels and inhibit the blood flow needed to achieve an erection. Molybdenum can prevent impotence and sexual difficulties. (See page 218.)
Zinc is required for the healthy functioning of the reproductive organs, and should be included in a varied, healthy diet. (See page 221.)
L-tryptophan may help to prevent feelings of anxiety from causing sexual difficulties. (See page 227.)

Mind–Body Healing
Therapy, or relaxation techniques, may be beneficial if anxiety is an issue. (See pages 68–69.)

In traditional Chinese medicine, Gou Ji (cibot root) is used to treat erection problems.

EJACULATION PROBLEMS

In most cases, ejaculation problems are psycho-sexual in origin, and not due to any physical abnormality. There are two main problems: premature ejaculation and absence of ejaculation. Premature ejaculation is very common and refers to the occurrence of the male orgasm before physical contact, at the time of penetration, or very soon after. Premature ejaculation is usually a feature of early sexual experience or performance anxiety. The absence of ejaculation is rare but can occur as a result of overindulgence, inadequate stimulation of the penis, or age-related loss of penile sensitivity. Some men experience a "retrograde," or dry, ejaculation as a result of genetics, illness, medication, surgery, or damage to the valves of the urethra that control the flow of semen.

SYMPTOMS
• Premature ejaculation • Absence of ejaculation

TREATMENT
Ayurveda
Sandalwood may relieve anxiety, and has an anesthetic effect on the area which can reduce premature ejaculation. (See page 179.)

Chinese Herbalism
Cibot root may work well. (See opposite.)
Problems associated with anxiety may be treated with Ren Shen (ginseng), Dang Gui (Chinese angelica), Bai Shao (white peony root), and Chai Hu (thorowax). (See pages 82, 159, and 160.)

Herbalism
Drink skullcap and valerian as a tea 3 times daily to calm. (See pages 181 and 195.)
Linden may ease anxiety and tension. (See page 191.)
Damiana and saw palmetto tone the male reproductive system and restore nerves. (See pages 183 and 192.)

Aromatherapy
A relaxing blend of essential oils of lavender, geranium, and bergamot in sweet almond oil or peach kernel oil may be used in the bath at times of great stress and anxiety. (See page 47.)

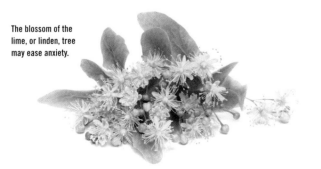

The blossom of the lime, or linden, tree may ease anxiety.

PRIAPISM

Priapism is the name given to prolonged and painful erection in the absence of sexual interest. It is caused by failure of the blood to return from the penis to the circulation after a period of sexual activity. This may be because of a disturbance in the nervous system's control of blood flow, due to a disease of the spinal cord or brain. It may also be caused by clotting due to leukemia or sickle-cell anemia, inflammation of the prostate, bladder stones, or urethritis.

SYMPTOMS
• Erection lasting more than 4 hours or erection in the absence of desire • Penile pain

TREATMENT
Ayurveda
Angelica can improve circulation. (See page 82.)
Black pepper increases blood circulation and feeds the nervous system. (See page 164.)
Calamus oil massage will improve circulation in the area. (See page 75.)
Cayenne pepper is analgesic and warming. (See page 98.)

Chinese Herbalism
Gui Zhi (cinnamon twigs) may be useful when the yang qi has failed to move fluids through channels. (See page 104.)
Dang Gui (angelica) will reduce pain and invigorate blood circulation. (See page 82.)

Herbalism
Herbs that encourage circulation include:
Broom (*Cytisus scoparius*), which tones the arteries.
Ginger, hawthorn tops, and rosemary, which are also stimulating. (See pages 114, 175, and 200.)
Lavender and vervain, which are calming, and can be sipped during an attack to ease symptoms. (See pages 143 and 196.)

Aromatherapy
Local massage with rosemary or peppermint will help normalize the blood flow in the area. (See pages 152 and 175.)
Massage the area with diluted juniper, marjoram, myrrh, or tea tree, which will act as a tonic. (See page 47.)

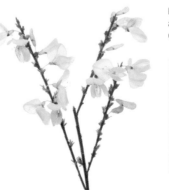

Broom tones the arteries, which can ease priapism.

> **CAUTION**
> Long-sustained erection can be dangerous as there is a risk of thrombosis, which may cause permanent loss of erectile function.

DISORDERS OF THE ENDOCRINE SYSTEM

THYROID PROBLEMS

The thyroid gland, found in the neck, is responsible for controlling the level of activity of the body. The condition of having an overactive gland is called hyperthyroidism, while an underactive gland is hypothyroidism. Occasionally thyroid disease forms part of a wider disease process, including diabetes and rheumatoid arthritis. Other causes of thyroid disease include iodine deficiency, which may exist from birth and features in mental retardation, enlargement of the thyroid gland (goiter), inflammation, and, rarely, cancer.

SYMPTOMS
In an overactive thyroid:
• Palpitations • Weight loss • Increased appetite • Anxiety
• Mood swings • Insomnia • Goiter • Sensitivity to heat
• Sweating • Twitching or trembling • Infrequent menstruation
• Untreated hyperthyroidism may lead to heart failure
In an underactive thyroid:
• Fatigue • Weight gain • Menstrual problems • Sensitivity to cold
• Slow movements and thoughts • Depression • Constipation
• No sweating • Loss of hair • Puffy face • Coronary artery disease
• Untreated hypothyroidism may lead to coma

TREATMENT
Chinese Herbalism
Hyperthyroidism is believed to be caused by heat in the liver, and marine plants and seaweed are prescribed. (See page 234.)

Herbalism
Bugleweed (*Lycopus virginicu*) is excellent, and should be drunk 3 times daily for hyperthyroidism.
Bladderwrack helps to regulate the function of the thyroid gland. Take 3 times daily, in any form. (See page 129.)

Nutrition
Nutritional deficiencies (for example, zinc, Vitamin A, selenium, and iron) and a toxic overload are thought to be the main factors involved in the onset of hypothyroidism.
Eat organic vegetables and seafood.
Garlic is a rich source of iodine, which can help regulate thyroid function. (See page 79.)

Curly kale is a rich source of vitamin A and calcium.

GOITER

Goiter is an enlargement of the thyroid gland, visible as a swelling on the neck, and is fairly common. In order for the thyroid to produce hormones it requires iodine in the diet for their synthesis. If there is insufficient iodine in the diet the gland increases its activity and swells, resulting in a goiter. The nontoxic enlargement of the thyroid due to insufficient iodine is common and easily remedied by eating more fish and iodized salt, thereby increasing iodine intake. Conditions of which goiter is a feature are: Grave's disease, where the thyroid is overactive and enlargement is accompanied by excessive hormone production; Hashimoto's thyroiditis, where the thyroid is underactive due to antibodies to thyroid hormone; sub-acute thyroiditis, which is probably a viral infection that causes inflammation and pain; dyshormonogenesis, a genetic enzyme deficiency which interferes with normal hormone synthesis; and tumors of the thyroid gland, which may be benign or malignant.

SYMPTOMS
• Swelling at the front of the neck, from a small lump to a very large mass • Difficulty in swallowing or breathing in severe cases
• Overactive thyroid, or underactive thyroid (see left)

TREATMENT
Herbalism
Bladderwrack can help goiter caused by an underactive thyroid. (See page 129.)
Bugleweed (*Lycopus virginicu*) is used to treat an overactive thyroid.

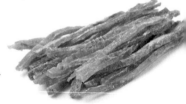

Both salt and fish may help to regulate the thyroid gland. Salted fish, shown here, may be a tasty addition to your diet.

Aromatherapy
Clary sage has a balancing effect on hormones, and since it is now believed that an underactive thyroid may be linked to an excess of female hormones, this may be a useful oil. (See page 178.)

Homeopathy
The following remedies, taken twice daily for up to 2 weeks, should improve the condition:
Spongia, for a long-standing condition, where there is a hard lump. (See page 185.)
Calcarea, for a pale, chilly, overweight person. (See page 213.)
Nat. mur., made from rock salt, is a possible homeopathic remedy for thyroid problems. (See page 154.)

Nutrition
Increase your intake of salt, fish, shellfish, and bladderwrack to ensure adequate iodine. (See page 216.)

DIABETES

The most common form of diabetes is diabetes mellitus. It is caused by a lack of, or insufficient, insulin (the hormone produced by the pancreas), as a result of which the body is unable to process glucose. This causes a high level of glucose in the blood, and low absorption of the vital energy-producing glucose by the tissues. In Type I (insulin-dependency) diabetes, the sufferer produces little or no insulin and requires lifelong monitoring. Blood sugar levels can swing wildly between hypoglycemia (featuring strange feelings, abnormal behavior, and a risk of coma) and hyperglycemia (causing overproduction of ketones, and coma). Type I usually first appears in those who are under the age of 35, particularly adolescents, and develops rapidly. Type II, maturity-onset diabetes, is thought to be caused by the body's cells' lack of response to insulin. It usually affects people aged 40 and over, and there is an association with obesity and pregnancy. The onset of Type II is gradual and may go unnoticed for some time.

SYMPTOMS
• Excessive thirst • Excessive urination • Weight loss • Fatigue, weakness, and apathy • Hunger • Bad breath
Complications include:
• Nerve damage, causing damage to the eye muscles and double vision • Damage to blood vessels affecting the eyes, sometimes causing blindness; kidneys; and circulation in the legs • Organic impotence • Arterial disease • Gangrene

TREATMENT
Ayurveda
For Type II diabetes, boil and cut one karalla, also known as bitter melon (*Momordica charantia*), into pieces and eat with the seeds every morning and evening. Do not take karalla during pregnancy.

Chinese Herbalism
Treatment aimed at nourishing the spleen, kidneys, and stomach would use Chinese yam (*Dioscorea polystachya*), lotus seed (*Nelumbo nucifera*), and mulberry (*Morus alba*).

Herbalism
Fenugreek seed works to control blood sugar levels. Drink daily. (See page 191.)
Alfalfa should be taken daily. (See page 150.)

Nutrition
Onions and garlic lower blood sugar levels. (See pages 78 and 79.)
Brewer's yeast contains chromium, which helps to normalize blood sugar levels. Take 2–3 tablespoons daily. (See page 229.)

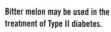

Bitter melon may be used in the treatment of Type II diabetes.

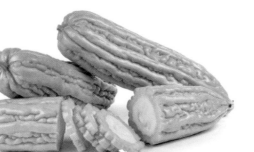

ADDISON'S DISEASE

Addison's disease is a disorder of the adrenal glands which leads to insufficient output of cortisol and aldosterone – the steroid hormones which help the body to react to stress and control water balance, respectively. The disease is caused by an inflammation followed by atrophy of the outer layer (cortex) of the adrenal gland. This in turn is caused by abnormal action of the immune system in which it behaves toward the gland tissue as though it were foreign. Addison's is therefore known as an autoimmune disease. Addison's disease is usually due to damage by an autoimmune reaction, tuberculosis, or fungal infections. Addison's disease is rare, and generally has a slow onset and chronic course, with symptoms developing gradually over months or years. Acute episodes, called Addisonian crises, can be brought on by infection, injury, or other stresses, and they occur because the adrenal glands cannot increase their production of steroid hormones which normally help the body to deal with stress. The condition was invariably fatal before hormone treatment became available in the 1950s.

SYMPTOMS
• Weakness • Fatigue • Low blood pressure • Excessive urination • Dehydration • Skin discoloration, as the pituitary gland attempts to compensate for insufficient adrenal output by overproducing a hormone which stimulates the pigment cells

TREATMENT
Herbalism
Treatment would be individual. It would include herbs to stimulate the endocrine system, and herbs to boost the immune system.

Aromatherapy
Oils that strengthen the adrenal system include: rosemary, ginger, and lemongrass. (See pages 118, 175, and 200.)

Homeopathy
Treatment would be constitutional; however, the following treatments may help:
Silicea, for when your feet are sweaty and smelly, cold weather makes the symptoms worse, and you feel really exhausted. (See page 220.)
Nat. mur., for when you have constipation, dry lips, a craving for salt, and symptoms which are made worse by sun. (See page 154.)

CAUTION
Be aware of the risk of a sudden worsening of symptoms, called an adrenal crisis, which happens if levels of cortisol fall significantly. An adrenal crisis is a medical emergency, which should be treated in hospital immediately.

HYPOGLYCEMIA

Hypoglycemia is a condition in which there is an abnormally low level of glucose in the blood. It is extremely dangerous because the brain is dependent on a constant supply of glucose. The most common cause of hypoglycemia is a relative insulin overdose by diabetics (i.e. the actual amount of insulin taken may be correct, but the intake of carbohydrate or the amount of exertion may have used up the supply too quickly). Excessive exercise and insufficient carbohydrate may, in fact, lead to hypoglycemia in non-diabetics. There are two main types of hypoglycemia: organic and functional. Any endocrine malfunction in the pancreas and adrenal glands, as well as the pituitary, thyroid, or sex glands, may result in organic hypoglycemia. Functional hypoglycemia is a temporary condition of markedly lowered blood sugar, most commonly occurring 2–3 hours after a meal high in carbohydrates.

SYMPTOMS
• Headache • Faintness • Rapid pulse and palpitations • Profuse sweating • Mental confusion and loss of memory • Irrational and disorderly behavior • Slurred speech • Numbness, temporary paralysis • Fits and, eventually, potentially fatal coma

TREATMENT
Traditional Home and Folk Remedies
Onions and garlic will help to regulate blood sugar levels. Eat raw or cooked, as often as possible. (See pages 78 and 79.)

Chinese Herbalism
Shan Yao (Chinese yam) and Lian Zi (lotus seed) will help to normalize blood sugar levels.

Flower Essences
Take Rescue Remedy if you feel an attack coming on. It will calm you and help to reduce the severity. (See page 158.)

Nutrition
Take extra Vitamin C and B-complex tablets, chromium (to regulate blood sugar levels), magnesium, potassium, zinc, and manganese. (See pages 206–209, 210, 214, 217, 218, and 221.)
For mild cases of low blood sugar, caused by overexertion, have some food or drink that contains sugar, such as fruit juice. Then eat some "starchy" carbohydrate food, such as a sandwich.

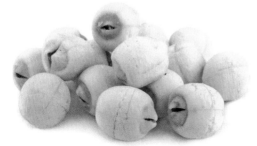

Traditional Chinese medicine suggests lotus seeds for the treatment of hypoglycemia.

OBESITY

Obesity is the excessive storage of energy in the form of fat, and applies to a bodyweight that is more than 20 percent over the recommended maximum for a person's height. The main cause of obesity is excessive calorie intake, but other factors include a low basal metabolic rate, genetics, emotional problems, metabolic disorders such as thyroid problems, and steroids or insulin.

TREATMENT
Ayurveda
Treatment would be aimed at addressing an addiction to food, accompanied by marma puncture and a diet modified to your dosha type. (See page 22.)

Chinese Herbalism
Increase your intake of foods that are bitter, pungent, astringent, and hot, which will encourage your body to eliminate waste more efficiently. Cut down on salty, sweet, and sour foods.

Traditional Home and Folk Remedies
Drink a glass of freshly squeezed grapefruit juice every morning to cleanse, break down fats, and suppress appetite. (See page 109.)

Herbalism
Bladderwrack may encourage the metabolism. (See page 129.)
Nettles are good diuretics and generally help the metabolism. Try drinking nettle tea before meals. (See page 194.)

Nutrition
A healthy diet should contain small amounts of fat and sugar; plenty of fruits, vegetables, and wholegrain starchy foods; and some milk, dairy, meat, fish, and other protein. (See page 58.)
Bee pollen stimulates the metabolism and helps to curb appetite. Take up to 1 teaspoon daily. (See page 228.)
Brewer's yeast will help to reduce various cravings for food and drink. (See page 229.)
Chromium supplements will help to ensure that your blood sugar levels are stable, and regulate appetite. (See page 214.)

Mind–Body Healing
It is recommended that adults do 150 minutes of at least moderate-intensity activity every week. Doing anything is better than nothing: start off with 10 minutes of brisk walking every day.

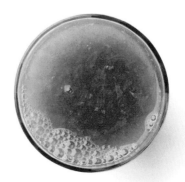

A daily glass of grapefruit juice will suppress the appetite and help break down fats.

GOUT

Gout is an acute disease of the joints. It is caused by the deposition of chalky crystals around the joints, tendons, and other body tissues when there is an abnormally high level of uric acid in the body. Severe inflammation and tissue damage result, and possibly structural damage to the kidneys and stone formation. Gout affects more than 1 million Americans, mostly men between the ages of 40 and 50. Primary gout appears to involve a hereditary factor.

SYMPTOMS
• First sign of gout is usually excruciating pain and inflammation of the innermost joint of the big toe (or, less frequently, the ankle, knee joint, hand, wrist, or elbow) • Attacks last for days or weeks and then subside • Usually there are recurrences, until gout is a constant presence

TREATMENT
Chinese Herbalism
Painful joints are said to be caused by wind cold, and some of the most useful herbs to relieve cold and damp include Gui Zhi (cinnamon), Dang Gui (angelica root), and wild ginger. (See pages 82, 104, and 200.)

Traditional Home and Folk Remedies
Raw apple and cucumber juice will help to reduce the severity and incidence of attacks. (See pages 116 and 148.)

Herbalism
Drink plenty of water and cleansing infusions such as celery seed tea. (See page 84.)
Bring down the acute inflammation with a compress made of crushed cabbage leaf. (See page 92.)
Nettle tea is helpful in preventing attacks. (See page 194.)

Aromatherapy
Rub a few drops of lavender and frankincense, mixed in a little grapeseed oil, into the affected joints. (See pages 90 and 143.) Pine, rosemary, or juniper oils, which increase circulation, can be added to the bath or foot bath to ease the condition. Rub them neat into the affected joints. (See pages 142, 163, and 175.)

Homeopathy
Homeopathic treatment would be constitutional, but in an attack one of the following remedies may be appropriate:
Lycopodium, for symptoms that are worse between 4 and 8 p.m. (See page 147.)
Urtica, for joints that feel hot and itchy. (See page 194.)
Arnica, for painful joints which feel bruised. (See page 86.)

Nutrition
A good diet is the key. Eat plenty of fresh, green vegetables and avoid sugary drinks and snacks, as well as high-protein foods such as red meat and seafood. (See pages 58–59.)
Eat food containing plenty of vitamin C (or take supplements of 1g. daily). (See page 210.)
Avoid alcohol, which increases uric acid, but drink plenty of water. Charcoal tablets may help to reduce the levels of uric acid in the body. (See page 230.)

Mind–Body Healing
Regular exercise to maintain a healthy weight is important, but choose activities such as swimming, which do not put too much strain on the joints. (See page 70.)

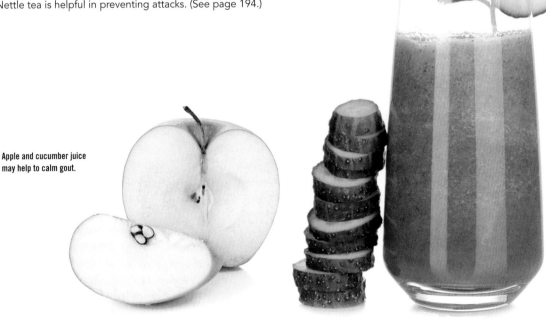

Apple and cucumber juice may help to calm gout.

DISORDERS OF THE IMMUNE SYSTEM

HIV AND AIDS

HIV is the human immunodeficiency virus, which makes the immune system unable to fight off infections. HIV is believed to be responsible for AIDS (acquired immune deficiency syndrome). Once acquired, HIV remains in the body for life, although there may be no symptoms for years. HIV may be contracted from transfusion of contaminated blood, from infected blood passing through the skin barrier via a deep graze, from a needle puncture, in the womb or at birth, by breastfeeding, or through unsafe sex. When the immune system reaches a particular stage of deterioration due to HIV, certain bacteria that are usually kept in check by healthy immune functioning are able to thrive (opportunistic infections). AIDS is diagnosed when one or more of these infections is present, but AIDS is not a disease in itself. Although there is no cure for HIV, today's pharmaceutical medications enable most people with the virus to live a long and healthy life.

SYMPTOMS
• Flu-like symptoms when HIV first enters the system (seroconversion)
Once HIV has begun to work on the immune system:
• Night sweats and fevers • Exhaustion • Weight loss • Diarrhea
• Thrush and herpes • Mouth ulcers and bleeding gums
Conditions associated with AIDS:
• Neurological problems • Fits and confusion • Yellow skin
• Swollen painful joints • Kaposi's sarcoma, a rare form of skin cancer characterized by raised purple blotches • Eye infections, particularly cytomegalovirus (CMV), which can lead to blindness
• Gut infections • Pneumocystis carinii pneumonia (PCP)

TREATMENT
Chinese Herbalism
Tonic herbs, such as Huang Qi (astragalus), Ren Shen (ginseng), and *Ganoderma* mushrooms will help your overall constitution. (See pages 87 and 160.)
Salvia, or sage, and Bai Shao (peony) will improve the blood and help promote good circulation. (See pages 159 and 177.)
Dang Gui (Chinese angelica) can restore energy and stimulate white blood cells and antibody formation. (See page 82.)

Herbalism
Treatment will always be tailored to the individual, but there are a number of herbs that can be used to boost immunity, including:
Garlic, to prevent infections of all kinds, including those that have now become immune to antibiotics. (See page 79.)

Licorice, to enhance recovery, stimulating the formation and efficiency of white blood cells and antibodies. It is also useful in preventing stress. (See page 132.)
Echinacea, for treatment of chronic and acute infections – it cleanses the blood and lymphatic system, stimulating production of white blood cells and antibodies. (See page 122.)
Ginseng, to boost immunity and encourage the body to deal efficiently with stress, as well as stimulating white blood cell production. (See page 160.)

Aromatherapy
Antiviral oils include tea tree, niaouli, eucalyptus, and thyme, which can be used in any form. Lymphatic massage is particularly recommended for stimulating the immune system. (See page 47.)
Lavender, tea tree, and bergamot stimulate production of white blood cells, and are active against one or more bacteria and viruses. (See pages 107, 143, and 150.)
Mood-enhancing and uplifting oils, such as bergamot, lavender, geranium, rose, sandalwood, and ylang ylang, may be useful. (See pages 94, 107, 143, 161, 174, and 179.)

Homeopathy
Your homeopath will suggest improved nutrition, fresh air, exercise, and rest, which can restore the ability of the immune system to cope. Homeopathic remedies will be prescribed in conjunction with this advice.

Nutrition
Include a variety of vegetables each day, with wholegrain cereals like brown rice and wholewheat bread, fruit, pulses (beans and lentils), and a few nuts and seeds for their oils. (See pages 58–59.)
A daily multivitamin and multimineral preparation – especially one containing high amounts of the antioxidant nutrients – acts to boost immune activity. (See pages 60 and 65.)
Vitamin C stimulates immunity and is antiviral. (See page 210.)
Acidophilus will encourage the healthy bacteria in your gut, which will help to fight off infections and infestations. (See page 142.)
Zinc stimulates the immune system, and acts as an antiviral agent. (See page 221.)

Mind–Body Healing
A diagnosis of HIV can be upsetting, and feelings of anxiety or depression are common. You are likely to be referred to an HIV clinic, which will offer counseling.
You may also like to make contact with support groups, local and online, which can offer friendship as well as advice. (See page 69.)
Relaxation and exercise will help to boost your mood and keep your body healthy. What was right for you before diagnosis will probably still be right for you, from yoga to team sports. (See page 70.)

> **CAUTION**
> Consult with your healthcare practitioner before taking any herbal remedies, as they may interfere with prescription drugs. The suggested remedies may help to manage the condition, but they are not intended as substitutes for the care of a registered physician.

GLANDULAR FEVER

Glandular fever, or infectious mononucleosis as it is also known, is caused by the Epstein-Barr virus (a herpes virus). The virus multiplies in the white blood cells, eventually harming the immune system's efficiency. Glandular fever is usually transmitted via saliva, hence its nickname of the "kissing disease." While symptoms may last for only six weeks, recovery is slow, and fatigue and low energy levels may linger for months. The disease occurs most commonly in adults 15–30 years old, but one attack confers immunity.

SYMPTOMS
• Flu-like symptoms, including fever, sore throat, headache • Fatigue and lethargy • Swollen lymph glands in the neck, armpits, and groin • Rash of small, slightly raised red spots • Chest pain, with breathing difficulty and cough • Enlarged spleen and possibly damaged liver, causing jaundice

TREATMENT
Chinese Herbalism 🥣
Tonic herbs, such as Huang Qi (astragalus), Ren Shen (ginseng), and *Ganoderma* mushrooms will help your overall constitution. (See pages 87 and 160.)
Salvia, or sage, and Bai Shao (peony) will improve the blood and help promote good circulation. (See pages 159 and 177.)
Dang Gui (Chinese angelica) can restore energy and stimulate white blood cells and antibody formation. (See page 82.)

Traditional Home and Folk Remedies ✋
Apply apple cider vinegar to the neck glands daily. Drink it in a cup of warm water to encourage healing. (See page 204.)
Ginseng acts to balance the glands. Chew the fresh or dried root, or add the powder to hot herbal teas. It will prevent fatigue and stimulate you. (See page 160.)

Herbalism 🌿
Herbs to promote healing include cleavers (*Galium aparine*), echinacea, and nettles, all of which stimulate immune activity as well as fighting infection. (See pages 122 and 194.)
Take lemon balm, oats, and skullcap, if depression accompanies the fever. (See pages 89, 152, and 181.)
Infusions of yarrow and elderflower will help to control fever and also induce sweating. (See pages 74 and 178.)

Aromatherapy 💧
Essential oils can be used in the bath, or in massage, which also has therapeutic benefits. Oils to consider are eucalyptus, lavender, rosemary, and tea tree, which will encourage immune activity and fight the virus. (See pages 124, 143, 150, and 175.)

Homeopathy 💊
Constitutional treatment is recommended, but Calcarea may be useful, taken up to 6 times daily, for 2 days. (See page 213.)

Flower Essences ⚘
Flower essences are often used by practitioners to help you cope with the physical and emotional effects of glandular fever.
Olive will help if you feel exhausted both physically and mentally. (See page 156.)
Wild mustard controls feelings of depression that have no identifiable cause. (See page 184.)
Gorse will help with feelings of hopelessness. (See page 192.)

Nutrition ✖
Take extra vitamin C (citrus fruit juices will be refreshing), B-complex (whole grains, protein, and fresh vegetables), and zinc (shellfish, meat, eggs, mushrooms, and brewer's yeast). (See pages 206–209, 210, and 221.)
Evening primrose oil will help to encourage healing. (See page 231.)
Royal jelly will help fight feelings of fatigue and depression, and stimulate the immune system. (See page 234.)
Eat plenty of foods containing antioxidants, such as blueberries, elderberries, cranberries, and artichokes. (See page 65.)

A traditional Chinese medicine practitioner may prescribe *Ganoderma* mushrooms, also known as Lingzhi.

ALLERGIES

An allergy is the immune system's abnormal response to contact with a specific substance. The system overreacts when faced with foreign substances or organisms – allergens – and deals with them as if they were harmful, as it would with invading bacteria, for example. The result is an allergic reaction, also known as a histamine reaction (histamine being the substance produced in response to attack). Common allergens include certain foods, grass pollens, spores, fabrics, drugs, household chemicals, and stress. Some of the most common allergic responses are urticaria (see page 258), dermatitis (see page 256), asthma (see page 288) and hay fever/rhinitis (see page 278). An estimated 35 million people in the United States suffer from various allergies, some of which are mistaken for the common cold.

SYMPTOMS
• Sneezing • Runny nose • Wheezing • Excess catarrh • Urticaria
• Anaphylactic shock (sometimes fatal), causing breathing difficulty, edema, constriction of air tubes, and heart failure

TREATMENT

Ayurveda
Cleansing and detoxification will be followed by a varied diet of organic foods. Herbal preparations to boost immunity may be appropriate, including harithaki (*Terminalia chebula*), also called myrobalan, which helps in cases of eczema; bitter orange for respiratory allergies; and stramonium. (See page 106.)

Chinese Herbalism
Bi Van Pian, also called "nose inflammation pills," for wind cold or wind heat to the face, indicated by sneezing, itchy eyes, facial congestion and sinus pain, acute and chronic rhinitis, and nasal allergies.
Yu Ping Feng San, or "Jade screen," helps prevent hay fever and guards against allergies.
Cang Er Zi Tang, or xanthium powder, for allergic rhinitis, with thick yellow catarrh or blocked nose.

Traditional Home and Folk Remedies
Eat the local honey if you suffer from hay fever. (See page 203.)
Honey and apple cider can be drunk in a glass of warm water to restore and prevent allergies. (See pages 148 and 203.)
Drink nettle tea to increase resistance. (See page 194.)
Apply nettle tea to skin, or use Urtica Urens cream or homeopathic remedy for urticaria. (See page 194.)

Herbalism
Echinacea acts as a natural antibiotic while building the immune system. Take three times daily, as an infusion, or a few drops of tincture in a glass of warm water, during attacks or when you are run down. (See page 122.)
Other useful herbs include chamomile, elderflower, red clover (*Trifolium pratense*), and yarrow. (See pages 74, 149, and 178.)

Add a small amount of ginseng powder to herbal drinks to overcome the tendency to allergic attacks, such as hay fever. (See page 160.)
Herbs to boost immunity include garlic, angelica, borage, and wild yam. (See pages 79, 82, and 121.)
Strengthen the weakened area with tonic teas, 2 cups taken over a period of time: the sinuses with elderflower tea; the stomach with chamomile, linden, and a warming digestive like cardamom; the skin with chamomile washes and rosemary in the bath. (See pages 122, 149, 175, 178, and 191.)

Aromatherapy
Place a few drops of Roman chamomile in a vaporizer or on a light bulb to treat an allergic reaction, including asthma. (See page 149.)
Lemon balm, in the bath or a vaporizer, soothes and reduces a reaction's severity. (See page 152.)
Lavender essential oil, in a light carrier oil, can be massaged into the chest or other affected area to reduce spasm and generally boost immunity. (See page 143.)

Homeopathy
Remedies will be prescribed according to your individual case, so see a registered practitioner to ensure the prescription is exact.
Urtica, for urticaria. (See page 194.)
Apis, for bee stings. (See page 203.)

Flower Essences
If suffering a sudden allergic reaction, take Rescue Remedy. (See page 158.)

Nutrition
Take steps to boost immunity, by increasing intake of magnesium, B vitamins, zinc, vitamin A, iron, and vitamin C. (See pages 206–209, 210, 215, 217, and 221.)
A diet high in protein will help to build immunity, while roughage from fruit, vegetables, nuts, seeds, and pulses will encourage the growth of beneficial bacteria in the gut, which helps the body to resist infection. (See page 58.)
Acidophilus, taken daily, will work to encourage bowel health. (See page 142.)
Evening primrose oil and blackcurrant seed oil are rich sources of essential fatty acids, which can prevent allergies. (See page 231.)
Pollen supplements are useful for preventing allergies, in particular hay fever. (See page 228.)

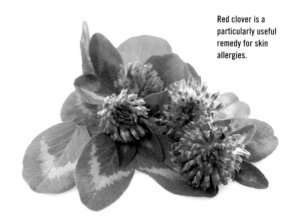

Red clover is a particularly useful remedy for skin allergies.

HODGKIN'S DISEASE

Hodgkin's disease (or Hodgkin's lymphoma) is a cancer that attacks the lymphatic tissue and the lymph nodes in particular. As the tissue becomes more and more damaged, relatively minor infections may become life-threatening. Late in the disease's development the bone marrow may also be affected. The cause of Hodgkin's is unknown, although it is thought that cancer-causing viruses are involved. In the United States, about 30 people out of every million have this ailment; it is more common in males between the ages of 20 and 40, although both sexes can suffer from the condition. Untreated, Hodgkin's disease is invariably fatal. (See also "Cancer," page 375.)

SYMPTOMS
• Painless enlargement of lymph nodes, which acquire a rubbery feel • Liver and spleen enlargement • Anemia • Fever • Appetite and weight loss • Night sweats
Possible secondary effects caused by pressure on other structures from enlarged nodes:
• Neurological damage • Obstruction to veins • Difficulty in swallowing and breathing • Jaundice

TREATMENT
Aromatherapy
Extra treatments to try are fennel, garlic, juniper, and rose, which can be used in the bath or in a vaporizer to detoxify the body. (See pages 79, 128, 142, and 174.)
Tea tree and lavender essential oils strengthen the body's defenses. (See pages 143 and 150.)
Oils that strengthen the action of the adrenals include geranium and rosemary, along with peppermint and thyme. (See page 47.)

Nutrition
Eat as much fresh fruit and vegetables as you can, paying particular attention to those containing antioxidants. (See page 251.)
Reduce your intake of animal fats and avoid processed foods.
A deficiency of vitamin C has been found in conjunction with certain tumors. Ensure you get plenty in your diet. (See page 256.)
Vitamin A can protect against cancer in smokers to some degree. (See page 252.)
Vitamin E is said to have anti-cancer properties. Ensure that you get plenty in your diet or take supplements. (See page 257.)

> **CAUTION**
> Orthodox treatment is essential for Hodgkin's disease.

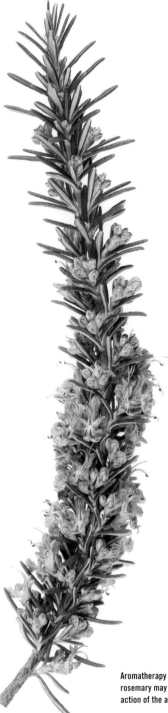

Aromatherapy oils such as rosemary may strengthen the action of the adrenal glands.

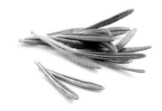

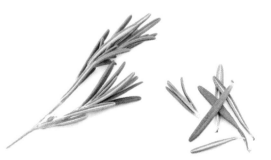

DISORDERS OF THE MUSCULOSKELETAL SYSTEM

OSTEOPOROSIS

In osteoporosis (meaning porous bones) the bones lose their density, becoming fragile and brittle. This is caused by alterations, with age, of the amounts of the various growth and sex hormones which control chemical changes in the bones, leading to progressive calcium and protein loss. Osteoporosis affects far more women than men, and may be triggered or accelerated by a sedentary lifestyle, loss of activity, a low-calcium diet, smoking, heavy alcohol consumption, hereditary factors, or prolonged lack of estrogen. An overactive thyroid gland, chronic liver disease, and prolonged use of corticosteroids all predispose a person to osteoporosis.

SYMPTOMS
• Loss of height from shrinkage of the spinal bones
• Sudden breakage of a bone in the spine, with severe pain and disfigurement • Reduced ribcage movement, causing shortness of breath and pain • Wrist, forearm, neck, or hip fractures resulting from minor stumbles or falls

TREATMENT
Chinese Herbalism
The condition is believed to be caused by kidney deficiency, and can be treated with Gou Ji (cibot rhizome), Gu Sui Bu (drynaria tuber), and Du Zhong (eucommia bark). (See page 124.) Gui Zhi (cinnamon twigs) will help to reduce pain. (See page 104.)

Herbalism
Drink a cup of comfrey leaf and bay leaf (*Laurus nobilis*) tea three times a day. (See page 186.)
If you are in pain, use analgesic herbs such as white willow, meadowsweet, or wild yam. (See pages 121, 127, and 177.)
Herbs that contain calcium include nettles, parsley, dandelion leaves, bladderwrack, and horsetail, which can be drunk as often as possible. (See pages 123, 129, 162, 188, and 194.)
Take estrogenic herbs, which discourage the loss of calcium from the bones, including calendula, ginseng, false unicorn root (*Chamaelirium luteum*), sage, hops (*Humulus lupulus*), blue cohosh (*Caulophyllum thalictroides*), wild yam, and licorice. (See pages 93, 121, 132, 160, and 177.)
Herbs that will encourage the digestion and absorption of minerals from your food include yellow dock root, rosemary, wormwood (*Artemisia annua*), and yarrow. (See pages 74, 175, and 176.)

Homeopathy
Constitutional treatment will be necessary, but Calcarea phos. may be useful to deal with bone pain. (See page 213.)

Nutrition
Recent evidence suggests that an increased intake of magnesium may help prevent the worst effects of osteoporosis. Magnesium sources include soybeans, nuts, and brewer's yeast. (See page 217.) Calcium can also be very helpful. Recommended doses are between 1,000mg. and 1,500mg. a day. (See page 213.) Vitamin D helps the body absorb calcium. (See page 210.) Increase your intake of foods containing boron, which reduces the body's excretion of calcium and magnesium, and increases the production of estrogen. (See page 212.)
Fluoride may be useful for preventing and treating the condition because it stimulates new bone formation. (See page 215.)

Mind–Body Healing
To guard against osteoporosis, at least 150 minutes of moderate-intensity aerobic activity, such as fast walking or cycling, is recommended per week. Weight-bearing and resistance exercises are very important for improving bone density. (See page 70.) If you have been diagnosed with osteoporosis, talk to your physician before starting a new exercise program.

USEFUL FACTS
• Osteoporosis is most common in white women after menopause. Bone mass reaches a peak in women between the ages of 30 and 45; between the ages of 55 and 70, a woman will have lost 30–40 percent of her bone mass.
• 50 percent of women between the ages of 45 and 75 suffer from some osteoporosis; 30 percent of these suffer from serious bone deterioration.
• Osteoporosis is aggravated by a variety of factors, including smoking, excessive alcohol consumption, and a sedentary lifestyle.
• A dowager's hump is an abnormal curvature of the spine in the upper back. Typically affecting older women, the curvature is a result of collapse of the spinal column, caused by osteoporosis.

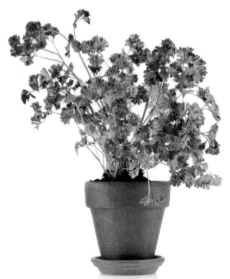

Drink an infusion of parsley as a herbal remedy for osteoporosis. Its high calcium content will be of benefit.

RHEUMATISM

Rheumatism is a very general term applied to aches, pains, and stiffness in bones and muscles, occurring as a result of viral infection, food allergy, emotional stress, or an underlying joint disease. The following may all come under the umbrella term rheumatism: fibrositis (see page 352); hyperthyroidism (see page 338); myositis, in which inflammation of muscles causes pain and weakness, developing from a bacterial or viral infection; polymyalgia rheumatica, featuring pain and stiffness in the shoulders, neck, back, and arms, possibly due to a blood disorder; and vitamin D deficiency, which causes bone pain and muscle weakness.

SYMPTOMS
• Aching in bones and muscles • Stiffness of movement

TREATMENT

Ayurveda
Ginger, coriander, and aloe vera (when there are hot pains) can be used to treat rheumatism. (See pages 80, 113, and 200.)
Angelica is warming for stiffness and discomfort. (See page 82.)
Barberry, taken as a tea or applied as a compress. (See page 90.)
Basil and camphor relieve rheumatism. (See pages 103 and 156.)
Rub calamus oil into the affected joints to improve circulation and drainage. (See page 75.)

Chinese Herbalism
The condition is thought to be caused by qi stagnation, excess wind, damp, and heat. Chinese herbalists use Huai Niu Xi (achyranthes root) and Huang Bai (cork tree bark). (See page 162.)

Traditional Home and Folk Remedies
Chew a tiny quantity of horseradish leaves, which is said to prevent attacks. (See page 86.)

Herbalism
Useful herbs, which may be taken internally or applied as a compress, include feverfew, meadowsweet, and white willow. (See pages 127, 177, and 187.)
Use a little cayenne pepper oil to warm the area and reduce pain and stiffness. (See page 98.)
A poultice of slippery elm may be of benefit. (See page 193.)
An infusion of celery seed may help reduce the level of acid in the blood, which is a contributory factor. (See page 84.)

Aromatherapy
Bergamot and myrrh reduce inflammation. Use in the bath, or massage the local area. (See pages 107 and 112.)
There are many oils that can reduce swelling and inflammation and encourage the healing process. Try massage with pine, lemon, or juniper, in a suitable carrier oil. (See pages 108, 142, and 163.)
Massage with oil of black pepper or eucalyptus can stimulate the circulation and relieve stiffness. (See pages 124 and 164.)
Lavender calms pain and helps to relieve stiffness. (See page 143.)

Flower Essences
Rub a little Rescue Remedy, or the cream, into the affected area. (See page 158.)

Nutrition
Many cases of rheumatism respond to a dietary change, and it is suggested that the following foods are eaten as often as possible to reduce muscular and joint inflammation: cabbage, celery, turnip, lemon, dandelion, and oily fish.
Drink plenty of water, which will flush the system and act as a detoxicant.
Eliminate members of the "nightshade" family of plants from your diet, as these can cause joint problems. These include potatoes, peppers, eggplant (aubergine), and paprika.
Evening primrose oil is a rich source of gamma-linolenic acid, which is necessary for the production of prostaglandins, which may have an anti-inflammatory effect. (See page 231.)

Mind–Body Healing
A good balance of rest and exercise is essential. Consult a physiotherapist for advice.

USEFUL FACTS
• Palindromic rheumatism is a disease that causes frequent and irregular attacks of joint pain, especially in the fingers, but leaves no permanent damage to the joints.
• Psychogenic rheumatism is common in women between the ages of 40 and 70, although men also contract this disease. Symptoms include complaints of pain in various parts of the musculoskeletal system that cannot be substantiated medically.
• One of the commonest forms of rheumatism is rheumatoid arthritis, affecting 1–3 percent of the population. Rheumatoid arthritis usually occurs between ages 35 and 40, but can occur at any age. It characteristically follows a course of spontaneous remissions and exacerbations, and in about 10–20 percent of patients remission is permanent.

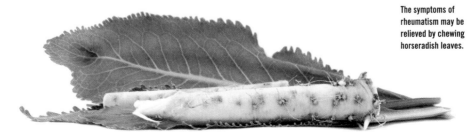

The symptoms of rheumatism may be relieved by chewing horseradish leaves.

FRACTURES

A fracture is a break or crack in a bone. It may occur as a result of excessive force through injury (particularly in sport), an accident such as a car crash, or disease. A simple fracture is one where the soft tissue overlying the broken bone is still intact; a compound fracture is one where the skin is damaged so that the fractured bone is exposed and therefore vulnerable to infection. Fractures caused by disease (such as osteoporosis, or a tumor or cyst) are known as pathological fractures. In such cases there is a weakening of bones that predisposes them to break more easily. An estimated 200,000 hip fractures occur in people over the age of 65 each year. The tendency to fracture increases with age.

SYMPTOMS
• Swelling • Pain and tenderness • Inability to move the affected part • Possibly a protruding bone, deformity, and discoloration

TREATMENT
Ayurveda
Aloe vera will help to encourage the healing of broken bones, and can be applied externally as a gel, or taken internally. (See page 80.)

Chinese Herbalism
Die Da Wan, or "bodily injury pills," and Imperial Ted Da wine resolve bruising, and promote healing in damaged tissue.

Herbalism
A comfrey poultice will encourage healing. Comfrey root can also be taken internally (in small amounts). (See page 186.)
Use an infusion of comfrey, horsetail, and mouse-ear (*Hieracium pilosella*) and apply locally (when the plaster cast has been removed) to help heal the bone. (See pages 123 and 186.)

Aromatherapy
Lavender in a vaporizer will help to relax and calm. (See page 143.)
Thyme, rosemary, and marjoram can be diluted and massaged into the area, or applied as a compress, to soothe pain and promote healing. (See pages 157, 175, and 190.)

Nutrition
Increase your calcium, magnesium, and phosphorus intake. (See pages 213, 217, and 219.)

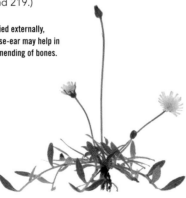

Applied externally, mouse-ear may help in the mending of bones.

CAUTION
If you suspect a fracture, see a physician immediately.

SPRAINS AND STRAINS

A sprain is the result of an overstretching or tearing of the ligaments which bind the joints together, caused by a sudden pull. Severe sprains may lead to dislocation of the affected joint (particularly common in the shoulder), and repeated injury of this nature can cause a loss of the ligaments' elasticity. The most commonly strained or sprained joint is the ankle, which is usually sprained as a result of going over on the outside of the foot so that the complete weight of the body is placed on the ankle. The back, fingers, knees, and wrists are also commonly sprained.

SYMPTOMS
• Swelling in the affected area • Pain, sometimes severe

TREATMENT
Chinese Herbalism
San Qi (notoginseng) is for swelling and pain. (See page 160.)

Traditional Home and Folk Remedies
Cider vinegar can be used as a compress to relieve pain and swelling. (See page 204.)
Apply a poultice of raw onions. (See page 78.)
Raise the affected limb and apply a cold compress as soon as possible. Strains should be bandaged with an elastic bandage, but take care not to bind too tightly and cut off circulation. Keep the limb elevated until some normal movement is possible.

Herbalism
Burdock can be taken internally as a tea, or applied as a poultice to the affected area. (See page 85.)
Ginger can be added to bath water or a foot bath, or applied as a compress to encourage healing. (See page 200.)

Aromatherapy
Use a little lavender oil in a foot bath, or on a cold compress applied to the area. Avoid massaging the area, which will increase inflammation. (See page 143.)
A compress of sweet marjoram and rosemary can be used to heal and to reduce inflammation. (See pages 157 and 175.)

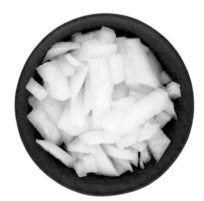

Apply a poultice of raw onions to a sprain.

NECK PROBLEMS

Constant movement of the neck, along with its position and the number of structures within it, makes it particularly vulnerable to problems, which include:

• Cervical osteoarthritis, in which the cartilage of the vertebrae of the neck wear away, most commonly in middle age, causing pain, stiffness, and sometimes tenderness to touch.
• Cervical rib, which is an abnormal floating rib or pair of ribs attached to the lowest vertebra of the neck, which can cause compression of various nerves and arteries.
• Cervical spondylosis, which is when neurological damage is caused in the neck region as a result of compression of the spinal cord or nerve roots by an outgrowth of bone. Sufferers develop a walking disorder (spastic gait) and weakness in the arm muscles.
• Locked neck, an overstrain of ligaments or muscle spasms caused by an awkward movement, often occurring during sleep.
• Neck rigidity, or stiffness and pain on movement caused by neck muscle spasms. This is also a classic symptom of meningitis.
• Neck swelling, which may be caused by tumors, allergy, bleeding, or inflammation. It can be extremely dangerous, seriously interfering with breathing. It may also affect swallowing.
• Torticollis (wry neck), which is an abnormality in the head's position caused by permanent twisting of the neck, due possibly to muscle damage sustained at birth, a whiplash injury, a visual problem, or shortening of the skin of the neck through scarring.

TREATMENT

Ayurveda

Barberry can be taken internally for pain. (See page 90.)
Mustard oil relieves muscular pains and stiffness. (See page 91.)
Turmeric and St. John's wort are also excellent for relieving stiffness, pain, and inflammation. (See pages 117 and 138.)

Chinese Herbalism

The cause of stiffness and "freezing" may be caused by weak yang qi, external cold and damp. Useful treatments include Gui Zhi (cinnamon twigs) and turmeric. (See pages 104 and 117.)

Traditional Home and Folk Remedies

Drink celery juice to ease nerve pain. (See page 84.)
Apply fresh horseradish to the affected area (do not leave on for long, or it will numb and burn). (See page 86.)
Apply bruised juniper berries to muscular swellings for effective relief. (See page 142.)
Local heat will help to relax tense muscles.

Herbalism

St. John's wort has sedative, painkilling properties. It can be drunk as an infusion or applied to the affected area in an oil. (See page 138.)
Valerian tea can reduce tension and help you to sleep. (See page 195.)
The following herbs reduce inflammation and relieve pain: Jamaican dogwood (*Piscidia piscipula*), St. John's wort, vervain, and white willow. (See pages 138, 177, and 196.)

Aromatherapy

A drop of juniper, mustard, or pepper oils, diluted in some carrier oil, can be massaged into the affected area. Wrap warmly afterward. (See pages 91, 142, and 164.)
Wintergreen oil (*Gaultheria procumbens*) is good for muscular pains: massage into the affected area.
Rosemary is stimulating and analgesic, and can be massaged into the area to relieve pain and stiffness. (See page 175.)
Take hot baths with a few drops of lavender, juniper, pine, or nutmeg to warm, reduce pain, and encourage the healing process. (See pages 142, 143, 153, and 163.)

Flower Essences

Rub Rescue Remedy cream into the affected area. (See page 158.)
Star of Bethlehem can be taken internally after an injury to reduce the effects of shock and trauma. (See page 158.)
Try olive, if the injury leaves you feeling exhausted and drained of spirit. (See page 156.)

Mind–Body Healing

Consult a physiotherapist for advice on what could be causing your neck problems, and forms of exercise that could help to prevent a recurrence.

CAUTION
A stiff neck accompanied by headache, nausea, vomiting, and abnormal sleepiness may indicate meningitis, and immediate medical attention is required.

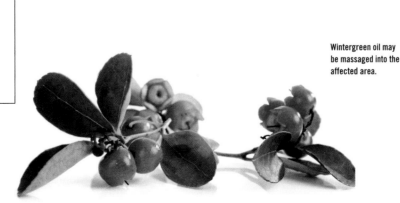

Wintergreen oil may be massaged into the affected area.

BACK PROBLEMS

Aches or pains in the back are due to mechanical disorders, which may cause or arise from damage to ligaments, muscles, vertebral joints, or disks. These may occur as a result of poor posture, lack of exercise, obesity, unaccustomed lifting or maneuvers, pregnancy, stress, or depression. Most back pain is caused by a muscle strain. Injuries are the second most common cause of pain. A slipped disk is another common cause. A slipped disk does not, in fact, slip, but it herniates when the outer layer of the disk degenerates and the soft interior material extrudes into the spinal column, causing pain and sciatica. Types of back pain vary according to the underlying cause.

SYMPTOMS
• Muscle spasms • Lower back pain, ranging from mild to excruciating • Stiffness • Referred pain or pins and needles in other areas

TREATMENT
Ayurveda
Aloe vera can be taken for inflammation, and applied externally for pain and inflammation. (See page 80.)
Massage the painful area with mustard oil to reduce pain and aching. (See page 91.)
Use cayenne externally for muscle soreness and stiffness. (See page 98.)

Chinese Herbalism
Teasel root (*Dipsacus* species), Ren Shen (ginseng), and Wu Jia Pi (acanthopanax) can be used to relieve pain. (See pages 74 and 160.)
Jing Jie (*Schizonepeta tenuifolia*) can be used to stop swelling and to kill pain.
San Qi (notoginseng root) can be used to relieve swellings and for general relief of pain. (See page 160.)

Traditional Home and Folk Remedies
It may be helpful to chew a small quantity of horseradish leaves every day to ease pain. (See page 86.)
A mustard poultice, applied to the area, will ease pain and reduce any congestion in the area. (See page 91.)

Herbalism
Massage cramp bark cream into the back. Or take cramp bark decoction, tincture, or capsules. (See page 197.)
Rub macerated comfrey or St. John's wort into the back to relieve pain. (See pages 138 and 186.)
The following herbs reduce inflammation and relieve pain: Jamaican dogwood (*Piscidia piscipula*), St. John's wort, vervain, and white willow. (See pages 138, 177, and 196.)

Aromatherapy
Relaxing in a warm bath to which lavender oil has been added can be very soothing. (See page 143.)
Pain due to fatigue or tension can be treated with a massage of ginger, juniper, marjoram, or rosemary; the same oils can be added to the bath. (See pages 142, 157, 175, and 200.)
Massage with ginger or black pepper can be used when there is acute pain. (See pages 164 and 200.)
Marjoram can help to treat the muscular problem in the longer term, as well as reducing pain. (See page 157.)
Bergamot and myrrh are anti-inflammatory: they are useful for massage or in the bath. (See pages 107 and 112.)

Homeopathy
Treatment would be constitutional, but Arnica may be useful for bruising and pain resulting from an injury. (See page 86.)

Mind–Body Healing
It was once thought that bed rest would aid recovery from a bad back, but it is now believed that people who keep gently active are likely to recover more quickly. In the long term, talk to your physician, personal trainer, or manual therapist about what exercise program will be right for you.
You may find it beneficial to receive treatment from a physiotherapist, osteopath, or chiropractor.

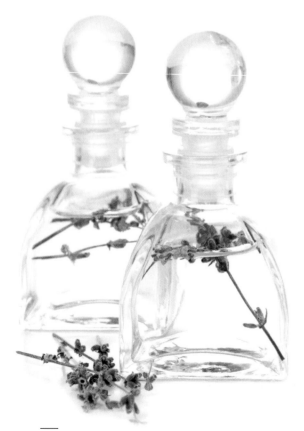

A relaxing bath with lavender oil can be extremely beneficial. It is one of the key oils for muscular pain.

LUMBAGO

Lumbago is the term used to describe any persistent or recurrent lower back pain. It is muscular in origin and usually concerns the large group of muscles surrounding the spine. Lumbago may vary in severity from a dull ache to severe pain; often it is experienced as a sudden excruciating pain on bending, on standing up from sitting, on twisting round, or on lifting heavy objects. It is generally brought on or exacerbated by cold, damp weather conditions, muscle strain, poor posture, obesity, and pregnancy. Lumbago is one of the most commonly reported complaints, and it generally becomes more frequent with age.

SYMPTOMS
• Dull to severe pain in the lower back • Sudden pain on bending or twisting

TREATMENT
Ayurveda
Saffron has antispasmodic properties. (See page 115.)

Chinese Herbalism
Apart from physical injury, the cause may be excess internal cold. Treatment would include tincture of achyranthes root (*Achyranthes bidentata*) and Wu Jia Pi (acanthopanax). (See page 74.)

Herbalism
Rub a little oil made from comfrey or St. John's wort into the affected area, to relieve the pain. (See pages 138 and 186.) The following herbs reduce inflammation and relieve pain: Jamaican dogwood (*Piscidia piscipula*), St. John's wort, vervain, and white willow. (See pages 138, 177, and 196.)

Aromatherapy
Add a little mustard, rosemary, and thyme oils to the bath to relieve pain. Hot baths are most effective. (See page 47.) Juniper, oregano (*Origanum vulgare*), pine, and rosemary poultices ease inflammation. (See pages 142, 163, and 175.)

Flower Essences
Agrimony is useful for those who make light of the pain and do not let it show in front of others. (See page 77.) Hornbeam, for weariness at the prospect of doing daily tasks that cause pain. (See page 96.)

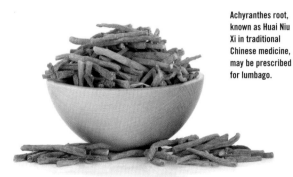

Achyranthes root, known as Huai Niu Xi in traditional Chinese medicine, may be prescribed for lumbago.

SCIATICA

Sciatica is the name given to the aching or pain along the route of the sciatic nerve. This is the largest nerve in the body, running from the spinal cord, through the buttock and the back of each leg. Sciatica is usually caused by pressure on the roots of the sciatic nerve, most commonly from a prolapsed disk (see "Back Problems," opposite), but other possible causes include pregnancy and childbirth, heavy lifting, stress, or a tumor. The pain varies from mild to more severe and "shooting" in nature.

SYMPTOMS
• Burning sensation in the back, buttocks, or leg • Muscle weakness • Numbness or pins and needles in the leg, foot, or toes • Muscle spasms in buttock or leg • Diminished reflexes in knees and ankles

TREATMENT
Ayurveda
Rub warming mustard oil into the affected area. (See page 91.)

Chinese Herbalism
Sciatica is believed to be caused by heat stagnation in the liver. Gou Teng (*Uncaria* species), known as cat's claw, may be useful. San Qi (notoginseng) can help with pain relief. (See page 160.)

Traditional Home and Folk Remedies
Add nettles to a warm bath to relieve the pain. (See page 194.) Celery juice or tea can alleviate sciatica. (See page 84.) Rub fresh lemon over the affected area. (See page 108.)

Herbalism
Apply bruised juniper berries to the affected area for pain relief. (See page 142.) Coltsfoot (*Tussilago farfara*) leaf or tincture can be used in a hot compress. Do not take internally. Try elderberry wine. (See page 130.)

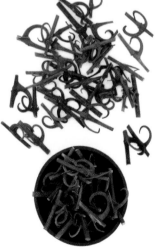

Gou Teng is a sciatica remedy.

Aromatherapy
Chamomile compresses or massage will lessen the pain. (See page 149.) Mix a few drops of juniper, mustard, or pepper essential oil in a little carrier oil and rub into the affected area. Cover with warm clothing. (See pages 91, 142, and 164.) Oregano and thyme can be added to the bath to relieve symptoms. (See page 190.)

Mind–Body Healing
Sciatica and other back pains may be eased by lying on the floor for 15 minutes. Prop the head up on a small pile of paperback books and keep the knees bent. Repeat daily.

FIBROSITIS

Fibrositis (or fibromyalgia) is a chronic stress- or occupation-induced condition in which a series of muscular spasms causes intermittent aches and pain, usually in the back and trunk. It seems to be triggered by cold weather conditions or emotional upset. Fibrositis is most common in middle-aged and elderly people, and may occur more often in anxious people, and in those who spend time sitting in a cramped position. Tender areas (there are nine specific spots) are felt on the affected muscles. Pain and stiffness may be felt in the neck, shoulders, chest, buttocks, knees, and back. In some cases the attacks are accompanied by exhaustion and disturbed sleep. Fibrositis is not considered to be a medical term, and some doctors refuse to recognize the condition because investigation usually fails to reveal any detectable reason for the symptoms.

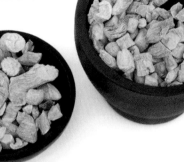
A traditional Chinese medicine practitioner may prescribe Ren Shen.

SYMPTOMS
• Aches and pain in muscles or tendons, usually in the back and trunk • Tenderness in particular spots on the affected muscles • Possibly stiffness

TREATMENT

Ayurveda
Barberry, taken as a tea or applied as a compress, treats fibrositis. (See page 90.)
Basil can provide pain relief. (See page 156.)
Rub calamus oil into the affected joints to improve circulation and drainage. (See page 75.)
Camphor can be rubbed into the affected area to warm and encourage healing. (See page 103.)

Chinese Herbalism
Gan Cao (licorice) is good for easing spasms in the legs. (See page 132.)
Bai Shao (white peony root) helps to prevent spasm in the feet and hands. (See page 159.)
Ren Shen (ginseng) will be useful as an overall tonic. (See page 160.)

Traditional Home and Folk Remedies
Apply compresses of apple cider vinegar to the affected area. Alternatively, use several cups of vinegar in bath water. (See page 204.)
Make a honey and vinegar drink, with 1 tablespoon of each in a cup of hot water, and drink. (See pages 203 and 204.)

Herbalism
A decoction of cramp bark taken 4 or 5 times a day should bring relief. Cramp bark can also be taken as a tincture or in capsule form. The ointment is useful for massaging into the affected area. (See page 197.)
Make a fresh peppermint poultice and apply to the area of spasm. (See page 152.)

Aromatherapy
Essential oil of lavender relieves pain and reduces inflammation. Use in the bath or in a gentle massage of the affected area. (See page 143.)
Chamomile, lavender, and rosemary are anti-inflammatory and pain-relieving, and are good for local massage or using in compresses. (See pages 143, 149, and 175.)
Black pepper, eucalyptus, marjoram, and benzoin oils, used in local massage, will improve the circulation in the area and reduce stiffness. (See pages 124, 157, 164, and 186.)

Homeopathy
Arnica may be helpful for muscles that feel bruised and are made worse by movement. (See page 86.)
Chamomilla may be useful for pain, stiffness, and bad temper. (See page 149.)

Flower Essences
Rub a little Rescue Remedy cream into the affected area to encourage healing and provide pain relief. (See page 158.)
Take Rescue Remedy during an attack to calm and restore. (See page 158.)
Try olive, if symptoms are causing exhaustion. (See page 156.)
Impatiens will be useful if the sufferer is feeling irritable and unwilling to slow down. (See page 140.)

Nutrition
Royal jelly may help to relieve symptoms. (See page 234.)
Take extra calcium, magnesium, and vitamin C, or make sure they are present in your diet, to encourage the health of the muscles and joints. (See pages 210, 213, and 217.)

Mind–Body Healing
Fibrositis is most common in those who spend time sitting in a cramped position. Contact a healthcare practitioner or physiotherapist for advice on exercise that may help to improve the condition.

ARTHRITIS

Athritis is an inflammation of the tissues of one or more joints, usually with pain, swelling, and redness. The two most common forms of arthritis are osteoarthritis and rheumatoid arthritis. Other disease processes and infections which cause arthritis include gout, psoriasis, tuberculosis, rubella, and gonorrhea. Osteoarthritis is a degenerative disorder in which the cartilage between the joints wears away. The body attempts to repair this damage by producing bony outgrowths at the margins of affected joints, but these cause pain and stiffness. It is usually age-related and affects the hips, knees, spine, and shoulders in particular. Rheumatoid arthritis is a chronic, progressive disorder. It most commonly arises between the ages of 30 and 40, affecting women more often than men, but the disease may start at any age. Its exact causes are not clear, but it is thought that there may be immunological (perhaps triggered by infection) and genetic factors. The synovial membrane lining the joint becomes inflamed, spreading over and eroding the cartilage, causing pain and stiffness. Anemia, joint infections and pericarditis are complications of rheumatoid arthritis.

SYMPTOMS
In osteoarthritis:
• Intermittent pain in affected joints, becoming more frequent
• Progressive movement limitation • Audible creaking • Swelling
In rheumatoid arthritis:
• Morning stiffness • Weakness and inflammation of the ligaments, tendons, and muscles • Eventual possible deformity of joints • Eye inflammation • Bursitis • Lethargy • Appetite and weight loss

TREATMENT
Ayurveda
Ginger, coriander, and aloe vera can be used to treat arthritis. (See pages 80, 113, and 200.)
Angelica is a good tonic and is warming. (See page 82.)
Take barberry as a tea or compress. (See page 90.)
Basil can provide relief from the pain of arthritis. (See page 156.)
Rub calamus oil into the affected joints to improve circulation and drainage. (See page 75.)
Camphor is indicated for the treatment of arthritis and rheumatism, and many other musculoskeletal problems. (See page 103.)

Chinese Herbalism
The source of the problem is considered to be wind damp. Painful joints are caused by wind cold. Arthritis with hot, swollen, but not painful, joints is considered to be caused by wind heat.
Treatment would include Gui Zhi (cinnamon twigs) to release qi; Dang Gui (angelica) and wild ginger to relieve cold and damp. (See pages 82, 104, and 200.)
Long Dan Cao (Chinese gentian) and Huang Bai (cork tree bark) can be used for wind heat. (See page 162.)
Gan Cao (licorice) and Huang Qin (Chinese skullcap) are recommended as anti-inflammatories. (See pages 132 and 181.)

Traditional Home and Folk Remedies
Eating nettles or drinking nettle tea is an old remedy for arthritis. The "stings" in stinging nettles contain histamine, which is anti-inflammatory. (See page 194.)
Vinegar and honey is another old remedy. (See pages 203 and 204.)
Apple cider or ginger root baths can reduce symptoms and encourage healing. (See pages 148 and 200.)
Apples are good detoxifiers. Eat daily to improve symptoms. (See page 148.)

Herbalism
Apply a poultice of slippery elm and cayenne to the affected joints. (See pages 98 and 193.)
Herbs that work to heal arthritis include feverfew, meadowsweet, celery seed, and white willow. They can be taken internally, or used externally, as required. (See pages 84, 127, 177, and 187.)
Bladderwrack capsules, tablets, or powder used regularly may prevent the progress of the disease. (See page 129.)
For aching joints, try a liniment made with tincture of comfrey and a few drops of black pepper essential oil. (See pages 164 and 186.)
Dandelion root and horsetail tea or tincture is recommended for degenerative arthritis. (See pages 123 and 188.)
For inflamed hand joints, take a decoction or tincture of devil's claw. (See page 135.)
Siberian ginseng is good for rheumatoid arthritis. (See page 160.)

Aromatherapy
Use juniper oil in the bath or in a massage oil blend. It is stimulating and antirheumatic. (See page 142.)
Massage petitgrain into the limbs for osteoarthritis. (See page 107.)
Lemon and cypress oils are detoxifying, and can be used in the bath and in massage to help the body eliminate poisons. (See pages 108 and 117.)
Chamomile, lavender, and rosemary are anti-inflammatory and pain-relieving; use in massage or compresses. (See page 47.)
Black pepper, eucalyptus, marjoram, and benzoin will improve the circulation in the area and reduce stiffness. (See page 47.)

Nutrition
There is some evidence to show that the antioxidants – vitamins A, C, and E, plus selenium – may have beneficial effects on arthritis. (See pages 206, 210, 211, and 219.)
Magnesium is required to form synovial fluid, which surrounds the joints, and an adequate intake will ensure health. (See page 217.)
Cod liver oil and evening primrose oil capsules are reported to help rheumatoid arthritis. (See pages 231 and 232.)

CAUTION
Bladderwrack should be avoided by anyone suffering from an overactive thyroid. Devil's claw should not be used during pregnancy; it is best avoided if you suffer from stomach acidity or ulcers. Do not use Siberian ginseng during pregnancy unless advised to do so by a qualified herbalist.

CRAMP

Cramp is a painful muscular spasm that occurs most frequently in the feet and legs, but can also affect the abdomen, arms, and hands (writer's cramp). Excess salt loss through sweating is the most common cause, and pregnancy, prolonged sitting or standing, strenuous or unaccustomed exercise, or lying in an unusual position may all be triggers. The muscle contraction is usually short-lived, lasting minutes only, but in some cases it may be prolonged, and repeated. Many elderly people suffer from night cramps. Some research indicates that a vitamin E deficiency may be partly to blame, and there may also be an imbalance of magnesium and calcium in the body.

SYMPTOMS
• Twitching, followed by severe pain and a sensation of contortion in the affected muscle

TREATMENT

Ayurveda
Yarrow is antispasmodic and can help to prevent and treat cramp. (See page 74.)
Aloe vera, taken internally and applied externally, can soothe muscular spasm. (See page 80.)
Basil, caraway, celery seed, garlic, and myrrh all help. (See pages 79, 84, 97, 112, and 156.)

Chinese Herbalism
Gan Cao (licorice) is good for spasm and cramps in the abdomen and legs. (See page 132.)
Bai Shao (white peony root) helps cramps in the feet and hands. (See page 159.)

Traditional Home and Folk Remedies
Apply compresses of apple cider vinegar to the affected area, and use several cups of vinegar in the bath. (See page 204.)
A pinch of salt and a sip of lemon juice before bed may prevent night cramps. (See page 108.)
Make a honey and vinegar drink, with 1 tablespoon of each in a cup of hot water, and drink. This works by distributing calcium throughout the bloodstream, which can reduce chronic cramp. (See pages 203 and 204.)

Herbalism
A decoction of cramp bark taken 4 or 5 times a day should bring relief. Cramp bark can also be taken as a tincture or in capsule form. The ointment is useful for massaging into the affected area. (See page 197.)
Make a fresh peppermint poultice and apply directly to the area affected by the spasm. (See page 152.)
Olbas Oil, sold in pharmacies, is effective for sports-induced muscle cramps and spasm.

Aromatherapy
Lavender is antispasmodic and can be usefully employed for cramp as a massage oil. (See page 143.)
Rub the affected area with geranium essential oil. (See page 161.)
Use lemon balm and chamomile oils for abdominal cramps, diluted in a light carrier oil. (See pages 149 and 152.)

Homeopathy
Take Mag. phos. (6c) every 5 minutes when cramp occurs. It is especially useful for writer's cramp and cramp that occurs after excessive exercise. For menstrual cramp, take Mag. phos. every 30 minutes. (See page 217.)
Cuprum metallicum, for the spasm and subsequent pain. (See page 214.)
Arnica, for cramps caused by muscle fatigue following prolonged exercise. (See page 86.)

Flower Essences
Rub a little Rescue Remedy cream into the affected area to encourage healing and provide pain relief. (See page 158.)
Take Rescue Remedy during an attack to calm and restore. (See page 158.)

Nutrition
Increase your intake of calcium if you are susceptible to cramp. Calcium tablets taken with vitamin C are said to prevent night cramps. (See pages 210 and 213.)
Vitamin D is essential for the absorption of calcium. (See page 210.)
Vitamin E supplements have been proved to help prevent night cramps. (See page 211.)
Increase your intake of salt and magnesium. (See page 217.)

Mind–Body Healing
To ease leg cramps, stretch and massage the affected muscle. If the cramp is in the calf, straighten the leg and lift the foot upwards, bending the ankle so the toes point toward the shin. Next, walk on your heels for several minutes.

One traditional remedy for cramp that works well is to take lemon with a pinch of salt. If taken before bed, it will help to prevent night cramps.

CAUTION
Seek medical advice if cramp in the chest occurs during or after exercise, as this may be angina.

RESTLESS LEGS

Restless legs is the term used to describe a condition associated with insomnia in which the legs ache and are constantly moved about in order to achieve comfort. It is thought to be due either to problems in the nervous system, or to hereditary factors. It is more common in older people and smokers, and it may be triggered by cold, damp weather conditions or overexertion of muscles. There is also an association with diabetes, vitamin B and iron deficiency, excess caffeine intake, and withdrawal from drugs.

SYMPTOMS
• Tickling sensation under the skin • Burning or prickling sensation
• Aching and jerking • Restlessness relieved by movement

TREATMENT
Ayurveda
Warming herbs such as mustard (seeds and oil) and turmeric may be recommended. (See pages 91 and 117.)
Black pepper stimulates circulation and the nervous system. (See page 164.)
Camphor stimulates the nervous system and body tissues. (See page 103.)
Cumin is useful for nervous conditions and is generally warming. (See page 116.)

Chinese Herbalism
Restlessness is thought to be caused by yin or blood deficiency, and a possible treatment is lotus seed sprouts, also called Lian Zi.

Herbalism
A chamomile infusion or compress can help dispel the condition. (See page 149.)
Valerian root works on the nervous system and can help to calm. (See page 195.)
Bruised cloves can be added to any tea to relieve nervous conditions. (See page 125.)

If you have trouble sleeping, try using sedative oils such as chamomile or ylang ylang. They may be inhaled safely from a vaporizer (pictured) as you sleep.

Aromatherapy
Benzoin, bergamot, and frankincense have a calming action on the nervous system and can be used in the bath, in a vaporizer, or in local massage to ease. (See pages 90, 107, and 186.)
If you have trouble sleeping, try using a few drops of chamomile, lavender, marjoram, and ylang ylang, which are hypnotic. (See pages 95, 143, 149, and 157.)

Homeopathy
Sepia, for twitching which is worse during the day, and better for taking exercise. (See page 182.)

Flower Essences
Rescue Remedy cream can be rubbed into the muscles of the legs, as required, to calm. (See page 158.)

Nutrition
Vitamin E will help to control the condition. (See page 211.)
Iron or vitamin B deficiency may be at the root of the condition, so ensure that you include plenty in your diet. (See pages 206–209 and 215.)
Take zinc, for trembling, twitching feet, and restless legs, even while sleeping. (See page 221.)
Cut consumption of stimulants, such as caffeine, alcohol, and tobacco.

Mind–Body Healing
Keep the affected muscles warm, and take plenty of hot baths.

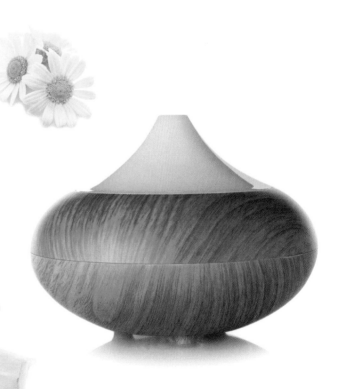

BURSITIS

Bursitis is inflammation of a bursa (a small fluid-filled sac). Bursas act in a protective capacity, reducing friction around joints. The membrane lining a bursa may increase fluid production in response to infection, injury, prolonged pressure, or rheumatic disease, causing the bursa to swell. This may occur in any of the large joints of the body, such as the ankle or shoulder, and is commonly associated with bunions at the joint between the big toe and the foot. The build-up of calcium deposits on tendons associated with a joint is a frequent precipitating cause. Constant kneeling is a trigger for bursitis, causing a condition known as "housemaid's knee."

SYMPTOMS
- Restricted movement in the affected joint, caused by swelling
- Pain and tenderness

TREATMENT

Ayurveda
Ginger, coriander, and aloe vera can be used to treat bursitis. (See pages 80, 113, and 200.)
Angelica is a good tonic and is warming. (See page 82.)
Barberry, taken as a tea or applied as a compress, can be used to treat pain and inflammation. (See page 90.)
Rub calamus oil into the affected joints to improve circulation and drainage. (See page 75.)

Chinese Herbalism
Gan Cao (licorice) and Huang Qin (Chinese skullcap) are excellent anti-inflammatories. (See pages 132 and 181.)
Gui Zhi (cinnamon twigs), Dang Gui (angelica), and Fang Feng (ledebouriella root) may be helpful. (See pages 82, 104, and 144.)

Traditional Home and Folk Remedies
Eating nettles, or drinking nettle tea, is a traditional remedy for pain and inflammation. The "stings" in stinging nettles contain histamine, which is anti-inflammatory. (See page 194.)
Apple cider foot baths or ginger root baths can help to reduce symptoms and encourage healing. (See pages 148 and 200.)
Hot or cold compresses on the area will help to disperse swelling. (See page 205.)

Herbalism
Apply a poultice of slippery elm and cayenne to the affected joints. (See pages 98 and 193.)
Herbs that work to heal bursitis include feverfew, meadowsweet, celery seed, and white willow. They can be taken internally, or used externally, as required. (See pages 84, 127, 177, and 187.)
For relief of aches and pains, try a liniment made with tincture of comfrey and a few drops of black pepper essential oil. (See pages 164 and 186.)
For improving inflamed joints, take a decoction or tincture of devil's claw. (See page 135.)
Siberian ginseng is a beneficial herb. (See page 160.)

Aromatherapy
Use juniper oil in the bath or as part of a massage oil blend. It has stimulating and antirheumatic qualities. (See page 142.)
Chamomile, lavender, and rosemary are anti-inflammatory and relieve pain. Use on a compress or for local massage. (See pages 143, 149, and 175.)
Black pepper, eucalyptus, marjoram, and benzoin will improve the circulation in the area and reduce stiffness. (See page 47.)

Homeopathy
Apis, for burning, stinging pain made worse by heat. (See page 203.)

Mind–Body Healing
Rest the joint, avoiding strenuous activities, until symptoms improve. Wear padding to protect the joint from further injury. Contact your physician, personal trainer, or physiotherapist for advice on an exercise regime that will not worsen your condition.

The condition commonly known as "housemaid's knee" is an example of bursitis around the kneecap. It is often caused or aggravated by constant kneeling. Massage with chamomile, lavender, or rosemary oils.

TENDINITIS

Tendinitis is an inflammation and thickening of the tendons, usually caused by an injury or overuse of the muscles. There is some association with bursitis (see opposite), and indeed the diagnosis is often difficult to make. Bursitis is characterized by a dull pain, whereas the pain of tendinitis is sharp.

SYMPTOMS
• Sharp pain and limited movement in the affected area
• Swelling • Pins and needles and numbness

TREATMENT
Ayurveda
Turmeric is anti-inflammatory. Use externally, as an infused oil, or take internally, 3 times daily, between meals. (See page 117.)

Traditional Home and Folk Remedies
Apply a vinegar compress to reduce inflammation. (See page 204.)
Wrap a bruised wet plantain leaf around the affected area to reduce swelling and stiffness. (See page 165.)

Herbalism
Apply a poultice of slippery elm and cayenne to the affected joints. (See pages 98 and 193.)
Feverfew, meadowsweet, celery seed, and white willow can be taken internally or used externally, as required. (See pages 84, 127, 177, and 187.)
For aching joints, try a liniment of tincture of comfrey and a few drops of black pepper essential oil. (See pages 164 and 186.)
For inflamed joints in the hand, take a devil's claw decoction or tincture. (See page 135.)

Aromatherapy
Chamomile, lavender, and rosemary are anti-inflammatory and pain-relieving. Use in local massage or compresses. (See pages 143, 149, and 175.)
Black pepper, eucalyptus, marjoram, and benzoin improve the circulation in the area and reduce stiffness. Use as cold or warm compresses. (See pages 124, 157, 164, and 186.)

Nutrition
The following nutrients in the diet help to encourage healing of the soft tissues: vitamin C, beta-carotene, zinc, selenium, and vitamin E. (See pages 206, 210, 211, 219, and 221.)
Bromelain, a digestive enzyme derived from the stems of pineapples, is an anti-inflammatory agent.

Dampen and bruise a plantain leaf, then wrap it round the affected area to reduce swelling.

BUNIONS

A bunion (or hallux valgus) is an inflammation of the soft tissue at the base of the big toe due either to ill-fitting shoes or an inherited weakness. Women are more prone to bunions than men, and there is also an association with flat feet. A bunion pushes the big toe outward at the base and in toward the other toes at the top. In some cases a bunion is so large it may distort the sufferer's shoe. Bunions are also known as bursitis (see left).

SYMPTOMS
• Pain and discomfort in the affected foot • The bunion is aggravated by continuous and prolonged pressure

TREATMENT
Ayurveda
Cedarwood can be used as a rub. (See page 100.)
Camphor can be used externally to ease the pain. (See page 103.)
St. John's wort can be taken internally and also used externally in the treatment of bunions. (See page 138.)
Mustard, used in a foot bath, will reduce pain and inflammation, and encourage healing. (See page 91.)

Chinese Herbalism
Ginger is a useful anti-inflammatory agent. (See page 200.)
Other herbs to try, for external use, include: San Qi (notoginseng), for general relief of pain and swelling, and Jing Jie (*Schizonepeta tenuifolia*) for inflammation, stiffness, and pain. (See page 160.)

Traditional Home and Folk Remedies
High-heeled shoes and shoes with narrow toes are especially bad for the feet. Go barefoot as often as is practical, walking on a variety of surfaces to exercise the small bones in the feet. Practice picking up small objects, such as marbles, with the toes.

Herbalism
Treatment to ease inflammation and swelling includes compresses of marshmallow, flaxseed, comfrey, and slippery elm. (See pages 81, 145, 186, and 193.)
Chamomile infusions, taken internally, will help. (See page 149.)

Aromatherapy
Add a drop of lemon balm or chamomile to massage oil and rub gently. (See pages 149 and 152.)

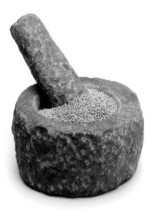

Make a warming mustard foot bath to reduce pain and inflammation. Crush some mustard seeds in a pestle and mortar and add to a bowl of warm water (as hot as is comfortable).

CHILDHOOD AILMENTS
SLEEP PROBLEMS

All babies and children need different amounts of sleep, and most of them experience some difficulty sleeping at some point. Common causes of sleep problems in babies are diaper rash, teething, colic, illness, being too hot or cold, or simply being wakeful. Older children may be worried about something at school, or a stressful event in the family home. Illness usually disrupts sleep patterns in some way. Some children experience night terrors, which may cause the child to waken suddenly, screaming and confused.

Babies will enjoy a gentle massage to help them drift off to sleep.

SYMPTOMS
• Difficulty falling or staying asleep • Tiredness or irritability during the day • Exhaustion and frustration for the parent

TREATMENT
Traditional Home and Folk Remedies
A little brewer's yeast, mixed with honey and warm milk, makes a soothing bedtime drink for children from the age of four upwards. (See pages 203 and 229.)

Herbalism
Vervain is a gentle sedative, and can help children fall asleep, particularly if they are fighting against it. (See page 196.)
Linden will calm nervous, sensitive children. (See page 191.)
Motherwort can be useful for calming a frightened child or baby. (See page 144.)
A crying baby may be soothed with an infusion of chamomile, offered an hour or so before bedtime or on waking. (See page 149.)
A strong infusion of chamomile, hops (*Humulus lupulus*), lavender, or linden can be added to a warm bath to soothe and calm a baby or child. (See pages 143, 149, and 191.)
Tincture of catmint (*Nepeta faassenii*), added to a little honey, can be given to a distressed child as and when required. Honey should not be given to infants under 12 months old. (See page 203.)

Aromatherapy
A few drops of chamomile, geranium, rose, or lavender can be added to the bath. (See pages 143, 149, 161, and 174.)
Lavender oil, on a handkerchief tied near the cot or bed, will help your baby or child to sleep. (See page 143.)
Lavender or chamomile can be used in a vaporizer in your child's room. (See pages 143 and 149.)
A gentle massage before bedtime, with a little lavender or chamomile blended with a light carrier oil, may ease any tension. (See pages 143 and 149.)

> **CAUTION**
> If you are concerned about the cause of your child's sleep problems, see your physician.

Flower Essences
White chestnut will be helpful for children with overactive minds. (See page 76.)
A distressed child or baby can be given Rescue Remedy, which will calm him or her. (See page 158.)
Rock rose may help with night terrors. (See page 135.)
Aspen is useful for anxiety for no identifiable cause. (See page 168.)
Walnut will be useful for change, such as a new baby, school, or house. (See page 141.)
A few drops of mimulus will soothe a child who is afraid of the dark. (See page 153.)

Nutrition
Avoid cold-energy foods such as bananas and cucumbers, which can cause colic and digestive problems.
A warm glass of goat's milk will encourage sleep without causing any digestive disturbance.
Older children may suck a zinc lozenge before bedtime to help them to go to sleep. (See page 221.)

Mind–Body Healing
Children (as well as teenagers and adults) will benefit from a period of quiet relaxation before bedtime, involving a bath, reading, dimmed lights, cuddling, and a good night kiss.
Avoid excitement, and electronic gadgets, within an hour of lights out. For additional tips on getting your baby to sleep, including establishing a calming bedtime routine, contact your healthcare practitioner.
If your child wakes at night, try to get them back into their own bed with as little fuss as possible. Leave, then promise to return with another kiss. Do so, then repeat the routine as needed until they are asleep. Consistency is key.
If you are concerned that something is upsetting your child, try to talk it through if they are willing, well before bedtime if possible.

HYPERACTIVITY

A hyperactive child has an excessively high energy level, being restless, inattentive, and easily frustrated. There are often prolonged tantrums, and fidgeting. Intelligence is common among hyperactive children, but there is such a short attention span that they often do not do well at school. Psychiatrists have labeled the problem attention-deficit hyperactivity disorder, or ADHD. (Some children display attention-deficit disorder, or ADD, without hyperactivity.) ADHD appears in children before the age of four, but its signs are often missed until the child attends school. Intolerance of certain foods, especially milk, wheat, and corn, produces ADHD in some children.

SYMPTOMS
• Restlessness • Inattentiveness • Tantrums • Fidgeting

TREATMENT
Herbalism 🌿
Herbs to support a stressed nervous system include vervain and skullcap. (See pages 181 and 196.)
Oats act as a tonic to the nervous system. (See page 89.)
Borage (*Borago officinalis*) and licorice will work to address an overworked adrenal gland. (See page 132.)

Aromatherapy 🜄
If the child can be persuaded to lie for a few minutes, both mother and child may benefit from the peace and calm of a massage. Use a little lavender or Roman chamomile oil. (See pages 143 and 149.)
Neroli, rose, and sandalwood essential oils have a calming action on the nervous system. (See pages 106, 174, and 179.)

Nutrition ⊗
Include plenty of vitamin B-complex, vitamin C, zinc, and essential fatty acids in the diet, which help behavioral problems. (See pages 206–209, 210, 221, 231, and 232.)

Mind–Body Healing 🖐
Ensure your child gets plenty of exercise during the day: sports, or running around the park, can help your child wear themself out and get a good night's sleep. See also "Sleep Problems" opposite.

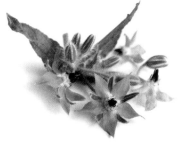

The adrenal gland is overworked by stress: borage helps redress the balance. Consult with your physician before giving any herbal remedy to a child, and always administer with care.

> **CAUTION**
> If you suspect ADHD, contact your physician. Help and advice may be needed to manage the condition and to ensure your child gets any extra help they may need at school.

BEDWETTING

Bedwetting is not considered to be a problem until your child is at least five years old. Many children, boys in particular, are slow in getting the message that they should get up to use the toilet at night, but that is no reflection of the state of their health, mental or otherwise. If a child sleeps heavily it may take longer for night dryness, but many children manage it by two or three years of age. Bedwetting in children who have already established a pattern of dry nights is usually caused by stress of some sort, like moving house, changing schools, or family fighting. Children who have never been dry at night may suffer from immature nerves and muscles controlling bladder function. Other medical causes include diabetes, urinary infection, a structural abnormality, nutritional deficiencies, and food allergies.

SYMPTOMS
• Bedwetting in children over the age of five, either habitual or during a period of stress or illness

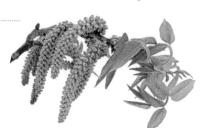

Walnut flower essence may help to stop bedwetting resulting from changes to routine.

TREATMENT
Herbalism 🌿
Offer St. John's wort and horsetail teas throughout the day, sweetened with honey, to soothe an irritable bladder and encourage control of the bladder. (See pages 123 and 138.)
If the bedwetting stems from an emotional upset, vervain and lemon balm relax and soothe. (See pages 152 and 196.)

Aromatherapy 🜄
Massage oil of chamomile into the lower back and tummy while settling your child down to sleep. (See page 149.)

Flower Essences 🌱
Try wild rose if your child drifts through life. (See page 174.)
Walnut will help if the bedwetting is brought on by change, such as a new house, school, or baby. (See page 141.)
Chestnut bud, if the child does not seem to learn from the experience. (See page 76.)
Star of Bethlehem, if bedwetting is related to a trauma or shock. (See page 158.)
Mimulus, when the problem is linked to fear. (See page 153.)

Mind–Body Healing 🖐
Practical considerations aside, bedwetting is only a problem if you suspect an underlying health or anxiety problem, or if it bothers your child, which may be the case if they are worried about attending sleepovers or camps. If so, contact your physician for advice. They can advise on whether there may be a physical cause, or whether this is just a stage that your child will grow out of with a little time and patience. If the bedwetting has begun in a usually dry-at-night child, consider any possible emotional causes.

CRADLE CAP

Cradle cap (seborrheic eczema) is common during the first three months of life and is characterized by a thick encrusted layer of skin on the baby's scalp. Yellow scales form in patches, especially on the top of the head. In severe cases, cradle cap can last for up to three years. Like dandruff, cradle cap is a condition in which the seborrheic glands are overactive, and it is often associated with seborrheic dermatitis, a skin condition in which there are red, scaly areas on the forehead, among other places.

SYMPTOMS
• Yellow scales of skin on a baby's scalp

TREATMENT
Traditional Home and Folk Remedies
Very gently, massage olive oil into the scalp each evening, and then shampoo away in the morning. (See page 156.)
Mash an avocado, apply to the scalp, and then gently rinse. Softly rub the skin of the avocado across the head to moisten and heal. (See page 161.)
Over-washing will make the condition worse. Gently brush away loosened crusts with a soft brush. Try not to loosen crusts that have not pulled away on their own, as bleeding and infection may result.

Herbalism
Rinse the scalp after washing with an infusion of meadowsweet, which is anti-inflammatory and will reduce itching. (See page 127.)
Burdock may also be used to rinse the scalp after washing your baby's hair. (See page 85.)

Aromatherapy
Gently massage a few drops of lavender or lemon oil, mixed in a light carrier oil, into the scalp before bedtime. Rinse gently each morning. (See pages 108 and 143.)

Flower Essences
Rock rose is useful if the itching causes distress. (See page 135.)
Add 2 drops of Rescue Remedy to the rinse water, and use after a shampoo. (See page 158.)

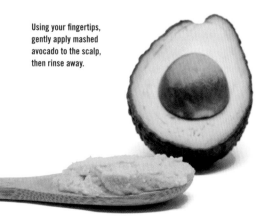

Using your fingertips, gently apply mashed avocado to the scalp, then rinse away.

STICKY EYE

Sticky eye is a mild infection of the eyes that causes a yellowish discharge and crusting. It is most common in the first week of life, and is usually the result of a foreign object entering the eye during birth, or from the blood or amniotic fluid. This condition is not serious and usually rights itself without treatment. In an older child, sticky eyes are usually a sign of conjunctivitis, which is a condition in which the conjunctiva of the eye becomes infected (see page 269). It may indicate a blocked tear duct.

SYMPTOMS
• Yellow discharge and crusting around the eyes, with no other signs of injury or infection

TREATMENT
Traditional Home and Folk Remedies
Apply cold bread to closed eyes to reduce the inflammation and soothe itching. (See page 202.)
Boil fennel seeds to make an eyewash for conjunctivitis and sore and inflamed eyes. (See page 128.)
Honey water can be used to cleanse the eye: it acts to destroy any infection, soothe, and encourage healing. (See page 203.)

Herbalism
Infusions of the following herbs can be taken internally to ease the condition: echinacea (which boosts the immune system and acts as a natural antibiotic), euphrasia, and golden seal (*Hydrastis canadensis*). (See pages 122 and 125.)
Apply infusions of chamomile, elderflower, euphrasia, and golden seal externally. (See pages 125, 149, and 178.)
Soak a chamomile tea bag and hold to the eyelids to soothe. Use it to gently clean the eyes (a new bag for each eye). (See page 149.)
Distilled rosewater or diluted witch hazel can help. (See page 134.)

> ### CAUTION
> If you suspect an eye infection or injury, contact a physician. Always use very weak herbal infusions for babies and toddlers: one-fifth of the dose for adults. Children should have half doses between the ages of 6 and 12.

A soaked chamomile tea bag will clean and soothe the eye.

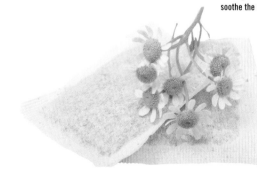

EARACHE AND MIDDLE EAR INFECTIONS

Earache may be caused by inflammation of the lymph nodes in the neck, or by another illness like mumps. There may be an ear infection in the inner, middle, or outer parts of the ear. Occasionally a boil can crop up in the outer ear, which can be very painful. The most common ear infections in children are middle ear infections. These are usually caused by the transmission of infection from the nose or throat by the Eustachian tube. Because this tube is short and small in babies and young children, it is easily blocked, and infection does not have far to travel to the middle ear itself. Ear infections can cause a great deal of pain, and the pressure may burst the eardrum, causing a discharge. Earache is also occasionally a sign of dental problems. If untreated, ear infections may become chronic. The tendency to ear infections is now believed to be inherited. Researchers have also linked recurrent middle ear infections in young children to food allergies.

SYMPTOMS
• Pain • Possibly discharge • Possibly fever • Possibly sore throat
• Malaise

TREATMENT

Traditional Home and Folk Remedies
Witch hazel can be added to a teaspoon of oil of St. John's wort and dropped into the ear. This will take away the pain and inflammation. (See pages 134 and 138.)
Crush fresh garlic and mix with a little honey, then swallow, to encourage the body to fight off the infection. Honey should not be given to infants under 12 months old. (See pages 79 and 203.)
Drink honey and lemon, or a little cider vinegar in some warm water, to help rid the body of catarrh and strengthen immunity. (See pages 108, 203, and 204.)
Blackcurrant tea will help to boost the immune system and to reduce catarrh.

Herbalism
Echinacea can be taken to boost the immune system and clear the pus. (See page 122.)
Apply a hot compress or poultice to the neck and ears using mullein or St. John's wort, which are anti-inflammatory. (See pages 138 and 195.)
Give chamomile tea to drink, to soothe pain and distress. (See page 149.)
A few drops of tincture of myrrh or golden seal (*Hydrastis canadensis*) can be added to a light oil, warmed, and dropped into the ear canal. (See page 112.)
Soak a large cotton ball with a few drops of warmed garlic oil and press gently into the ear canal. (See page 79.)

Aromatherapy
A few drops of neat lavender oil can be placed in the ear on a large cotton ball (never poke a cotton bud or any other object into the ear). (See page 143.)
Gently massage the neck and head around the ear with oil of mullein or lavender in a light carrier oil. (See pages 143 and 195.)
Tea tree or lavender oil can be used in a vaporizer for their antiseptic properties. (See pages 143 and 150.)
Use a few drops of lavender oil on a handkerchief by the bed to help your child to stay calm and to sleep. (See page 143.)

Homeopathy
Give Chamomilla when the child is inconsolable and the pain is made worse if the child is in a draft. (See page 149.)

Flower Essences
Rub a little Rescue Remedy (stock or cream) into the painful parts just below the ears to stop the child panicking and to reduce inflammation. (See page 158.)
Rescue Remedy or rock rose taken internally will ease panic. (See pages 135 and 158.)
Olive can be used during recuperation. (See page 156.)

Nutrition
Make sure your child's diet is rich in foods containing vitamin C and zinc, which boost the immune system and help to treat infection. (See pages 210 and 221.)

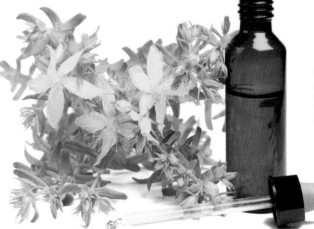

Use a clean dropper to administer St. John's wort, along with witch hazel, to relieve pain and inflammation.

CAUTION
Untreated ear infection may scar the eardrum and cause permanent hearing damage. Infection can also spread from the ear to other parts of the head, which may be life-threatening.

GLUE EAR

Glue ear is a chronic condition affecting a large number of children. It is characterized by a thick, often smelly, mucus which builds up in the middle ear, due to Eustachian tube obstruction. It impairs hearing, and causes the eardrum to perforate, allowing the mucus to be discharged. Glue ear is common in children who have frequent colds or other infections, which block the Eustachian tube (see "Middle Ear Infection" on page 272 and "Outer Ear Infection" on page 273). There is some indication that overuse of antibiotics may encourage the condition, and many children have excess or chronic catarrh (see page 277) which may be linked to food allergies or intolerance. Usually both ears are affected, and it is often accompanied by enlarged adenoids and frequently occurs with viral upper respiratory infections, such as the common cold. The first and often the only sign of glue ear is some degree of deafness.

SYMPTOMS
• Hearing loss • Inattention • Possibly frequent ear infections
• Possibly snoring due to enlarged adenoids

TREATMENT

Chinese Herbalism
Herbs to reduce inflammation and mucus (phlegm) would be Sheng di Huang (Chinese foxglove root) or Yuan Zhi (Chinese senega root). (See pages 166 and 172.)

Traditional Home and Folk Remedies
Drink lemon and honey or cider vinegar to clear the mucus and to strengthen the immune system. (See pages 108, 203, and 204.)
Garlic is excellent at shifting catarrh. Offer as garlic perles, or chop fresh garlic and serve with a teaspoon of honey. (See page 79.)
Blackcurrant tea is excellent for catarrh and will encourage healing of the ear.

Herbalism
Chamomile and echinacea are antiseptic, and can be taken internally or added to a foot or hand bath to reduce subsequent infection and to relieve unpleasant symptoms. (See pages 122 and 149.)
Clean away discharge outside the ear with a warm infusion of antiseptic herbs, such as chamomile or golden seal (*Hydrastis canadensis*). (See page 149.)
Herbal remedies which will boost the immune system include chamomile, echinacea, and peppermint. (See pages 122, 149, and 152.)
Herbs to help clear the catarrh include elderflowers, euphrasia, golden rod (*Solidago canadensis*), and hyssop. (See pages 125, 139, and 178.)
Herbs that work to reduce catarrh include golden rod (*Solidago canadensis*), ground ivy (*Glechoma hederacea*), and elderflower. (See page 178.)

Aromatherapy
Dilute essential oils of lavender, chamomile, eucalyptus, or rosewood in a light carrier oil, warm, and massage around the ear and neck. (See pages 83, 124, 143, and 149.)
A steam inhalation of eucalyptus, chamomile, or lavender can help to reduce catarrh and ease accompanying symptoms. (See pages 124, 143, and 149.)
Apply a hot compress to the nose, ears, and throat made using diluted essential oils of lavender, rosewood, or chamomile. (See pages 83, 143, and 149.)

Nutrition
Chronic infection can be caused by a build-up of catarrh (see page 277). Reduce consumption of dairy produce and any other possible allergens, including wheat. Contact a nutritionist for advice on how to maintain a healthy diet without these allergens.
Take cod liver oil and vitamin C to boost the immune system. (See pages 210 and 232.)

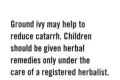

Ground ivy may help to reduce catarrh. Children should be given herbal remedies only under the care of a registered herbalist.

CAUTION
Severe inattention among children under two years could well be due to partial deafness caused by glue ear. It is essential that this is investigated in order to avoid long-term speech, comprehension, and intellectual impairment.

COLDS

Small children are more susceptible than adults to the viruses causing colds and flu because their immune systems are immature. Do not be surprised if your child seems to contract every cold he or she comes into contact with. Symptoms of a cold include a running nose, headache, and sometimes a cough. There may be a mild fever and a feeling of general malaise. Most colds run their course within 7–10 days. Some colds may be symptoms of allergy (particularly when the mucus remains clear) or common childhood illnesses and fevers, or part of a pattern of symptoms associated with asthma or cystic fibrosis. Recurrent colds (almost constantly suffering) may indicate a lowered immune capacity, which can be treated by complementary remedies.

SYMPTOMS
• Running nose • Headache • Sometimes a cough • Possibly a mild fever • Feeling of general malaise

TREATMENT

Traditional Home and Folk Remedies
Blackcurrant tea is excellent for catarrh and infections.
Eat plenty of fresh garlic and onions to reduce catarrh and cleanse the blood. Garlic is also antibiotic and boosts the immune system. (See pages 78 and 79.)
Hot lemon and honey will help to clear catarrh, prevent a secondary infection (such as tonsillitis or bronchitis), and soothe discomfort. Honey should not be given to infants under 12 months old. (See pages 108 and 203.)

Herbalism
Elderflowers, drunk as an infusion, will reduce catarrh and help to decongest. (See page 178.)
Peppermint is another decongestant and will also work to reduce a fever. (See page 152.)
Eucalyptus, rosemary, and thyme will help to clear congestion and work as antiseptics, which may help to prevent a secondary infection of the tonsils or bronchi (bronchitis). (See pages 124, 175, and 190.)
Chamomile will soothe an irritable child and help him or her to sleep. Chamomile also has antiseptic action, which will help to rid the body of infection, and it works to reduce fever and feverish symptoms. (See page 149.)

Try adding a strong infusion of chamomile or yarrow to the bath. (See pages 74 and 149.)
Mullein or comfrey can be drunk or used as a compress around the neck to soothe a sore throat. (See pages 186 and 195.)
Herbs to strengthen the immune system, including echinacea, can be taken throughout a cold. (See page 122.)

Aromatherapy
Place your child's head over a steaming bowl of water with a few drops of essential oil of cinnamon. Place a towel over their head to make a tent, and let them sit there for 4 or 5 minutes to ease congestion. (See page 104.)
Massage a few drops of pine or eucalyptus, blended in a light carrier oil, into the chest area. (See pages 124 and 163.)
Try a few drops of lavender or tea tree oil in a warm bath to encourage healing and open up the airways. (See pages 143 and 150.)
Use chamomile, cloves, lavender, pine, lemon, and thyme together or separately in a room vaporizer to help ease symptoms and promote healing. (See pages 108, 125, 143, 149, 163, and 190.)

Homeopathy
Offer Nat. mur., which may help with very watery colds. (See page 154.)
Ferr. phos. may help with hot colds. (See page 215.)
Try Euphrasia for colds affecting the eyes. (See page 125.)

Flower Essences
Rescue Remedy will soothe any distress. (See page 158.)
Olive will help with fatigue. (See page 156.)
Willow will help if the child feels sorry for him or herself. (See page 177.)

Nutrition
Serve your child plenty of foods with vitamin C and zinc, which will help discourage a cold and reduce its duration. (See pages 210 and 221.)

Serve your child plenty of foods rich in vitamin C.

COUGHS

Coughing expels foreign bodies and irritating mucus from the trachea and airways of the lungs. The membranes lining the whole respiratory tract are very sensitive and react to inhaled particles or infection by producing mucus, which is then coughed up. The color of the mucus or phlegm indicates the nature or the degree of irritation or infection. There are many types of coughs, some of which accompany a cold, while others are caused by chemicals, other infections, like ear and tonsil infections, excess catarrh, inflammation of the airways, and many other things. A chronic cough is one that lasts for more than 10 days, or one that recurs frequently.

TREATMENT

Traditional Home and Folk Remedies

Fresh garlic should be eaten as often as possible to cleanse the blood, improve the immune response, and encourage healing. (See page 79.)

Give your child lots of honey, which has antibacterial action and will also soothe a sore throat. Do not give honey to infants under 12 months old. (See page 203.)

Blackcurrant tea will ease the pain of a sore throat and help to reduce catarrh.

Ginger, added to meals, will help to get rid of any lingering catarrh. (See page 200.)

Pineapples are traditionally used for expelling excess catarrh.

Lemon and honey will soothe a sore throat and ease a tickly cough. (See pages 108 and 203.)

Herbalism

Aniseed and fennel will warm the system and help to shift a cough. (See page 128.)

Cayenne pepper can be added to food (a few grains) to stimulate the body's immune defenses and clear the wet secretions from the lungs. (See page 98.)

For fever, try infusions of chamomile, catmint (*Nepeta faassenii*), hyssop, and yarrow. (See pages 74, 139, and 149.)

Comfrey helps expel mucus from the lungs and airways. Mix 10 drops of the tincture with warmed honey. Serve by the teaspoonful. Do not give honey to infants under 12 months old. (See pages 186 and 203.)

Thyme can be infused and used to treat a wet cough. (See page 190.)

When the mucus is tough to shift, try strong infusions of ginger and fennel or thyme. (See pages 128, 190, and 200.)

Aromatherapy

Use lavender, myrrh, eucalyptus, or thyme in a vaporizer. (See pages 112, 124, 143, and 190.)

A few drops of oil of thyme, pine, cinnamon, clove, or eucalyptus can be used in combination or on their own in a foot bath to ease congestion. (See pages 104, 124, 125, 163, and 190.)

Add a few drops of eucalyptus and sandalwood to a carrier oil or some petroleum jelly, and rub into the chest and upper back. (See pages 124 and 179.)

Myrrh can be massaged into the body in the same way, to reduce mucus. Or put a few drops on a handkerchief and tie it to the bed. (See page 112.)

Lavender oil on a handkerchief or pillow will encourage sleep and aid the healing process. (See page 143.)

Homeopathy

Spongia is excellent for croup (see page 365) and for a loud, crowing cough. (See page 185.)

Drosera, for a tickling cough which is worse when lying down. (See page 121.)

Chamomilla will soothe an inconsolable child, who is better for being held. (See page 149.)

Flower Essences

Use Rescue Remedy when your child experiences distress, or panics because breathing is difficult. Rescue Remedy may also help your child to sleep. A few drops can be taken internally or applied to pulse points. (See page 158.)

Olive is good for a child who is overwhelmed by fatigue. (See page 156.)

Nutrition

Plenty of fluids and bed rest will make it easier for your child to shift a cough. Offer fluids alone for the first couple of days, and then just light meals. Avoid dairy produce altogether until the catarrh has shifted.

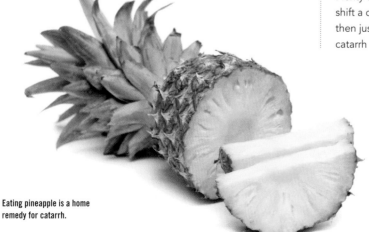

Eating pineapple is a home remedy for catarrh.

CAUTION

If a cough is accompanied by a high fever and your child has difficulty breathing, see your physician immediately. If a cough does not improve within a few days, see your physician.

CROUP

Croup is an acute inflammation and narrowing of the air passages, especially the larynx, in young children. The disorder is caused by various viruses, particularly the para-influenza virus, or by bacteria. The primary symptoms are coughing, hoarseness, and noisy, difficult breathing, which can sometimes be alleviated with steam inhalations. The characteristic cough of croup is a definite loud bark or whistle, caused by inflammation of the vocal cords. Infectious croup occurs mainly in the winter, when the larynx (voice box) or trachea (windpipe) become inflamed and swollen after what seems to be simply a cold. Other causes include allergy or the inhalation of a foreign body. Because the larynx swells and blocks the passage of air, breathing can be very difficult, which can panic a child.

SYMPTOMS
• Loud barking or whistling cough
• Hoarseness • Difficulty breathing

TREATMENT
Traditional Home and Folk Remedies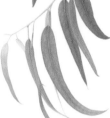
Offer a hot honey and lemon drink to ease the symptoms. Honey has strong antibacterial properties and will be useful if the cause of the croup is bacterial infection. Do not give honey to infants under 12 months old. (See pages 108 and 203.)
A little cider vinegar mixed with a mug of warm water can be sipped to ease symptoms. (See page 204.)
Blackcurrant tea is helpful and restorative.
Take your child into the bathroom, shut the door, and run the hot taps to create steam. Alternatively, fill a bowl with boiling water and gently place your child's head over it, covered by a towel. Steam will open the airways and reduce symptoms.
Raise the upper end of the cot or bed so that breathing is easier.

A few drops of eucalyptus oil can be placed on a handkerchief by the child's cot or bed.

Herbalism
Infuse lavender or chamomile in a bowl of hot water, then ask your child to lean over it, to help breathing. (See pages 143 and 149.)
Infuse some chamomile and catmint (*Nepeta faassenii*) and give small sips before bedtime and during an attack. (See page 149.)

Aromatherapy
Essential oils of eucalyptus, lavender, pine, chamomile, thyme and cinnamon can be added to a vaporizer or foot bath. (See page 47.)
A few drops of eucalyptus or lavender can be placed on a handkerchief by the child's bed. (See pages 124 and 143.)

> **CAUTION**
> Contact your physician if you suspect croup. If your child turns blue, call a physician immediately.

THRUSH

Thrush, or candidiasis, is a fungal, or yeast infection of the *Candida albicans* fungus, which is very common in those with immature immune systems, or those with immune systems that are compromised or very stressed. Thrush takes many forms, the most common of which are oral and that which develops in the diaper area.

SYMPTOMS
In oral thrush:
• Sore, white, raised patches in the mouth
In the diaper area or skin folds:
• Itchy red rash with a white top

TREATMENT
Herbalism
Echinacea, to boost the immune system, will help to prevent chronic thrush and help the body to fight infection. (See page 122.)
Oral thrush may be helped by preparing a mouthwash solution with lavender, lemon, or peppermint in spring water. Rinse the child's mouth, without swallowing, or dab a few drops on the affected areas. (See pages 108, 143, and 152.)

Aromatherapy
Use tea tree oil in a vaporizer in your child's room, to boost the immune system and act as an antifungal agent. (See page 150.)
Extremely dilute lavender oil or tea tree oil can be dabbed onto patches in the mouth and on the bottom. Avoid the genitals. (See pages 143 and 150.)

Homeopathy
Treatment will be constitutional, but Capsicum may be useful for sore, hot patches. (See page 98.)

Flower Essences
Apply a little Rescue Remedy cream to the affected area (externally) and a few drops of diluted stock remedy to sores in the mouth. (See page 158.)
Olive can be useful if outbreaks are linked to exhaustion. (See page 156.)

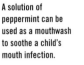

A solution of peppermint can be used as a mouthwash to soothe a child's mouth infection.

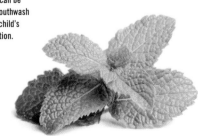

TEETHING

Your baby's first teeth will probably appear at about six months of age, and there may be problems with teeth coming through until the age of two or three. Most babies experience some discomfort, which can range from quite mild, which may make them clingy and fractious, to severe, accompanied by dribbling, loosened stools, and sleeping problems.

SYMPTOMS
• Sore red gums around the new tooth • Chewing on hands or objects • Increased saliva and dribbling • Flushed cheeks • Irritability • Disturbed sleep • Loss of appetite

TREATMENT
Traditional Home and Folk Remedies
Give your baby a cold licorice root to gnaw on. Make sure the root is too large to be a choking hazard, and hold it securely in your own hands. (See page 132.)
Cold raw carrots are useful teethers, but watch your baby carefully to make sure he or she doesn't bite off a piece and choke on it. (See page 120.)

Herbalism
Syrup made from the marshmallow root will soothe inflamed gums. Add a few teaspoons to your baby's normal meals. (See page 81.) Offer infusions of chamomile or fennel to calm and to soothe. (See pages 128 and 149.)

Aromatherapy
Put a few drops of lavender oil on the bedclothes to help your baby to sleep. Essential oils of chamomile and lavender can be added to the bath water to calm a distressed baby. (See pages 143 and 149.) Rub the gums with a little chamomile oil mixed with a teaspoon of honey. However, honey should never be given to infants under 12 months old. (See pages 149 and 203.)
Clove oil also acts as a local anesthetic, and a minute amount can be diluted and rubbed into the gums. (See page 125.)

Flower Essences
Rub a little diluted Rescue Remedy into the gums, or apply to pulse points if your baby is crying inconsolably. A few drops at nighttime will calm your baby, enabling him or her to sleep. (See page 158.)

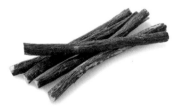

Try a piece of licorice root as a teether for your baby. Supervise them as they chew.

CAUTION
Vomiting is not a symptom of teething. See your physician if your baby seems unwell. Care should always be taken when administering herbal remedies to babies and young children. Most physicians advise that herbal teas should not be given to babies under 6 months old.

VOMITING AND DIARRHEA

There are many causes of vomiting and diarrhea in children, including infections such as gastroenteritis, eating rich or fatty foods (or, indeed, overeating), emotional upsets, and food poisoning. These conditions are not usually serious, unless they recur. Gastroenteritis is usually present if there is fever of 38°C (100°F), vomiting, lack of enthusiasm for feeds, and torpor. Occasionally diarrhea is due to too early reintroduction of milk after an attack of gastroenteritis. Remember that children can dehydrate quickly, so make sure they drink plenty of liquids.

SYMPTOMS
Symptoms of dehydration are:
• Sunken eyes • Dry mouth • Few tears when crying • Dark yellow urine • Fewer wet nappies

TREATMENT
Traditional Home and Folk Remedies
Milk and honey are excellent for treating food poisoning. Do not give honey to children under 12 months old. (See page 203.)
Mustard is a natural emetic and can be taken internally, mixed with a few teaspoons of warm water. (See page 91.)
Garlic boosts immunity, cleanses the blood, and is a natural antibiotic, so is excellent in bacterial infection. (See page 79.)
Give fresh lemon juice, warmed and mixed with a little honey, to cleanse the gut. (See pages 108 and 203.)
Drink blackcurrant juice, as a gut astringent.
Raw apple that has gone brown is useful for settling an upset stomach. Offer in small quantities. (See page 148.)

Herbalism
Meadowsweet or marshmallow syrup can help with vomiting. (See pages 81 and 127.)
Chamomile and vervain can be taken internally to soothe a child who is distressed by the vomiting. (See pages 149 and 196.)
Try ginger, crushed or decocted, to ease nausea. (See page 200.)

Nutrition
Following an attack of vomiting or diarrhea, offer lots of live yogurt and very ripe bananas to restore the proper bacterial balance of the gut. An acidophilus tablet can be taken for the same purpose. These are available in vanilla flavor. (See page 142.)

CAUTION
Babies and children can very easily become dehydrated by vomiting or diarrhea, and it is important that you seek medical treatment urgently if you spot the symptoms. See your physician if there is blood in the vomit or feces. If vomiting lasts longer than 1–2 days, and diarrhea longer than 5–7 days, see your physician. Contact them earlier if you are concerned.

COLIC

Colic is characterized by apparently unending frantic crying, usually at around the same time of day or night. The legs are drawn up to the abdomen, and the baby appears to be in severe pain. Excessive crying causes the baby to swallow air, which can exacerbate the problem and lead to abdominal bloating. The cause is unknown, but colic may be caused by contractions of the colon, an allergy to something in the formula (if bottle-fed) or the mother's diet (if breastfed), or simply excessive air which is gulped in through repeated bouts of crying. The most common form of colic is three-month colic, typically coming on in the evening and lasting anything from a few minutes to several hours. Burping or laying the baby over the knee or shoulder usually has little effect.

SYMPTOMS
• Bouts of crying, usually in the afternoon or evening, in an otherwise healthy baby • Red, flushed face, without fever
• While crying, clenched fists, drawn-up knees, or arched back
• For the parent, possibly stress and exhaustion

TREATMENT
Traditional Home and Folk Remedies
During bouts of crying, try holding your baby gently against your chest and shoulder, while walking or dancing lightly: the movement may soothe, and bring up any wind.
Caraway water can be diluted and given to even a very young baby in a sterilized bottle. Offer a few sips just before a feed. Do not offer too much, as it may interfere with breastfeeding. (See page 97.)

Herbalism
Relaxing herbs can be used in the bath, or infused, cooled slightly and taken by bottle. Chamomile, lemon balm, and linden are the most effective. (See pages 149, 152, and 191.)
A warm bath with an infusion of dill, fennel, marshmallow, or lemon balm will soothe a colicky baby. (See pages 81, 128, and 152.)
Catmint (*Nepeta faassenii*), infused and diluted, can be added to your baby's bath water to relax any abdominal spasm.

Aromatherapy
Rub a little very dilute fennel oil into the abdomen before feeds to prevent colic. (See page 128.)
A gentle massage of the abdominal area with one or a blend of chamomile, dill (*Anethum graveolens*), lavender, or rose will help to ease symptoms and calm a distressed baby. (See page 47.)
If your baby is wakened by discomfort, place a handkerchief with a few drops of lavender oil by the bed. (See page 143.)
Try a few drops of lavender or chamomile oil in a warm bath, just before evening feeds. (See pages 143 and 149.)

Homeopathy
Chamomilla is useful for babies who seem better when they are held. (See page 149.)

Flower Essences
Rock rose is excellent for extreme fright in a baby. (See page 135.)
Rescue Remedy can be used to calm a baby and should therefore help to reduce any spasm. (See page 158.)
For the parent, elm may help to calm feelings of inadequacy. (See page 193.)
Olive will help a parent who is exhausted. (See page 156.)

Nutrition
If you are breastfeeding, avoid dairy produce for a few days to see if this helps. Other foods that should be avoided are very spicy foods, citrus fruits, gassy foods (beans, onions, cabbage, etc.), and sugar.

Mind–Body Healing
When a baby's crying seems unstoppable and you are feeling overwhelmed, put them down in a safe place, such as their cot. Remaining in sight if you prefer, carry out breathing exercises, or meditation, for a few moments. When you return to your baby, your calmness may calm baby. (See page 68.)
Caring for a colicky baby can be exhausting and stressful, so try to share the burden with a partner, family member, or friend. Contact your healthcare provider, who can offer advice and refer you to a support group if needed. Remember that colic is not your fault, and it always passes eventually.

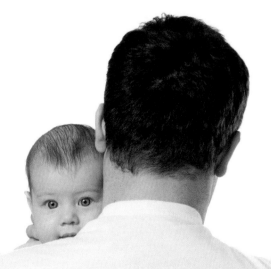

Try holding your baby against your shoulder and gently waltzing them.

CAUTION

Vomiting or diarrhea are not symptoms of colic and treatment must be sought immediately. Most physicians advise that herbal teas should not be given to babies under 6 months old. Consult with your physician or healthcare provider before administering herbal remedies to infants.

DIAPER RASH

Diaper rash is caused by contact with urine or feces, which cause the skin to produce less protective oil and therefore provide a less effective barrier to further irritation. It can also be caused by irritating chemicals in feces, not thoroughly rinsing soap or detergent out of diapers, and the chemicals contained in disposable diapers. The baby's buttocks, thighs, and genitals become sore, red, spotty, and weepy in areas touched by diapers. In boys, the foreskin may become inflamed, making urination painful. The rash may become secondarily infected with the *Candida* fungus if the baby has been given antibiotics or if breast milk has antibiotics in it, or if the mother has oral or genital thrush.

A natural disinfectant, tea tree oil can be added to rinse water to get diapers extra clean.

SYMPTOMS
• Red patches in the diaper area • Possibly spots, pimples, or blisters • Possibly, discomfort and distress

TREATMENT
Traditional Home and Folk Remedies
Rub the skin of an avocado on the rash to encourage healing. (See page 161.)
Wash the bottom with a little diluted cider vinegar and allow it to dry before putting on the diaper. (See page 204.)
Live yogurt can be spread on the diaper area to soothe, and to prevent thrush in the folds of the skin. (See page 142.)
Egg white can be painted on the sore bottom and allowed to dry before putting on a diaper. This will encourage the skin to heal and prevent further irritation.
Avoid using soap on the diaper area. Rinse carefully with clean water at each diaper change. Frequent diaper changes are suggested, and using a disposable diaper liner may help to reduce irritation. Allow your baby to go for as long as possible with a bare bottom, to allow it to dry and heal. Give plenty to drink.

Herbalism
Calendula ointment can be rubbed onto the diaper area to soothe and to reduce inflammation. (See page 93.)
Wash the diaper area with infusions of marigold, rosemary, or elderflower. (See pages 93, 175, and 178.)
Powdered golden seal (*Hydrastis canadensis*) can be applied to a clean diaper area before putting on the new diaper.
If your baby is over 6 months old, give soothing drinks, such as diluted chamomile tea, to reduce the acidity of the urine. (See page 149.)

Aromatherapy
Add a few drops of tea tree to the rinse cycle of your machine when using cloth diapers to disinfect. (See page 150.)
A few drops of lavender or rose oil in a peach kernel carrier oil can be gently rubbed into the diaper area. Use this blend to protect against diaper rash as well. (See pages 143 and 174.)
A drop of oregano or thyme oil, in a light carrier oil, can be used to discourage thrush. (See page 190.)

Homeopathy
Calendula ointment can be applied to the diaper area. (See page 93.)

Flower Essences
Rescue Remedy cream may be gently massaged into the affected area to reduce inflammation and ease pain or itching. A few drops of Rescue Remedy on pulse points will calm a distressed baby. (See page 158.)

> **CAUTION**
> Any diaper rash that does not heal within a week or so should be seen by a physician.

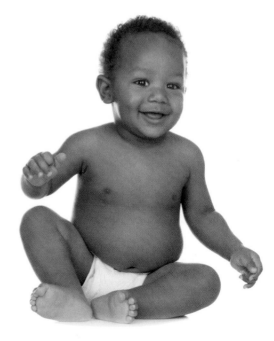

THREADWORMS

An infestation of threadworms in the digestive system is quite common, particularly in young children. Threadworms, which are tiny, white threadlike worms which infest the rectum, are not dangerous, although they do disturb sleep. Worms can sometimes be seen around the anus, or in the feces. They cause itching around the anus, and sometimes mild, colicky abdominal pain. Worms are usually acquired at school or nursery, by accidental ingestion of worm eggs carried under the fingernails and on the hands of other children. They may also be acquired by eating under-cooked, infected meat, by contact with soil or water contaminated by worm larvae, or by accidental ingestion of worm eggs from soil contaminated by infected feces.

SYMPTOMS
• Itching around the anus (and, in girls, the vagina), particularly at night • Soreness from scratching • Disturbed sleep • Possibly loss of appetite and bedwetting

TREATMENT
Traditional Home and Folk Remedies
Raw garlic, which is toxic to worms and parasites, can be eaten, or a small piece, wrapped in some gauze, can be inserted into the anus. (See page 79.)
Give 5 lemon pips, ground and mixed with honey, daily for 5 days. (See pages 108 and 203.)

Herbalism
Cayenne pepper and senna can be combined; the former stuns the worms and the latter encourages them to be expelled. Mix in a little live yogurt, to avoid irritating the digestive tract. (See pages 98, 99, and 142.)

Aromatherapy
Rub a little black pepper oil, very diluted in grapeseed oil, into the abdominal area. (See page 164.)

Flower Essences
Rescue Remedy for distress caused by discomfort. (See page 158.)
Crab apple, if your child feels unclean. (See page 148.)

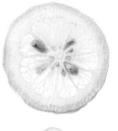

Grind lemon pips with honey for worm treatment.

> **CAUTION**
> Repeat treatment after two weeks to expel the worms that were embryos at the first treatment. Treat the entire family. Encourage good hand hygiene, wash all towels and bed linen, and vacuum around beds.

CHICKEN POX

Chicken pox is a contagious viral infection, which features headache, fever and malaise, with spots starting usually on the trunk and spreading to most parts of the body, including the mouth, anus, vagina, and ears. They appear as pimples, which fill with fluid to become blisters. Eventually the spots dry up and form a scab. Spots are very itchy and it is important that the child does not scratch, as scarring and bacterial infection can result. The incubation period is 10 to 14 days, and sufferers are contagious from just before the spots appear. Although chicken pox is not usually serious, it can be life-threatening to children with depressed immune systems. There is a chicken pox vaccine.

SYMPTOMS
• Red rash of spots or blisters • Tiredness and malaise • Fever • Feeling sick • Loss of appetite • Headache • Aching muscles

TREATMENT
Chinese Herbalism
The illness is believed to be caused by wind and heat invasion. Hong Hua (safflower), Sheng Ma (cimicifuga), and Jin Yin Hua (honeysuckle) may be used. (See pages 75, 97, and 146.)

Traditional Home and Folk Remedies
Add baking soda to the bath to ease itching. (See page 202.)

Herbalism
A witch hazel compress can be applied directly to the spots, or a little added to the bath, to ease discomfort. (See page 134.)
Tincture of comfrey or elderflower can be applied directly to the spots to encourage healing and to relieve the itching. (See pages 178 and 186.)
Add burdock infusion to your child's bath. (See page 85.)
Crushed peppermint leaves, applied to the spots, relieve symptoms. (See page 152.)

Aromatherapy
A few drops of Roman chamomile can be used in the bath to soothe. (See page 149.)
Lavender can be dabbed directly on spots to ease the itching and encourage healing. Lavender also has an antibacterial action, which will help prevent a secondary infection. (See page 143.)

> **CAUTION**
> Contact your physician to confirm the diagnosis of chicken pox. When fever lasts for more than a couple of days, or there is an obvious chest infection accompanying the rash, see your physician. Very rarely, chicken pox pneumonia can occur as a secondary infection. A mother with chicken pox may transmit the virus to her baby during the last days of her pregnancy. If you are pregnant and have come into contact with chicken pox but have not either had the illness or been vaccinated, contact your physician immediately, as you may need antiviral medication.

COMMON AILMENTS IN THE ELDERLY

DEPRESSION

Many elderly people feel a sense of worthlessness as they age: they feel that they no longer matter to others, that their dependency is problematic, and that they have lost any sense of purpose or usefulness. Often this is exacerbated by inadequate social intercourse, and lack of mental stimulation. A feeling of isolation develops, and withdrawal and depression are common responses to the loss of control that old age often brings.

SYMPTOMS
• Irritability or aggression • Bewilderment • Disorientation
• Possibly, fecal incontinence

TREATMENT

Ayurveda
Detoxification treatment would be followed by specific oral medication to balance the three doshas. Treatment is always individual. (See page 20.)

Chinese Herbalism
Depression is believed to be caused by stagnation of the liver qi, and may be treated with Dang Gui (angelica), Bai Shao (white peony root), Gan Cao (licorice), and Chai Hu (thorowax root). (See pages 82, 132, and 159.)

Traditional Folk and Home Remedies
Clove tea, or bruised cloves added to teas such as chamomile or peppermint, are able to lift mild depression. (See page 125.)
Drink sage tea, and add fresh sage to food. (See page 177.)

Agrimony flower essence may be useful for someone who tries to bury their sadness and worries.

Herbalism
The best antidepressant and nervine (with specific action for nerves) herbs include: lemon balm, borage, linden, oats, rosemary, and vervain. These can be taken as teas, added to the bath, or taken as tablets or tinctures. (See pages 89, 152, 175, 191, and 196.)
Ginseng is an antidepressant herb and will help with other problems accompanying old age, such as confusion, memory problems, and a weakening system. (See page 160.)

Aromatherapy
Antidepressant oils include: bergamot, chamomile, clary sage, jasmine, geranium, lavender, lemon balm, neroli, orange, rose, sandalwood, and ylang ylang. These may be blended or used singly in massage (which will also be very therapeutic), or in the bath or a vaporizer. (See page 47.)
Basil, chamomile, juniper, marjoram, and tea tree will act as a tonic, and can be used in any of the same ways. (See page 47.)

Flower Essences
Cherry plum, for fear of doing dreaded things, and of doing violence to oneself or others. (See page 170.)
Agrimony, for deeply held emotional tensions that are hidden from others. (See page 77.)
Gorse, for feelings of great hopelessness. (See page 192.)
Gentian, for relief of feelings of despondency. (See page 130.)
Wild mustard, for blacker and deeper feelings that seem to have no identifiable cause. (See page 184.)

Nutrition
Do not include an excessive amount of vitamin D, zinc, copper, or lead in the diet. (See pages 210, 214, and 221.)
Ensure you have an adequate intake of vitamin C and the B vitamins, which help the health of the mind and nervous system. (See pages 206–209 and 210.)
Calcium, potassium, and magnesium may also need to be supplemented. (See pages 213 and 217.)
Take plenty of the antioxidant nutrients, which help to delay some of the effects of aging. (See page 65.)
Some therapists may recommend using the amino acid tryptophan. (See page 227.)

Mind–Body Healing
Regular exercise, even for the chair-bound, will help to boost mood. For the more physically active, joining a walking group or dance class may be fun. (See page 70.)
More company, in the form of visits from family and friends, or by joining art or craft classes, will help to lift the spirits. Contact a physician for a referral to a counselor if needed. (See page 69.)

CONFUSION

One of the most common problems among elderly people is confusion. This may be a symptom of dementia (see right), hypothermia (very common among old people, who tend to economize on fuel and heating), or acute brain syndrome (caused by pneumonia, circulatory problems, or drug side-effects). Most often, however, it is a consequence of being cut off from the mainstream of life. Without visitors and possibly with no access to daily news, one day seems very much like another.

SYMPTOMS
• Self-neglect • Forgetfulness • Lack of orientation, particularly in terms of time • Bewilderment • Agitation • Depression • Hallucinations (in acute brain syndrome)

TREATMENT

Ayurveda
Henbane (*Hyoscyamus niger*) may be suggested, but it should be taken only under the close care of a registered practitioner, as well as lemon or lime juice. (See pages 105 and 108.)

Chinese Herbalism
Treatment might address deficient kidney essence, and useful herbs include Tu Su Zi (dodder seeds), Sang Shen (mulberry; *Morus alba*), and black ginger seed. (See page 118.)

Traditional Folk and Home Remedies
Ginseng powder, added to herbal teas, will improve memory and help with symptoms of confusion and agitation. (See page 160.) Gotu kola can revive memory and focus the mind. Add a small amount to your tea for a few days running, but discontinue use occasionally. (See page 101.)

Herbalism
Rosemary is a tonic, particularly for the elderly, as it improves concentration. Use fresh, or drink an infusion. (See page 175.) Orange blossom, particularly in the form of neroli oil, works on the nervous system and effectively counteracts nervous exhaustion, confusion, and depression. (See page 106.)

Aromatherapy
Geranium oil regulates the nervous system, and helps fight confusion, panic, and anxiety. (See page 161.)

Flower Essences
White chestnut, for a mind plagued by repetitive thoughts. (See page 76.)
Scleranthus, if you suffer from indecision and cannot make up your mind. (See page 180.)

Mind–Body Healing
Keeping up interest in a subject, doing regular crosswords or Sudoku, or reading novels will help to keep the mind sharp.

SENILE DEMENTIA

Senile dementia is a form of chronic organic brain disease in which there is progressive loss of intellectual power due to shrinkage (atrophy) and deterioration of the brain in old age. The onset is subtle and is sometimes only identified retrospectively by slight personality changes. The risk of dementia increases with age, but not all older people will get dementia. Most dementias are irreversible, but people with dementia can function better with treatment of other medical or sensory problems, and optimal social and environmental support. Stimulation and activity can help people with dementia.

SYMPTOMS
In the early stages:
• Insomnia • Restlessness
• Loss of interest • Forgetfulness, particularly of recent events
• Impaired judgment and reasoning
In the later stages:
• Progressive memory loss, until only events in the distant past may be remembered
• Mood swings • Inablility to follow instructions
• Repetitive conversation • Delusions • Apathy and indifference
• Failure to feed and warm oneself, which leads to dependency
• Incontinence

In traditional Chinese medicine, mulberry fruit may be prescribed for dementia.

TREATMENT

Chinese Herbalism
Dementia may be treated with herbs such as Gou Qi Zi (Chinese wolfberry). (See page 147.)
Treatment might be aimed at deficient kidney essence, and herbs to address this include Sang Shen (mulberry; *Morus alba*) and Tu Su Zi (dodder seeds). (See page 118.)

Aromatherapy
Basil and rosemary oils can be used in the bath, or in a massage, diluted in a little carrier oil, to clear the mind and stimulate mental activity. (See pages 156 and 175.)
Chamomile, lemon balm, rosemary, marjoram, and lavender strengthen the nervous system. (See page 47.)
Tea tree acts as a general tonic. (See page 150.)

Nutrition
Ensure that your diet contains plenty of vitamins B and C, as well as zinc and magnesium. (See pages 206–209, 210, 217, and 221.)
Lecithin, which contains phosphatidyl choline, improves memory when taken daily. (See page 233.)
Take supplements that contain all 22 amino acids to improve brain function. (See pages 222–227.)

Mind–Body Healing
Contact a physician or other registered healthcare provider for advice on how to stay well and independent for longer.

FALLS AND ACCIDENTS

Cataracts and other vision problems, unsteadiness, slower reflexes, dizziness, stiffness, and muscle weakness all contribute to the vulnerability of elderly people, making them more prone to falls and accidents. Often a stumble that would be little more than an inconvenience to a younger person is a serious hazard to the elderly, causing physical disability and, sometimes, emotional complications. This may be partly explained by problems such as osteoporosis (see page 346); delicate skin, prone to bruising and tearing more easily than previously; and slower healing processes, causing long periods of disability and despondency. (See also "First Aid," pages 376–379.)

SYMPTOMS
- Broken bones • Muscular injuries • Bruises and tears
- Immobility, leading to despondency

TREATMENT

Ayurveda
Harithaki (*Terminalia chebula*) can help for conditions related to impaired vision, which can help to prevent accidents.

Herbalism
Use witch hazel on a cold compress for bruises. (See page 134.)
Calendula cream will help healing of sprains, cuts, and bruises. (See page 93.)
Compresses of herbs like hyssop, lavender, or fennel will reduce swelling and bruising. As an injury heals, essential oil of rosemary can be applied as a compress to encourage the circulation and, through that, the healing process. (See pages 128, 139, 143, and 175.)
Rosemary is a tonic, particularly for the elderly, as it stimulates and nourishes the nervous system and will help keep you alert. (See page 175.)
Orange blossom, particularly in the form of neroli oil, is an effective nervine tonic (for the nervous system), which can help prevent accidents that are caused by a lack of concentration, and general confusion. (See page 106.)

Aromatherapy
Oils that refresh and invigorate will help focus the mind, which prevents accidents. Use one or more of the following in the bath: rosemary, peppermint, geranium, eucalyptus. (See page 47.)
Basil oil also clears the mind and stimulates mental activity. (See page 156.)
Bergamot, chamomile, lavender, marjoram, and rosemary will help to ease pain in the event of an accident. Do not apply to broken skin, but use in a vaporizer or in massage, avoiding the affected areas. (See pages 107, 143, 149, 157, and 175.)

Homeopathy
Arnica aids healing in someone who is constantly falling or having accidents. Follow it with Symphytum (made from comfrey), for fractures, to promote healing. (See pages 86 and 186.)
Calendula will help heal deep and painful wounds. (See page 93.)
Hypericum, for wounds that are characterized by shooting nerve pains. (See page 138.)

Flower Essences
Rescue Remedy can be used after an accident and in cases of shock. (See page 158.)

Nutrition
Ensure that you have a good intake of vitamin C and zinc, and B vitamins, which feed the nervous system. (See pages 206–209, 210, and 221.)
Vitamin E will help healing. (See page 211.)

Mind–Body Healing
Keeping physically and mentally active, perhaps with enjoyable hobbies, will help to prevent accidents. If despondency leads to depression during long periods of healing, see the advice for "Depression" on page 245.

Hyssop has wound-healing properties and is useful on a cold compress.

TRIGEMINAL NEURALGIA

Trigeminal neuralgia is a condition in which sudden nerve impulse discharges occur in the sensory nerve of the face on one side. These discharges cause severe pain and may be triggered by chewing, swallowing, or sometimes speaking. Usually there are repeated attacks over a period of some weeks, and the periods in between tend to become shorter. The cause of trigeminal neuralgia is unclear, but it is unusual under the age of 50.

SYMPTOMS
• Excruciating pain lasting from a few seconds to one or two minutes • Feeling of being on edge in anticipation of the next attack • Tic caused by the wincing of the facial muscles (hence trigeminal neuralgia is also known as tic douloureux)

TREATMENT
Chinese Herbalism
Treatment would be aimed at addressing wind, damp, and heat which have entered the meridians. Long Dan Cao (Chinese gentian) and Qing Hao (*Artemisia annua*), also known as oriental wormwood, may be useful.

Traditional Home and Folk Remedies
Celery juice or celery tea will help to ease the pain of neuralgia. (See page 84.)
Rub lemons on the affected area for relief. (See page 108.)
Rub peppermint oil into the affected area. (See page 152.)
Clove oil can be used where pain is experienced inside the mouth. (See page 125.)
A compress of warm cider vinegar can bring relief. (See page 204.)

Herbalism
Drink rosemary and lavender infusions to relieve the pain. (See pages 143 and 175.)
Rub in cayenne-infused oil. (See page 98.)
Warm chamomile compresses, applied to the affected area, will ease inflammation and pain. (See page 149.)

Aromatherapy
Massage essential oil of eucalyptus, lavender, or chamomile into the affected area, or add the infused herbs to the bath. (See pages 124, 143, and 149.)
A compress of rosemary essential oil will invite the circulation to the area, which will encourage healing. (See page 175.)
Blend 1 drop each of mustard and pepper oils in some grapeseed oil, and massage into the affected area. (See pages 91 and 164.)

Nutrition
Vitamins B1, B2, and biotin help nerve health. (See pages 206, 207, and 212.)
Take extra vitamin E and chromium. (See pages 211 and 214.)

INCONTINENCE

Incontinence, or involuntary urination, is extremely common among the elderly and usually has a physical cause. In men this may be prostate disease, and in women a prolapse of the bladder. Urinary infections or damage to the nervous system, such as acute or chronic brain disease, may also be responsible. Fecal incontinence is less common. It may be caused by constipation (if watery feces escape around the obstruction) or depression. Both types of incontinence are very distressing. Fecal incontinence should be treated according to the cause (see "Constipation," "Senile Dementia," "Depression," and "Gastroenteritis"). Treatments for urinary incontinence are offered below.

SYMPTOMS
• Leaking of urine • Distress

TREATMENT
Chinese Herbalism
Treatment would address kidney yang deficiency with internal cold, and the best herb to use is golden lock (Jin Suo Gu Jing Wan), taken as a tea.
If the condition accompanies prolapse, treatment will be given for deficient qi, using central qi pills. These will help with the control of fecal and urinary incontinence.

Herbalism
The seeds of the ginkgo biloba plant act as a tonic to the kidneys and bladder, and have been used for incontinence and excessive urination. (See page 131.)
Horsetail has toning and astringent properties, making it useful for treating incontinence and frequent urination. (See page 123.)

Homeopathy
Treatment would be based on the cause of the incontinence, but some of the following might be useful:
Ferr. phos., for an inability to control the bladder, with pain and a frequent urge to urinate. (See page 215.)
Sepia, for incontinence related to weak pelvic floor muscles. (See page 182.)

Flower Essences
A number of flower remedies will help with negative emotions and distress. Some to try are:
Sweet chestnut, for feelings of despair. (See page 100.)
Agrimony, if you hide behind a cheerful face. (See page 77.)
Crab apple, if you feel unclean. (See page 148.)

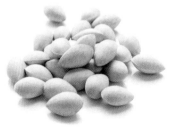

Ginkgo biloba seeds help to treat incontinence. The plant comes from China.

CHRONIC ILLNESSES

CHRONIC FATIGUE SYNDROME

Chronic fatigue syndrome (CFS) is also known as post-viral fatigue syndrome and myalgic encephalitis (ME), and its cause is the subject of controversy: it is thought by some to be caused by a viral infection (possibly herpes, polio, or Epstein-Barr), while others hold that it may be a psychological or neurological disorder, and others still that it is the result of damage to the immune system. Research has confirmed variations in basic bodily functions of people with CFS. There are recurrent acute attacks and rarely a full return to health in between. Symptoms may persist for years, aggravated by periods of stress or exertion.

SYMPTOMS
• Profound fatigue • Fever • Headache • Nausea and dizziness
• Muscle pain • Weight fluctuation • Sleep disturbance
• Depression • Memory loss

TREATMENT
Ayurveda
Complete detoxification will help, along with oral preparations to strengthen the immune system and balance the doshas. Cluster fig (*Ficus racemosa*) and ginger may be useful to stimulate. (See page 200.)

Chinese Herbalism
CFS is believed to be caused by weakness of qi, deficient blood, and damp heat, and herbal treatment would be given accordingly, probably in conjunction with acupuncture. Dang Gui (Chinese angelica) can restore energy and stimulate white blood cells and antibody formation. (See page 82.)

Herbalism
Herbs that address the immune system, such as echinacea, will be most useful. (See page 122.)
Ginseng and ginkgo biloba will encourage energy. (See pages 122 and 160.)
Rosemary and sage wines act as an excellent tonic when you are run down and tired. (See pages 175 and 177.)
Licorice can enhance recovery and stimulate the formation of white blood cells. (See page 132.)
Astragalus can increase energy levels and resistance to disease. (See page 87.)

Aromatherapy
Use uplifting oils, such as bergamot, rose, and neroli, in a massage or in the bath. (See pages 106, 107, and 174.)
Tea tree and niaouli will strengthen the immune system. Use these in a massage or in the bath. (See pages 150 and 151.)

Rosemary is stimulating, and can be added to the bath, used in massage, or put in a vaporizer while you are working. (See page 175.)

Homeopathy
Homeopathic treatment would be constitutional, based on individual needs, but China may be taken every 12 hours, for a few days, while waiting for constitutional treatment. (See page 103.)

Flower Essences
Wild mustard, for depression, when you feel gloomy for no known reason. (See page 184.)
Olive, when you are exhausted on all levels. (See page 156.)
Rock rose, for feelings of terror at the thought that you will never get better. (See page 135.)
Crab apple, if you feel unclean or impure on any level. (See page 148.)
Hornbeam for exhaustion at the thought of doing anything. (See page 96.)

Nutrition
A B-complex vitamin tablet will help to ensure the health of the nervous system and give you more energy. (See pages 252–255.)
Some sufferers have food allergies that may exacerbate or even cause the condition. Try an elimination diet to see if you are allergic to anything – in particular, dairy produce and wheat.
Chronic yeast infection may be at the root of the condition. Taking an acidophilus supplement, or eating plenty of live yogurt, will help fight the infection. (See page 142.)
Evening primrose oil, taken over three months, has proved to be a useful treatment for CFS. (See page 231.)

Mind–Body Healing
Both cognitive behavioral therapy and exercise therapy (a slow increase in activity, in line with the sufferer's abilities) may prove beneficial. (See page 69.)

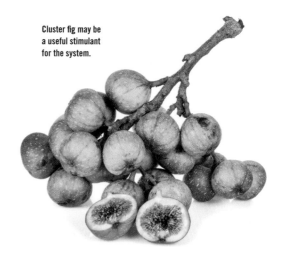

Cluster fig may be a useful stimulant for the system.

CANCER

Cancer is a chronic disease that may occur anywhere in the body, beginning with a malignant tumor which may be either a carcinoma or a sarcoma. Carcinomas arise in the lining of the skin and internal organs. Sarcomas arise from solid tissues such as muscle, bone, lymph glands, blood vessels, and other connective tissues. Both are invasive: a cell becomes cancerous, divides, and forms an abnormal mass which grows until the healthy cells are outnumbered. The mass then spreads into adjacent tissues and structures, often destroying them. Secondary cancers occur if an invading cancer grows through the wall of a blood vessel so that the blood then carries cancerous cells to other parts of the body. A tumor of low malignancy may take months or years to cause problems, whereas a high-malignancy tumor may have spread widely before the sufferer is aware of it. Conventional treatments for cancer become more effective year by year: contact your physician as soon as you notice a change in your body. The remedies suggested below will help to bolster the sufferer through conventional treatment.

SYMPTOMS

It is impossible to enumerate all the symptoms of all cancers here, but awareness of signs that a change has occurred is important. They may have a harmless explanation, but include:
• Unusual bleeding or discharge, especially from the vagina or rectum • A lump or thickening in the breast or elsewhere
• A wound that does not heal • Persistent change in bowel habits
• Persistent hoarseness or coughing • Persistent indigestion or difficulty in swallowing • Change in the size or shape of a wart or mole • Unexplained weight loss • Nagging pain in the chest

TREATMENT

Chinese Herbalism

Treatment will be aimed at supporting the immune system and reducing the harmful effects of chemotherapy and radiotherapy.
Ren Shen (ginseng) protects the immune system and helps to restore vitality. (See page 160.)
Dang Gui (Chinese angelica) will protect the liver, restore energy and stimulate white blood cells and antibodies. (See page 82.)
Huang Qi (astragalus) will act as a tonic, support the nervous system, and invigorate the immune system. (See page 87.)

Herbalism

Chamomile, valerian, and linden will calm the nervous system. (See pages 149, 191, and 195.)
Echinacea can be used to promote healing. (See page 122.)
Cleavers (*Galium aparine*), red clover (*Trifolium pratense*), and burdock will boost the immune system. (See page 85.)
St. John's wort is an antidepressant and restorative. (See page 138.)
Several herbs are believed to have anticancer properties, and might be used in conjunction with conventional medical treatment: yellow dock, garlic, nettle, myrrh, cleavers, thyme, calendula, and plantain. (See pages 79, 93, 112, 165, 176, 190, and 194.)

Aromatherapy

An aromatherapy massage will restore the body's equilibrium. However, do not massage the body immediately prior to or just after chemotherapy because it can encourage the spread of cancer cells through the body. In the early stages of cancer, use aromatherapy oils in the bath or in a vaporizer only.
Geranium and rose, for lifting depression. (See pages 161 and 174.)
Rosemary, bergamot, and sandalwood, for fatigue. (See page 47.)
Fennel, for nausea. (See page 128.)

Flower Essences

Mimulus is particularly good for feelings of fear. (See page 153.)
Rock rose is useful if you feel helpless and experience terror or panic. (See page 135.)
Olive will help if you feel exhausted on all levels. (See page 156.)
Sweet chestnut is for when you feel there is no way out. (See page 100.)
Gorse will help with feelings of hopelessness. (See page 192.)

Nutrition

Eat as much fresh fruit and vegetables as you can, particularly those containing antioxidants. (See page 251.)
Reduce animal fats and avoid processed foods.
A deficiency of vitamin C has been found in conjunction with certain tumors. Ensure you get plenty in your diet. (See page 256.)
Vitamins A and E are said to be beneficial in fighting cancer. (See page 257.)

Mind–Body Healing

Ask your physician to put you in touch with a local support group, or to refer you to a counselor or other professional who can offer practical and emotional support. Although maintaining a positive frame of mind may bolster you through treatment, constantly showing a brave face to the world can be exhausting, so make sure you are able to express your feelings when you need to.
During chemotherapy or radiotherapy, you may find relaxation techniques useful: consider breathing, meditation, or visualization. (See page 68.)

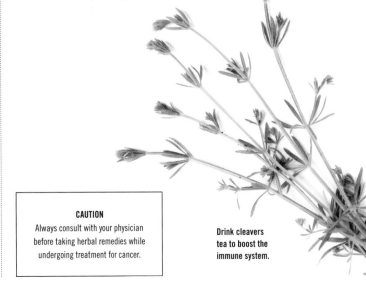

> **CAUTION**
> Always consult with your physician before taking herbal remedies while undergoing treatment for cancer.

Drink cleavers tea to boost the immune system.

FIRST AID

BITES AND STINGS

Insect bites and stings are common, and may cause discomfort, but unless you suffer from an allergic reaction, the best course of treatment is to soothe the pain and reduce swelling. The stinging insects inject a toxin through a stinger at the tail end of the abdomen. The reaction is usually local, but if the sting occurs in the mouth or throat, swelling can cut off the air supply and cause death by asphyxiation. Death can occur in individuals who are hypersensitive to bee venom. Animal bites should always be cleaned carefully and seen by a doctor. Dogs and other animals can transmit the infectious disease rabies through bites. Symptoms include fever and convulsions.

SYMPTOMS
• In most cases, discomfort and localized swelling

TREATMENT

Ayurveda
Aloe vera can be applied to the bite or sting to soothe; it also has anti-inflammatory and antiseptic properties. (See page 80.)
Bitter orange is anti-inflammatory and bactericidal. Rub ghee on the affected area. (See page 106.)
Place a slice of raw onion on the bite or sting for natural relief. (See page 78.)
Cedar is a natural insect repellent. Spray around the room in an atomizer half full of water. (See page 100.)

Traditional Home and Folk Remedies
Do not remove a bee sting with tweezers, as that can inject more venom: scrape a credit card over the sting to dislodge it.
The juice of a spring onion or a cucumber can be applied to stings to soothe and reduce inflammation. (See pages 78 and 116.)
The juice of daikon radish is useful for spider bites.
Bathe stings in a bowl of water with several teaspoons of baking soda. (See page 202.)
Apply garlic and onion to ant bites, and cucumber juice to ease the discomfort. (See pages 78, 79, and 116.)

Make a compress from a pad of cotton wadding soaked in lemon juice or cider vinegar and apply to a wasp sting. (See pages 108 and 204.)
Granulated sugar can be used to prevent a bite wound from scarring. Apply a poultice of sugar to the wound, after it has been cleaned, and bandage it with gauze.

Herbalism
Marigold petals are useful on a bee sting. (See page 93.)
Calendula cream will reduce swelling. (See page 93.)
The leaves of sage or rue (*Ruta graveolens*) can be macerated and applied to spider, scorpion, or jellyfish stings. (See page 177.)
Cover bites and stings with a wet, macerated plantain leaf. When it dries, replace with a wet leaf. (See page 165.)
Witch hazel is useful on mosquito bites. (See page 134.)

Aromatherapy
Use neat lavender oil on stings to reduce swelling and discomfort. (See page 143.)
A drop of tea tree oil can be rubbed into an insect bite or sting. (See page 150.)
A few drops of geranium oil, added to water, can be used to clean a bite wound and encourage it to heal. (See page 161.)
Prevent insect bites by diluting essential oils of eucalyptus or citronella in half a mug of water, and then gently applying to exposed areas, avoiding the eyes and mouth. Use cider vinegar in the same way. (See pages 119, 124, and 204.)

Homeopathy
Clean stings with pure tincture of Hypericum. (See page 138.)
Take Arnica for bruising. (See page 86.)

Flower Essences
Rescue Remedy, diluted in a few ounces of cool water, or the cream, can be applied to the sting or bite. Take orally for shock, pain, or distress, or apply to pulse points. (See page 158.)

Daikon radish may be used for mild spider bites.

BLISTERS

A blister occurs when a small area of the skin becomes raised and swollen by an accumulation of blood serum beneath it. If a blister is punctured the flesh beneath it becomes open to infection. It is therefore essential that it is kept clean and dry in order to heal effectively. Blisters can be caused by a number of things, including injuries – such as burns, scalds, or chafing (in new or ill-fitting shoes, for example) – insect bites, or infections. Some diseases will produce blisters, including chicken pox, herpes, eczema, and impetigo, and the disease can be transmitted by the virus particles inside the blisters.

SYMPTOMS
• Small pockets of fluid in the upper layers of skin • Fluid is usually clear, but blisters may be filled with blood or pus, if infection is present

TREATMENT
Ayurveda
Aloe vera juice can be applied to the blister to encourage healing. (See page 80.)
Barberry can be used for an infected blister. (See page 90.)
Apply a basil oil poultice to the area. (See page 156.)

Traditional Home and Folk Remedies
Boiled and mashed carrots can be applied to blisters to help healing, and this is particularly good for infection. (See page 120.)
Use roasted onions, applied as a poultice, particularly for blisters that have become infected. (See page 78.)
Peach pit tea is recommended to heal blisters. (See page 280.)
Ice will reduce inflammation, itching, or pain. (See page 205.)
Bathe the blister with cold, salty water, which will discourage infection and help the blister to dry out. (See page 205.)
You can apply surgical spirit, and then petroleum jelly, to areas that may be susceptible to blisters caused by chafing.
Cover blisters in the daytime to prevent damage and infection. Remove bandages at night to allow them to dry out.

Herbalism
Calendula cream can be applied to a blister to promote healing. (See page 93.)
Witch hazel, applied neat to a blister, will quickly relieve pain and swelling, and encourage healing. (See page 134.)

Use ice to ease swelling and pain.

CAUTION
Try not to burst a blister, which will leave the skin open to infection. See your physician if blisters become very painful and inflamed, or if blisters appear for no reason.

MILD SHOCK

Injury and emotional upset can lead to mild shock, when the sufferer is temporarily pale, frightened, and shaky. However, severe injury or emotional trauma can lead to a potentially dangerous medical condition called shock, in which the blood fails to circulate properly. In serious cases of shock, the brain and other organs can be deprived of oxygen. Causes of shock include extreme pain, severe vomiting or diarrhea, blood infection, or violent allergy.

SYMPTOMS
In mild shock:
• Temporary shakiness • Paleness • Tearfulness
In severe shock, which is a medical emergency:
• Pale, cool, clammy skin • Rapid pulse and breathing
• Nausea or vomiting • Enlarged pupils • Weakness
• Dizziness or fainting • Change in mental state or behavior

TREATMENT
Chinese Herbalism
Ginger and black pepper are warming and will help to restore circulation in cases of mild shock. (See pages 164 and 200.)

Traditional Home and Folk Remedies
Encourage the sufferer to sit down with a cup of warm, sweetened tea. (See page 94.)

Herbalism
Sip chamomile tea to calm. (See page 149.)
Add a little powdered ginseng to warm water with honey and lemon to restore. (See pages 108, 160, and 203.)

Aromatherapy
Lavender, lemon balm, or peppermint can be dropped on a handkerchief and held under the nose. (See pages 143 and 152.)

Homeopathy
Take Arnica, for any bruising, mild injury, or upset. (See page 86.)

Flower Essences
Four drops of Rescue Remedy can be taken internally or applied to the temples and pulse points, to reduce the effects of shock and ease a feeling of panic. (See page 158.)
Rock rose is suitable if you are experiencing terror or panic. (See page 135.)
Try mimulus for fear. (See page 153.)

CAUTION
Only mild shock should be treated with natural remedies. In cases of severe shock, call for an ambulance.

CUTS AND ABRASIONS

Minor cuts and abrasions should be cleaned with a mild antiseptic or with cooled, previously boiled water to ensure that they do not become infected. More serious cuts, wider than 2in. (5cm.) or with damage to the structures below, should be seen by a physician.

SYMPTOMS

• Bleeding should stop within a few minutes • Healing should begin within a few days

Signs of an infected wound include:

• Discharge or pus coming from the wound • Redness, swelling, and warmth in the affected area • Fever • Increasing rather than decreasing pain

TREATMENT

Ayurveda ✵

Aloe vera can be applied to cuts and grazes to encourage healing, reduce inflammation and prevent infection. (See page 80.)

Yarrow improves blood clotting and may be useful for deeper wounds. (See page 74.)

Myrrh can be used to clean the wound. (See page 112.)

Traditional Home and Folk Remedies ✋

Direct pressure should be applied to the bleeding area, and maintained until the flow of blood ceases.

Lemon juice is an excellent styptic, and can be diluted and applied directly to a clean wound. (See page 108.)

Use a peach pit tea compress on infected wounds. (See page 280.)

Sugar is said to prevent scar tissue. Press a few teaspoons of granulated sugar into a clean wound and dress with gauze. Rinse the wound carefully and dress again. Repeat up to five times daily, but take care not to disturb the clotting action.

Herbalism ✿

Cayenne pepper is a useful styptic, and a minute quantity can be applied to a clean wound to stop any bleeding. (See page 98.)

A few drops of marigold tincture in fresh, warm water can be used to clean the wound. This will help to prevent infection and encourage healing. (See page 93.)

Echinacea can be diluted and used directly on the wound to prevent infection. (See page 122.)

Comfrey ointment can be used on wounds that have become inflamed. (See page 186.)

Use a witch hazel compress on wounds. (See page 134.)

Tincture of myrrh is an antiseptic. Apply a few drops to bandages before dressing. (See page 112.)

> **CAUTION**
> If you are unable to stop the bleeding, seek emergency medical attention. Do not offer food or drink. See your physician if a wound becomes infected.

BURNS AND SCALDS

A burn is an injury to the tissue of the body caused by heat, chemicals, or electricity. Serious burns must be seen by a physician as an emergency, but minor burns and scalds (not those caused by corrosive substances) can be treated at home. Always cool a burn by letting cool water run over it until the pain has stopped. Do not apply anything to the burn until it is cooled. "Wet" burns should be dressed with a fabric, like gauze, which will "breathe." Change the dressing regularly.

SYMPTOMS

Serious burns, which require immediate attention by a physician, are:

• Deep, or larger than the person's hand • Cause charred or white skin • Cause blistering • Are caused by chemicals or electricity

TREATMENT

Ayurveda ✵

Aloe vera cools and prevents infection. (See page 80.)

Onions may be used directly on the skin for relief. (See page 78.)

St. John's wort can be used directly on the burn to cool and soothe. (See page 138.)

Traditional Home and Folk Remedies ✋

After washing, apply Hypericum lotion (about 10 drops of mother tincture, in a cup of water). (See page 138.)

Crush blueberries and extract the juice. Keep in the refrigerator or freezer to use on burns or scalds in the case of an emergency.

Honey can be applied directly to a burn to facilitate healing and to help prevent infection. (See page 203.)

Raw potatoes can be placed on a cooled burn. (See page 184.)

Herbalism ✿

A few drops of echinacea tincture in a liter of water, poured over the burn, will help to prevent infection. (See page 122.)

Marigold tincture, applied sparingly to a dressing, is a useful healing agent. (See page 93.)

Aromatherapy ⟳

Lavender oil is ideal for burns and can be applied neat (use sparingly). (See page 143.)

A few drops of geranium oil in a liter of cooled boiled water can be poured over a burn or scald to aid healing. (See page 161.)

Keep blueberry juice in the freezer to use on burns or scalds.

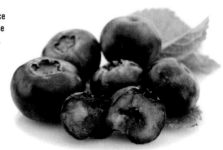

HEAT EXHAUSTION

Heat exhaustion, which leads to the medical emergency of heatstroke, is usually caused by the excessive loss of water from the body that is the result of intensive heat. It is a mild form of shock. If heat exhaustion is not treated, heatstroke ensues, in which sweating ceases and the body temperature may be 105°F (40.5°C) or higher. Heatstroke is a disorder that occurs when body-temperature regulating mechanisms are overwhelmed by excessive heat or fail in otherwise tolerable heat.

SYMPTOMS

Symptoms of mild heat exhaustion:
• Heavy sweating • Intense thirst • Headache • Dizziness
Additional symptoms of heatstroke, which is a medical emergency:
• No sweating • Vomiting • Fever • Physical collapse
• Fast breathing or pulse

TREATMENT

Ayurveda

Add the juice of a lime or lemon to half a glass of soda water and sip in small doses.

Chinese Herbalism

Fresh ginger, Gui Zhi (cinnamon twigs), and peppermint may be useful. (See pages 104, 152, and 200.)

Traditional Home and Folk Remedies

Sip a little fresh cucumber juice to cool. (See page 116.)

Herbalism

Small sips of fresh ginger tea, made with root ginger, will help to ease the symptoms. (See page 200.)
Teas of rock rose flowers or wild rose flowers, with a little honey, will be helpful. (See pages 135, 174, and 203.)

Flower Essences

Rescue Remedy should be offered as soon as possible to treat shock. (See page 158.)
Olive will help in the aftermath. (See page 156.)

> **CAUTION**
> Only very mild cases of heat exhaustion can be treated with natural remedies. Fluid must be replaced as soon as possible, and, in severe cases, intravenously. Find a cool place and sit down until any dizziness subsides. If you suffer from dizziness that lasts for more than an hour or from vomiting, see your physician.

Add a little lime juice to water, than take frequent small sips.

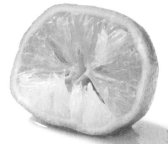

FOOD POISONING

Food poisoning is usually caused by eating food or drinking water that has been contaminated with bacteria, often the salmonella strain. Gastroenteritis (see page 301), an inflammation of the digestive system, can also result. Extra care should be taken in food poisoning during pregnancy and in children and the elderly.

SYMPTOMS

• Diarrhea • Fever • Vomiting • Possibly pain in the abdomen

TREATMENT

Ayurveda

Lemon juice will help to cleanse. (See page 108.)
Strong spices like cayenne, curry powder, and turmeric have preventive properties against food poisoning. (See pages 98 and 117.)
Combine 1 teaspoon of black pepper, 2 cloves of garlic, 1 tablespoon of cumin seeds, and a little salt in 4 cups of water. Boil until the liquid has reduced to 2 cups, and drink three times daily to cleanse and treat diarrhea. (See pages 79, 116, and 164.)

Traditional Home and Folk Remedies

Drink plenty of cool fresh water, and avoid any food for at least 24 hours.
Add plenty of honey to a cup of warm water and sip for its antibacterial and immune-enhancing properties. (See page 203.)
Chew ginger root to help ease the nausea. (See page 200.)
Cider vinegar, drunk with some warm water, will encourage vomiting to expel the poisons. (See page 204.)
When the vomiting has ceased, ripe bananas can be eaten to help restore the bacterial balance in the gut. Live yogurt will have a similar effect. (See page 142.)

Herbalism

Make a tea of comfrey root and meadowsweet to treat infection and relieve symptoms. (See pages 127 and 186.)
Arrowroot (*Maranta arundinacea*) or slippery elm tea can be sipped during the worst symptoms to soothe the digestive tract, and afterward to help restore bowel health. (See page 193.)
Licorice tea will help to flush out the toxins. (See page 132.)
Fresh garlic, or garlic capsules, should be taken to reduce infection. (See page 79.)
Chamomile, drunk as a tea, will ease digestion and reduce inflammation. (See page 149.)

Aromatherapy

Tea tree, garlic, eucalyptus, and juniper work to kill bacteria, and can be added to a cool bath or placed on a burner. (See page 47.)

> **CAUTION**
> Any case of food poisoning that lasts longer than 48 hours should be seen by a physician. All cases of salmonella should be reported to the medical authorities.

REFERENCE

CHAPTER FOUR

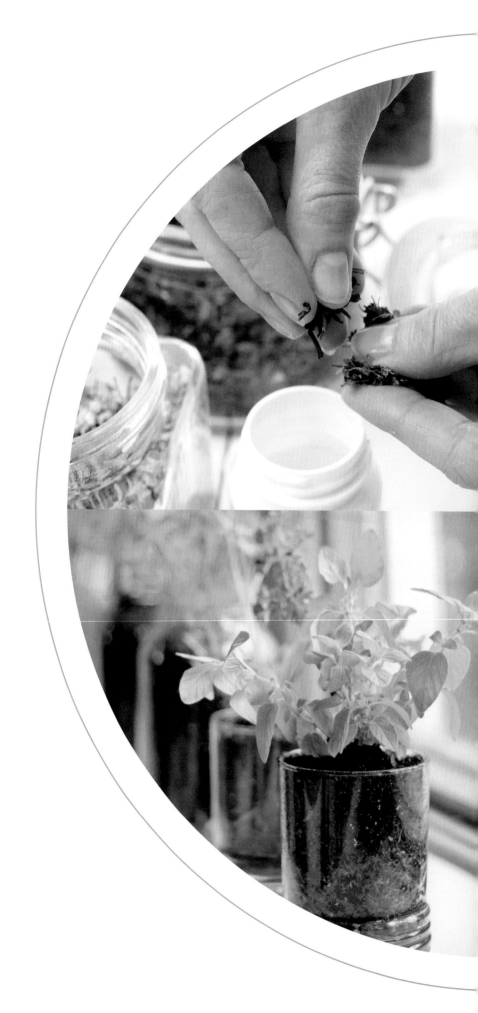

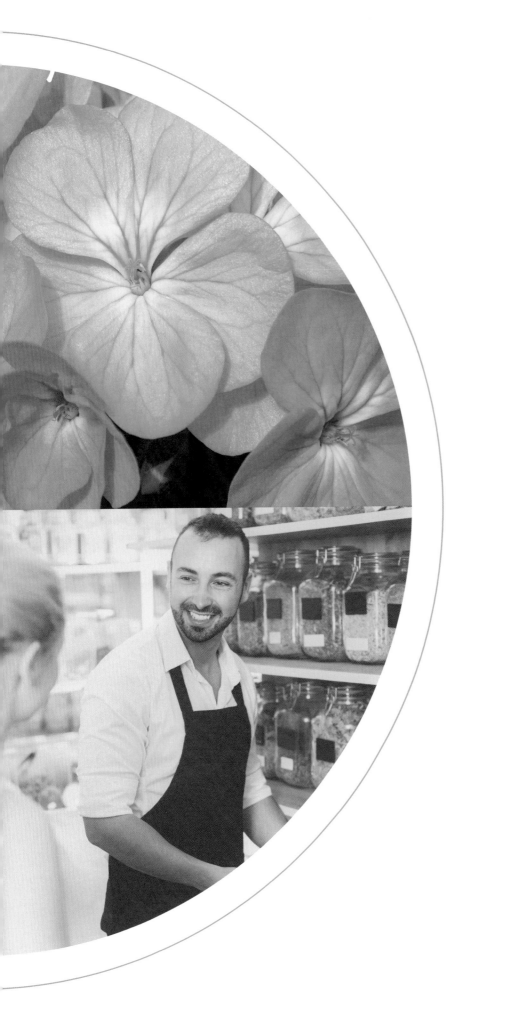

USEFUL RESOURCES

If you are keen to use herbal remedies, you will need to know how best to find and source your natural ingredients. If you enjoy gardening, you can take pleasure in growing your own fresh herbs while enjoying their aroma. With a little knowledge and time, searching for wild herbs is also an option. There are also plenty of options for buying natural ingredients from shops or online.

GROWING HERBS
—

There is something special about growing your own herbs and being able to pick the leaves or snip the stems whenever you need a fresh supply of natural ingredients. One of the benefits of herb-growing is that you do not need a huge garden to do so – or even a garden at all. Many herbs can be successfully grown in small pots on a windowsill. As long as they have good light and are regularly watered, indoor growing works well. Out in the garden, herbs can be grown in between other plants or in their own dedicated herb bed. Many herbs have the bonus of attracting bees and butterflies.

Herbs can be grown from seed, cuttings, or simply from the herb pots commonly available at grocery stores. Bear in mind that some herbs, such as rosemary, tend

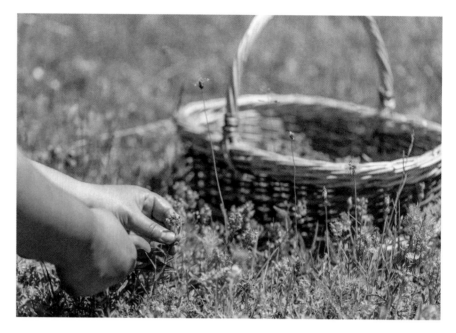

Use the photographs presented in this book to identify herbs in the wild.

to be slow growers, so you might want to start with an established plant or cutting rather than grow from seed. Good herbs to grow from seed include parsley, basil, and coriander, while sage and mint can grow well from cuttings.

Once you have established plants, remember that some herbs, such as sage and rosemary, thrive all year round, while others are seasonal. To make the most of seasonal herbs, you can pick them, dry them, and store them for future use so you always have your favorites to hand.

To dry herb leaves and stems, collect and tie them in small bunches and hang to dry in a warm space. When the leaves are brittle, they are ready. Crumble them gently into clean dark glass jars or pottery pots with airtight lids and keep them out of direct sunlight. To dry flowers, spread the flower heads on trays and place in a warm room, before decanting them into dark glass jars. For lavender flowers, dry them in bunches, tied loosely with a paper bag.

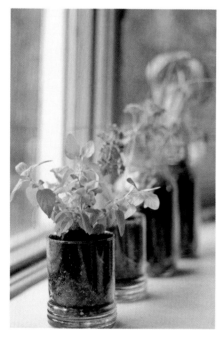

A windowsill herb garden can be a year-round source of healing remedies.

GATHERING HERBS IN THE WILD
—

If you have access to countryside, parks, or open spaces, you could look for suitable herbs growing in the wild. Herbs such as wild garlic, nettle, and mint often grow profusely in the wild. However, make sure you know exactly what you are looking for and are able to properly identify the plants. If you are at all uncertain you have found the right herb, do not take any chances.

It is polite to not pick masses of herbs from one area and to check that the land and plants do not belong to someone else before you pick. Avoid wild herbs that grow right next to busy roads, as they can pick up the effects of car exhaust fumes. Also try to avoid areas where you know the plants may have been exposed to pesticides or herbicides.

SHOPPING FOR INGREDIENTS ONLINE
—

These days you can buy a lot of natural ingredients and herbal products online, so you are no longer restricted to what you are able to obtain locally. However, online shopping does bring with it a few downsides. Sadly some sellers are less reputable than others, and items are not always as they seem. There is the risk that products might not be 100 percent pure, are not the strength they say, or contain unexpected ingredients.

If you are buying fresh plants such as herbs online, be aware that they can be grown using different methods, which can affect the concentration of the plant and its efficiency as a healing remedy. Ideally, look for organically grown herbs that have not been exposed to pesticides.

To reduce your risk of falling foul of disreputable sellers, always buy from online stores you know and trust. Look for product brands that you are familiar with, or research them first to make sure they sell quality items.

SHOPPING FOR INGREDIENTS IN STORES
—

When you are shopping for ingredients in stores, take the same discerning approach you use for buying online. Take time to read labels and look at the strength of the products. There will always be some products that are less expensive than others, but they may not match the strength or have been produced as effectively as the more expensive ingredients.

For example, essential fatty acid oils such as omega-3 can be extracted using various methods. The heat extraction method is quick and easy, but it can degrade the product. In contrast, cold-pressed extraction methods take longer, but provide a much better product. So although two omega-3 oil products might seem the same except for their price, the one that is cold pressed and more expensive is better value overall than the cheaper heat-extracted version.

If you have questions about a specific natural health product, ask in store. Many specialist natural health stores will have staff equipped to answer your question. If they cannot help, contact the product manufacturer, by phone, email, or social media.

When shopping in stores, ask for help from knowledgeable sales staff.

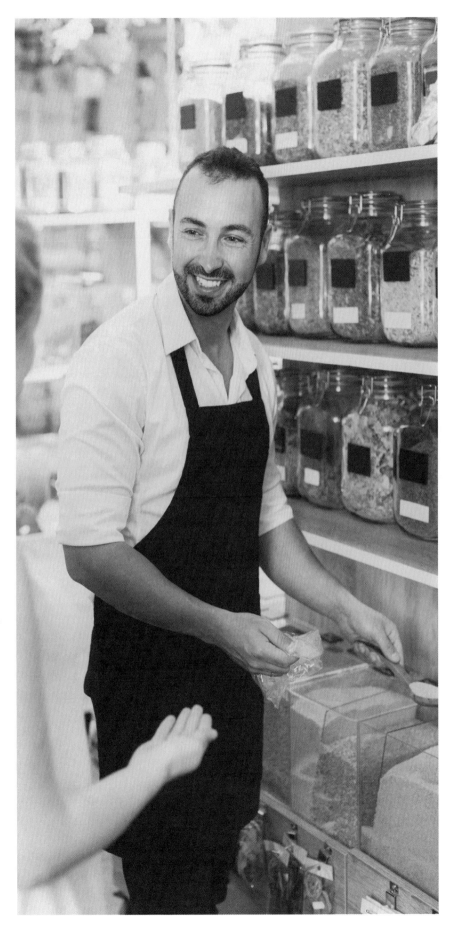

FINDING A PRACTITIONER

WHERE TO START
—

If you have decided to try a natural health therapy or are interested in joining an exercise class, it is always beneficial to find a professional for treatment or learning. In the case of natural medicine, it is especially important that you see a professional who is fully trained and qualified. Natural medicine can be powerful and you want to ensure you receive the best care and the correct medicines for your needs.

For therapeutic exercise, it is best to learn from a professional so that you get the positions and moves right. You will get the best health benefits from doing the exercises correctly from the start and this will reduce your risk of injury.

When you are looking for a qualified practitioner, you can either start your search by asking around for word-of-mouth recommendations, or use the search facility online. Local magazines and lifestyle publications often have ads for therapists working in your area, or you could ask at a local health food store or gym to see if anyone has left business cards with their details.

Online it is common to find searchable directories of practitioners, but make sure you are looking on a reputable site. The websites of the key professional organizations or associations representing each natural therapy are the perfect place to start your search (see pages 386–391). Many of them insist that members need to be highly trained to even join the organization, so you can be sure that the people listed really are qualified and experienced in what they do.

Whatever type of natural therapist you are looking for, remember that it is fine to ask questions about their background and training. Most should be only too happy to share details with you. Working with a therapist can often be a personal experience, so it is also good to "shop around" and continue your hunt until you find someone you feel comfortable with.

AYURVEDA
—

The National Ayurvedic Medical Association (NAMA) classes professionals registered with them as either Health Counselors, Ayurveda Practitioners, or Ayurvedic Doctors, depending on the amount of training and knowledge they have, with the last mentioned having the highest level of training.

The Association of Ayurvedic Professionals of North America (AAPNA) has members located all over the world and has several levels for classifying professionals. These are registered Ayurvedic Lifestyle Consultants (RALC), Ayurvedic Practitioners (RAP), Advanced Ayurvedic Practitioners (RAAP), or Master Ayurvedic Specialists (RMAS). As previously, the last mentioned is the highest level of accreditation. You can tell what level someone is by looking for the letters after their name.

TRADITIONAL CHINESE MEDICINE
—

If you are looking for a practitioner of traditional Chinese medicine, which can include Chinese herbalism and acupuncture, organizations such as the American Association of Acupuncture and Oriental Medicine (AAAOM) and the American TCM Association hold details of practicing members.

HERBALISM
—

To find a trained herbalist, check out the American Herbalists Guild. They hold a list of practitioners who meet their criteria for Registered Herbalist and you can search by state and province.

AROMATHERAPY
—

The National Association of Holistic Aromatherapy (NAHA) has three main levels of membership available to practicing aromatherapists (Certified, Professional Aromatherapist, and Clinical Aromatherapist) and provides a searchable directory of members. For members who have websites, look out for their NAHA level badge on their site, so you can see at a glance what their experience is. Other good organizations to be aware of that professional aromatherapists could be registered with are the Aromatherapy Registration Council and the Alliance of International Aromatherapists.

HOMEOPATHY
—

Homeopaths registered with the North American Society of Homeopaths can use the letters RSHom(NA) after their name, indicating that they are part of the internationally recognized organization. The society holds a membership directory that can be searched to find someone appropriate in your area. Another useful organization that offers a search for qualified practitioners is the American Institute of Homeopathy, which has been established for over 100 years.

NUTRITIONISTS
—

If you are looking for a qualified nutritionist, a good starting point is the American Nutrition Association (ANA). Nutritionists registered with the ANA are able to obtain the status of Registered Nutrition Professional or Nutritional Professional, Registered and use the letters NPR after their name. The Academy of Nutrition and Dietetics is one of the largest organizations of food and nutrition professionals. They have Registered Dietician Nutritionists (RDN) and Nutrition and Dietetic Technicians (NDTR) on their membership lists and can help you find an expert.

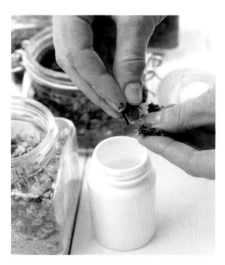

Although it is possible to make your own herbal remedies, a consultation from a registered herbalist may be beneficial for chronic problems.

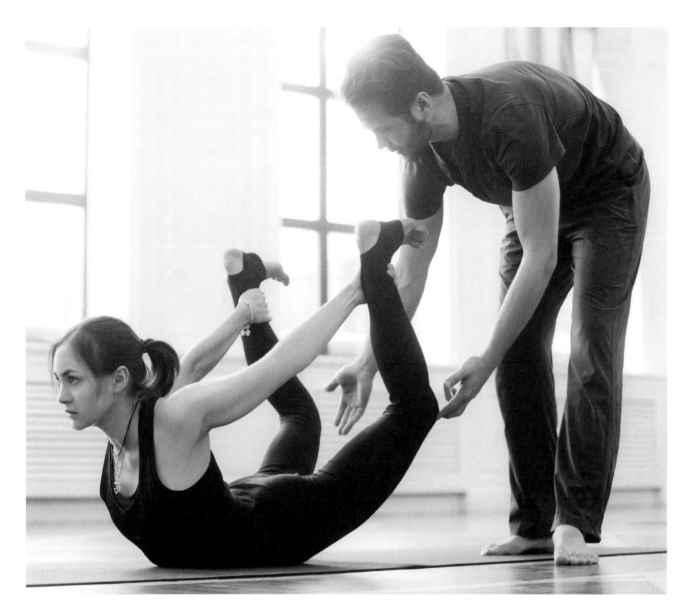

COUNSELORS AND PSYCHOTHERAPISTS

—

Counseling is usually a brief treatment that centers around behavior patterns. Psychotherapy works with clients for a longer period and draws from insight into emotional problems. Psychotherapy is conducted by professionals such as a psychiatrist, psychologist, or counselor. While a psychotherapist is qualified to provide counseling, a counselor may not have the necessary training to provide psychotherapy.

Counselors often specialize in a variety of different areas, but one organization that brings them all together is the American Counseling Association. The American Psychological Association is also a useful

Find a qualified yoga instructor using local recommendations or by contacting an internationally recognized association.

organization, as you can find members by specialty. If you would prefer to see a psychotherapist, the American Psychotherapy Association can help you find a suitable therapist. Alternatively, contact your healthcare provider for a recommendation.

YOGA

—

To find a qualified yoga professional for an expert exercise class, the Yoga Alliance is an internationally recognized association. Their members must meet Yoga Alliance Registry Standards and it is clear what level individuals have reached. Their free search facility helps identify qualified yoga

professionals worldwide. The International Association of Yoga Therapists has a long history of working with experienced yoga teachers and therapists and can also provide help if you are looking for a therapist.

PILATES

—

To find a qualified teacher of Pilates, the Pilates Method Alliance is one of the world's largest professional associations of Pilates teachers. The Pilates Teacher Association also has members worldwide. Both organizations offer the chance to search online for a suitable teacher near you. Members of the United States Pilates Association have all been classically trained in Pilates and follow the original approach of Pilates founder Joseph Pilates.

ADDRESSES AND WEBSITES

AYURVEDA

—

North America

Association of Ayurvedic Professionals of
North America (AAPNA)
aapna.org
567 Thomas Street
Suite 400
Coopersburg, Pennsylvania 18036
U.S.A.

The Ayurvedic Institute
www.ayurveda.com
11311 Menaul NE
Suite A
Albuquerque, New Mexico 87112
U.S.A.

Banyan Botanicals
www.banyanbotanicals.com
6705 Eagle Rock Ave. NE
Albuquerque, New Mexico 87113
U.S.A.

Maharishi Ayurveda Products International
(MAPI)
www.mapi.com
1680 Highway 1 North
Suite 2200
Fairfield, Iowa 52556
U.S.A.

National Ayurvedic Medical Association
(NAMA)
www.ayurvedanama.org
8605 Santa Monica Boulevard, #46789
Los Angeles, California 90068-4109
U.S.A.

Australasia

Australasian Association of Ayurveda
www.ayurved.org.au
77 Canterbury Road
Blackburn
Victoria 3130
Australia

Europe

Ayurvedic Professionals Association
apa.uk.com
23 Green Ridge
Brighton
BN1 5LT
U.K.

British Association of Accredited Ayurvedic
Practitioners
www.britayurpractitioners.com
5 Blenheim Road
North Harrow
Middlesex HA2 7AQ
U.K.

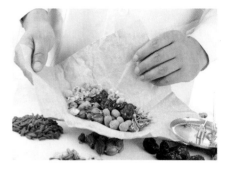

CHINESE HERBALISM

—

North America

Acupuncture Foundation of Canada
www.acupuncturecanada.org
895 Don Mills Road Tower II
Suite 109
North York
Ontario M3C 2W3
Canada

American Association of Acupuncture and
Oriental Medicine (AAAOM)
www.aaaomonline.org
P.O. Box 96503 #44114
Washington D.C. 20090-6503
U.S.A.

American TCM Association (ATCMA)
www.atcma-us.org

Dr. Shen's Herbs
drshen.com
1071 San Pablo Ave.
Albany, California 94706
U.S.A.

World Federation of Chinese
Medicine Societies
en.wfcms.org

Australasia

Australian Acupuncture and Chinese
Medicine Association Ltd
www.acupuncture.org.au
Unit 1
55 Clarence Street
Coorparoo
Queensland 4151
Australia

Chinese Medicine Board of Australia
www.chinesemedicineboard.gov.au

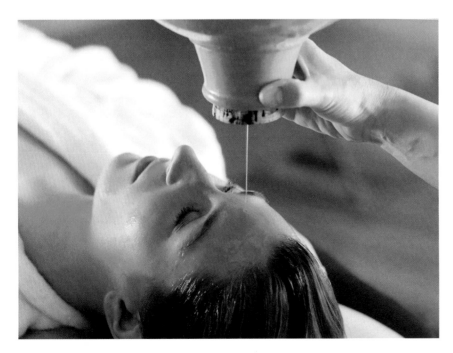

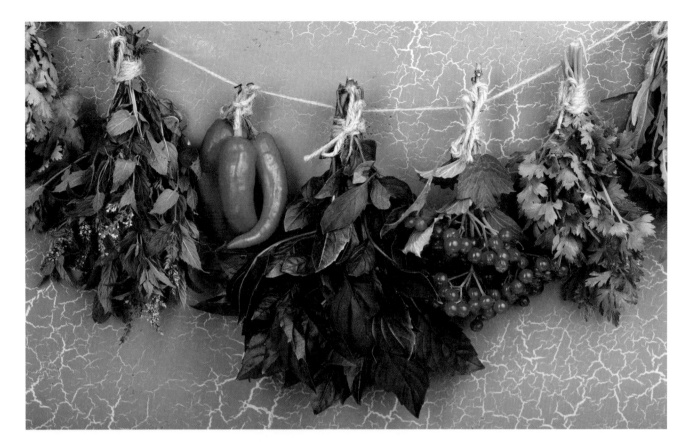

New Zealand Chinese Medicine and
Acupuncture Society
www.chinesemedicine.org.nz
PO Box 17318
Greenlane
Auckland 1546
New Zealand

Europe

British Acupuncture Council (BAC)
www.acupuncture.org.uk
63 Jeddo Road
London W12 9HQ
U.K.

G. Baldwin and Co.
www.baldwins.co.uk
171–173 Walworth Road
London SE17 1RW
U.K.

Register of Chinese Herbal Medicine
rchm.co.uk
Suite 5
Sackville Place
44–48 Magdalen Street
Norwich NR3 1JU
U.K.

HERBALISM

—

North America

American Herb Association
ahaherb.com
P.O. Box 1673
Nevada City, California 95959
U.S.A.

American Herbalists Guild
www.americanherbalistsguild.com
P.O. Box 3076
Asheville, North Carolina 28802-3076
U.S.A.

Canadian Council of Herbalist
Associations (CCHA)
herbalccha.org
35 des Bouleaux
Ste-Anne-des-Lacs
Quebec J0R 1B0
Canada

The Growers Exchange
www.thegrowers-exchange.com
11110 Sandy Fields Road
Charles City, Virginia 23030
U.S.A.

Monterey Bay Spice Company
www.herbco.com
241 Walker Street
Watsonville, California 95076
U.S.A.

Mountain Rose Herbs
www.mountainroseherbs.com
P.O. Box 50220
Eugene, Oregon 97405
U.S.A.

Australasia

National Herbalists Association of
Australia (NHAA)
www.nhaa.org.au
P.O. Box 696
Ashfield
New South Wales 1800
Australia

New Zealand Association of Medical
Herbalists (NZAMH)
nzamh.org.nz
P.O. Box 12582
Chartwell
Hamilton 3248
New Zealand

Europe

British Herbal Medicine Association (BHMA)
bhma.info
P.O. Box 583
Exeter EX1 9GX
U.K.

College of Practitioners of Phytotherapy
(CPP)
thecpp.uk
Oak Glade
9 Hythe Close
Polegate
East Sussex BN26 6LQ
U.K.

The Herb Society
www.herbsociety.org.uk
P.O. Box 196
Liverpool L18 1XE
U.K.

National Institute of Medical Herbalists
(NIMH)
www.nimh.org.uk
Clover House

James Court
South Street
Exeter EX1 1EE
U.K.

AROMATHERAPY

—

North America

Alliance of International
Aromatherapists (AIS)
www.alliance-aromatherapists.org
3000 South Jamaica Ct.
Suite 145
Aurora, Colorado 80014
U.S.A.

The Aromatherapy Institute and Research
aiprograms.org
3530 Forest Lane
Suite 306
Dallas, Texas 75229
U.S.A.

Aromatherapy Registration Council (ARC)
aromatherapycouncil.org

Aromatics International
www.aromatics.com
247 Westgate Way
Florence, Montana 59833
U.S.A.

Eden Botanicals
www.edenbotanicals.com
3820 Cypress Drive #12
Petaluma, California 94954
U.S.A.

National Association of Holistic
Aromatherapy (NAHA)
naha.org
P.O. BOX 27871
Raleigh, North Carolina 27611-7871
U.S.A.

The Pacific Institute
of Aromatherapy
www.pacificinstituteofaromatherapy.com
P.O. Box 6723
San Raphael, California 94903
U.S.A.

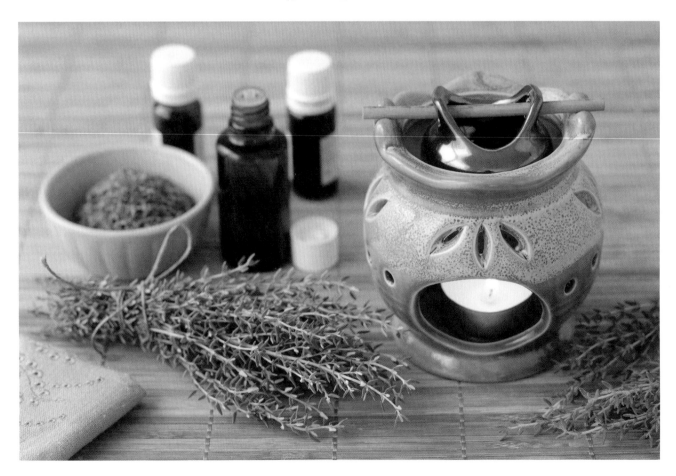

Australasia

International Aromatherapy and Aromatic
Medicine Association (IAAMA)
www.iaama.org.au
P.O. Box 5058
Brassall
Queensland 4305
Australia

New Zealand Register of Holistic
Aromatherapists (NZROHA)
www.aromatherapy.org.nz
P.O. Box 18399
Glen Innes
Auckland 1743
New Zealand

Europe

The Aromatherapy Council
aromatherapycouncil.org.uk

International Federation of Aromatherapists
(IFA)
www.ifaroma.org
146 South Ealing Road
Ealing
London W5 4QJ
U.K.

International Federation of Professional
Aromatherapists (IFPA)
www.aromatherapy-studies.com
82 Ashby Road
Hinckley
Leicestershire LE1O 1SN
U.K.

HOMEOPATHY
—
North America

American Institute of Homeopathy
www.homeopathyusa.org
c/o Sandra M. Chase, M.D. DH.t.
10418 Whitehead St.
Fairfax, Virginia 22030
U.S.A.

Boiron
shop.boironusa.com
6 Campus Boulevard
Newtown Square, Pennsylvania 19073-3267
U.S.A.

Canadian Society of
Homeopaths (CSOH)
www.csoh.ca
101–1001 West Broadway
Unit 120
Vancouver BC V6H 4E4
Canada

North American Society of Homeopaths
(NASH)
homeopathy.org
P.O. Box 115
Troy, Maine 04987
U.S.A.

Australasia

Australian Homeopathic Federation
www.homeopathyoz.org
PO Box 7108
Toowoomba South
Queensland 4350
Australia

New Zealand Homeopathic Society
homeopathy.ac.nz
P.O. BOX 67 095
Mt. Eden
Auckland 1349
New Zealand

Europe

The British Homeopathic
Association (BHA)
www.britishhomeopathic.org
CAN Mezzanine
49–51 East Rd
London N1 6AH
U.K.

The Royal London Hospital for Integrated
Medicine
www.uclh.nhs.uk/OurServices/OurHospitals/
RLHIM
60 Great Ormond Street
London WC1N 3HR
U.K.

FLOWER ESSENCES
—
North America

Bach Foundation International Register
www.bachcentre.com/found/rp_list.php

Bach Original Flower Remedies
www.nelsonsnaturalworld.com/en-us/us/
our-brands/bachoriginalflowerremedies
Nelson Bach USA Ltd.
21 High Street
Suite 302
North Andover, Massachussetts 01845
U.S.A.

Flower Essence Society
www.flowersociety.org
P.O. Box 459
Nevada City, California 95959
U.S.A.

Australasia

Martin and Pleasance
www.martinandpleasance.com/brands/
bach-original-flower-remedies
7 Rocklea Drive
Port Melbourne
Victoria 3207
Australia

Europe

The Bach Centre
www.bachcentre.com
Mount Vernon
Bakers Lane
Brithwell-cum-Sotwell
Oxfordshire OX10 0PX
U.K.

Nelsons Natural World
www.nelsonsnaturalworld.com/en-gb/uk
Nelsons House
83 Parkside
London SW19 5LP
U.K.

NUTRITION
—
North America

Academy of Nutrition and Dietetics
www.eatright.org
120 South Riverside Plaza
Suite 2190
Chicago, Illinois 60606-6995
U.S.A.

American Nutrition Association (ANA)
americannutritionassociation.org

Canadian Association
of Natural Nutritional Practitioners
cannp.ca
335 St. Andrews Street East
Fergus
Ontario N1M 1R3
Canada

Swanson Health Products
www.swansonvitamins.com
P.O. Box 2803
Fargo, North Dakota 58108-2803
U.S.A.

Vitamin World
www.vitaminworld.com
4320 Veterans Memorial Highway
Holbrook, New York 11741-9002
U.S.A.

Australasia

Australasian College of Nutritional and
Environmental Medicine (ACNEM)
www.acnem.org
P.O. Box 298
Sandringham
Victoria 3191
Australia

Europe

British Association for Applied
Nutrition and Nutritional
Therapy (BANT)
bant.org.uk
27 Old Gloucester Street
London WC1N 3XX
U.K.

Holland and Barrett
www.hollandandbarrett.com
Samuel Ryder House
Barling Way
Eliot Park
Nuneaton
Warwickshire CV10 7RH
U.K.

Nutrition Therapy Education
Commission (NTEC)
www.nteducationcommission.org.uk
B.M. Box 3304
London WC1N 3XX
U.K.

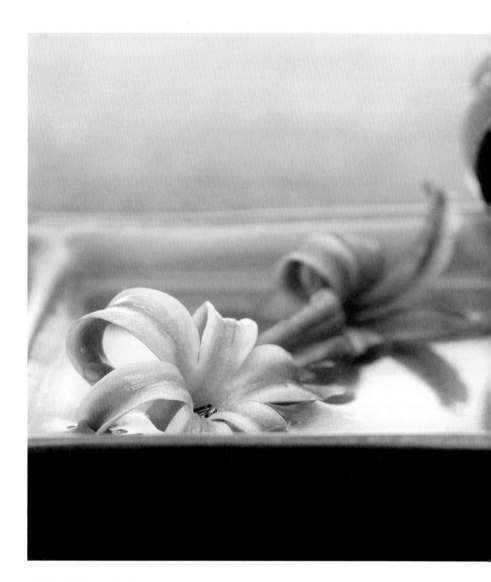

MIND–BODY HEALING

—

North America

American Counseling Association
www.counseling.org
6101 Stevenson Ave., Suite 600
Alexandria, Virginia 22304
U.S.A.

American Holistic Health Association
ahha.org
P.O. Box 17400
Anaheim, California 92817-7400
U.S.A.

American Holistic Nurses Association
www.ahna.org
2900 S.W. Plass Court
Topeka, Kansas 66611-1980
U.S.A.

American Psychological
Association (APA)
www.apa.org
750 First St. NE
Washington, D.C. 20002-4242
U.S.A.

American Psychotherapy Association
www.americanpsychotherapy.com
2750 E Sunshine St.
Springfield, Missouri 65804
U.S.A.

Canadian Integrative Medicine
Association (CIMA)
www.cimadoctors.ca
P.O. Box 80
3351 Piercy Road
Denman Island
British Colombia VOR 1TO
Canada

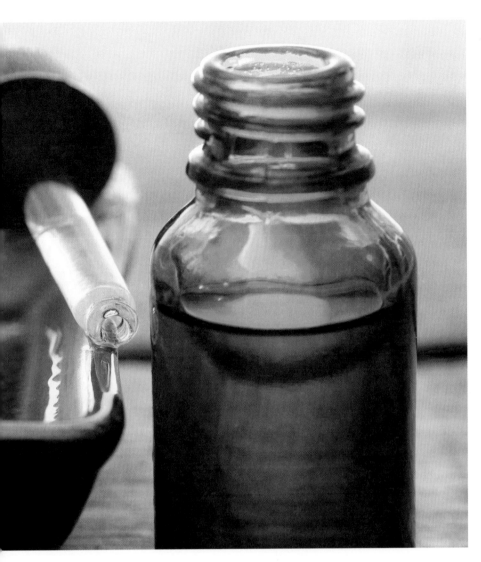

International Association
of Yoga Therapists (IAYT)
www.iayt.org
P.O. Box 251563
Little Rock, Arkansas 72225
U.S.A.

Pilates Method Alliance (PMA)
www.pilatesmethodalliance.org
1666 Kennedy Causeway, Suite 402
North Bay Village, Florida 33141
U.S.A.

Pilates Teacher Association (PTA)
www.pilatesteacherassociation.org

United States Pilates Association
unitedstatespilatesassociation.com
1500 East Broward Blvd., Suite 250
Fort Lauderdale, Florida 33301
U.S.A.

Yoga Alliance
www.yogaalliance.org
1560 Wilson Blvd. #700
Arlington, Virginia 22209
U.S.A.

Australasia

Australian Psychological Society (APS)
www.psychology.org.au
P.O. Box 38
Flinders Lane
Victoria 8009
Australia

New Zealand Association of
Psychotherapists
nzap.org.nz
P.O. Box 57025
Mana, Porirua 5247
New Zealand

Pilates Method Alliance (PMA)
www.pilatesmethodalliance.org

Psychotherapy and Counselling
Federation of Australia
www.pacfa.org.au
290 Park Street
North Fitzroy
Victoria 3068
Australia

Yoga Alliance
www.yogaalliance.org

Europe

British Association for Counselling
and Psychotherapy (BACP)
www.bacp.co.uk
BACP House
15 St. John's Business Park
Lutterworth LE17 4HB
U.K.

British Wheel of Yoga
www.bwy.org.uk
25 Jermyn Street
Sleaford
Lincolnshire NG34 7RU

Pilates Method Alliance (PMA)
www.pilatesmethodalliance.org

Pilates Teacher Association (PTA)
www.pilatesteacherassociation.org
9 Church Street
Troon KA10 6AU
U.K.

Royal College of Psychiatrists
www.rcpsych.ac.uk
21 Prescot Street
London E1 8BB
U.K.

Yoga Alliance Professionals
www.yogaallianceprofessionals.org
The Clocktower
Bush House Cottages
Edinburgh Technopole
Milton Bridge
Midlothian RH26 0BA
U.K.

FURTHER READING

Ayurveda
—

Ayurveda (Idiot's Guides)
Sahara Rose Ketabi and Dr. Deepak Chopra
Alpha, 2017

The Ayurveda Way
Ananta Ripa Ajmera
Storey Publishing, 2017

*The Complete Illustrated Guide
to Ayurveda*
Gopi Warrier and Dr. Deepika Gunawant
Element Books, 2000

The Everyday Ayurveda Cookbook
Kate O'Donnell
Shambhala, 2015

The Handbook of Ayurveda
Dr. Shantha Godagama
North Atlantic Books, 2004

Quantum Healing
Dr. Deepak Chopra
Bantam Books, 2015

Chinese Herbalism
—

*Chinese Herbal Medicine: Modern
Applications of Traditional Formulas*
Chongyun Liu and Angela Tseng
CRC Press, 2004

The Chinese Medicine Bible
Penelope Ody
Sterling, 2012

*Routledge Handbook of
Chinese Medicine*
Vivienne Low and Michael Stanley-Baker
Routledge, 2018

*Using Traditional Chinese Medicine to
Manage Your Emotional Health*
Zhang Yifang
Shanghai Press, 2013

*Your Guide to Health with Food and Herbs:
Using the Wisdom of Traditional Chinese
Medicine*
Yao Yingzhi and Zhang Yifang
Shanghai Press, 2012

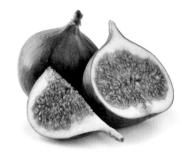

Traditional Home and Folk Remedies
—

*The Country Almanac of Home
Remedies*
Brigitte Mars and Chrystle Fiedler
Fair Winds Press, 2014

The Doctors Book of Home Remedies
The Editors of Prevention Magazine
Rodale Books, 2010

The Natural Home Remedies Guide
Karen Sullivan
Thorsons, 2017

Natural Remedies for Kids
Kate Tietje and Bob Zajac
Fair Winds Press, 2015

*The People's Pharmacy Quick and Handy
Home Remedies*
Joe and Terry Graedon
National Geographic, 2011

*Vinegar Socks: Traditional Home Remedies
for Modern Living*
Karin Berndl and Nici Hofer
Hardie Grant, 2015

Herbalism
—

*Backyard Medicine: Harvest and
Make Your Own Herbal Remedies*
Julie Bruton-Seal and Matthew Seal
Skyhorse Publishing, 2009

The Complete Herbal Tutor
Anne McIntyre
Gaia Books, 2010

The Complete Herbs Sourcebook
David Hoffman
Sterling, 2013

The Herbal Apothecary
J.J. Pursell
Timber Press, 2015

Herbal Recipes for Vibrant Health
Rosemary Gladstar
Storey Publishing, 2008

*Herbal Remedies: A Practical Beginner's
Guide to Making Effective Remedies
in the Kitchen*
Christopher Hedley and Non Shaw
Parragon, 2002

Aromatherapy
—

*Aromatherapy: A Complete Guide to the
Healing Art*
Kathy Keville and Mindy Green
Crossing Press, 2008

*The Complete Book of Essential Oils and
Aromatherapy*
Valerie Ann Worwood
New World Library, 2016

The Encyclopedia of Essential Oils
Julia Lawless
Conari Press, 2013

Essential Oils
Susan Curtis and Fran Johnson
DK, 2016

The Heart of Aromatherapy
Andrea Butje
Hay House, 2017

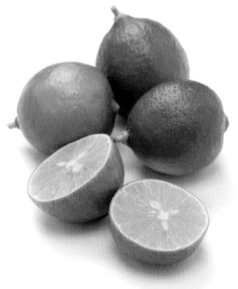

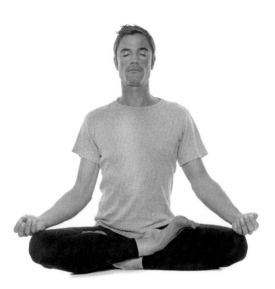

Homeopathy

—

The Complete Homeopathy Handbook
Miranda Castro
St. Martin's Griffin, 1991

Encyclopedia of Homeopathy
Andrew Lockie
DK, 2006

Homeopathy: An A–Z Home Handbook
Alan Schmukler
Llewellyn Publications, 2006

Flower Remedies

—

Bach Flower Remedies Form and Function
Julian Barnard
Lindisfarne Books, 2004

The Bach Remedies Workbook
Stefan Ball
Random House, 2005

Collected Writings of Edward Bach
Dr. Edward Bach
CreateSpace Independent Publishing
Platform, 2016

Flower Essences Plain and Simple
Linda Perry
Hampton Road Publishing, 2017

Heal Thyself
Dr. Edward Bach
Random House, 2004

Nutrition

—

The Complete Guide to Nutrients
Dr. Michael Sharon
Carlton Books, 2014

Healing Foods
Dorling Kindersley
DK, 2013

Prescription for Nutritional Healing
Phyllis A. Balch C.N.C.
Avery, 2010

Raw Energy
Stephanie L. Tourles
Storey Publishing, 2009

The Real Vitamin and Mineral Book
Shari Lieberman and Nancy Pauling Bruning
Avery, 2007

Superfoods
David Wolfe
North Atlantic Books, 2009

Vitamins and Minerals
Sara Rose
Bounty Books, 2016

*The Wisdom and Healing Power
of Whole Foods*
Patrick Quillen
Nutrition Times Press, 2009

Mind–Body Healing

—

*B.K.S. Iyengar Yoga: The Path to
Holistic Health*
B.K.S. Iyengar
DK, 2013

*Breathe: The Simple, Revolutionary
14-Day Program to Improve Your Mental
and Physical Health*
Belisa Vranich
St. Martin's Griffin, 2016

*The Massage Bible: The Definitive Guide to
Soothing Aches and Pains*
Susan Mumford
Sterling, 2009

*Mindfulness: An Eight-Week Plan for Finding
Peace in a Frantic World*
Mark Williams, Danny Penman
and Jon Kabat-Zinn Ph.D.
Rodale Books, 2012

*The Mind Illuminated: A Complete
Meditation Guide*
Culadasa (John Yates Ph.D.), Matthew
Immergut and Jeremy Graves
Touchstone, 2017

Pilates: Body in Motion
Alycea Ungaro
DK, 2002

Yoga Body and Mind Handbook
Jasmine Tarkeshi
Sonoma Press, 2017

GLOSSARY

A
—

abortifacient
an agent that causes the early expulsion of a fetus

abscess
a self-contained pocket of pus that results from a bacterial infection, and causes inflammation of the local area

absolute
a highly concentrated viscous, semi-solid, or solid perfume, usually obtained by alcohol extraction from the concrete

acute
of sudden onset and brief duration

adaptogen
an agent that modulates hormones

adaptogenic
an agent that adapts itself to respond to the body's needs: for example, lavender is adaptogenic and will relax you if you need to be relaxed, or invigorate you if you are tired

adenoids
lymphatic tissue at the back of the nose

adrenal
the adrenal glands are a pair of endocrine glands, each located on the top of one of the kidneys, which secrete hormones that regulate the functions of other organs and systems into the bloodstream

adrenaline
a substance secreted by part of the adrenal gland that increases the heart rate in response to stress

aerophagia
excessive swallowing of air, which may be a response to stress or a consequence of eating too quickly

aggravation
the exacerbation of symptoms that can occur when taking some natural remedies, particularly in the case of chronic ailments

agni
meaning "fire," or the forces which break down substances consumed; in Indian medicine, considered to be metabolism

agoraphobia
fear of open or crowded places

alcohols
a group of chemical compounds with antiseptic, antiviral, and uplifting properties

aldehydes
chemicals that have a sedative and sometimes anti-inflammatory effect

aldosterone
the steroid hormone which helps the body to control water balance

-algia (suffix)
meaning "pain in;" for example, arthralgia, pain in the joints

allergen
a substance that causes an allergic reaction

allergy
an abnormal response by the body to a food or foreign substance

allopathic
Western medicinal treatment, based on treating symptoms rather than the underlying condition

alopecia
hereditary hair loss

alterative
corrects disordered body functions, works according to the needs of the body. Often used in the same way as "adaptogenic"

ama
in Ayurveda, a toxic substance believed to gather in the weak parts of the body and cause disease. Ama occurs when the metabolism is impaired due to an imbalance of agni

amenorrhea
absence of menses (menstrual periods)

analgesic
pain-relieving

anaphrodisiac
reduces sexual desire

anaphylaxis
an extreme allergic reaction to a foreign substance. Subsequent exposure can produce an overwhelming body reaction called anaphylactic shock

anemia
deficiency in either quality or quantity of red corpuscles in the blood

anodyne
painkilling

anorexia nervosa
psychological problem causing extreme loss of appetite, drastic weight loss, and, sometimes in severe cases, death

anosmia
loss of the sense of smell. It can be either temporary or permanent

antacid
a remedy or medicine that reduces stomach acidity

anthelmintic
a vermifuge, destroying or expelling intestinal worms

anthraquinone
a powerful laxative which can cause diarrhea and intestinal cramps

antiallergic
an agent that helps to reduce allergic reactions

antiarthritic
an agent that combats arthritis

antibacterial
acts against bacteria, an agent that prevents bacteria forming, e.g. penicillin

antibilious
an agent that helps remove excess bile from the body

antibiotic
an agent that prevents the growth of, or destroys, bacteria

antibody
a chemical produced by the body's immune system to attack what it considers to be an invader, e.g. a bacterium, virus, or allergen

anticarcinogenic
an agent that acts to prevent or treat the development or spread of cancer

anticatarrhal
an agent that helps remove excess catarrh from the body

anticonvulsant
an agent that helps arrest or prevent convulsions

antidepressant
an agent that relieves depression

antidiarrheal
an agent that prevents or treats diarrhea

antidote
the term used to describe substances that nullify the effect of a prescribed remedy

anti-emetic
an agent that reduces the incidence and severity of nausea or vomiting

antifungal
an agent that works to prevent the spread and incidence of fungal conditions

antihistamine
an agent that prevents or treats a histamine reaction (see "Allergies," page 344)

antihypertensive
an agent that works to lower blood pressure

anti-infective
any agent that works to prevent or halt the spread of infection

anti-inflammatory
reducing inflammation

antimicrobial
acts against infection, particularly bacterial infection

antioxidant
a substance that prevents cell degeneration and decay

antiseborrheic
helps to control the production of sebum from sweat glands

antiseptic
helps to counter infection, by fighting bacteria

antispasmodic
prevents contractions of the muscles, or alleviates spasms and cramp

antiviral
inhibits the spread of viruses

aperitif
a stimulant to the appetite

aphrodisiac
increases or stimulates sexual desire; said to be a sexual stimulant that increases vitality

aromatherapy
the therapeutic use of essential oils

aromatic
a substance with a strong aroma or smell

arteriosclerosis
hardening of the arteries

articulation
range of movement of the joints

asthma
spasm of the bronchi in the lungs, narrowing the airways

astringent
constricts the blood vessels or membranes in order to reduce irritation, inflammation, and swelling, has a binding and contracting effect, usually on the mucous membrane, to give it a protective coating against irritants or infective organisms, also one of the six tastes in Ayurveda, found in potatoes, beans, and witch hazel

athma
in Indian medicine, the unique, individual spirit which occupies the body and which is transferred to another body after death

atopic
persons with allergies are often called atopic. The common atopies include hay fever; asthma; infantile eczema, which is an itchy skin lesion; contact dermatitis, which is a skin inflammation caused by poison ivy or a variety of chemicals that may contact the skin; and perhaps some food or drug allergies

aura
every person, animal, and plant is said to have a visible aura, or magnetic field. These are said to indicate the state of health, emotions, mind, and spirit

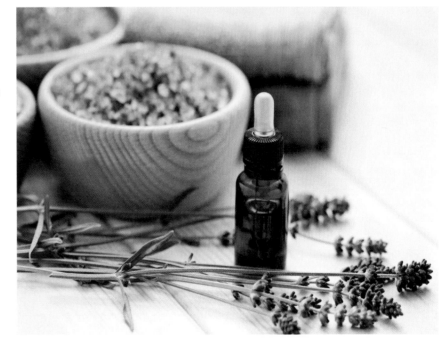

autogenic discharge
sensations or muscle movements that accompany the release of stored tensions

autoimmune disorder
occurs when the body creates antibodies against itself and attacks healthy cells

B
—
bactericidal
an agent that destroys bacteria (a type of microbe or organism)

balsam
a resinous semi-solid mass or viscous liquid exuded from a plant, which can be either a pathological or a physiological product. A "true" balsam is characterized by its high content of benzoic acid, benzoates, cinnamic acid, or cinnamates

balsamic
a soothing medicine or application having the qualities of a balsam

benign
of a tumor, not cancerous or otherwise dangerous

bile
thick, oily fluid excreted by the liver, bile helps the body digest fats

biliousness
disorder of bile production (to excess)

biofeedback
a process using electronic monitoring of a bodily function in order to train a person to gain voluntary control of that function

bioflavonoids
also called vitamin P, bioflavonoids are widely found in food plants, where they impart color to flowers, leaves, and stems. There are at least 500 naturally occurring varieties, and they are said to strengthen or preserve the integrity of the veins, among other things

biopsy
removal of fluid or tissue from the body for examination

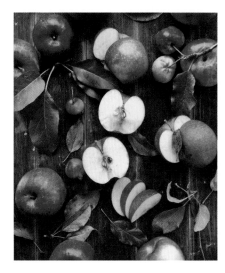

bitter
a tonic component that stimulates the appetite and promotes the secretion of saliva and gastric juices by exciting the taste buds/ one of the six Ayurvedic tastes; found in barks, tannins, and resins

blepharospasm
a twitch or tic in which there is spasmodic closure of one or both eyes

Blood
in Chinese medicine, "Blood" has a specialized meaning

bronchio-dilator
a substance which dilates the bronchi, the tubes of the lungs

bursa
a small fluid-filled sac

C
—
calcul
a kidney stone

calmative
a sedative agent

Candida
Candida albicans, a fungus affecting the mucous membranes and skin, causes thrush

carbuncle
a bacterial infection of the skin, an interconnected group of boils that have many perforations, through which pus drains

carcinogenic
an agent that can cause cancer; cancer-causing

carcinoma
a cancerous tumor

cardiac
pertaining to the heart

cardioactive
an agent that stimulates heart activity

cardiotonic
having a stimulating effect on the heart

carminative
settles the digestive system and relieves flatulence

cathartic
an agent that purges the body, usually the intestine, and cleanses the system

cautery
burning tissue in the body

centesimal scale (c)
in homeopathy, the scale that measures the potency of remedies in hundredths. One drop of mother tincture is mixed with 99 drops of water or alcohol to make a remedy of 1c potency. This remedy is then diluted with a further 99 drops of water or alcohol to make a remedy of 2c potency. The sequence is repeated: 200c is usually the highest dose. The more the remedy is diluted, the more powerful it becomes

cephalic
remedy for problems relating to the head

cerebrovascular accident (CVA)
another term for stroke

chakras
in Eastern medicine, circles which are thought to be found along the mid-line of the body, in line with the spinal column

channels
invisible pathways in which qi (or chi) travels; also called meridians. They appear in and on the body

chelated

of mineral supplements, means that the mineral is combined with amino acids to make assimilation more efficient

chi (or qi)

the life force of the body, which circulates through its meridians or channels

chlamydia

a sexually transmitted disease caused by parasitic bacteria

cholagogue

an agent that stimulates the secretion and flow of bile into the duodenum

cholesterol

a steroid alcohol found in nervous tissue, red blood cells, animal fat, and bile. Excess can lead to gallstones

chronic

persisting for a long time, a state showing no change or very slow change

cicatrizant

an agent that promotes healing by the formation of scar tissue

coagulate

an agent that acts to clot or thicken the blood

cognitive behavioral therapy

a type of psychotherapy in which negative patterns of thought are challenged with the aim of altering unwanted behavior patterns or treating mood disorders

complementary

the term used to describe alternative forms of medical treatment – emphasizing the fact that they support rather than replace orthodox medicine

compress

a lint or pad that is soaked in hot or cold substances and applied to the body for relief of swelling and pain, or to produce localized pressure

concomitant

in homeopathy, a symptom coming at the same time, but not directly related to, the main complaint

concrete

a concentrated, waxy, solid, or semi-solid perfume material prepared from previously live plant matter, usually a hydrocarbon type of solvent

congestion

abnormal accumulation of blood

constitutional

homeopathic term relating to the physical and mental constitution of a person, including hereditary factors and underlying health issues

contraindication

any factor in a patient's condition that indicates that treatment would involve a greater than normal risk and is therefore not recommended

cordial

a stimulant and tonic

corticosteroids

adrenal cortico hormones. There are two classes of corticosteroids. The glucocorticoids such as cortisone primarily affect carbohydrate and protein metabolism. They have limited use in the treatment of many immunologic and allergic diseases, such as arthritis. The mineralocorticoids such as aldosterone principally regulate salt and water balance. Synthetic steroids include anti-inflammatory drugs, oral contraceptives, and a synthetic adrenal steroid used to treat Addison's disease

cortisol

the steroid hormone which helps the body to react to stress

coryza

profuse discharge from the mucous membranes of the nose – "common cold"

counseling

the provision of professional assistance and guidance in resolving personal or psychological problems

counter-irritant

an application to the skin that relieves deep-seated pain, usually applied in the form of heat; see also rubefacient

D
—

dan tien

energy centers in the body. In traditional Chinese medicine there are considered to be three: an upper (between the eyebrows), a middle (in the center of the trunk), and a lower (the lower abdomen). Qi is stored here

decimal scale (x)

in homeopathy, the scale that measures the potency of remedies in tenths. One drop of mother tincture is mixed with nine drops of water or alcohol to make a remedy of 1x potency. This remedy is then diluted with a further nine drops of water or alcohol to make a remedy of 2x potency. The sequence is repeated. The more the remedy is diluted, the more powerful it becomes

decoction

a herbal preparation, where the plant material (usually hard or woody) is boiled in water and reduced to make a concentrated extract

decongestant

an agent for the relief or reduction of congestion, e.g. congestion of the mucous membranes

decongestive

relieves or reduces mucus congestion

deficient

condition in Chinese medicine, any disorder that is caused by the body's inability to maintain balance, through improper function of the zangfu

degenerative

a condition in which there is irreversible and progressive decomposition

demulcent

an agent that protects mucous membranes and allays irritation

depurgative

cleanses the blood

detoxificant/detoxifier

an agent that acts to detoxify, or remove toxins from the body

detoxification
external and internal cleaning of the body, the removal of toxins from the body

dhatus
in Indian medicine, seven essential tissues which make up the body

dialogue
discussion on how habitual ideas and emotions can affect your mind, body, and spirit

diaphoretic
an agent that causes sweating

digestive
an agent that promotes or aids the digestion of food

digoxin
a glycoside isolated from the dried leaves of the foxglove plant. It is prescribed to millions of patients suffering from cardiac problems such as rapid atrial fibrillation or heart failure

dina chariya
a daily program recommended by Ayurveda for healthy living

discharge
an excretion or substance evacuated from the body

diuretic
an agent that aids production of urine, promotes urination, or increases flow, reducing the fluid level of the body

DNA
deoxyribonucleic acid, a chemical which makes up our chromosomes

doshas
the three basic constitutional types in Indian medicine – vátha, pitta, and kapha – which are known as the "tridoshas"

douche
a substance used internally to cleanse or treat the vagina

drawing
draws poisons out from boils and from abscesses etc.

dysfunction
abnormal functioning of a system or organ within the body

dysmenorrhea
severe pains accompanying the menstrual period

dyspepsia
difficulty with digestion associated with pain, flatulence, heartburn, and nausea

dyspnea
labored or difficult breathing

E
—

ectomorph
one of three basic body types, characterized by thinness and weakness

ectopic
a pregnancy that occurs at a site other than inside the uterus, such as in the Fallopian tube, on the ovary, or at sites outside the abdomen, is termed ectopic

edema
a painless swelling caused by fluid retention beneath the skin's surface

EFAs
essential fatty acids

effleurage
slow, rhythmic massage

eight principal patterns
in Chinese medicine, the system of organizing diagnostic information according to the principles of yin, yang, interior, exterior, cold, hot, excess, and deficiency

emetic
an agent that induces vomiting

emmenagogue
an agent that induces or assists menstruation

emollient
an agent that softens and soothes the skin

Empty Heat
Internal Heat in the body resulting from a yin deficiency

endocrine
the endocrine system consists of specialized glands located in different parts of the body. These glands secrete chemical substances called hormones, which transfer information from one set of cells to another

endometriosis
a common disease in women of reproductive age. It involves tissues of the endometrium, the inner lining of the uterus. During the menstrual cycle, built-up endometrial tissues normally are shed if pregnancy does not occur. In many women some endometrial cells escape from the womb into the pelvic cavity, where they attach themselves and continue their hormone-stimulated growth cycle. They may also migrate to remote parts of the body

endomorph
one of the three basic body types, characterized by roundness, fatness, and heaviness

endorphins
a group of chemicals manufactured in the brain that influence the body's response to pain

engorgement
congestion of a part of the tissues, or fullness (as in the breasts)

enuresis
bedwetting

enzyme
complex proteins that are produced by the living cells and catalyze specific biochemical reactions

epidural
epidural anesthesia involves depositing anesthetic into the epidural space of the vertebral canal

epigastric
above the navel

epigastrium
the area above the navel

episiotomy
an incision made in the perineum (the area between the anus and the vagina) to prevent tearing while delivering a baby

esophagitis
inflammation of the lining of the esophagus

essence
the pure energy extracted from food that is transformed into qi by the body. Also the integral part of a plant, its life force, as used in flower remedies, herbalism, and aromatherapy

essential oil
a volatile and aromatic liquid (sometimes semi-solid) which generally constitutes the odorous principles of a plant. It is obtained by a process of expression or distillation from a single botanical form or species. A pure, concentrated essence taken from the plant; said to be its life force

esters
chemical compounds that are fungicidal and sedative

estrogen
a hormone produced by the ovary and necessary for the development of female secondary sexual characteristics

etiology
the science of the cause of illness and disease

excess condition
a condition in which qi, blood, or body fluids are imbalanced, accumulating in parts of the body

expectorant
promotes the removal of mucus from the respiratory system

expectoration
coughing up

external
in Chinese medicine, any factors influencing the body from the outside

exudative
a substance or agent that causes something to exude; for example, a warm compress

would cause infection or pus to exude from a boil or wound

F
—
fast
abstention from all or most foods for a given period

febrifuge
an agent that combats fever

febrile
feverish

feces
excrement, stools

fever
elevation of body temperature above normal (98.4°F/36.8°C)

five elements
the system in Chinese medicine based on observations of the natural world. Built around the elements of fire, water, wood, metal, and earth

fixative
a material that slows down the rate of evaporation of the more volatile components in the composition of a perfume

fixed oil
the name given to a vegetable oil obtained from plants that, in contradistinction to essential oils, is fatty, dense, and nonvolatile, such as olive or sweet almond oil

flavonoids
antioxidants which act on the immune system

fomentation
a hot compress

four levels
the system of diagnosis in traditional Chinese medicine

friction
small circular movements often used in massage

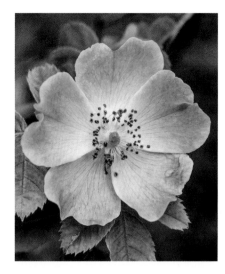

fu
hollow yang organs in the body

fungicidal
an agent that combats fungal infection

fungicide
attacks fungal infestations

G
—
galactagogue
an agent that increases the secretion of milk

gan
sweet, used to assign taste to Chinese herbs

ganglion
swelling within a tendon or joint, also a group of nerves

gas exchange
the exchange of water carbon dioxide in the blood for fresh oxygen, it takes place in the alveoli of the lungs

generals
in homeopathy, symptoms relating to the whole person that can be expressed "I am…"; compare particulars

germicidal
destroys germs or micro-organisms such as bacteria

ghee
milk or butter fat, clarified by boiling and used in Indian cooking

giardiasis
an infectious parasite that attacks the gastrointestinal tract

giennial
a plant that completes its life-cycle in two years, without flowering in the first year

gliadin
a protein from wheat and rye cereals

gluten
a protein from wheat and other cereals

gum
"true" gum is little used in perfumery, being virtually odorless. However, the term "gum" is often applied to "resins," especially with relation to turpentines, as in the Australian "gum tree." Strictly speaking, gums are natural or synthetic water-soluble materials, such as gum arabic

gunas
in Ayurvedic medicine, characteristics which can be attributed to all matter, organic and inorganic, and to thoughts and ideas

H
—

halitosis
bad breath

hallucinogenic
causes visions or delusions

harmonize
to balance, or encourage something, such as the body, to work in harmony, with all systems at optimum level

hematoma
a collection of blood

hemorrhage
loss of blood

hemorrhoids
piles, anal varicose veins

hemostatic
stops the flow of blood, a type of astringent that stops internal bleeding or hemorrhaging

hepatic
relating to the liver, an agent that tones the liver and aids its function

herniate
to rupture, or burst out, a slipped disk herniates

holistic
aiming to treat the individual as an entity, incorporating body, mind, and spirit, from the Greek word holos, meaning whole

homeopathy
medical therapy devised by the 19th-century German doctor Samuel Hahnemann, based on the premise that like cures like, sick people are given minute doses of a remedy that will cause the symptoms of their disease, which may help the body to cure itself

homeostasis
the tendency of the internal environment of the body to remain constant in spite of varying external conditions

hormone
a product of living cells that produces a specific effect on the activity cells remote from its point of origin

humors
the four body fluids (blood, phlegm, choler, and melancholy) which are believed to determine emotional and physical disposition, in Chinese medicine

hybrid
a plant originating by fertilization of one species or subspecies by another

hypercalcemia
calcium deposits in the kidneys

hyperglycemia
a condition characterized by an abnormally high level of glucose (sugar) in the bloodstream

hyperhidrosis
excessive sweating caused by overactive sweat glands

hypermetropia
long-sightedness

hyperparathyroidism
secretion of parathyroid hormone resulting from a tumor, enlargement, or cancer of the thyroid glands

hypertension
raised blood pressure

hypertensive
raises blood pressure

hypnotherapy
the use of hypnosis as a therapeutic technique

hypnotic
causing sleep

hypoglycemia
a condition characterized by an abnormally low level of glucose (sugar) in the bloodstream

hypotension
low blood pressure, or a fall in blood pressure below the normal range

hypotensive
lowers blood pressure

I
—

immunodeficiency
a deficiency of immune activity

immune-stimulant
an agent that stimulates immune activity, and the immune system

immunosuppressive
an agent or condition that suppresses the immune system, and normal or excessive immune activity

incontinence
partial or complete loss of control of urination

infection
multiplication of pathogenic (disease-producing) micro-organisms within the body

inflammation
protective tissue response to injury or destruction of body cells characterized by heat, swelling, redness, and usually pain

infusion
liquid obtained from steeping a herb in hot or cold water

inhalant
a remedy or drug that is breathed in through the nose or mouth

insecticidal
an agent that repels or kills insects

insomnia
inability to sleep

internal
refers to aspects of disharmonies that arise within the body, in Chinese medicine

-itis
(suffix) "inflammation of"; for example, arthritis, inflammation of the joints

J
—

jin ye
body fluids – jin refers to the lighter fluids, and ye refers to the denser ones

jing
the essence of all life in the body – the energy that governs our development

jingluo
Chinese term for the channels, or meridians, which run invisibly through the body, carrying the qi, or life force

K
—

kapha
the moon force, which is a basic life force or element in Ayurvedic medicine

ketogenic diet
a diet which is high in fat and very low in carbohydrates

ketones
chemical compounds that ease congestion and aid the flow of mucus

ku
bitter, a term used to describe the taste of Chinese herbs

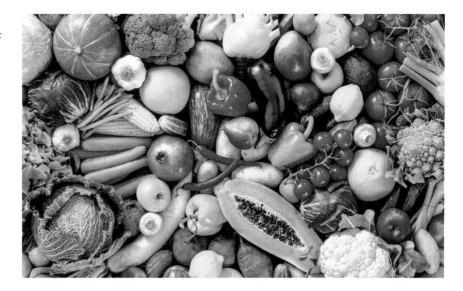

kundalini
an energy which is believed to travel upwards through the chakras, promoting spiritual knowledge

L
—

lactagogue
a substance which encourages the production of milk in the breasts

laxative
a substance that provokes evacuation of the bowels

legume
a fruit or vegetable consisting of one carpel, opening on one side, such as a pea. Also called a pulse

lesion
a term used to describe an abnormality in or damage to the body

leucocyte
white blood cells responsible for fighting disease

leukorrhea
vaginal discharge

liniment
a warming rub, often made by mixing tinctures with herbal infused oils

lithotrophic
dispels stones

liverishness
a term used to describe inadequate liver function

lymph
a colorless fluid which contains mainly white blood cells, which are collected from the tissues of the body and transported through the lymphatic system

lymphatic
pertaining to the lymphatic system. A lymphatic remedy would encourage the flow of lymph

M
—

macerate
soak or pound until soft

mahabbutas
a Sanskrit term for the elements

malas
in Indian medicine, waste products of the body, including feces, urine, and sweat

malignant
cancerous and possibly life-threatening

mammograph
an X-ray technique used to aid in the diagnosis of breast cancer in women

MAOI
a type of antidepressant drug known as monoamine oxidase inhibitors

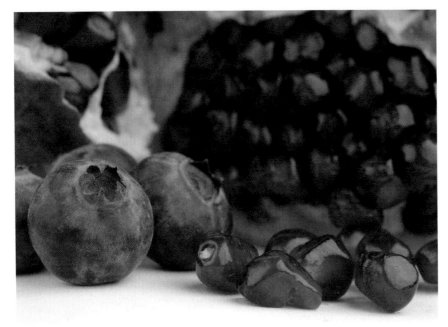

mantra
a syllable, word, or phrase which may
be spoken aloud and repeated as an aid
to meditation

marma puncture
in Ayurvedic medicine, the technique of
inserting a needle into the marma points
for certain treatments

marmas
in Ayurvedic medicine, energy points in
the body where two or more important
functions meet

marrow
in traditional Chinese medicine, the
substance that makes up the brain and
spinal column

materia medica
a branch of science dealing with the
origins and properties of remedies,
a complete description of remedies
suggested in therapies such as
homeopathy and herbalism

medicated oil
an oil produced by steeping herbs
or flowers for one or more months,
then straining

meditation
exercising the mind in contemplation, with
the aim of calming the thoughts

meninges
the membranes that cover the brain and
spinal cord

menopause
the normal cessation of menstruation,
a life change for women

menorrhagia
an excess loss of blood occurring
during menstruation

mentals
in homeopathy, symptoms relating to the
mental state, mood, and ideas

meridians
in traditional Chinese medicine,
channels that run through the body,
beneath the skin, in which the life
force, or qi, is carried. There are
14 main meridians running to and
from the hands and feet to the body
and head

mesomorph
one of the three basic body types,
characterized by a muscular physique
and prominent bone structure

metabolism
the complex process that is the fundamental
chemical expression of life itself, and the
means by which food is converted to energy
to maintain the body

metrorrhagia
bleeding that occurs in the middle of the
menstrual cycle

microbe
a minute living organism, especially
pathogenic bacteria, viruses, etc.

micronutrients
vitamins, minerals, and other health-giving
components of our food, such as amino
acids, fiber, enzymes, and lipids

micturation
involuntary leakage of urine during
coughing, sneezing, laughing, or
muscular effort

modality
in homeopathy, the factor that makes
symptoms better or worse

mother tincture
in homeopathy or flower remedies,
the source remedy, which is diluted to
make the therapeutic dosages prescribed
by practitioners

moxa
dried mugwort, which is burned on the
end of needles or rolled into a stick, and
then heated in moxabustion. It is said to
warm the qi in the body in order to
increase its flow

moxabustion
see moxa

moxides
a group of chemical compounds with
expectorant properties

mucilage
a substance containing gelatinous
constituents that are demulcent

mucilaginous
a substance that encourages the body
to create more mucus

mucolytic
a substance that thins mucus

mucous membranes
surface linings of the body, which
secrete mucus

musculoskeletal
anything pertaining to the muscles and bones (skeletal system) of the body

myopia
short-sightedness

N
—

narcotic
an agent that induces sleep, intoxicating or poisonous in large doses

nasya
in Ayurveda, inhalation of oils

naturopathy
treatment based on using natural agents and forces to bring about a cure. The naturopath tends to rely on natural products such as herbs and vitamins, rather than on synthetic drugs and surgery, and may also employ manipulation (such as osteopathy) and electrical treatments

nervine
strengthening and toning to the nerves and nervous system

noradrenaline
a hormone secreted by the adrenal gland

nosode
in homeopathy, a remedy made from a diseased source, for example, tuberculinum, made from tissue infected with tuberculosis

nutritive
a substance that promotes nutrition

nystagmus
abnormal, jerky movements of the eyes

O
—

occupational therapy
the use of particular activities, professional advice on lifestyle, and provision of physical aids, to help with recuperation from physical or mental illness

oja
in Indian medicine, the ultimate vital energy that runs through the system

oleo gum resin
a natural exudation from trees and plants that consists mainly of essential oil, gum, and resin

oleoresin
a natural resinous exudation from plants, or an aromatic liquid preparation extracted from botanical matter using solvents. It consists almost entirely of a mixture of essential oil and resin

onycholysis
detachment of the nail from its bed

oophorectomy
removal of the ovaries

opacification
becoming opaque

orchitis
inflammation of the testes

orthodox
a term used to describe conventional medicine

overbreathing
breathing too quickly and too shallowly

P
—

palindromic
something which can be read the same when taken in reverse order

palpation
examination with the hands

panacea
a cure-all

panchakarma
in Ayurveda, internal cleansing, which consists of five forms of therapy, including vomiting, purging, two types of enema, and nasal inhalation. It is said to prevent disease and to rebalance vitality

parainfluenza
a type of cold virus

parasiticide
prevents and destroys parasites

paronychia
an infection of the soft tissue around the nail, usually as a result of repeated minor injury, causing pain, swelling and inflammation. Pus may sometimes appear at the edge of the nail

particulars
in homeopathy, symptoms relating to a part of the person that can be expressed "My..."; compare generals

parturient
encouraging the onset of labor

pasteurized
heat treated to destroy harmful micro-organisms

pathogenic
referring to any disease-causing agent

peculiars
in homeopathy, strange, rare, and peculiar symptoms which relate to the individual and are not common in illness

peptic
a term applied to gastric secretions and areas affected by them

percussion
vigorous drumming massage

pericarditis
inflammation of the pericardium of the heart

perineal
pertaining to the perineum, the area between the anus and the genital organs

periodontitis
loosening of a tooth, often caused by gingivitis

peristalsis
rhythmic movement of the gut to push food along the intestinal tract

pessary
a treatment that is inserted into the vagina or anus

petrissage
kneading massage movement

pharmacopeia
an official publication of drugs in common use in a given country

phenols
a group of chemical compounds with bactericidal and stimulating properties, they can be irritants

phlegm
in traditional Chinese medicine, a disharmony of the body fluids produces either external (or visible) phlegm or internal (or invisible) phlegm, thick, shiny mucus produced in the respiratory passage

photosensitivity
a sensitivity to light

phototoxic
a substance that becomes poisonous on exposure to light

phthalides
chemicals which have a sedative effect and can ease insomnia

physical therapy
also known as physiotherapy; the treatment of disease or injury through massage, heat treatment, and exercise

phytotherapy
the treatment of disease by plants, herbal medicine

Pilates
a system of exercises, some using apparatus, designed to improve physical strength, flexibility, and posture, and to enhance mental awareness

pitta
in Ayurvedic medicine, the sun force, or one of the three basic life forces or elements controlling all physical and mental processes

placebo
a medicine or procedure prescribed for the psychological benefit to the patient rather than for any physiological effect

plasma
the clear, yellowish fluid part of blood or lymph in which cells are suspended

polyphenols
antioxidants which have beneficial effects on the circulatory system

postnatal
following delivery of a baby, after pregnancy; also called postpartum

potencized
diluted to homeopathic prescription

potency
the dilution of a homeopathic remedy; the higher the number, the higher the strength, and the greater the dilution

potentiate
in homeopathy, to shake a remedy to increase its potency

poultice
the therapeutic application of a soft moist mass (such as fresh herbs) to the skin to encourage local circulation and to relieve pain

prakruti
in Ayurvedic medicine, a person's individual constitution, determined by their "dosha" type

prana
the vital energy that runs through our bodies, in Ayurvedic medicine, also known as our life force

pranayama
the breathing exercises associated with yoga

priapism
prolonged penile erection, usually without sexual desire

progesterone
a female sex hormone that prepares the uterus for the fertilized ovum and maintains pregnancy

prolapse
the sinking or falling-down of an organ – usually the term refers to the vagina or uterus

prophylactic
preventive of disease or infection

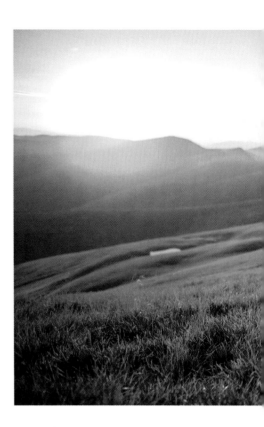

prostaglandins
hormone-like substances that occur in tissues and organs of the human body. They affect several body systems, including the central nervous, cardiovascular, gastrointestinal, urinary, and endocrine systems

prostatitis
inflammation of the prostate gland

proving
the process used in homeopathy for testing a remedy; it can occur when the wrong remedy is prescribed and taken over a period of time, and the symptoms of the condition it is aimed at manifest themselves

psychogenic
symptoms or conditions of mental rather than physical origin

psychosomatic illness
the manifestation of physical symptoms resulting from a mental state

psychotherapy
the use of psychological methods, usually based on regular personal interaction, to help a person overcome psychological problems

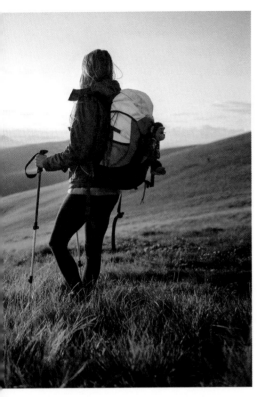

purgative
an agent stimulating evacuation of
the bowels

purines
nitrogenous compounds in nucleic
acids found in foods including caffeine,
anchovies, fish roe, sweetbreads and other
organ meats. People who have difficulty
metabolizing purines may be prone to gout

purulent
containing pus

purvakarma
in Ayurveda, a cleansing process involving
oil and steam bath therapy

pustular
referring to elevated skin containing pus

pyorrhea
any condition characterized by discharge
of pus

Q
—

qi (chi)
the essential energy of the universe which
is fundamental to all elements of life.

It runs through the whole body in channels
or meridians

qi ni
rebellious qi, which moves in the
wrong direction

qi xian
sinking qi, which is too deficient to perform
its holding function

qi zhi
stagnant qi that is sluggish and not
moving efficiently

R
—

rajasic
in Ayurveda, energy-producing

rasayana
the branch of Ayurveda which
involves rejuvenation

RDA
recommended daily allowance

RDI
recommended daily intake

rectification
the process of redistillation applied
to essential oils to rid them of
certain constituents

referred pain
pain that is felt in a different part of the
body from the area that is actually affected

regulator
an agent that helps balance and regulates
the functions of the body

rejuvenative
to invigorate, bring back to life or to the
optimum level of functioning, to give new
youth or restore vitality

relaxant
a substance that promotes relaxation (either
muscular or psychological)

remedy picture
in homeopathy, the collection of symptoms
that characterize a remedy

remission
a period in which the symptoms of a disease
abate or lessen

ren
the Chinese meridian that runs down the
front of the body, from the lower lip to
behind the genitalia

resin
a natural or prepared product, either
solid or semi-solid in nature. Natural
resins are exudations from trees,
such as mastic; prepared resins are
oleoresins from which essential oil has
been removed

resolvent
an agent that disperses swelling or effects
absorption of a new growth

restorative
an agent that helps strengthen and
revive the body systems, usually
strengthening and promoting wellbeing
after illness

rhinitis
inflammation (often chronic) of the mucous
membranes lining the nasal passage

rhizome
an underground plant stem lasting more
than one season

Rishis
wise and holy men of ancient India who
meditated and acquired the knowledge
that was codified as Ayurveda

RNA
ribonucleic acid, or RNA, is needed in
all organisms in order for protein synthesis
to occur. It is also the genetic material of
some viruses, which are referred to as
RNA viruses

rubefacient
a mild irritant which causes redness of
the skin

S
—

salpingitis
infection of the Fallopian tubes

salty
one of the six Ayurvedic tastes, found in rock salt, seaweed, sea salt, and vegetables

salve
a mixture of beeswax with vegetable oil used to preserve herbs and spices

samagni
in Ayurvedic medicine, a balanced appetite, when digestion, absorption, and metabolism function efficiently

san jiao
the triple warmer/heat/burner which is a process organ in the Chinese zangfu system

Sanskrit
ancient Indian language, sacred to Hinduism. Ayurveda was written in Sanskrit

saponins
chemicals which may affect red blood cells

sclerosis
hardening of tissue due to inflammation

seborrheic
involving the sebaceous glands, which secrete sebum into the hair follicles and onto most of the body surface

sebum
an oily, lubricating and protective substance

sedative
an agent that reduces functional activity; calming

self-limiting
a condition that lasts a set length of time and usually clears of its own accord

septic
putrefying due to the presence of pathogenic (disease-producing) bacteria

serotonin
a neurotransmitter in the brain which regulates and induces sleep, and is also said to reduce sensitivity to pain

shad rasa
the six basic food tastes identified by Ayurveda: sweet, acidic, salty, pungent, bitter, and astringent

shen
in Chinese medicine, an important aspect of mind or spirit, the spirit of the person

shiatsu
a type of massage that works on pressure points of the body

shock
sudden and disturbing mental or physical impression, also a state of collapse characterized by pale, cold, sweaty skin, rapid, weak, thready pulse, faintness, dizziness, and nausea

sialogogue
an agent that stimulates the secretion of saliva

six stage patterns
a Chinese diagnostic system

soft tissues
tissues of the body, including muscles, tendons, ligaments, and organs

soporific
an agent that induces sleep, sleep-inducing

sour
one of the six Ayurvedic tastes; found in fats, amino acids, fermented products, fruits, and vegetables

spasm
sudden, violent, involuntary muscular contraction

specific
remedy effective for a particular ailment

spermatorrhea
leaking of sperm

spermicidal
an agent or substance which acts to kill sperm

splenomegaly
abnormal enlargement of the spleen

spondylosis
progressive disease of the spine

sputum
spit

stagnant
when the flow of chi, or qi, is blocked in the meridians

STD
sexually transmitted disease

steroids
fat-soluble organic compounds that occur naturally throughout the plant and animal kingdoms and play many important functional roles

stimulant
increases activity in specific organs or systems of the body, warms and increases energy

stomachic
an agent that stimulates the functioning of the stomach

stroma
connective tissue that forms the foundation of the breast

stye
an infection of the follicle of an eyelash or of a sebaceous gland of an eyelid

styptic
an astringent agent that stops or reduces external bleeding

suan
sour, a description of taste for Chinese herbs

subclinical symptoms
symptoms which are not gross enough to be considered precursors to or evidence of clinically diagnosed disease

subfertility
below-normal fertility

succussion
the shaking method used in preparing homeopathic remedies

sweet
one of the six Ayurvedic tastes, found in sugar, carbohydrates, and dairy products

symptom picture
homeopathic term for the overall pattern of

symptoms characterizing each
individual patient

symptomatology
the study and interpretation of symptoms

symptoms
perceived changes in, or impaired function
of, body or mind indicating the presence of
disease or injury

synovial
referring to the fluid that bathes the joints

synthesization
to become synthesized, or amalgamated

T
—

tachycardia
an unduly rapid heartbeat

talking therapy
a method of treating psychological
disorders or emotional difficulties that
involves talking to a therapist or counselor,
in individual or group sessions

TCM
Traditional Chinese medicine

tenesmus
a spasm of the rectum where one feels the
need to defecate without being able to

terpenes
chemical constituents with anti-inflammatory
and bactericidal properties

tincture
a herbal remedy prepared in an
alcohol base

tisane
a type of herbal infusion, usually drunk as
a tea

tissue salt
an inorganic compound essential to the
growth and function of the body's cells

tonic
restores tone to the systems, balances, and
nourishes; strengthens and enlivens the
whole or specific parts of the body

tonification
a process in Chinese medicine that
involves strengthening and supporting
the Blood and qi

tonify
to tone or balance, in traditional
Chinese medicine, to strengthen
and support

topical
local application of cream, ointment,
tincture, or other medicine

topical irritant
a substance that irritates the skin

torticollis
wry neck

toxin
a substance that is poisonous to the body

trauma
a physical injury or wound, also an
unpleasant and disturbing experience
causing psychological upset

trigeminal nerve
a nerve that divides into three and supplies
the mandibular (jaw), maxillary (cheek),
ophthalmic (eye), and forehead areas

tuber
a swollen part of an underground plant
stem of one year's duration, capable of
new growth

type
a term used by Bach and other flower
remedy therapists to describe a person's
general personality and approach to life.
Also used by homeopaths to refer to a
constitutional picture which relates to a
particular remedy

U
—

ulcer
slow-healing sore occurring internally
or externally

ureteric
referring to the ureter, the tube that carries
urine from the kidneys to the bladder

urethral
referring to the urethra, the canal that
carries urine from the bladder out of
the body

uterine tonic
a substance that has a toning effect on
the whole reproductive system, in particular
the uterus

V
—

vaginitis
inflammation or infection of the vagina

vasoconstrictor
an agent that causes narrowing of the
blood vessels

vasodilator
an agent that dilates the blood vessels and
so improves circulation

vátha
the wind force in Ayurvedic medicine – one
of the three basic life forces or elements
that must be in balance for physical and
mental processes to be balanced

Vedic
relating to the Vedas, the ancient, sacred
literature of Hinduism

vermifuge
an anthelmintic remedy that kills worms and
intestinal parasites

verruca
a plantar wart

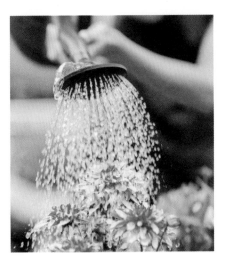

vesicant
causing blistering to the skin

vibrational medicine
any medicine which treats the body on a vibrational or "energy" level, such as homeopathy and flower essence therapy, based on the theory that we are all dense bodies of energy, and by taking substances that adjust that energy, we can effect a cure

virulent
extremely infective, or with a violent effect

volatile
unstable, evaporates easily

vulnerary
an agent that helps heal wounds and sores by external application; assists in the healing of wounds by protecting against infection and stimulating cell growth

vulval
relating to the vulva

W
—

warming
any agent which warms the body, usually by increasing circulation or the flow of qi

wei qi
defensive qi, which protects the body from invasion by external pathogenic factors. It flows just beneath the skin

X
—

xian
salty; a description of taste for Chinese herbs

xin
acrid, a description of taste for Chinese herbs

xu
deficiency, a common disharmony in Chinese medicine

Y
—

yang
one aspect of the complementary aspects in Chinese philosophy; reflects the active, moving, and warmer aspects

yin
one aspect of the complementary aspects in Chinese philosophy; reflects the passive, still, reflective aspects

yin/yang
Chinese philosophy that explains the interdependence of all elements of nature. These contrasting aspects of the body and mind must be balanced before health and wellbeing can be achieved. Yin is the female force, and yang is the male

ying qi
nutritive aspects of qi that nourish the body

yoga
a Hindu spiritual discipline, part of which, including breathing control, meditation, and the adoption of bodily postures, is practiced for health and relaxation

yuan qi
original or source qi; this aspect of qi is passed on from our parents

Z
—

zanfu zhi qi
qi of the organs, the qi that nourishes the organs of the body

zangfu
the complete yin and yang organs of the body; in traditional Chinese medicine, the term for internal organs (different from those of Western medical science)

zheng qi
normal or upright qi; qi that circulates through the channels and the organs of the body

zong qi
gathering qi; the qi that gathers in the chest area through the coming together of gu qi and kong qi

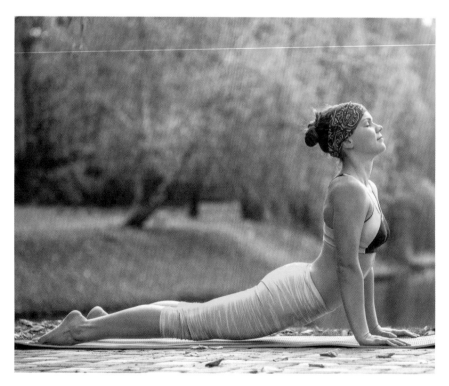